Pathophysiology:
A Clinical Approach

SECOND EDITION

Pathophysiology: A Clinical Approach

Carie A. Braun, PhD, RN
Associate Professor of Nursing
College of St. Benedict
St. John's University
St. Joseph, Minnesota

Cindy M. Anderson, PhD, RN, WHNP-BC, FAAN
Associate Professor
College of Nursing
University of North Dakota
Grand Forks, North Dakota

 Wolters Kluwer | Lippincott Williams & Wilkins
Health

Philadelphia • Baltimore • New York • London
Buenos Aires • Hong Kong • Sydney • Tokyo

Acquisitions Editor: David B. Troy
Associate Product Manager: Erin M. Cosyn
Product Director: Tanya M. Martin
Marketing Manager: Allison Powell
Senior Designer: Paul Fry
Artists: Dragonfly Media Group, Mark Miller
   Anatomical Chart Company
   Imagineering
Compositor: MPS Limited, a Macmillan Company
Printer: C&C Offset

351 West Camden Street
Baltimore, MD 21201
530 Walnut Street
Philadelphia, PA 19106

The publisher is not responsible (as a matter of product liability, negligence, or otherwise) for any
injury resulting from any material contained herein. This publication contains information relating to general principles of medical care that should not be construed as specific instructions for
individual patients. Manufacturers' product information and package inserts should be reviewed
for current information, including contraindications, dosages, and precautions.

Printed in China

Library of Congress Cataloging-in-Publication Data

Braun, Carie.
 Pathophysiology : a clinical approach/Carie A. Braun, Cindy M. Anderson. — 2nd ed.
  p. ; cm.
 Includes bibliographical references and index.
 ISBN 978-1-60547-304-8
 1. Physiology, Pathological. 2. Health—Miscellanea. I. Anderson, Cindy Miller. II. Title.
 [DNLM: 1. Pathology. 2. Physiology. QZ 4]
 RB113.B73 2011
 616.07—dc22

                2010038801

*The publishers have made every effort to trace the copyright holders for borrowed material. If they
have inadvertently overlooked any, they will be pleased to make the necessary arrangements at the
first opportunity.*

To purchase additional copies of this book, call our customer service department at **(800) 638-3030**
or fax orders to **(301) 223-2320**. International customers should call **(301) 223-2300**.

Visit Lippincott Williams & Wilkins on the Internet: http://www.LWW.com. Lippincott
Williams & Wilkins customer service representatives are available from 8:30 a.m. to 6:00 p.m., EST.

           06 07 08 09 10
        1 2 3 4 5 6 7 8 9 10

This edition is dedicated to all of those pathophysiology students who believed wholeheartedly in this project and gave countless hours of their time to provide substantial criticism and advice.

—Carie A. Braun

To my students who provide a constant source of enthusiasm and motivation;

to Dr. Carie Braun, a kindred spirit whose vision provided the inspiration for this project;

to my nursing colleagues, especially Dr. Jody Ralph, for their innovation and dedication to student learning;

to my husband Kevin and daughters Rachel, Amy, and Michelle who have given me unconditional support, motivation, and love.

—Cindy M. Anderson

Preface

This second edition represents the growing interest in and acceptance of applied conceptual learning in pathophysiology. The vast majority of pathophysiology textbooks choose a traditional body systems approach to learning, which focuses more on anatomy than physiology, and does not fully recognize that diseases cross multiple body systems. This text teaches pathophysiology through the lens of conceptually-based body functions (physiologies) and what happens when function is altered through injury or disease. Rather than learning only about a limited (or vast) number of diseases by body systems, the conceptual approach taken here illustrates pathophysiological concepts through carefully selected diseases, called clinical models. Because students learn through application, they start to think about pathophysiology in a way supportive of clinical decision-making, by recognizing signs and symptoms and etiology and tying this to the pathophysiologic concepts to predict the functional changes in the body. As a result, this text serves as an important learning tool for students in the health professions.

The most obvious change in this edition is the title. The title change is reflective of the increased emphasis on applying pathophysiologic concepts to any disease process. The most substantial internal revision is the use of modules to better engage students with the text. The module approach was suggested by student focus groups as an effective way to break up long chapters into manageable pieces that could be more easily read and retained. We have reconfigured this edition by adding one chapter. Previously, altered reproductive function was integrated. This time around, altered reproductive function gains status as a separate chapter. This was primarily at the request of reviewers who wanted more visibility for this concept.

Faculty and student reviewers have been the impetus for other improvements as well. We have added more clinical models, case studies, practice exam questions, and photographs as part of the comprehensive art program. These are all designed to promote application and to appeal to the visual learner. Information about age, race, gender, and ethnicity as contributing factors to disease are now integrated within the text, rather than presented as separate features.

At its core, this edition continues to emphasize student learning, application of knowledge, active learning strategies, critical thinking, and evidence-based practice through the many features and learning resources that accompany this text. We are excited about the opportunity to share this learning tool and continue to welcome your valuable feedback!

Learning Resources

The supplemental material that accompanies this book provides numerous opportunities for students to reinforce their learning. The book comes with a CD-ROM that contains pathophysiology animations to help visual learners understand some of the most important concepts. Also included on the accompanying CD-ROM are several games similar in style to the game show Jeopardy! to help students review chapter content.

Students can also purchase the study guide, a supplement tailored specifically to the approach and content of *Pathophysiology*. It contains test-taking strategies, concept-mapping exercises, case studies, and quiz questions to further ensure comprehension.

Instructors' resources are available on CD-ROM or via the Web site (http://connection.lww.com/BraunAnderson). Included in the instructors' resources are the following valuable assets:

- PowerPoint presentations by chapter
- Test generator
- Image bank

- Additional case studies
- Answers to chapter exercises
- Additional learning activities
- Conversion tools

Detailed lesson plans are also available to help instructors transition from a standard body-systems approach to the conceptual approach presented here.

Pathophysiology: A Clinical Approach represents a paradigm shift in thinking and learning about pathophysiology focused on functional alterations in health. We recognize that learning pathophysiology can be challenging. The goal of this text is to show how fascinating these challenges can be.

User's Guide

In today's health care careers, a thorough understanding of pathophysiology is more important than ever. *Pathophysiology: A Clinical Approach* not only provides the conceptual knowledge you will need, but also teaches you how to apply it. This User's Guide introduces you to the features and tools of this innovative textbook. Each feature is specifically designed to enhance your learning experience, preparing you for a successful career as a health professional.

Take a few minutes to look through the text and get acquainted with its organization. The table of contents of *Pathophysiology: A Clinical Approach* is structured around 16 core concepts of altered human function. The categories, devised by a group of educators, were selected by analyzing and clustering human health conditions with high prevalence, incidence, and severity. Clusters were formed by looking at the common impacts and ultimate results of different groups of diseases on the human body.

This novel approach shows you how diseases are rarely confined to one body system and challenges you to build on previously gained knowledge. An integrative study at the end of the book emphasizes the practical nature of the material by helping you apply the complex pathophysiologic concepts that you have learned to a common condition—diabetes mellitus.

Next, take a look at the chapters themselves. We've included some important tools to help you learn about pathophysiology and apply your new knowledge:

LEARNING OBJECTIVES

Highlight important concepts—helping you organize and prioritize learning.

CONCEPT MAPS

Visually illustrate the important interrelationships of key concepts.

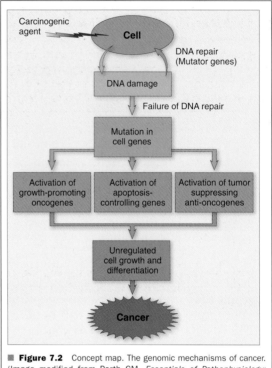

■ **Figure 7.2** Concept map. The genomic mechanisms of cancer. (Image modified from Porth CM. *Essentials of Pathophysiology: Concepts of Altered Health States*. Philadelphia: Lippincott Williams & Wilkins; 2003, with permission.)

From the Lab

Rheumatoid factor (RF), a substance that can be found in the blood, synovial fluid, and synovial membranes, signifies that antibodies (IgM, IgG, or IgA) are acting against other antibodies (mainly IgG). RF is present in the vast majority of patients that have RA and can also be found in a variety of other conditions. The presence of RF in RA often signifies more severe disease.

FROM THE LAB

Explain common laboratory procedures and results.

STOP *and Consider*

What can you do to improve or strengthen your first line of defense?

STOP AND CONSIDER

Challenge you to think beyond the information presented in the textbook as you proceed through the chapter.

Research Notes

Salt transport depends on the recycling of potassium in the thick ascending limb of the loop of Henle. The genetic alterations associated with Bartter syndrome contribute to the loss of potassium channel secretory activity, accounting for the alteration in electrolytes characteristic of the syndrome.[12]

RESEARCH NOTES

Highlight new findings and demonstrate how research can be incorporated into clinical practice.

SUMMARY

Provides a concise review of the chapter, highlighting the key points you should understand after reading the chapter.

Summary

- Cellular homeostasis depends on the proper functioning of cellular components, with direct effects on tissues and organs.
- Cellular adaptations to stress, injury, and damage form the basis of all disease.
- Alterations in cell size (atrophy and hypertrophy), cell number (hyperplasia), and cell structure (metaplasia and dysplasia) cause changes in tissue function and impact the entire person.
- Most cellular adaptations are necessary for cell survival.
- When damage exceeds the ability of the cell to adapt to a stressor, cell death by apoptosis or necrosis results.
- The clinical models presented in this chapter illustrate the applications of the concepts of cellular adaptation, including atrophy, hypertrophy, hyperplasia, metaplasia, dysplasia, apoptosis, and necrosis.

CASE STUDIES

Case studies and related questions help you build critical thinking skills and apply the chapter material to real-world clinical scenarios. You are encouraged to search the Internet for relevant journal articles and Web sites to confirm your predictions.

Case Study 12.1

A couple seeks reproductive counseling for inability to achieve a pregnancy after 14 months of unprotected intercourse. After multiple diagnostic tests with both individuals, the male partner is determined to have a moderately decreased sperm count and motility. Upon physical examination of the scrotum, enlargement of scrotal veins is determined, described by the clinician as feeling like "a bag of worms." The condition is termed varicocele.

1. Outline the process that has occurred in his body.
2. What were the risk factors that he demonstrated?
3. What would you expect for clinical manifestations?
4. What additional diagnostic tests could be used?
5. What treatment measures would you anticipate?

PRACTICE EXAM QUESTIONS

Provide practice and review for the types of questions to expect on an exam.

Practice Exam Questions

1. Which of the following is an example of a strong acid?
   a. Albumin
   b. Inorganic phosphorus
   c. Sodium
   d. Lactate

2. An anion gap of 16 can be calculated by which of the following scenarios?
   a. Sodium 146, chloride 102, bicarbonate 26 mEq/L
   b. Sodium 140, chloride 102, bicarbonate 26 mEq/L
   c. Sodium 136, chloride 122, bicarbonate 30 mEq/L
   d. Sodium 148, chloride 100, bicarbonate 28 mEq/L

3. Fluid loss in response to hypervolemia is promoted by:
   a. Stimulating secretion of ADH, promoting urinary sodium and water elimination
   b. Inhibiting the secretion of aldosterone, promoting urinary sodium and water elimination
   c. Lowering mean arterial pressure
   d. Administering osmotically active fluids

4. Which of the following ions is most closely related to water movement?
   a. Potassium
   b. Sodium
   c. Chloride
   d. Calcium

5. A pH of 7.5 is defined as:
   a. Alkalosis
   b. Acidosis
   c. Acidemia
   d. Alkalemia

6. Which compartment contains the greatest amount of body water?
   a. Transcellular
   b. Plasma
   c. Interstitial
   d. Intracellular

7. Which of the following transport mechanisms is associated with movement of water across a semipermeable membrane?
   a. Diffusion
   b. Osmosis
   c. Facilitated diffusion
   d. Active transport

8. Which one of the following conditions will most likely result in edema?
   a. Intravascular filtration pressure greater than interstitial filtration pressure
   b. Intravascular reabsorption greater than interstitial reabsorption
   c. Intravascular oncotic pressure greater than interstitial oncotic pressure
   d. Increased lymphatic reabsorption

9. An example of anion exchange includes:
   a. Sodium and hydrogen exchange
   b. Sodium and chloride exchange
   c. Bicarbonate and chloride exchange
   d. Hydrogen and bicarbonate exchange

10. Hypokalemia is often associated with which one of the following conditions?
    a. Metabolic alkalosis
    b. Metabolic acidosis
    c. Hyperchloremia
    d. None of the above

11. Metabolic acidosis may be associated with
    a. Increased chloride levels
    b. Increased metabolic acids
    c. Decreased bicarbonate
    d. All of the above

12. Ascites is the primary mechanism of body fluid imbalance in which of the following conditions?
    a. Salt-losing tubulopathy
    b. Cirrhosis
    c. AIDS
    d. Isonatremic dehydration

13. Hyperlactatemia due to drug treatment is a complication in which of the following conditions?
    a. Salt-losing tubulopathy
    b. Cirrhosis
    c. AIDS
    d. Isonatremic dehydration

14. Hypokalemia is a hallmark of which one of the following conditions?
    a. Salt-losing tubulopathy
    b. Cirrhosis
    c. AIDS
    d. Isonatremic dehydration

15. Hypotonic fluid loss may result in:
    a. Hyponatremic dehydration
    b. Isonatremic dehydration
    c. Hypernatremic dehydration
    d. None of the above

DISCUSSION AND APPLICATION

Helps you gauge your understanding of what you have learned.

Discussion and Application

1. What did I know about altered cellular proliferation and differentiation prior to today?

2. What body processes are affected by altered proliferation and differentiation? What are the expected functions of those processes? How does altered proliferation and differentiation affect those processes?

3. What are the potential etiologies for altered cellular proliferation and differentiation? How does altered proliferation and differentiation develop?

4. Who is most at risk for developing altered cellular proliferation and differentiation? How can altered proliferation and differentiation be prevented?

5. What are the human differences that affect the etiology, risk, or course of altered cellular proliferation and differentiation?

6. What clinical manifestations are expected in the course of altered cellular proliferation and differentiation?

7. What special diagnostic tests are useful in determining the diagnosis and course of altered proliferation and differentiation?

8. What are the goals of care for individuals with altered cellular proliferation and differentiation?

9. How does the concept of altered cellular proliferation and differentiation build on what I have learned in the previous chapters and in previous courses?

10. How can I use what I have learned?

BONUS WEB SITE

Inside the front cover of your textbook, you will find your personal access code. Use it to log on to thePoint—the companion Web site for this textbook. The Web site includes the following features to help you reinforce and review your knowledge:

- Pathophysiology animations
- A quiz bank of additional review questions to help you study for exams

Visit http://thepoint.lww.com/product/isbn/9781605473048 to kickstart your pathophysiology success today!

As you can see, all the chapter features are designed to hone critical thinking skills and judgment, build clinical proficiency, and promote comprehension and retention of the material by applying pathophysiologic knowledge, rather than merely memorizing facts and figures.

Reviewers

The publisher and authors gratefully acknowledge the many professionals who shared their expertise and assisted in developing this textbook, helping us refine our plan, appropriately targeting our marketing efforts, and setting the stage for subsequent editions. We are grateful to the following reviewers:

Jeanne Calvert, MS
Associate Professor, Biology
University of St. Francis
Ft. Wayne, Indiana

Karen Chandra, RN, MSN, MBA
Nursing Department
Harper College
Palatine, Illinois

Thomas Chartrand, DC
Associate Lecturer, Clinical Lab Sciences
University of Wisconsin—Milwaukee
Milwaukee, Wisconsin

William Hill
Anishinabek Educational Institute
North Bay, Ontario, Canada

Kathleen Holbrook, BS
Director, A&H Training Corporation
Latham, New York

Joseph Inungu, MD, PhD
Professor
School of Health Sciences
Central Michigan University
Mt. Pleasant, Michigan

John Knesel
Associate Professor, Biology
University of Louisiana at Monroe
Monroe, Louisiana

Lori Knight, CCHRA(C)
Instructor, Health Information Services Program
Saskatchewan Institute of Applied Science and Technology (SIAST)
Regina, Saskatchewan, Canada

Jeffrey Kushner
Associate Professor
Department of Integrated Science and Technology
James Madison University
Harrisonburg, Virginia

Treena Lemay, BScN
Professor, Health and Community Studies
Algonquin College
Pembroke, Ontario, Canada

Vikki McCleary, PhD
Assistant Professor, Physician Assistant Program
School of Medicine & Health Sciences
University of North Dakota
Grand Forks, North Dakota

Irene L. E. Mueller, EdD
HIA Program Director and Assistant Professor
Health Sciences
Western Carolina University
Cullowhee, North Carolina

Stephanie Olsen
Instructor, Health Information
SAIT Polytechnic
Calgary, Alberta, Canada

David Reff, BS, DDS
Program Director, Dental Assisting and Dental Hygiene
Apollo College
Boise, Idaho

Kristine Scordo, PhD, RN, CS, ACNP
Director, Acute Care Nurse Practitioner Program
Wright State University
Dayton, Ohio

Rachel Smetanka, PhD
Assistant Professor, Biology
Southern Utah University
Cedar City, Utah

J. Steve Smith, MD
Professor
Medical Technology Program
University of West Florida
Pensacola, Florida

Catherine Thompson, PhD, MS, PT
Assistant Professor, PT Education
Rockhurst University
Kansas City, Missouri

David Weissman, MD
Associate Professor, Pathology
Robert Wood Johnson Medical School
New Brunswick, New Jersey

Jean Zorko, MS
Assistant Professor
Stark State College of Technology
Canton, Ohio

Acknowledgments

We would like to acknowledge David Troy, Matt Hauber, Erin Cosyn, and the rest of the team at LWW for believing in a clinical approach.

—**Carie A. Braun**

—**Cindy M. Anderson**

Contents

Expanded Contents

Chapter 1

Introduction to Pathophysiology

LEARNING OBJECTIVES

1. Define and use the key terms listed in this chapter.
2. Discuss the value of prerequisite science courses as a foundation for learning pathophysiology.
3. Differentiate individual versus population-focused care.
4. State and give examples of the three levels of prevention upon which interventions are based.
5. Describe the relevance of gender, age, race, ethnicity, locale, and socioeconomic status to pathophysiology.
6. Explain the significance of evidence-based practice to pathophysiology.

Defining Pathophysiology

What is pathophysiology? **Pathophysiology** is the study of the functional changes that occur in the body as a result of an injury, disorder, or disease. Applying pathophysiology combines what we know about **pathology**, the study of changes in cells and tissues as a result of injury or disease, and **physiology**, the mechanisms of human body functioning. Pathophysiology is often referred to as a study of the mechanisms of disease.

When you study pathophysiology, you must recognize the obvious interdependence on altered structure and function. **Structure** is how the human body is put together, including the component parts and location of those parts. This is often learned in a course in human anatomy. **Function** is concerned with how these component parts operate together. This is most often discovered in a course in human physiology. In addition, preparation in other health science topics such as human biology, microbiology, and chemistry is helpful. Pathophysiology builds on previous learning and applies that learning to discern what happens to both structure and function in the human body in the face of injury, disorder, and disease.

Understanding Pathophysiology

PATHOGENESIS

The first step to understanding pathophysiology is to recognize and use key terms appropriately. First, consider the onset of the disease. **Disease** is the functional impairment of cells, tissues, organs, or organ systems. In this text, the term disease is often used broadly to include injuries, disorders, illnesses, and even **syndromes**, defined as a specific condition with a recognizable, predictable pattern. The origination and development at the point of disease onset are referred to as its **pathogenesis**, literally the disease beginning. The pathogenesis is bordered by when the disease process first begins to the point when the actual disease presents itself. For example, in diabetes mellitus, pancreatic beta-islet cell destruction can begin years before the onset of diabetes. The pathogenesis is concerned with factors at the onset of pancreatic beta-islet cell destruction, the progression of cell destruction, and the point of developing signs of diabetes mellitus. Although we may not know what exactly triggered the original beta-islet cell destruction, we can still understand the pathogenesis by studying cellular and tissue changes in those who develop the disease. Many times this occurs in individuals with specific **risk factors**, or

Box 1.1 Examples of Risk Factors

The presence of one or more of these select risk factors increases a person's chances for developing coronary artery disease:

- Elevated blood cholesterol level
- Elevated blood pressure
- Cigarette smoking
- Family history/genetic predisposition
- Obesity
- Sedentary lifestyle

vulnerabilities. An example of a set of risk factors for coronary artery disease is provided in Box 1.1. Modifiable risk factors are those that can be changed by the individual. For example, dietary intake, weight, and smoking are risk factors that are modifiable, whereas genetic composition or gender is not. The goal in studying pathogenesis is often to prevent disease from occurring. When prevention is not possible, understanding the pathogenesis can facilitate early diagnosis and intervention to avoid complications and improve quality of life.

ETIOLOGY

At the very beginning of the disease process there is an **etiology**, or precise cause of disease. Sometimes the etiology is identifiable, as with the inhalation of a viral microorganism that causes influenza in the airways. In this case, the etiology is traced to a specific **pathogen**, or disease-causing microorganism. Sometimes the etiology is unknown or **multifactorial** (having more than one genetic and/or environmental causing events), such as with cardiovascular disease or many cancers. When there is no known etiology, the disease is termed **idiopathic**.

Nosocomial disease is the result of exposure to infection in the health care environment. For example, a nosocomial illness is one where a child gets varicella (chickenpox) while a patient in the hospital. The child did not have varicella when they were admitted but were exposed while hospitalized and contracted the disease. Health care professionals have an important obligation to prevent the spread of disease in the health care setting through appropriate hand hygiene and infection control measures. **Iatrogenic** diseases are those that are the inadvertent result of medical treatment. For example, a patient who develops a urinary tract infection from the placement of a catheter, a tube in the bladder, has an iatrogenic disease.

STOP *and Consider*

Would you consider iatrogenic and nosocomial diseases to be medical errors?

CLINICAL MANIFESTATIONS

Clinical manifestations are the presenting signs and symptoms of the disease. More specifically, the **signs** of a disease are the observable or measurable expressions. For example, in herpes simplex (a cold sore), a sign would be redness with raised, clear, fluid-filled vesicles on the individual's lip. The signs are considered the "objective" manifestations that can be seen or measured by the health care professional. The **symptoms** are indicators that are reported by the ill individual and are considered the "subjective" manifestations. Symptoms of herpes may include tingling or discomfort at the site of the vesicles or a feeling of lethargy, or tiredness. These symptoms are difficult for the health care provider to observe or to measure. In addition, patients may describe **precipitating factors**, or triggers, that promote the onset of clinical manifestations. Examples of precipitating factors that promote shortness of breath and coughing in asthma are listed in Box 1.2.

Signs and symptoms can be local or systemic. **Local** refers to those manifestations that are found directly at the site of disease and are confined to that specific area. Examples of local manifestations are confined redness, swelling, bruising, or pain. **Systemic** manifestations present throughout the body and are not confined to one area, such as with fever, lethargy, generalized body aching, or high blood pressure. Timing is also important in classifying disease processes and clinical manifestations. **Acute** manifestations or diseases are those that begin abruptly and last a few days to a few months. The common cold is a good example of an acute disease. There is a noticeable onset, the disease lasts

10 to 14 days, and there is complete resolution. **Chronic** diseases, however, generally last longer than 6 months and are **insidious**, or gradual, in onset. With chronic disease, the person can have **remissions**, or symptom-free periods, and **exacerbations**, or flaring of symptoms. **Subacute** is a term used to describe diseases that fall somewhere between acute and chronic in duration and severity.

Some conditions are completely **asymptomatic**; that is, the person does not have any noticeable symptoms even though diagnostic tests may indicate that the disease is present. Screening tests, such as Pap smears, breast mammograms, or blood pressure measurements, are invaluable for detecting diseases that are asymptomatic.

DIAGNOSIS AND TREATMENT

Health care providers cluster the presenting clinical manifestations and laboratory and diagnostic tests to determine a **diagnosis**, or label, for the disease. A recognizable cluster of clinical manifestations can be diagnosed as a syndrome, such as with Down syndrome. You are probably very familiar with many different medical diagnoses and syndromes. The clinical models in this text use the medical diagnosis to identify the various conditions. Some health professionals use different diagnostic categories to describe disease processes. For example, nursing professionals use **nursing diagnoses** to describe the human response to illness, such as altered fluid balance and ineffective airway clearance. Depending upon the health profession that you are studying, you may find that there are other terms used to diagnose your patients.

The **prognosis** for a patient is the forecast or prediction of how the individual will proceed through the disease process. An excellent prognosis indicates that the individual will most likely recover completely. A poor prognosis signifies increasing risk for **morbidity**, a negative outcome with disease complications that impact the quality of life, and possibly **mortality**, or death. Prognosis is often based on health statistics across populations where the rates of survival and outcomes of others with similar diseases help predict the individual patient's outcome.

The treatment of disease is dependent upon the etiology and clinical manifestations. Treatment is aimed at eliminating or reducing the cause of disease and thereby eliminating or reducing the clinical manifestations. For example, in a burn injury, treatment is aimed at removing the source of the burn and then cooling the skin and protecting the body from infection. Figure 1.1 details the relationships between many of these terms.

Box 1.2 Examples of Precipitating Factors

Individuals with asthma often report one or more of these precipitating factors that lead to an asthma exacerbation:

- Exercise
- Cold weather
- Upper respiratory infection
- Stress
- Dust
- Pollen
- Animal dander
- Mold

Applying Pathophysiology

INDIVIDUAL HEALTH

You will undoubtedly spend much of your health professional career caring for individuals. In whatever setting you choose to practice, the focus must be on the whole person, defined by that individual's perception of health and illness. **Health**, defined as the perceived wholeness of body, mind, and spirit, and **illness**, a state that results in suffering or distress, are on a dynamic continuum. The continuum implies that individuals perceive themselves anywhere along the line of extremely healthy to extremely ill. There are varying degrees of health and varying degrees of illness. Dynamic means the patient's perceptions of how healthy or ill he or she is can change from day to day, month to month, or year to year. Effective communication with your patients can determine where they perceive themselves along this continuum and how you can best help them maintain or return to optimal health.

● **STOP** *and Consider*

Are you healthy or ill? How do you know? What characteristics describe someone who is healthy? When does a person often become labeled as ill? Think about a situation where a person was diagnosed with an illness but considered themselves to be healthy. How about when a person does not have a diagnosis but considers themselves to be ill?

In other science coursework, you have probably talked about the concept of homeostasis. **Homeostasis** is a dynamic balance in the body marked by the appropriate and effective response to stimuli, thereby keeping the body in a steady state. Although it often happens at a cellular level, homeostasis is an important body goal and is often reflected in the patient's perception of the health–illness continuum. Throughout this text, you will develop a greater appreciation for the response systems in the body that allow homeostasis to continue. You will also learn what happens when stressors present excessive and insurmountable challenges to homeostasis.

An important thing to keep in mind when caring for individual patients is that people should not be defined by their pathophysiology. Calling a patient by his or her disease state ignores the holistic physical, spiritual, emotional, and psychological components that comprise all of us. Health professionals should avoid calling patients "diabetics" or "the skull fracture in room 202" and replace these labels with "the woman with diabetes" or "the patient in room 202 with a skull fracture." After all, if the overall goal is high-quality holistic health care, this can only begin in a genuinely caring environment (Fig. 1.2).

POPULATION HEALTH

Your role as a health professional also requires that you consider the health of populations. Focusing on **epidemiology**, the study of disease in populations, has many advantages such as the following:

1. Recognition of where a disease is most widespread
2. Recognition of who is most affected by the disease
3. Discovering why the disease is presenting in that population

Figure 1.2 People first. A practitioner listens to a patient. The focus needs to be on the *patient*; the health problem is always secondary. (From Carter PJ, Lewsen S. *Lippincott's Textbook for Nursing Assistants: A Humanistic Approach to Caregiving.* Philadelphia, PA: Lippincott Williams & Wilkins; 2005, with permission.)

4. Discovering how to reduce the spread of disease, reduce morbidity, or eradicate the disease in that population

Health statistics are an important aspect of population-focused health care. **Incidence** is the rate of occurrence of a disease at any given time. Incidence represents the probability that a disease will occur in a certain population. For example, the incidence of Down syndrome, or the chance that one will be born with Down syndrome, is approximately 1 in 733.[1] Prevalence is the number or percentage of a population that is affected by a particular disease at a given time. As an example of prevalence, 400,000 people in the United States are currently living with Down syndrome.[1]

When the incidence and **prevalence** of a disease are predictable and stable, this is termed **endemic**. A dramatic increase in disease incidence in a population is called an **epidemic** and represents a rate considerably above the endemic rate. When an epidemic spreads across continents, the disease is considered to be a **pandemic**. The World Health Organization (WHO) is an important epidemiology resource and provides a yearly guide to health statistics inclusive of its 193 member states. The annual World Health Reports detail mortality and life expectancy rates across the globe and provide incidence and prevalence statistics for numerous diseases. For example, in the 2008 report, the 10 leading causes of death worldwide were listed as heart disease, stroke, lower respiratory infections, chronic obstructive pulmonary disease, HIV/AIDS, diarrheal diseases, tuberculosis, cancers, road traffic accidents, and prematurity and low birth weight.[2] Decreasing the incidence and prevalence of these conditions can have the greatest impact on the health of populations around the world.

● **STOP** *and Consider*

Take out the newspaper and look for current reports related to health. What are the epidemic conditions currently present in your geographic area? What is being reported around the world? Do you notice any pandemic condition reports?

DISEASE PREVENTION

Prevention of disease is a critical role for the health professions. Disease prevention is most often discussed in three levels: primary, secondary, and tertiary.

1. **Primary prevention**. Primary prevention prohibits a disease condition from occurring. An example is wearing a bike helmet to prevent a head injury.
2. **Secondary prevention**. Secondary prevention is the early detection and treatment of disease through screening. An example is performing breast or testicular self-examination every month for early cancer detection.
3. **Tertiary prevention**. Tertiary prevention is rehabilitation of a patient after detection of disease. Tertiary prevention focuses on preventing complications or progression of the condition; for example, applying physical therapy and occupational therapy interventions to improve gross and fine motor function after a stroke.

● **STOP** *and Consider*

What activities do you participate in which would count as primary prevention? How about secondary prevention? Identify other examples of tertiary prevention.

▨ Evidence-Based Practice

Evidence-based practice is a way of caring for others that is cognizant of the most current research and knowledge in the health professions. The Research Notes feature of this text highlights some of the current research on the various pathophysiologic concepts and diseases. However, evidence-based practice goes beyond one piece of research and encompasses the totality of what is known through research and the knowledge and practices of clinical experts.

Health professionals must be prepared to work effectively with people of all races and cultures. This requires a conscientious respect for human health variations. Evidence-based practice and epidemiology provide a framework for determining those most likely to be afflicted with certain diseases based on gender, age, race, locale, socioeconomic factors, or

Research Notes

The Human Genome Project has been instrumental in stimulating research interest in the area of human diversity and disease. Research is underway to determine the variability in DNA sequence patterns among populations in Africa, Asia, and the United States.[3] These studies aim to identify "DNA regions" associated with complex diseases, such as cancer, diabetes, heart disease, and certain types of mental illness. These DNA regions will identify those who are more likely to develop these complex diseases based on their genetic structure. This information will provide additional clues to the human factors that increase the risk and development of disease.

ethnicity. Recognizing differences based on these factors will help promote effective prevention measures. Health professionals must always balance what is known from an epidemiologic standpoint with what is unique to each human based on his or her life situation, avoid stereotyping, and be ready to identify and assist all patients in promoting health.

Pathophysiology is arguably one of the most important subjects that you will ever study as a student in the health professions. Your patients will rely on you to recognize health problems and act accordingly. Decisions about pharmacologic treatments, surgical interventions, health-promotion measures, nutritional interventions, and even genetic counseling are dependent upon your learning in this course.

Functional Concepts of Altered Health

The information contained in this book represents a journey into the world of conceptual learning. A **concept** is a general idea that can be applied to similar situations. In other words, a conceptual approach in pathophysiology clusters current knowledge about human health and disease and

---

Box 1.3 Functional Concepts of Altered Health

Basic alterations in cells and tissues
Inflammation
Immunity
Infection
Genetic and developmental disorders
Altered cellular proliferation and differentiation
Altered fluid/electrolyte and acid/base balance
Altered neuronal transmission
Altered sensory function and pain perception
Altered hormonal/metabolic processes
Altered reproductive function
Altered ventilation and diffusion
Altered tissue perfusion
Altered nutrition
Altered elimination
Degenerative changes in aging

---

organizes that knowledge into meaningful and useful ideas. These ideas are referred to as functional alterations in health. Box 1.3 lists the select functional alterations upon which this text is based.

A conceptual approach dictates learning general disease processes and then applying these processes to specific conditions. It is impossible to detail every disease condition. A conceptual approach supplies you with the tools to be more effective at figuring out what is known and how this applies to that which is unknown. The effective application of that knowledge to the health care setting is the destination.

Summary

- Pathophysiology is the study of the mechanisms of disease and focuses on the physiology of altered health states, specifically the functional changes that accompany a particular injury, syndrome, or disease.
- Those studying pathophysiology are concerned with the etiology, pathogenesis, and clinical manifestations of disease; this involves the analysis of cellular, tissue, organ, and body system changes that occur in a disease state.
- Health professionals cluster signs and symptoms (also called clinical manifestations) to formulate a diagnosis, or label, for the disease condition. Appropriate interventions can then be applied, with respect to human diversity, to provide high-quality health care and to promote optimal health outcomes.
- Epidemiology is a science that deals with the study of disease trends in populations; epidemiologists identify the incidence and prevalence of diseases worldwide, including the presence of endemic, epidemic, and pandemic conditions. A major goal of understanding disease is to effectively apply the three levels of prevention whenever possible.

Case Study 1.1

Kim is a 10-year-old girl who presents to the urgent care clinic with a 14-day history of nasal stuffiness, copious amounts of green nasal drainage, fever, generalized headache ("my whole head hurts"), facial pain above and below the eyes, and fatigue. Kim reports that her younger sister recently had a "bad cold"; no one else in the family is currently ill.

Kim's medical history is significant for seasonal allergies, usually flaring up this time of the year. Kim has been using her antihistamine medication to block the seasonal allergies, but this treatment has not been effective. Kim's mother reports that Kim is "constantly stressed out and puts way too much pressure on herself." Kim says that her biggest concern is missing the school musical; she is the lead and the opening production is in 2 days. Upon physical examination, Kim has an oral temperature of 100.4°F. The practitioner taps gently above and below Kim's eyes; her sinuses are tender when touched. The lymph glands along her neck are enlarged and tender. Kim undergoes sinus radiographs (X-rays). The radiographs indicate fluid accumulation in the frontal and maxillary sinuses. Kim is diagnosed with sinusitis, related to a persistent upper respiratory infection. Kim is prescribed a 3-week course of antibiotics to treat the sinus infection.

1. *Would you define Kim as healthy or ill? Explain.*
2. *What risk factors does Kim have that could have led to the development of the sinusitis?*
3. *What is the etiology of Kim's sinusitis? Would the sinusitis be considered either nosocomial or iatrogenic? Explain.*
4. *Identify the symptoms that Kim reports.*
5. *Identify the signs leading to the diagnosis of sinusitis.*
6. *How would you categorize this illness: acute or chronic? Explain.*
7. *Which of the manifestations are local and which are systemic?*
8. *What is the prognosis for Kim?*
9. *What aspects related to human diversity and disease would be important to consider with regard to Kim?*
10. *What additional dimensions of the health history would you need to explore to provide holistic health care?*

■ Case Study 1.2

Jay is a public health worker and is charged with developing an immunization tracking program for residents of his county aged birth to 21 years. Jay is primarily interested in measles vaccination rates. There has been a major increase in measles diagnoses in young children and adolesecents from the years 2005 to 2010 (10 cases in the county in 2005 up to 20 cases in 2010). The current chance of county residents being diagnosed with measles before the age of 21 is 1 in 200,000. Jay is interested in understanding why this increase occurred over such a short period of time.

1. *Explain how you can look at this scenario from both an individual perspective and a population perspective.*
2. *What is the level of prevention indicated in the case study? How could the other levels of prevention be represented within this scenario?*
3. *What are the incidence and prevalence of measles in this case study? Would this situation be considered endemic, epidemic, or pandemic? Explain.*
4. *What are some of the possible explanations for the major increase in measles cases?*
5. *What could be some of the ways to track immunizations within the county system?*
6. *Explain how evidence-based practice would have a role in Jay's work.*

Practice Exam Questions

1. You are expecting your first child and are told that the child has a 1 in 800 chance of being born with a congenital anomaly. This statistic refers to the:
   a. Incidence
   b. Prevalence
   c. Epidemic
   d. Diagnosis

2. You decide that it has been too long since your last physical examination, so you schedule an appointment for a routine health screening. You have a blood cholesterol level checked and it is within the expected range. This activity represents which level of prevention?
   a. Primary prevention
   b. Secondary prevention
   c. Tertiary prevention
   d. None of these

3. At your health screening, you describe the following: achiness, lethargy, and vague abdominal discomfort. These are categorized as:
   a. Local manifestations
   b. Systemic manifestations
   c. Signs
   d. Symptoms

4. The study of functional alterations in human health because of an injury, disease, or syndrome describes which of the following?
   a. Pathology
   b. Pathophysiology
   c. Physiology
   d. Morphology

5. A patient wants to know what has caused his illness. This information is termed the:
   a. Etiology
   b. Pathogenesis
   c. Epidemiology
   d. Nosocomia

6. Joe has many risk factors for the development of lung cancer. Which of these is NOT modifiable?
   a. Smoking
   b. Family history of lung cancer
   c. Working in an asbestos-filled area
   d. Poor nutritional intake

7. Which of the following terms indicates the dynamic steady state that the body strives to achieve everyday?
   a. Homeostasis
   b. Mortality
   c. Morbidity
   d. Health

8. Which of the following contributes to evidence-based practice and high-quality patient care?
   a. Primary research
   b. Clinical expertise
   c. Meta-analysis studies
   d. All of these contribute

9. Cancer is on the rise across the globe. Which term describes this phenomenon?
   a. Epidemic
   b. Endemic
   c. Pandemic
   d. Morbidity

10. Your grandmother is diagnosed with congestive heart failure and is told that she has 6 months to live. This prediction is referred to as her:
    a. Prognosis
    b. Diagnosis
    c. Morbidity rate
    d. Prevalence

Discussion and Application

1. What did I know about pathophysiology prior to today?

2. How does the study of pathophysiology build on what I have learned in previous courses?

3. How can I use what I have learned?

RESOURCES

World Health Organization Health Statistics:
http://www.who.int

Healthy People 2020 Outlines the Health Goals for the United States:
http://www.healthypeople.gov

United States National Health Statistics:
http://www.cdc.gov/nchs/

Canadian Health Statistics:
Accessible at: http://www.statcan.gc.ca

REFERENCES

1. National Down Syndrome Society (2009). About Down syndrome: Down syndrome fact sheet. Available at: http://www.ndds.org. Accessed February 25, 2009.
2. World Health Organization (2008). World health statistics 2008. Available at: http://www.who.int/whosis/whostat/EN_WHS08_Full.pdf. Accessed February 25, 2009.
3. US Department of Energy Human Genome Program (2008). Genomics and its impact of science and society: The Human Genome Project and beyond. Available at: http://www.ornl.gov/sci/techresources/ Human_Genome/publicat/primer2001/5.shtml. Accessed February 25, 2009.

Altered Cells and Tissues

LEARNING OBJECTIVES

1. Define and use the key terms listed in this chapter.
2. Discuss the changes in cells and tissues after injury.
3. Compare and contrast cellular structural adaptations to injury.
4. Identify maladaptive cellular responses to injury.
5. Recognize health conditions that can precipitate maladaptive cellular responses.
6. Describe diagnostic tests and potential treatment strategies relevant to cellular and tissue alterations.
7. Apply cellular adaptations and maladaptations to select clinical models.

INTRODUCTION

When considering health and disease, what comes to mind first? The answer may be organs and organ systems. **Organs**, fully differentiated body parts with specialized functions, are more familiar and are used more often in discussion about health and disease. Although most people can describe a heart, brain, or liver, it is harder to describe the tissues and cells that determine organ structure and function. **Tissues** are groups of different cell types that combine to form a specific function. Like organs, the four major tissue types in the body (epithelium [skin], connective tissue [including blood, bone, and cartilage], muscle, and nerve) are familiar. **Cells**, the basic units that make up tissues, are the sites where changes in structure and function lead to symptoms and diseases in individuals. This chapter discusses the responses of cellular structure and function caused by stress, injury, or damage. Many of the concepts introduced here are expanded in subsequent chapters. Developing an understanding of these responses will help the student to translate these adaptations to the signs and symptoms of disease states that result from cellular injury.

Review of Cellular Structure and Function

The cell is the smallest component of the living individual. The structural components of the cell and the function of its components contribute to the integrity of the cell and the individual. Consequently, cell damage or injury can affect the functioning of organs, body systems, and overall health.

Cellular Components

The component parts of the cell provide structure and determine functional capacity. Physiologic functioning at the cellular level is critical to proper functioning of tissues and organs and to the health of the individual.

CELLULAR MEMBRANE

Each cell is surrounded by a **plasma membrane**, which protects the cell by creating a barrier that separates the intracellular components from the extracellular environment surrounding it. The plasma membrane represents an organized structure composed of lipids, carbohydrates, and proteins arranged in a **bilayer** (two interconnected layers). The **lipid bilayers** are mainly made up of **phospholipids** (phosphate [PO$_4^-$] bound to lipid). The phosphate connected to the lipid structure is known as the "head." The lipid structure is known as the "tail" due to its shape. The heads are **polar** or **hydrophilic** (having affinity to water). The lipid tails, composed largely of cholesterol, are **nonpolar** or **hydrophobic** (lacking an affinity to water). Two of these lipid layers align so that the nonpolar tail portions are intertwined and the polar heads line both the outer and inner surface of the cell. **Glycolipids** (carbohydrate bound to lipid) also make up the lipid bilayer but are present in smaller numbers than phospholipids. The barrier created by the lipid bilayer prevents the unintentional passage of water-based substances by the hydrophobic cell surface. The cell membrane allows for transfer of ions and molecules into and out of the cell for homeostasis, containment of the essential organelles and structures inside the cell, and communication of cellular signals between the cell and the external environment.

Proteins are often suspended in the plasma membrane, acting as receptors that bind substances, including hormones. Proteins that pass through the membrane are known as **transmembrane proteins**, allowing communication and transport

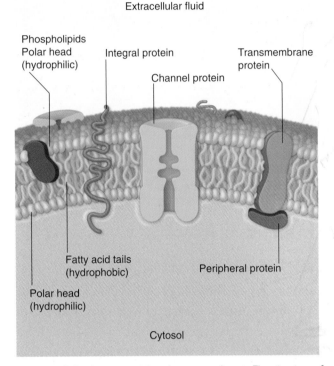

■ **Figure 2.1** Structure of the plasma membrane. The structure of the plasma membrane shows the arrangement of polar heads in contact with both the extracellular fluid and cytosol, and the nonpolar tails forming the center of the lipid bilayer. The embedded membrane proteins, including channel, transmembrane, peripheral, and integral proteins, are shown related to their relationship with the plasma membrane.

between the extracellular and intracellular environments. **Integral proteins** are a specific type of transmembrane protein that, because of the tight binding to lipid tails, becomes part of the membrane itself. Integral proteins often form **channel proteins** that allow for the transport of ions (atom with an electrical charge) across the plasma membrane. Peripheral proteins project into either the intracellular or the extracellular environment, excluding the ability to promote transport functions. Figure 2.1 shows the structure of the lipid bilayer and proteins of the plasma membrane.

CYTOPLASM AND ORGANELLES

The cytoplasm contains the organelle structures essential for cellular survival. **Cytoplasm** is a colloidal substance surrounding the cell nucleus composed of water, proteins, fats, electrolytes, glycogen, and pigments. **Organelles** are structures within a cell that perform a distinct function; these structures include the following:

- **Endoplasmic reticulum**
  - A complex network of tubules, producing proteins and fats
  - Important in the regulation of ions within the cell
  - Types
    - Rough
      - Synthesis of proteins via bound ribosomes
      - Production of lysosomal enzymes (acid hydrolases)
    - Smooth
      - Synthesis of lipids, lipoproteins, and steroid hormones
      - Regulation of intracellular calcium
- **Golgi apparatus**
  - Membranous structure
  - Prepares substances produced by the endoplasmic reticulum for secretion out of the cell
- **Lysosome**
  - Small sacs surrounded by membrane
  - Digests cellular debris with hydrolytic enzymes
  - Important in the metabolism of particular substances
- **Peroxisomes**
  - Membrane-enclosed sacs smaller than lysosomes
  - Contain enzymes called oxidases that neutralize **oxygen free radicals** (atoms carrying an unpaired electron and no charge)
  - Promote survival of the cell by neutralizing harmful substances potentially damaging to the cell
- **Proteosomes**
  - Large organelles that recognize abnormally folded or formed proteins
  - Involved in **proteolysis** (breakdown of protein)
- **Mitochondria**
  - Principal producer of cellular energy source, **adenosine triphosphate (ATP)**
  - Contain the cytochrome enzymes of terminal electron transport necessary for the production of ATP
  - Contain enzymes needed for the citric acid cycle, fatty acid oxidation, and oxidative phosphorylation

Enclosed by a structure called the nuclear envelope, the **nucleus** of the cell contains **deoxyribonucleic acid (DNA)**, which controls cell **reproduction** (see Chapter 6). Each cell contains 23 pairs of **chromosomes**, coiled structures of chromatin forming an individual's genetic code. The **genes**, individual units of inheritance, are located on the chromosomes containing DNA. Genes determine cell protein characteristics. The membrane surrounding the nucleus contains "pores" providing access for protein products to move from the nucleus to the cytoplasm of the cells.

CYTOSKELETON

The **cytoskeleton** is composed of tubule and filament structures that contribute to cell shape, movement, and intracellular transport. The main cytoskeleton components include:

- Microtubules
  - Thin protein structures composed of tubulin
- Microfilaments
  - Thin
    - Comprise the protein actin
  - Intermediate
    - Comprise filaments with diameter size between thin and thick filaments
  - Thick
    - Comprise the protein myosin

Cellular Function

Functions common to all cell types include:

- Transportation
- Ingestion
- Secretion
- Respiration
- Communication
- Reproduction

Specialized cellular function is determined by cell type. Examples of specialized functions of cells are movement in muscle cells and conduction in nerve cells.

CELLULAR MECHANISMS OF TRANSPORTATION

The semipermeable character of the cell membrane allows for the transport of some substances but acts as a barrier to others. For cells to obtain the nutrients and other substances needed for survival, they must develop functional mechanisms for the passage of substances through the cell membrane. The movement of substances is often classified according to the amount of energy required in the act of transport.

Passive Transport

Substances may enter the cell passively, meaning that little energy is required by this process. **Diffusion**, or movement of particles from an area of higher concentration to lower concentration

(**concentration gradient**), is an example of passive transport. Electrical charge in particles can also promote movement across the cell membrane. Particles become uniformly distributed, achieving a state of equilibrium. Small particles and lipid-soluble gases, including carbon dioxide and oxygen, are common examples of substances involved in this type of transport. The ability and rate of particles to diffuse through the membrane are affected by the particle size and by the size of the **membrane pore**, the membrane passage between the extracellular and intracellular environments.

Membranes may be impermeable to particles, but most allow movement of water (see Chapter 8). **Osmosis** is the process by which water passively moves across the semipermeable cell membrane. A concentration gradient promotes movement of water from areas of low particle concentration to high particle concentration. The pressure generated by this process is known as **osmotic pressure**.

The movement of some substances across the cell membrane requires **facilitated diffusion**, or the use of transport proteins. Substances are unable to cross the membrane because of their large size or hydrophilic characteristics that require transport proteins to promote passage. Glucose is an example of a large substance needing transport proteins to allow movement across the lipid bilayer. Facilitated diffusion is also important in the movement of ions through channels of integral proteins, bypassing the lipid-soluble portion of the cell membrane. Ion channels are often classified according to the type of triggers that prompt opening and closing. Categories of ion channels include:

- Leak channels: Open without need for stimulation
- Gated channels: Open and close in response to stimuli
    - Voltage-gated; stimulated by change in **membrane potential** (charge inside a cell membrane in relation to the surrounding extracellular fluid)
- Ligand-gated; stimulated by receptor–ligand binding
- Mechanically gated; stimulated by vibration, stretching, and pressure

Active Transport

Active transport requires energy when transporting particles across the cell membrane. Diffusion moves particles passively along the concentration gradient, whereas active transport moves particles against its concentration or its electrochemical gradient. A common example of this type of transport mechanism is the movement of sodium out of the cell across the membrane with the assistance of the

A. Diffusion

B. Osmosis

Water

C. Facilitated Diffusion

D. Active Transport

■ **Figure 2.2** Mechanisms of cellular membrane transport. **A:** Particles move across the semipermeable membrane to achieve equal distribution during diffusion. **B:** Water flow is regulated by osmotically active particles in osmosis. **C:** Transport proteins are required for particles to move across the membrane in facilitated diffusion. **D:** ATP drives movement of particles across the membrane in active transport.

sodium-potassium (Na$^+$/K$^+$)–ATPase pump. Energy is required for transport because the concentration of sodium outside the cell is far greater than inside the cell. This pump also moves extracellular potassium across a large concentration gradient to the intracellular space. This process requires the direct use of energy in the form of ATP, also known as **primary active transport**. When movement of a second substance depends on energy derived from the active transport of the primary substance, the process is known as **secondary active transport**. Systems in which substances are transported in the same direction are known as **cotransport** or **symport**. Movement of substances in opposite directions is considered **countertransport** or **antiport** movement. Figure 2.2 describes mechanisms of cellular membrane transport.

INGESTION

The cellular plasma membrane serves an important function as a barrier to the external environment; however, specific processes allow the cell to **ingest** substances necessary for its own use into the cytoplasm. **Endocytosis** is the process used to transport large substances into cells. Two categories of endocytosis are pinocytosis and phagocytosis. **Pinocytosis** is the ATP-requiring process of ingesting small vesicles. **Phagocytosis** is the process of ingesting large particles such as cells, bacteria, and damaged cellular components, resulting in the release of *oxygen free radicals*. Phagocytosis is critical in the defense of the body from foreign invaders (see Chapter 5). Any alteration in the ability of the cell to ingest substances required for survival or in

the demand on cells to ingest substances can result in the cellular foundation of disease.

SECRETION

Carbohydrates are combined with proteins in the Golgi apparatus to form large glycoproteins to be **secreted**, the process of release of metabolic products from cells. The Golgi apparatus works with the endoplasmic reticulum to package products into vesicles, then directs their delivery within the cell and outside the cell. The vesicles move from the Golgi into the cytoplasm and then out of the cell via the cell membrane, a process known as **exocytosis**. Lysosomes are formed by the Golgi apparatus and are responsible for digestive functions within the cell. Substances such as proteins, carbohydrates, damaged cellular structures, and pathogens are broken down for removal or recycling by hydrolytic enzymes, called acid hydrolases, contained within the lysosomes. Figure 2.3 illustrates the concepts of endocytosis and exocytosis.

RESPIRATION

The cell's survival depends on the availability of ATP produced by cellular respiration as a source of energy for all cellular functions. Cellular **respiration** is a series of metabolic processes that transforms fuel molecules into energy (in the form of ATP) and waste products. **Anaerobic respiration** is the process of ATP production that occurs without oxygen. The chemical reactions of oxidation and reduction between oxygen and nutrient products such as glucose is called **aerobic respiration**. **Glycolysis**,

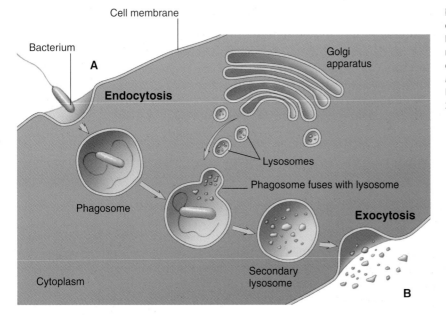

Figure 2.3 Vesicular transport. A: Objects enter the cell by the process of endocytosis. B: Vesicles bind to the plasma membrane and release their contents through a process called exocytosis. (Image from Premkumar K. *The Massage Connection: Anatomy and Physiology*. Baltimore, MD: Lippincott Williams & Wilkins; 2004, with permission.)

the process of breaking down glucose in the cytosol of the cell, occurs in the absence of oxygen, releasing only a small amount of energy. This anaerobic reaction leads to a small amount of ATP (2 molecules for each molecule of glucose metabolized) and the production of waste products, including lactic acid. Aerobic respiration occurs in metabolic pathways in the mitochondria. When oxygen is present, the products from glycolysis in the cytoplasm enter into the citric acid cycle and oxidative phosphorylation. These aerobic pathways produce a total of 38 molecules of ATP for each molecule of glucose metabolized. The waste products produced in aerobic respiration include carbon dioxide, water, and heat, all readily metabolized.

COMMUNICATION

The proteins required for cell function are a product of the cell itself, formed by genes in response to cellular needs. These products include proteins used for cell structure and cell function and enzymes used to stimulate chemical reactions. Impaired proteolytic enzyme activity, often a result of a genetic mutation, has been linked to the development of disease, including diabetes, cataracts, multiple sclerosis, and Duchenne muscular dystrophy.[1] **Feedback mechanisms** regulate gene activation to tightly control the production of proteins and to prevent cell damage caused by overproduction or underproduction.

Optimal function of tissues requires cell-to-cell communication. The message, or signal, transmitted from one cell to another cell influences cellular behavior and plays a role in determining function. The target cell is able to communicate through a special protein known as a **receptor**. Receptors can be present on the cell membrane (membrane bound) or within the cell (intracellular). Signaling molecules, or **ligands**, bind to receptors in a specific way, similar to a key turning a lock. When a ligand binds to a receptor, the target cell begins the process of communication known as a **signal transduction pathway**. The tightness, or strength of binding, is also referred to as **binding affinity**. The binding of an extracellular ligand to a membrane-bound receptor begins a cascade of signaling events that alters cell behavior. For a ligand to bind to an intracellular receptor, it must be able to diffuse across the plasma membrane and enter the cell.

Ligand–receptor binding that results in signal transduction with a local effect is known as **paracrine signaling**. The ligands involved in paracrine signaling (**local mediators**) exert a rapid local response. A wider range of impact occurs when signal transduction affects cell behavior within the entire organism (**endocrine signaling**). The ligands involved in endocrine signaling are called **hormones**. These hormones can influence cell behavior on a larger scale. Because of the dependence on the required processes and blood flow needed to carry the hormones through the body where they can bind with receptors, this pathway is often slower and longer lasting than the one that is involved with paracrine signaling. Hormone influences in the body are discussed in detail in Chapter 11.

REPRODUCTION

Reproduction of cells is another function operating under genetic control. Genes control the growth of cells, timing of the division of cells, and differentiation of cells. The rate of cell growth is specific to each cell type and is regulated to meet the constantly changing needs of the individual. Cell size is determined primarily by the amount of functional DNA in the cell. Without DNA reproduction, cells can grow only to a particular size before they stop growing.

Cell division occurs at different times depending on the cell type and on the signals sent to the cell for division. **Proliferation** is the increase in cell number. **Differentiation**, or changes in physical and functional properties of cells, directs the cell to develop into specific cell types. As all cells contain identical genetic material, this process explains why one cell contributes to the development of one tissue while another can develop into a different tissue. This process occurs by the repression of certain genes in a cell and the expression of others in the same cell. Alterations in the proliferation and differentiation of cells are described in detail in Chapter 7.

Module 2

Cellular Adaptation and Response to Stress

Cells are consistently challenged with stressors that can lead to altered function. Cellular structures must adapt their function when faced with damage and injury for the cell to survive. Potentially damaging conditions faced by cells include changes in oxygenation, temperature, molecular toxins, and electrolytes. The two responses of the cell to these stressors are **adaptation** or **death**. Mechanisms

■ **Figure 2.4** Adaptive cell changes. Normal cells adapt to stress by altering size, number, or type/structure. (Asset provided by Anatomical Chart Company.)

that promote cellular adaptation result from signals that cause changes in gene function. The ways in which these cells respond form the cellular basis of disease (Fig. 2.4). Cellular responses include changes in size, number, and structure.

● **STOP** *and Consider*

What would happen if cells did not have the ability to adapt to stressors? What are the implications in health and disease?

▨ Atrophy

Atrophy is the decrease in the size of a cell and can occur for several reasons. A decrease in the functional demand on a cell prompts a decrease in cell size. This type of decrease often occurs when a limb is immobilized in a cast and active muscle movement is impaired. The lack of muscle movement reduces demand on muscle cells, leading to decreased cell size. Muscle cell atrophy causes reduction in the muscle itself due to the large

numbers of cells affected. A decreased oxygen supply to the cell, or **ischemia**, can also contribute to a decrease in cell size. Ischemia can occur secondary to a blockage in the arterial blood supply, which reduces the delivery of oxygen. Although cells may have the ability to adapt to a chronically reduced oxygen supply via atrophy, a complete lack of oxygenation is more likely to result in irreversible cell death.

Many cells depend on specialized signals to maintain function. Atrophy is often the response of these cells when signals are removed. The sources of these signals are often hormones, which target specific cell types. A similar event occurs when neural signals are removed from cells dependent on them for normal functioning. Chronic nutritional deprivation and the process of aging also result in decreased cell size, which translates into decreased organ size. Atrophy also can occur as a response to the removal of hormonal signals that stimulate growth, resulting in **involution**, or decreased size, of tissues and organs. Atrophy may result in the manifestation of clinical signs and symptoms stemming from the decrease in size and function of the organ involved.

Spinal muscular atrophy results from disuse caused by impaired neural innervation to muscle tissue. Signals to muscle cells are decreased due to degeneration of motor neurons of the spinal cord. The decreased stimulation of muscle cells because of loss of neural signaling causes atrophy, resulting in weakness of voluntary muscles. The loss of function associated with the atrophic cell and tissue changes highlights many conditions characterized by atrophy.

● STOP *and Consider*

From this discussion of atrophy caused by decreased trophic signals of hormones, what other tissue types can be similarly affected?

Hypertrophy

Hypertrophy is an increase in cell size. Cells often respond with hypertrophy from an increase in **trophic**, or growth, signals. Signals stimulating an increase in sex hormones are responsible for the development of hypertrophied reproductive cells during puberty as well as in the breast cells during pregnancy that allow mothers to make and deliver breast milk. Increased demand can also contribute to hypertrophy. Strength-building exercise often results in an increase in muscle cell size and muscle mass.

Hypertrophy of the adenoid tissue is a common and familiar condition. **Adenoid hypertrophy** is caused by enlargement of lymphoepithelial adenoid tissue in the back of the nasal area and can result in obstruction of the nasal passage. The increased functional demand required of the lymph tissue in filtering out infectious agents in the upper respiratory tract can lead to an increase in lymphoid and epithelial cell size. The most common effects of adenoid hypertrophy are snoring, bad breath, and stuffy nose. More serious consequences of adenoid hypertrophy can affect respiratory function, with manifestations of sleep apnea, pulmonary hypertension, or heart failure.

Hyperplasia

Hyperplasia is an increase in the number of cells. Like hypertrophy, hyperplasia can also be caused by hormone signaling and an increase in workload. Because some of the same conditions cause both hyperplasia and hypertrophy, they are often seen together. For example, the uterus responds to the increase in hormone levels of estrogen during monthly menstrual cycles by increasing the number of cells. Also, when people are exposed to high alti-

■ **Figure 2.5** Breast tissue adaptation to trophic signals. **A:** Puberty (hyperplasia). **B:** Pregnancy (hypertrophy). **C:** Menopause (atrophy). (Asset provided by Anatomical Chart Company.)

tudes, adaptation to this stressor includes an increased production of red blood cells to maximize the hemoglobin's oxygen-carrying ability. This "increased workload" to oxygenate stresses the cell to produce this adaptation.

Adaptation of cells and tissues to hormonal signals is a dynamic process. One cell or tissue type can undergo a series of adaptations in response to varied signals over a lifetime. This process is clearly illustrated in the adaptations of the ductal tissue of the breast over a woman's lifetime, as in Figure 2.5. The hormonal changes of puberty induce hyperplastic changes in the breast, noted by increased size of the functional lobular and ductal tissue. Hormones secreted during pregnancy promote hypertrophic changes in breast tissue to support production and delivery of breast milk. When hormone production ceases during **menopause**, atrophic changes associated with decreased breast size are noted. These changes result from the intensity of trophic signals induced by the hormones, which promote the genetic basis of these adaptations.

Metaplasia

Metaplasia refers to the changing of one cell type to another. This is one way that cells can adapt to a persistent stressor. In the case of a person with gastroesophageal reflux disease (GERD), the cells of the esophagus are exposed to the acidic contents of the stomach. Over time, these cells often change from a squamous epithelium cell type to a glandular cell type. A similar situation occurs when cells that line the bronchial tubes of the lungs are exposed to cigarette smoke over a period of time. This exposure leads to cell adaptation to this stressor by the development of squamous metaplasia, in which the columnar cells turn into squamous cells in the cell's attempt to survive the exposure to toxins (Fig. 2.6). When the stressor that caused these cell changes is removed, cells often return to their normal state. In the presence of a persistent stressor, cells may develop changes that lead to pathologic changes.

■ **Figure 2.6** Squamous metaplasia in the transformation zone in the cervix.The proliferating cells displace the glandular epithelium. The metaplastic cells mature into glycogen-rich squamous cells. (Image from Rubin E, Farber JL. *Pathology*. 4th ed. Philadelphia, PA: Lippincott Williams & Wilkins; 2005, with permission.)

Dysplasia

Dysplasia refers to the actual change in cell size, shape, uniformity, arrangement, and structure. As with metaplasia, dysplasia is often a cell's response to a chronic and persistent stressor and is likely to resolve when the stressor is removed. Dysplasia is caused by abnormal differentiation of dividing cells and is considered a problem in regulating cell growth. When cell reproduction occurs, the DNA may be reproduced with **mutations**, or changes in the material that makes up the chromosomes. These mutations are often repeated as more cells divide and proliferate. Although these cells are not cancerous, they may appear as an early change that can progress to cancer. Figure 2.7 depicts the progression from normal cells (A) to mild dysplasia (B) to severe dysplasia (C).

Bronchopulmonary dysplasia (BPD) is a condition in which stressors prompt cellular alterations that lead to chronic, irreversible tissue changes. Some infants require high concentrations of oxygen and mechanical ventilation at birth, often because of respiratory distress and the inability to maintain adequate levels of tissue oxygenation. BPD is caused by forceful mechanical ventilation with high oxygen concentrations during the early newborn period of life. The bronchial and alveolar tissues of the lungs become thickened, reducing the ability to take air into the

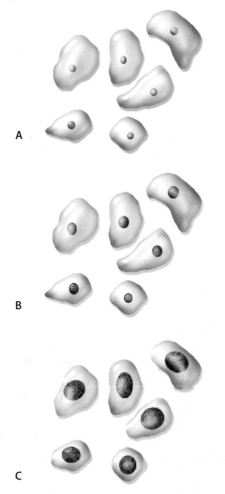

■ **Figure 2.7** Cellular changes in dysplasia. **A:** Large squamous cells with small nuclei. **B:** Nucleus increasing in size and darkening in color. **C:** Markedly enlarged and darkened nucleus with abnormal chromatin. (Asset provided by Anatomical Chart Company.)

lungs, oxygenate tissues throughout the body, and excrete waste products, including carbon dioxide. The damage is the likely result of the combination of cellular stressors and the susceptibility to damage in the developmentally immature lung tissue.

● **STOP** *and Consider*

What are the common characteristics of the different mechanisms of cellular adaptation? What are the differences?

Module 3

Cellular Injury and Death

As discussed earlier in the chapter, in the process of cellular adaptation, exposure to stressors can cause changes in both cell structure and function. Many of the adaptations that cells make allow the cell to survive. If the stressor is too great or lasts too long, the cell may lose its ability to adapt, resulting in death.

Conditions such as ischemia can be overcome if the exposure is not too great and does not last too long. Other conditions, such as **oxidative stress**, radiation, chemicals, and pathogens (bacteria and viruses) can cause cell injury, followed by cell death if the damage is too great.

Mechanisms of Cell Death

The changes in cell and organelle structure and function prevent the cell from returning to a normal condition. Cellular damage that overwhelms the capability for recovery results in cellular death. The two major ways in which cells die are by the processes of apoptosis and necrosis.

APOPTOSIS

Apoptosis can be both a physiologic and a pathologic cell response to cellular signals. Apoptosis is often referred to as "cellular suicide." It is programmed cell death prompted by a genetic signal and is designed to replace old cells with new. Cells are programmed for death for many reasons, including damaged genetic material or mutation, old age of the cell, and an attempt to decrease the actual number of cells. Death occurs in the cell because of enzyme reactions in the cell that change the structure, and therefore function, of the organelles and other cell components.

This process is common during the development of the embryo when cells grow and develop into well-defined organs and systems. Embryonic hands begin as outgrowths in the shape of buds, progressing to webbed, flattened, paddle shapes by the fifth week of development. Cartilage and bone development is followed by bone ossification during the seventh week, along with the transformation of the webbed hand into digits through the process of apoptosis by the eighth week. Alterations in this process of apoptosis during embryologic development can lead to the manifestation known as **syndactyly**, the fusion or incomplete separation of digit soft tissue.

NECROSIS

Necrosis, another mechanism of cell death, is different from apoptosis. Cell death by necrosis is a disorderly process associated with inflammation (see Chapter 3). **Necrosis** is death of cells related to cell injury. Injury causes damage to cellular structures, including the mitochondria, depleting ATP. Without ATP to energize cellular processes, organelles and cells swell disrupting the plasma cell membrane barrier. The loss of the cell membrane barrier allows the spilling of the cell contents from within the cell. Enzymes are released that dissolve the cell

Figure 2.8 Necrosis. Diabetic foot with necrosis of the digits. (Image provided by Stedman's, with permission.)

components, which in turn trigger white blood cells to respond and digest the cellular debris through phagocytosis. The result is local inflammation and death of cells. When overgrowth of infectious agents is combined with decreased blood flow, necrosis can occur (Fig. 2.8).

Causes of Cell Injury and Death

Injury to cells stems from a variety of sources of stress (Fig. 2.9). **Infection** from bacteria, viruses, protozoa, or fungi can initiate damage to cells (see Chapter 5). **Physical injury** from mechanical, thermal, or chemical sources can cause damage to the structure of a cell and affect cell function. **Mechanical injury** can be caused by impact of a body part causing direct injury, such as falling off a skateboard or a bike. **Thermal injury** is caused by extremes of temperature, as occurs with burns and frostbite. Toxins can also cause harm to cells. These toxins can be **endogenous** (from within the body system). For example, when a person has an allergic reaction, toxins are released from within the body, which cause cell damage and associated symptoms (see Chapter 4). Toxins can also be **exogenous** (from the external environment). A common exogenous toxin is alcohol, which can damage the cells of the liver with prolonged exposure. Damage to cells can also result from **deficit injury**, in which the cell is deprived of oxygenation, hydration, and nutrition. This is commonly seen in conditions of ischemia (see Chapter 14), severe malnutrition, and eating disorders such as anorexia nervosa (see Chapter 15).

It may be helpful to remember the common causes of cell injury and death with the acronym TIPS:

- *Toxins* (chemical, pathogenic)
- *Infections*

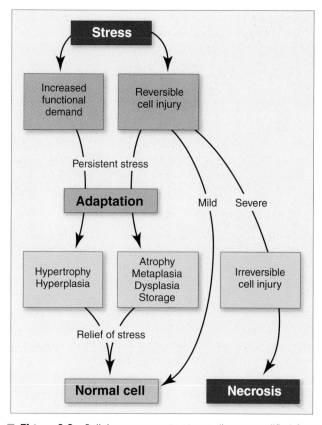

Figure 2.9 Cellular response to stress. (Image modified from Rubin E, Farber JL. *Pathology*. 4th ed. Philadelphia, PA: Lippincott Williams & Wilkins; 2005, with permission.)

- *Physical injury* (mechanical, chemical, thermal)
- *Serum deficit injury* (nutrition, hydration, oxygenation)

Cells can be damaged in a variety of ways that result in injury or death. Oxidative stress can be increased by many conditions, including biologic aging, infection, inflammation, ischemia, radiation, and use of chemicals and drugs. Oxidative stress involves exposure of cells to **reactive oxygen species (ROS)**, toxic oxygen molecules or radicals that are formed by the reaction between oxygen (O_2) and water (H_2O) during mitochondrial respiration. ROS species include superoxide (O_2^-), hydrogen peroxide (H_2O_2), the hydroxyl radical (OH), and peroxynitrite ($ONOO^-$). Cell damage can result from too many ROS or not enough available enzymes, including catalase, to convert these radicals to less harmful substances. Cellular damage resulting from ROS is known as **free radical injury**. ROS produces damage to cells, often by targeting DNA. Injury by ROS exposure has been implicated in many disease conditions, including heart disease, diabetes, cancer, and others. ROS scavengers, such as catalase, peroxidase, superoxide dismutase, and antioxidants, can work with detoxifying enzymes to limit cell damage (Fig. 2.10). The use of antioxidants, such as vitamin E, may reduce oxidative stress for many disease conditions.[2,3]

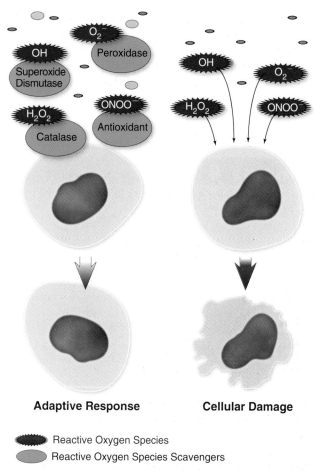

Adaptive Response **Cellular Damage**

⬤ Reactive Oxygen Species
⬭ Reactive Oxygen Species Scavengers

Figure 2.10 Cellular response to oxidative stress. Oxidative stress occurs as a result of increased reactive oxygen species (ROS), decreasing antioxidants, or inability to neutralize or repair damage caused by ROS with ROS scavengers.

⬤ **STOP** *and Consider*

Hydrogen peroxide (H_2O_2) is familiar to most people as a product to be used on cuts and scrapes. The solution that can be bought at the local grocery store contains 3% of H_2O_2, with the remaining 97% of the solution made up of water. When the solution is applied to a cut or scrape, the combination of H_2O_2 combines with the enzyme catalase, which is released from the damaged cells and blood. Catalase causes a chemical reaction, converting hydrogen peroxide into water (H_2O) and oxygen (O_2). The evidence of this reaction is the foam that is produced when the hydrogen peroxide is applied to the injury, releasing the oxygen gas.

$$H_2O_2 \xrightarrow{\text{catalase}} H_2O + O_2$$

Catalase works the same way in the cells of the body to scavenge ROS, minimizing oxidative damage.

Source: http://science.howstuffworks.com/question115.htm.

Damage to cells can result in disruption of metabolic processes that can prove fatal. The imbalance of electrolytes, ischemia caused by oxygen deprivation, and damage to DNA as a result of radiation injury are examples of events that may lead to accumulation of metabolites within the cell, causing further injury.

Clinical Models

The following clinical models have been selected to illustrate the concepts of cellular adaptation in health and disease. While reading the descriptions of these models, think about the stressors that can cause cellular adaptation, injury, and death, and the responses of the cells to the stressors. Consider the concepts of cellular adaptation as they apply to the specific conditions to assist in the understanding and application of these concepts.

Cerebral Atrophy

Cerebral atrophy describes the reduction in size of the cells in the cerebrum of the brain. The progressive reduction in the size of the neurons leads to the reduction in the brain tissue itself. Neurons are the functional cells in brain tissue and are responsible for conducting neural impulses within the brain and to other areas of the body. Many neurologic diseases are associated with loss of neuronal function due to atrophy, several of which are included as clinical models in this text (Fig. 2.11).

PATHOPHYSIOLOGY

Cerebral atrophy may be either a cause or consequence of a neurologic disorder. Decreased stimulation resulting from reduction in physical and intellectual activities may lead to atrophy of brain structures.[4,5] Individuals with low levels of B vitamins may experience increased brain atrophy, an example of deficit injury.[6]

Destruction of neurons and the loss of neurotransmitter production in one part of the brain may lead to atrophy of neurons in another region due to lack of stimulation. Conditions leading to reduced perfusion to the brain increase the risk of injury due to a deficit in oxygen and nutrient delivery. Neurotoxic injury resulting from ischemia, hyperthermia, inflammation, or trauma may exceed the ability of the neuron to recover, leading to neuronal death. Subcortical ischemic vascular disease reduces perfusion to the brain, with affected individuals manifesting decreased psychomotor speed, executive control, and global cognitive function.[6] Brain atrophy in multiple sclerosis is characterized by a loss of gray and white brain matter, leading to the manifestations involving motor deficits and cognitive impairment.[7] As neurons decrease in size, their physical relationship with other neurons changes. The close connections

Figure 2.11 Cerebral atrophy. MRI of the brain shows enlargement of the ventricles and deepening of the sulci, evidence of cerebral atrophy.

between neurons are required for effective communication; as neurons atrophy, communication is further impaired as the distance between neurons increases. Because neurons are not able to replicate, death leads to permanent loss of cells and function.

CLINICAL MANIFESTATIONS

The manifestations of cerebral atrophy can be focal (localized to a particular region) or global (affecting the entire brain). Neurons in each area of the brain provide specific functions (see Chapter 9). As neurons atrophy, the function associated with those neurons becomes altered. Neuronal atrophy in the frontal and temporal lobes of the brain leads to cognitive impairment. Alzheimer's disease, a condition affecting memory and comprehension, is associated with atrophy of the hippocampus and cerebral cortex.[7] Movement disorders result from neuronal atrophy in the basal ganglia, responsible for production of the neurotransmitter dopamine.

The pattern of brain atrophy contributes to a wide range of manifestations related to degree of atrophy. Cerebral palsy is a condition that occurs due to neuronal insult during a critical time in brain development, during the prenatal, perinatal, or postnatal periods. Manifestations vary from mild to severe and may involve motor skills, coordination and balance, and seizure activity, reflecting the involved areas of the brain.

DIAGNOSIS

Brain atrophy is a pathologic finding related to a significant range of neurologic diseases. The first step in diagnosis is designed to determine underlying pathology in order to identify the specific condition and initiate appropriate treatment. Early diagnosis is critical in neurologic disease associated with brain atrophy due to the limited ability to restore function that has been lost by the time the diagnosis is made.

A careful history that includes signs and symptoms, including onset, duration, and severity, is the first step in the diagnostic process. The early manifestations of brain atrophy may be difficult to identify in the early stages due to the insidious and subtle development of signs. The signs of brain atrophy may be first observed by others rather than the affected individual who may be unable or unwilling to disclose symptoms.[8] Physical exam is needed to define specific neurologic deficits, needed to determine actual diagnosis. Specific measures of brain atrophy using nonconventional magnetic resonance imaging (MRI) techniques have become increasingly

common and are used in determination of location and severity of atrophy.[9] Combined, the strategies of history, physical exam, and imaging techniques aid in the diagnosis, prognosis, and treatment of conditions associated with brain atrophy.

TREATMENT

Treatment of individuals with brain atrophy is targeted toward prevention or slowing of continued pathology. When neurons are atrophied and damaged, recovery is severely limited due to the inability of neurons to replicate. Supportive care assists individuals in completing activities of daily living. Physical, speech, or occupational therapy is critical to promotion of optimal function. Pharmacologic therapies may be instituted to address impairment in neurologic signal transmission. Treatment is individualized based on the specific diagnosis and the type of brain atrophy involved, with a goal of maximizing function and minimizing continued pathology.

STOP *and Consider*

Why do age and developmental maturity affect the degree of brain atrophy that can be expected?

Cardiac Hypertrophy

Myocardial cells, or cardiac myocytes, differ from other cells because they do not continually divide and replace themselves. After the first 4 weeks of life, growth of the heart is achieved by hypertrophy of existing cardiac myocytes. Injury to these cells often results in permanent damage and chronic cardiac disease. **Cardiac hypertrophy**, or hypertrophic cardiomyopathy, is a disease of cardiac muscle that results from excessive workload and functional demand. The most common cause of sudden unexpected cardiac death in young individuals, primary hypertrophic cardiomyopathy, is most common among individuals less than 30 years of age.[10,11] The most common cause of secondary cardiac hypertrophy is increased blood pressure, imposing additional workload on the ventricle.

PATHOPHYSIOLOGY

Primary hypertrophic cardiomyopathy, without a specifically known cause, is often a result of an inherited non–sex-linked genetic autosomal-dominant trait. Secondary hypertrophy is often caused by an

■ **Figure 2.12** Hypertrophy of the left ventricle caused by hypertension. (Asset provided by Anatomical Chart Company.)

underlying condition that causes an increase in ventricle workload. Hypertrophy can occur in the right ventricle due to increased pressure in the pulmonary circulation or in the left ventricle due to increased pressure in the systemic circulation, as in hypertension. In systemic hypertension, the left ventricle of the heart may be forced to pump harder due to an increase in outflow pressure from a stiff aortic valve or increased pressure in the aorta. The wall of the left ventricle, responsible for the pumping of blood out of the aorta into the systemic circulation, becomes thickened and stiff as a result of the increase in myocardial cell size. The muscle becomes less effective at contracting despite the increased size of the myocardial cells. The lack of **compliance**, or stiffness, of the ventricle may prevent adequate filling and therefore may lower cardiac output. This rigidity of the ventricle combined with smaller chamber size eventually leads to "pump failure" and cardiac decompensation. This condition exemplifies the way in which increased workload produces a biochemical signal that causes a genetic response resulting in hypertrophy. Figure 2.12 illustrates hypertrophy of the left ventricle.

CLINICAL MANIFESTATIONS

The evidence of cardiac hypertrophy is variable in its expression. Some individuals do not develop symptoms, and others develop manifestations that severely limit function. Massive ventricular hypertrophy leads to the clinical manifestations of this condition. The left ventricle is the main pump of the heart, moving blood received from the lungs into the aorta, providing arterial circulation to the body. Impaired pumping in the left ventricle leads to decreased circulatory output and congestion or backflow of blood into the left atrium and the pulmonary circulation. Perfusion to the heart muscle itself is also affected, reducing delivery of oxygen to the myocytes and other cardiac cells. Symptoms of pump failure are based on its severity and can include shortness of breath, chest pain, and **syncope** (fainting). Syncope is of particular concern because its manifestation is a marker for sudden death. Cardiac hypertrophy can also lead to irregular heart rate and rhythm. As the cardiac myocytes enlarge, the physical relationship of cardiac conducting cells becomes altered, disrupting neurologic signaling in the heart tissue.

DIAGNOSIS

Preclinical diagnosis in primary cardiac hypertrophy can be achieved by genetic testing when a family history of the condition exists. For those identified with the associated genetic mutation, the earliest identification of manifestations of disease is paramount. In those with secondary cardiac hypertrophy, treatment of the primary pathology is critical to management of the progression of pathology. Routine screening to determine blood pressure, exercise tolerance, and the presence of ventricular arrhythmia can be done periodically to identify impaired cardiovascular function. Screening techniques can include:

- Electrocardiogram (EKG): Evaluates electrical activity of the heart
  - 12-Lead EKG: Identifies electrical defects while at rest
  - Ambulatory Holter EKG: Identifies arrhythmias during activities of daily living
- Two-dimensional echocardiogram: Ultrasound measurement of ventricle dimensions, heart valves, and blood vessels (aorta, pulmonary artery)
- Exercise stress testing: Determine cardiovascular response to exercise

On physical examination, a heart murmur during cardiac contraction is often heard. Resting left ventricular outflow obstruction is diagnosed when systolic pressure gradient reaches 30 mm Hg; it is considered moderate to severe when systolic pressure gradient reaches 50 mm Hg or exceeds 75 mm Hg, respectively. Obstruction of left ventricular outflow is often manifested by arrhythmia of the atria; bradyarrhythmia (abnormally slow heart rate);

systolic ejection murmur; or abnormal peripheral vascular response.

TREATMENT

Treatment strategies target symptom relief and prevention of sudden cardiac death. Primary cardiac hypertrophy should be treated at the earliest manifestation of disease. The secondary form of cardiac hypertrophy can be improved if the condition and the factors causing it are identified and treated before the cells undergo permanent damage. Treatment is geared toward relaxation of the ventricle and relief of the outflow obstruction that is increasing the ventricular workload. An example of this is use of antihypertensive medications to lower the resistance against which the left ventricle must pump when the hypertrophy is caused by underlying hypertension.

Pharmacologic treatment is initiated when clinical manifestations of the condition are present. Treatment includes pharmacologic management with drugs designed to relieve the resistance against which the left ventricle must pump. Blocking the effect of catecholamines and slowing the heart rate to allow filling of the ventricle during cardiac relaxation represent the first-line approach to treatment.[12] Beta-adrenergic receptor blockers are the drugs of choice. Their mode of action is through competition with catecholamines for available beta-adrenergic receptors, slowing heart rate, decreasing the risk of arrhythmia, and decreasing the risk of resistance against the left ventricle. Surgery to reduce left ventricular muscle mass or to repair heart valves may be needed, but complications from this treatment are significant. An alternative to surgery, alcohol ablation of the septum, causes necrosis of the interventricular septum by the injection of alcohol into a small arterial branch leading to the muscle source. This cutting-edge procedure is promising; however, long-term effects are not fully known.[13] Activity restrictions may be required to minimize the risk of sudden cardiac death, especially for young athletes involved in strenuous activities.

STOP *and Consider*

What is the benefit of causing necrosis of the interventricular septum in the treatment of cardiac hypertrophy?

STOP *and Consider*

The effect of cardiac hypertrophy involving the left ventricle was described in this clinical model. What would happen if hypertrophy involved the right ventricle?

Acromegaly

Acromegaly is a condition of hyperplasia prompted by hormone stimulation of excessive growth. The condition is derived from the Greek words for extremities (acro) and enlargement (megaly). The term acromegaly provides an accurate description of the most common clinical manifestations—abnormal growth of the hands and feet.

PATHOPHYSIOLOGY

A form of hyperpituitarism, secretion of excessive growth hormone (GH) from the pituitary gland causes exaggerated skeletal and organ growth occurring after **epiphyseal**, or long bone ossification site,

From the Lab

Several genetic mutations have been identified that result in alterations in proteins necessary for cardiac muscle contraction. In approximately half of families affected, the gene mutation affects production of the proteins myosin, troponin T, alpha-tropomyosin, cardiac myosin–binding protein C, or regulatory light chains of myosin. The abnormal proteins cannot function appropriately and contribute to the hypertrophic changes. Cells seen under a microscope are disordered, lacking the normal parallel alignment necessary to produce normal electrical conduction and contraction.

closure. The hypothalamus secretes two hormones that regulate GH secretion by the pituitary. Hypothalamic secretion of somatostatin has an inhibitory effect on the pituitary, decreasing secretion of pituitary GH. The stimulation of pituitary GH secretion is induced by hypothalamic production of growth hormone–releasing hormone (GHRH). GH binds to its receptor and begins signaling events in the cell, which induces a genetic response involving cell cycle control. This event stimulates *proliferation*, or rapid reproduction of cells, which leads to hyperplasia. The secretion of GH stimulates the production of another hormone, **insulin-like growth factor 1 (IGF-1)**, in the liver. The actions of IGF-1 promote growth in bones, cartilage, soft tissues, and organs. Normally, this increase in IGF-1 along with other regulatory hormones signals the pituitary to reduce the production of GH via the influence of somatostatin

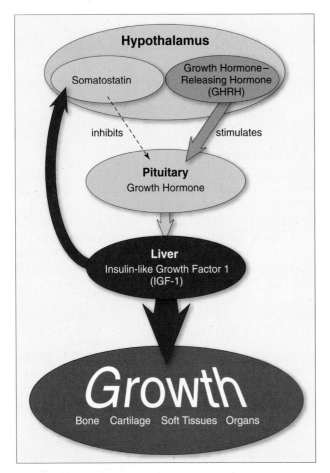

■ Figure 2.13 Feedback mechanism for growth stimulation. Regulation of growth hormone by growth hormone–releasing hormone *(GHRH)* promotes growth through the action of insulin-like growth factor 1 *(IGF-1)*. Increases in IGF-1 trigger an increase in somatostatin to inhibit growth. Dysregulation can result in gigantism or acromegaly.

(Fig. 2.13). When this negative feedback loop fails, GH secretion continues in an unregulated fashion. In more than 90% of these individuals, the oversecretion of GH can be attributed to the presence of a benign pituitary tumor called an **adenoma**.

Acromegaly is often confused with a similar condition known as **gigantism**, also a condition of hyperplasia characterized by excessive growth. The difference between this condition and acromegaly is the timing of GH excess. In gigantism, GH excess occurs prior to the closure of the epiphyseal growth plates of the long bones. For this reason, gigantism affects infants and children, increasing their height up to three times of the expected height for their age.

CLINICAL MANIFESTATIONS

Symptoms of acromegaly are related to excessive growth. Manifestations of acromegaly can include:

- Soft tissue swelling (difficulty getting rings on and off)

- Altered facial features
  - Prominence of jaw, brow, and nasal bone
  - Enlargement of tongue and lips
  - Increased spacing between teeth
- Pain and numbness in hands
- Deepening voice
- Snoring
- Skin changes
  - Coarse hair growth
  - Oily appearance
  - Sweating
  - Body odor
  - Development of skin tags
- Altered reproductive functioning
- Menstrual cycle alterations (women)
- Impotence (men)
- Breast discharge

Objective symptoms of skeletal growth include increased size of hands and feet, facial brow, jaw, and nasal bone, as well as increased spacing of teeth. Arthritis and carpal tunnel syndrome may also result from overgrowth of bone, cartilage, and soft tissue. Hyperplasia of the cells of sinuses and vocal cords may lead to a deepened voice and upper airway obstruction. Excessive sweating and skin odor may result from glandular hyperplasia. Skin may become thick and oily and develop skin tags. Menstrual disorders in women and sexual dysfunction in men may occur. Enlargement of organs, including liver, spleen, kidneys, and heart, may also result from hyperplasia and lead to serious health consequences, including diabetes, colon cancer, and cardiovascular disease. Acromegaly can induce both hyperplastic and hypertrophic changes in cardiovascular tissue. The hyperplastic cardiac changes in acromegaly eventually lead to cardiac hypertrophy and possibly heart failure if left untreated.[14] Suppression of GH and IGF-1 can reverse these changes, decreasing left ventricular mass and restoring cardiac function, highlighting the cells' adaptive responses. Figure 2.14 illustrates the clinical manifestations of acromegaly in men and women.

Acromegaly resulting from pituitary adenoma causes manifestations related to physical pressure on surrounding structures as the adenoma increases in size. Pressure on brain tissues affects associated nerves, leading to the development of headaches and impaired vision. The function of the pituitary itself can be altered because of adenoma compression, resulting in altered production of other pituitary hormones and contributing to the reproductive manifestations of acromegaly.

DIAGNOSIS

The diagnosis of this condition may be delayed because of the slow and insidious onset of clinical

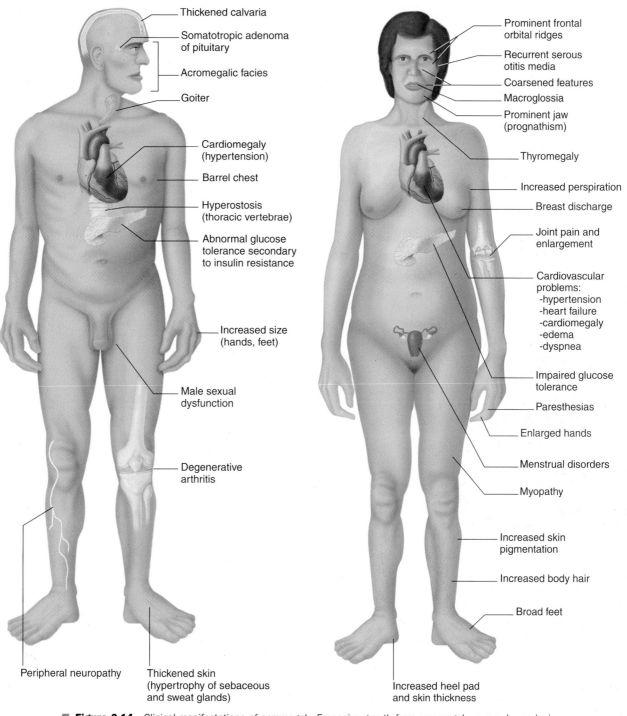

Figure 2.14 Clinical manifestations of acromegaly. Excessive growth from acromegaly causes hyperplasia and multiple clinical manifestations in both men (**A**) and women (**B**).

manifestations. Confirmation of the diagnosis of acromegaly depends on elevated levels of GH and IGF-1 in the blood. A specific method of GH measurement and follow-up is required to obtain accurate and reliable results (See From the Lab). Once acromegaly is diagnosed, the next step is to determine whether the cause is related to pituitary adenoma. The presence of a pituitary adenoma can be diagnosed with imaging techniques such as computerized tomography (CT) or MRI.

TREATMENT

Treatment is designed to reduce the overproduction of GH to reverse or reduce the effects of acromegaly. The chronic effects can be halted if the condition is identified early in its course before permanent cell injury occurs. Treatment options include:

- Drug therapy
- Radiation therapy
- Surgical removal of adenoma

Pharmacologic management of acromegaly is directed toward reduction in pituitary adenoma size and GH secretion. Drugs may be used as sole therapy or as a means to reduce the size of pituitary adenoma, improving prognosis for successful surgical removal. Drugs may also be used as adjuvant therapy after surgical removal of the adenoma, when complete cure is not attained. Three classes of drugs are the main agents for treatment of acromegaly: the GH inhibitors, dopamine agonists, and the somatostatin analogs. GH inhibitor pegvisomant (Somavert) works at the level of target cells, blocking GH from binding to receptors in body tissues. The dopamine agonists bromocriptine (Parlodel) and cabergoline (Dostinex) work at the level of the pituitary to reduce GH and subsequent IGF-1 secretion. The somatostatin analog octreotide (Sandostatin) induces an inhibitory effect on the pituitary, reducing GH and IGF-1 secretion. A long-acting release formulation allows less frequent dosing (once per month).

From the Lab

GH levels can be measured in the blood but are not reliable based on a single measurement due to the typical variations in secretion throughout the day. IGF-1 levels in the blood are more stable and therefore provide a more accurate result.[15] An additional accurate measurement of GH blood level is conducted after a glucose tolerance test. Ingestion of 75 g of glucose normally suppresses GH to less than 1 ng/mL. An elevated GH level 1 hour after the glucose injection points to the diagnosis of acromegaly.[16]

Radiation can be used as the primary treatment or in combination with pharmacologic and/or surgical management. Radiation of the pituitary is designed to promote cell death in the adenoma. Complications can include extension of the area of cell death to include healthy pituitary tissue, leading to subnormal secretion of other hormones, in addition to GH.

Surgical removal of the pituitary adenoma is also an effective management strategy. Prognosis is best when the adenoma is small, termed a microadenoma (less than 1 cm). Prognosis for successful surgery includes a primary tumor of less than 10 mm in diameter and a preoperative GH blood level of less than 40 ng/mL. Large tumors may require reduction in size using pharmacologic therapies prior to surgical intervention. Transsphenoidal hypophysectomy, a technique for adenoma removal through an incision

in the nose, immediately reduces symptoms attributed to both excessive hormonal stimulation of growth and those related to compression of surrounding tissues. Surgery is considered successful when GH blood levels are less than 2 ng/mL after a 75-g oral glucose load. Even after successful surgery, follow-up for recurrence is necessary.

● STOP *and Consider*

Why does GH excess in children produce manifestations that are different than those in adults?

◪ Cervical Metaplasia and Dysplasia

Cervical development is a dynamic process, evolving throughout the reproductive lifetime. The cells of the cervix respond to the hormonal environment, promoting adaptive and maladaptive responses.

PATHOPHYSIOLOGY

The epithelial cells of the cervix are arranged in a multilayer organization much like that of the skin. Actively dividing cells are located along the basal layer and are not usually found at the surface layer. The cervix is made up of two distinct cell types: squamous epithelium and columnar epithelium (Fig. 2.15). **Squamous epithelium**, the cell type lining the outside of the cervix and the vagina, is apparent on physical examination when the cervix is visualized.

Endocervix
Columnar epithelium

Internal os

External os

Squamocolumnar junction

Ectocervix
Stratified squamous epithelium

■ **Figure 2.15** Cell types comprising the transformation zone. The endocervix is lined by columnar epithelium. The ectocervix is lined with stratified squamous epithelium. The squamocolumnar junction marks the merging point of these two epithelial cell types. (Asset provided by Anatomical Chart Company.)

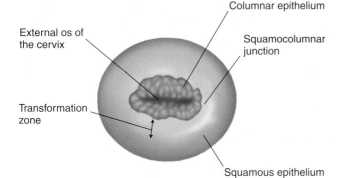

Figure 2.16 Transformation zone of the external cervical os. The transformation zone comprises the area distal to the squamocolumnar junction and is the site of squamous metaplasia. (Image from Bickley LS, Szilagyi P. *Bates' Guide to Physical Examination and History Taking*. 8th ed. Philadelphia, PA: Lippincott Williams & Wilkins; 2003, with permission.)

Columnar epithelium is the cell type lining the **endocervical canal**, the area between the external and internal cervical os. This cell type provides secretions that plug the canal with mucus and protect the uterus from pathogens that can ascend from the vagina.

The location at which these two cell types merge is known as the **squamocolumnar junction**. This area is dynamic throughout a woman's reproductive life, migrating and changing location on the cervix in response to stimuli, including hormones and pH. The area comprising the merging of these cell types is called the **transformation zone** (Fig. 2.16). As the transformation zone migrates from inside the endocervical canal to the outside of the cervix, or **ectocervix**, it can often be visualized on physical examination. High estrogen levels, as experienced in the luteal phase of the menstrual cycle and during pregnancy, promote the gradual transition of squamous epithelium to columnar epithelium. Low estrogen levels, as occur in menopause, cause the squamocolumnar junction to recede into the endocervical canal where it can no longer be visualized on physical examination. The adaptations that these cell types undergo are examples of metaplasia—the cellular response of changing from one type to another in the face of an environmental stressor.

Although the metaplastic changes of the cervix are not pathologic, the squamous epithelial cell component of the transformation zone is vulnerable to stressors, which may cause the cells injury or damage. The epithelium can be injured by several factors, including chronic infection, irritation, and trauma. The transformation zone represents the most likely site for the cellular response of dysplasia. Cells altered with dysplastic changes are characterized by an abnormal growth and a disordered process of differentiation (dividing cells are not

confined to the basal layer). Dysplastic cells are sloughed off the cervical surface prematurely and are often immature.

Changes in cellular structures, particularly in the nucleus, are apparent in dysplastic cervical cells. Alterations in the **chromatin**, genetic material made of DNA, are responsible for the darkened appearance of the cell nucleus and the abnormal differentiation of dividing cells. Cervical dysplasia is considered to be a precancerous condition. If identified and treated early, the damaged cervical cells can be replaced by normal cells, leading to full recovery. If left untreated, the cells may recover spontaneously or may progress into **malignancy** or cancer.

CLINICAL MANIFESTATIONS

There are no signs and symptoms of cervical dysplasia, emphasizing the importance of routine cervical cytologic screening for early detection. The presence of risk factors for cervical dysplasia should be considered when determining screening type and frequency. Risk factors include:

1. Early-onset sexual activity
2. Multiple (more than three) sexual partners
3. Exposure to **human papilloma virus (HPV)**
4. Smoking

The *human papilloma virus* is implicated as a common factor in the development of cervical dysplasia.[17] HPV enters the host cell and can be integrated into its genome. The changes in the DNA are translated into unregulated cellular reproduction and can potentially result in cancer, although not all strains of the virus are considered to be potentially **oncogenic** (cancer causing).

STOP *and* *Consider*

Can the prevalence of high-risk types of HPV vary geographically? Why is it important to determine the most common types of high-risk HPV in a particular region or geographic area?

DIAGNOSIS

Identification of cervical dysplasia is achieved through both screening and diagnostic testing.

Screening Tests

Routine screening of cervical cells is done to identify characteristics of cells. Cells from the ectocervix, ideally from the more vulnerable transformation zone, and from the endocervical canal are obtained

Table 2.1 Laboratory and Diagnostic Tests Used with Cervical Dysplasia

Lab or Diagnostic Test	Purpose of the Test	Procedure
Physical examination	Visual evaluation of cervix	Speculum examination of the ectocervix to detect transformation zone and general appearance
Cervical sampling	Obtaining a specimen for cytologic evaluation	Pap smear requiring the use of a spatula for ectocervical sample and a cytobrush for endocervical sample or liquid sampling also capable of determining human papilloma virus (HPV) type
Cervical assessment	Evaluation of the cervix and endocervical canal for evidence of dysplasia	Examination of the cervix with a colposcope; sampling of endocervical canal and biopsy of all lesions suspected of dysplasia
Diagnostic excisional procedure	Provide histologic sample of the transformation zone and endocervical canal for evaluation	Laser conization, cold-knife conization, large-loop electrosurgical excision procedure (LEEP), and loop electrosurgical conization comprise the surgical procedures employed to obtain specimens

for microscopic evaluation. Metaplastic and dysplastic changes can be determined with this screening method.[18] In addition to identification of cellular changes, some screening tests can determine whether an oncogenic form of HPV is present by DNA analysis. The results of these tests are used to determine treatment and follow-up plans (Table 2.1).

The Papanicolaou (Pap) smear, named for the originator Dr George Papanicolaou, has been the primary method of cervical screening since the early 1940s. Cells from the ectocervix and endocervix are collected during a pelvic examination. Placement of a speculum into the vagina allows viewing of the cervix. A collecting device, often referred to as a spatula, is placed on the transformation zone of the ectocervix, and superficial cells are collected by rotating the collection device. Cells from the endocervix are also collected during this procedure. In a conventional Pap smear, the cells are placed (smeared) on a glass slide and preserved with fixative for subsequent examination by a cytotechnologist or a pathologist. Cells collected from the cervix can also be placed in a vial of preservative solution for analysis using a newer method of Pap smear analysis, liquid-based Pap testing. The use of the liquid-based method of analysis may be indicated for determination of cervical cell infection with HPV.

Women at high risk for cervical dysplasia are encouraged to have annual Pap screenings for cervical dysplasia. Recommendations for screening for women at low risk include:

- Annually, until two negative results are obtained
- After two negative results, 1 year apart
  - Every 3 years for women who are sexually active
  - Every 3 years for women over 20 years of age

The results of the Pap smear screening are used in consideration of management and treatment strategies. Results of Pap screenings are reported using the Bethesda System as follows:

- Negative for intraepithelial lesion or malignancy
  - No signs of cancer or precancerous changes
  - Reactive cellular changes
    - May indicate adaptive responses to infectious agents
- Epithelial cell abnormalities
  - Epithelial cellular changes that may indicate cancer or a precancerous condition
  - Atypical squamous cells of undetermined significance (ASCUS)
    - Cellular changes not definitive
    - May indicate changes caused by infection or represent precancerous changes
    - May resolve spontaneously
    - May require HPV DNA testing to determine appropriate treatment
  - Low-grade squamous intraepithelial lesion (LGSIL)
    - May resolve spontaneously or develop into cancer
  - High-grade squamous intraepithelial lesion (HGSIL)
    - More likely than LGSIL to develop into a cancerous lesion
  - Squamous cell carcinoma
    - Cellular changes likely caused by invasive squamous cell cancer
- Glandular cell abnormalities
  - Atypical glandular cells of undetermined significance (AGUS)
    - Changes that cannot rule out cancer
  - Adenocarcinoma

Abnormal screening may indicate the need for HPV testing. Identification of high-risk HPV strains provides further information for determining treatment approaches. Analysis of cells for the presence and strain of HPV DNA indicates infection with the virus and identifies the risk status of the specific virus. Indications for HPV testing have been developed to identify those individuals at the greatest risk for the consequences of HPV infection. HPV testing is indicated for screening along with a Pap smear as an aid for treatment determination in all women with a slightly abnormal Pap smear result.

Diagnostic Tests

Diagnostic testing is performed based on cellular screening tests. Evaluation of tissue is completed to obtain an accurate diagnosis and to form the basis of treatment. One of the most common diagnostic tests is the colposcopy. Colposcopy allows a more careful visual observation of cervical changes and serves as a guide for biopsy site selection. An outpatient procedure, colposcopy is similar to a Pap smear in the approach of visualization of the cervix using a speculum. Rather than viewing the cervix with the naked eye, the tissue is magnified by a colposcope, a binocular-like device placed about 30 cm outside the opening of the vagina. An acetic acid solution is applied to the cervix, which causes areas to turn white (aceto–white), suggestive of dysplasia. Small, 1/8-inch tissue sections (punch biopsies) are taken from the whitened areas and sent to pathology for analysis. Further tissue is collected by endocervical curettage, providing a tissue sample from the endocervix. A narrow instrument (curette) is passed into the endocervix to obtain the sample, providing tissue for accurate diagnosis.

Biopsy results are reported as follows:

- Cervical intraepithelial neoplasia (CIN)
  - CIN 1
    - Mild dysplasia
    - Confined to the lowest third of epithelium
  - CIN 2
    - Moderate dysplasia
    - Lower two thirds of epithelium
  - CIN 3
    - Severe dysplasia
      - Extending to the upper third of the epithelium
      - Not full thickness
- Carcinoma in situ
  - Involves full thickness of the epithelium
- Squamous cell carcinoma
  - Invasive cancer of the squamous cells
- Adenocarcinoma
  - Invasive cancer of the glandular cells

High-risk HPV types are positively associated with increasing severity of cervical dysplasia.[19] At least 15 types of HPV are considered high risk due to their association with cervical cancer. In June 2006, the U.S. Food and Drug Administration (FDA) licensed Gardasil, the first vaccine that specifically prevents cervical cancer. Approved for use in females 9 to 26 years of age, Gardasil targets high-risk HPV types 16 and 18 for prevention of cervical cancer and HPV types 6 and 11 for prevention of genital warts. It is estimated that a vaccine against these types has the potential to prevent 71% of cervical cancers worldwide.[15]

TREATMENT

Treatment to remove superficial cells is accomplished by cryosurgery, a form of cold therapy that destroys mildly dysplastic cells. Liquid nitrogen is applied to the dysplastic cells on the ectocervix, identified by colposcopy via a probe placed in the desired area. Cone biopsy, also known as conization, is a surgical procedure that removes a cone-shaped area of cervical tissue in the area of the transformation zone. Traditional cone biopsy is done using a scalpel, or "cold knife." Large-loop electrosurgical excision procedure (LEEP) is similar but is done with a wire heated by an electrical current. After abnormal Pap smear and histologic findings are found, increased surveillance with Pap screening is accomplished to determine resolution of dysplasia. In cases of carcinoma, a hysterectomy may be indicated.

From the Lab

Interpretation of traditional Pap smears with cells viewed in a slide preparation is limited by the quality of the collection. Cells may be placed too thickly on the slide, obscuring some of the cells from view. Other cell types, such as bacteria, yeast, and white blood cells, can also prevent adequate viewing of the cervical cells of interest. Liquid-based cytology is a newer method of cervical cell processing that allow the cells collected to be placed in a fixative filled vial rather than on a slide. One advantage of this method is the ability of the cytotechnologist or pathologist to view cells more clearly. Cells of interest can be analyzed more easily because of removal of mucus, bacteria, yeast, and other cells. An additional benefit provided by liquid-based Pap preparations includes the ability to screen for HPV in cells with abnormal findings.

Environmental Toxins and Cardiovascular Disease

Results from numerous studies worldwide have provided an important link between exposure to airborne environmental toxins and pollution with the development of cardiovascular disease.

Environmental components of air pollution include carbon monoxide nitrates, sulfur dioxide, ozone, lead, and secondhand tobacco smoke. These toxic substances promote the development of physical cellular injury and contribute to disease and illness. Fine particles in air pollution are associated with an increase in mortality and with the development of cardiovascular disease caused by inflammation, atherosclerosis, and altered cardiac function. When the individuals smoked, these effects were additive.[20] The evidence is so strong that the American Heart Association included air pollution as a known risk factor for cardiovascular disease.[21]

PATHOPHYSIOLOGY

Cigarette smoking is one of the most common environmental pollutants known to cause cellular damage. The particulate matter from the tar and the gas in cigarette smoke contains free radicals, with toxicity potential ranging from seconds to months.[22] These toxins are present in both **mainstream** (active) and **sidestream** (passive or secondhand) **smoke**. When the toxin-containing smoke enters the lung, the free radicals (O_2^-, H_2O_2, and $ONOO^-$) promote the development of oxidative stress. This results in inflammation, release of cytokines, vascular dysfunction, and altered gene activation and contributes to the development of atherosclerosis. The resulting cellular damage increases an individual's risk of developing coronary heart disease.[23,24] Studies have demonstrated that even small exposures to these toxins can cause a significant increase in cardiovascular disease.[25]

CLINICAL MANIFESTATIONS

The manifestations of exposure to firsthand and secondhand smoke reflect the overall effects of pathology on the entire body. From cellular dysfunction to organ involvement, smoking affects nearly all body systems. According to a report by the U.S. Surgeon General,[26] the following findings represent the consequences of smoking on health.

- Smoking is harmful to every organ in the body
- Smoking causes many diseases, reducing the health of smokers

- Smoking cigarettes with reduced tar and nicotine does not offer any health benefit

Health consequences of smoking include aortic aneurysm, acute myeloid leukemia, cataract, cancer (cervical, kidney, pancreatic, stomach, bladder, esophageal, laryngeal, lung, oral, and throat), pneumonia, periodontitis, chronic lung diseases, coronary heart and cardiovascular diseases (including ischemic stroke), reproductive effects, and sudden infant death syndrome.

DIAGNOSIS

Smoking serves as both a causative and an additive factor in cardiovascular disease. History may reveal poor exercise tolerance due to impaired ability of the heart or blood vessels to meet the increased demands of activity. Dyspnea is a frequent complaint that may indicate either an underlying cardiovascular or a pulmonary condition. Cool, pale, and painful extremities may indicate the presence of a clot or the presence of peripheral vascular disease. Physical examination may reveal increased blood pressure and heart rate, and decreased cardiac output, and coronary blood flow. Laboratory studies may indicate markers of cardiovascular disease, including decreased HDL (high density lipoprotein, "good cholesterol") and increased LDL (low density lipoprotein, "bad cholesterol").

TREATMENT

Smoking cessation is the first step in the prevention of further complications. Smoking cessation is a challenge for many individuals. Tips provided by the U.S. Surgeon General (http://www.surgeongeneral.gov/tobacco/quits.pdf) for successful cessation include:

- Get ready
- Get support
- Learn new skills and behaviors
- Get medication and use it correctly
- Be prepared for relapse or difficult situations

Pharmacologic management includes the use of bupropion (Zyban), a norepinephrine/dopamine reuptake inhibitor FDA approved for use in smoking cessation. Nicotine replacement in several forms, including gum, inhaler, nasal spray, and skin patch, can be used to wean from the nicotine previously provided by smoking. Although some smoking-related damage may be reversible, treatment of the persistent health consequences of smoking is disease specific and may be required long term.

From the Lab

Cotinine, a nicotine metabolite, can be measured in the blood, urine, or saliva. Cotinine levels can provide an objective measurement of exposure to active or **passive smoke**. Since the early 1990s, cotinine levels in nonsmokers have decreased by more than 70% in adults, 58% in children, and 55% in adolescents, indicating lowered environmental smoke exposure.[27]

● **STOP** *and* *Consider*

Who is most at risk for illness related to second-hand smoke? What increases vulnerability to disease?

Summary

- Cellular homeostasis depends on the proper functioning of cellular components, with direct effects on tissues and organs.
- Cellular adaptations to stress, injury, and damage form the basis of all disease.
- Alterations in cell size (atrophy and hypertrophy), cell number (hyperplasia), and cell structure (metaplasia and dysplasia) cause changes in tissue function and impact the entire person.
- Most cellular adaptations are necessary for cell survival.
- When damage exceeds the ability of the cell to adapt to a stressor, cell death by apoptosis or necrosis results.
- The clinical models presented in this chapter illustrate the applications of the concepts of cellular adaptation, including atrophy, hypertrophy, hyperplasia, metaplasia, dysplasia, apoptosis, and necrosis.

Case Study 2.1

You are spending the winter skiing high in the mountains of Colorado. You notice that exertion while skiing makes you tired and that you do not have as much energy as you did before staying in the mountains. You realize that you are feeling this way because your body cannot take in as much oxygen at the higher altitude. One long-term adaptation your body must make is to increase the production of red blood cells to better oxygenate your tissues and cells. Based on the information in this chapter

and on additional readings, answer the following questions:

1. *What is the most likely stressor that will cause your cells to adapt?*
2. *What are the adaptations your cells likely to make to respond to the stressor?*
3. *What is the potential outcome if your cells are unable to adapt?*
4. *What lab tests can be used to identify the expected adaptations?*
5. *Can any treatments be used to support your body's adaptation?*

Log onto the Internet. Search for a relevant journal article or Web site that details oxygenation at higher altitude to confirm your predictions.

Case Study 2.2

A 56-year-old man arrived in the emergency room, complaining of chest pain. After evaluation, it was decided that he needed a coronary angiogram to determine if there were areas of blockage causing ischemia. One day after the angiogram, his renal function began to deteriorate. He was diagnosed with contrast-induced nephropathy.

1. *What is contrast-induced nephropathy?*
2. *What is the epidemiology of contrast-induced nephropathy?*
3. *What is the etiology of contrast-induced nephropathy?*
4. *What are the adaptations his cells likely to make to respond to the stressor?*
5. *How does the cellular injury manifest?*
6. *What can be done to prevent or treat nephrotoxic cellular injury in contrast-induced nephropathy?*

Log onto the Internet. Search for a relevant journal article or Web site that details cellular injury and adaptation resulting from contrast-induced nephropathy to confirm your predictions.

Practice Exam Questions

1. The organelle that is involved in cellular respiration and is linked to the development of oxidative stress is known as the:
   a. Endoplasmic reticulum
   b. Golgi apparatus
   c. Lysosome
   d. Mitochondria

2. Cells develop into tissues with specialized structure and function through the process of:
   a. Differentiation
   b. Proliferation
   c. Endocytosis
   d. Exocytosis

3. The cell's typical response to a decrease in trophic signal is:
   a. Atrophy
   b. Hypertrophy
   c. Hyperplasia
   d. Phagocytosis

4. Cell death by necrosis is:
   a. The cell's way of replacing aged cells with new cells
   b. Also known as programmed cell death
   c. Often a response to inflammation
   d. Commonly seen during the period of embryo development

5. You are caring for a female patient who has reported a noticeable decrease in breast size and muscle mass. Which of the following conditions and causes is the most likely explanation?
   a. Puberty
   b. Pregnancy
   c. Menopause
   d. Acromegaly

6. The changes seen in cells adapting to stressors that promote metaplasia:
   a. Are irreversible
   b. Can result in cancer
   c. Change from one cell type to another
   d. Show abnormal differentiation

7. Cellular atrophy results in
   a. Increase in tissue volume due to increase in cell number
   b. Increase in tissue volume due to increase in cell size
   c. Decrease in tissue volume due to decrease in cell size
   d. No change in tissue volume

8. Treatment of chronic conditions associated with cerebral atrophy
   a. Are effective at restoring neuronal function
   b. Are targeted toward slowing neuronal injury and atrophy
   c. Are best initiated when advanced signs and symptoms are evident
   d. Are not indicated

9. Which of the following hormones is secreted from the anterior pituitary?
   a. Growth hormone
   b. Somatostatin
   c. Growth hormone–releasing hormone
   d. Insulin-like growth factor 1

10. Which one of the following is a diagnostic test for cervical dysplasia?
    a. Liquid-based Pap cytology
    b. Conventional Pap cytology
    c. Cervical punch biopsy
    d. HPV testing

11. Which of the following reactive oxygen species is scavenged by catalase?
    a. Hydroxyl radical
    b. Peroxynitrite
    c. Superoxide
    d. Hydrogen peroxide

12. Which of the following terms describes cells that are enlarged, with darkened nuclei and abnormal chromatin?
    a. Hyperplastic
    b. Dysplastic
    c. Metaplastic
    d. Aplastic

Discussion and Application

1. What did I know about basic alterations in cells and tissues before today?

2. What body processes are affected by altered cellular and tissue adaptation? How do cellular and tissue adaptations impact those processes?

3. What are the potential etiologies for altered cellular and tissue adaptation? How do cellular and tissue adaptations develop?

4. Who is most at risk for developing altered cellular and tissue adaptation? How can these alterations be prevented?

5. What are the human differences that affect the etiology, risk, or course of altered cellular and tissue adaptation?

6. What are the clinical manifestations expected in the course of altered cellular and tissue adaptation?

7. What special diagnostic tests help to determine the diagnosis and course of altered cellular and tissue adaptation?

8. What are the goals of care for individuals with altered cellular and tissue adaptation?

9. How does the concept of altered cellular and tissue adaptation build on what I have learned in the previous chapter and in the previous courses?

10. How can I use what I have learned?

RESOURCES

American Heart Association. Diseases and Conditions: Cardiomyopathy:
http://www.americanheart.org/presenter.jhtml?identifier=4468
Retrieved April 12, 2009.

Center for Disease Control. Second National Report on Human Exposure to Environmental Chemicals:
http://www.cdc.gov/exposurereport
Retrieved April 12, 2009.

National Institute of Diabetes and Digestive and Kidney Diseases. Acromegaly:
http://endocrine.niddk.nih.gov/pubs/acro/acro.htm
Retrieved April 12, 2009.

National Institute of Neurological Disorders and Stroke. Cerebral atrophy:
http://www.ninds.nih.gov/disorders/cerebral_atrophy/cerebral_atrophy.htm
Retrieved April 10, 2009.

Ries LAG, Eisner MP, Kosary CL, et al. SEER Cancer Statistics Review, 1975–2005. Bethesda, MD; National Cancer Institute:
http://seer.cancer.gov/csr/1975_2005/
Retrieved April 12, 2009.

REFERENCES

1. Zatz M, Starling A. Calpains and disease. *N Engl J Med.* 2005;352(23):2413–2423.
2. Stone WL, Krishnan K, Campbell SE, et al. Tocopherols and the treatment of colon cancer. *Ann N Y Acad Sci.* 2004;1031:223–233.
3. Colcombe SJ, Erickson KI, Scalf PE, et al. Aerobic exercise training increases brain volume in aging humans. *J Gerontol A Biol Sci Med Sci.* 2006;61:1166–1170.
4. Gordon BA, Rykhlevskaia EI, Brumback CR, et al. Neuroanatomical correlates of aging, cardiopulmonary fitness level, and education. *Psychophysiology.* 2008;45:825–838.
5. Erickson KI, Suever BL, Prakash RS, et al. Greater intake of vitamins B6 and B12 spares gray matter in healthy elderly: a voxel-based morphometry study. *Brain Res.* 2008;1199:20–26.
6. Jokinen H, Kalska H, Ylikoski R. Longitudinal cognitive decline in subcortical ischemic vascular disease—the LADIS study. *Cerebrovasc Dis.* 2009;27:384–391.
7. Grassiot B, Desgranges B, Eustache F, et al. Quantification and clinical relevance of brain atrophy in multiple sclerosis: a review. *J Neurol.* 2009;256(9):1397–1412.
8. Apostolova LG, Thompson PM. Mapping progressive brain structural changes in early Alzheimer's disease and mild cognitive impairment. *Neuropsychologia.* 2008;46:1597–1612.
9. Maron BJ, Ackerman MJ, Nishimura RA, et al. Task Force 4: HCM and other cardiomyopathies, mitral valve prolapse, myocarditis, and Marfan syndrome. *J Am Coll Cardiol.* 2005;45(8):1340–1345.
10. Nishimura RA, Holmes DR Jr. Clinical practice. Hypertrophic obstructive cardiomyopathy. *N Engl J Med.* 2004;350(13):1320–1327.
11. Elliott P, McKenna WJ. Hypertrophic cardiomyopathy. *Lancet.* 2004;363(9424):1881–1891.
12. Vitale G, Pivonello R, Lombardi G, et al. Cardiovascular complications in acromegaly. *Minerva Endocrinol.* 2004;29(3):77–88.
13. Matsukura T, Sugase M. Human papillomavirus genomes in squamous cell carcinomas of the uterine cervix. *Virology.* 2004;324(2):439–449.
14. Whincup PH, Gilg JA, Emberson JR, et al. Passive smoking and risk of coronary heart disease and stroke: prospective study with cotinine measurement. *BMJ.* 2004;329(7459):200–205.
15. Canadian Cancer Society. Canadian Cancer Statistics 2005. National Cancer Institute of Canada, Statistics Canada, Provincial/Territorial Cancer Registries, Public Health Agency of Canada; 2005.
16. Minuto F, Resmini E, Boschetti M, et al. Assessment of disease activity in acromegaly by means of a single blood sample: comparison of the 120th minute postglucose value with spontaneous GH secretion and with the IGF system. *Clin Endocrinol (Oxf).* 2004;61(1):138–144.
17. Finkelstein MM, Jerrett M, Sears MR. Traffic air pollution and mortality rate advancement periods. *Am J Epidemiol.* 2004;160(2):173–177.
18. Brook RD, Franklin B, Cascio W, et al. Air pollution and cardiovascular disease: a statement for healthcare professionals from the Expert Panel on Population and Prevention Science of the American Heart Association. *Circulation.* 2004;109(21):2655–2671.
19. Wright TC Jr, Cox JT, Massad LS, et al. 2001 Consensus Guidelines for the management of women with cervical cytological abnormalities. *JAMA.* 2002;287(16):2120–2129.
20. Munoz N, Bosch FX, Castellsague X, et al. Against which human papillomavirus types shall we vaccinate and screen? The international perspective. *Int J Cancer.* 2004;111(2):278–285.
21. Ambrose JA, Barua RS. The pathophysiology of cigarette smoking and cardiovascular disease: an update. *J Am Coll Cardiol.* 2004;43(10):1731–1737.
22. Pechacek TF, Babb S. How acute and reversible are the cardiovascular risks of secondhand smoke? *BMJ.* 2004;328(7446):980–983.
23. US Department of Health and Human Services. *The Health Consequences of Smoking: A Report of the Surgeon General.* Rockville, MD: US Dept of Health and Human Services, Centers for Disease Control and Prevention, National Center for Chronic Disease Prevention and Health Promotion, Office of Smoking and Health; 2004.
24. Lipshultz SE, Sleeper LA, Towbin JA, et al. The incidence of pediatric cardiomyopathy in two regions of the United States. *N Engl J Med.* 2003;348(17):1647–1655.
25. Center for Disease Control. *CDC's Second National Report on Human Exposure to Environmental Chemicals: Spotlight on Cotinine.* Rockville, MD: US Dept of Health and Human Services; 2003.
26. Gaziano JM. Vitamin E and cardiovascular disease: observational studies. *Ann N Y Acad Sci.* 2004;1031:280–291.
27. Pope CA III, Burnett RT, Thurston GD, et al. Cardiovascular mortality and long-term exposure to particulate air pollution: epidemiological evidence of general pathophysiological pathways of disease. *Circulation.* 2004;109(1):71–77.

Chapter 3

Inflammation and Tissue Repair

LEARNING OBJECTIVES

1. Define and use the key terms listed in this chapter.
2. Differentiate the three lines of defense.
3. Outline the process of acute inflammation, including the role of chemical mediators.
4. Describe the process of healing and repair after tissue injury.
5. Differentiate acute and chronic inflammation.
6. Identify the cardinal signs of inflammation.
7. Discuss treatment methods used for acute and chronic inflammation.
8. Apply concepts of acute and chronic inflammation to select clinical models.

INTRODUCTION

Think back to all of the injuries, even minor ones, that you have sustained in your lifetime. When did you last burn the roof of your mouth on a hot pizza, get a paper cut, or sprain your ankle? All of these activities, and many others, cause tissue trauma that requires healing. This chapter focuses on the inflammatory response, which occurs with any type of injury. Inflammation is critical for you to understand as a student in the health professions. All disease processes cause injury; healing can only occur with an effective inflammatory response. The *acute* inflammatory response is considered an expected body response to injury; *chronic* inflammation is presented as an altered inflammatory response due to unrelenting injury. The stages of tissue repair and complications that can occur during the healing process are also detailed in this chapter.

Review of Body Defense Mechanisms

Protection of the body depends on three major lines of defense, as depicted in Figure 3.1:

- The first line of defense relies on the protection of the skin and mucous membranes.
- The second line of defense is waged through an effective inflammatory response.
- The third line of defense is activated through the specificity of the immune response.

The skin and mucous membranes comprise a physical and chemical barrier to invasion and are considered the first line of defense. Skin allows a protective physical barrier against harmful substances in the external environment. Areas not covered by skin are protected by chemically coated

mucous membranes that help to neutralize or destroy many harmful invaders. Tears and saliva are examples of enzyme-filled fluids that bathe mucous membranes and offer essential protection to the eyes and oral cavity. Breaks in the skin and mucous membranes or loss of protective fluids allow microorganisms and other harmful agents to enter the body and threaten homeostasis.

STOP *and Consider*

What can you do to improve or strengthen your first line of defense?

The second line of defense, or inflammatory response, is activated when the first line of defense is inadequate. The inflammatory response is nonspecific; that is, the process of waging an inflammatory response is identical regardless of the cause of injury. The **immune response** is considered to be the third line of defense. The immune response wages a specific defense depending on the type of invader; this is the focus of Chapter 4.

STOP *and Consider*

What lines of defense are you enhancing by putting on an antibiotic ointment and covering a laceration with a band-aid?

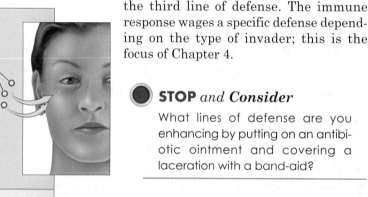

First line of defense
- Blink reflex occurs
- Lashes catch particles
- Tears wash particles away
- Enzymes in tears neutralize harmful substances
- Intact surrounding skin prevents entry of harmful substances

Harmful substances

Inadequate 1st line

Second line of defense
- Inflammatory mechanisms are activated
- Vasodilation and increased capillary permeability cause redness (erythema) and swelling
- Phagocytes move in to engulf and destroy harmful substances

Third line of defense
- Immune response is activated
- Immune cells recognize and destroy harmful substances

Adequate response   **Inadequate response**

Resolution   Disease spread

Figure 3.1 Lines of defense.

Acute Inflammation

Acute inflammation is triggered by tissue injury and is essential for healing. **Injury** is defined in the broadest sense to include any form of damage or alteration to cells or tissues. Injury can include invasion by microorganisms, cellular mutations, hypoxia or anoxia, nutritional deficiencies, and physical or chemical damage. The acute inflammatory response has three major goals:

1. To increase blood flow to the site of an injury, which is referred to as the **vascular response**
2. To alert the products of healing to attend to the site of injury, which is referred to as the **cellular response**
3. To remove the injured tissue and prepare the site for healing

The process of inflammation requires the ability to recognize the injury, activate a response, and appropriately shut down the response when the injury has passed. The result is either tissue repair or regeneration or the formation of scar tissue.

Vascular Response

Tissue injury requires a response at the level of the blood vessel near the site of the injury. Put simply, clotting and healing must occur. If the blood vessels are considered roads, injury requires that the roads be widened and expanded to allow for emergency vehicles to get to the scene of the accident. The objective is to attract sufficient products of clotting and healing to the site of injury and to prevent infection.

Anatomically, the structure of the blood vessels must change to accommodate this increase in emergency vehicle traffic.

1. The blood vessels **dilate**, or widen, to accommodate increased blood flow to the site of injury.
2. The lining of the blood vessel becomes more **permeable**, or loosens to allow cells to easily move from the vessel into the injured tissue.

Loosening of the blood vessel must occur with the basement membrane of the blood vessel and adjacent endothelial cells (Fig. 3.2). **Endothelial cells** form a tight junction within the inner lining of the blood and lymphatic vessels and the heart. Endothelial cells are connected to the basement membrane. The **basement membrane** is the outer membrane of the vessels, which separates the vessel from the

tissues of the body. The vessel walls are needed to confine blood cells and plasma, but with injury must be loosened to allow for movement of healing fluids and cells into damaged tissues.

Increased blood and fluid are needed at the site of the injury for two reasons:

1. Blood is composed of cells active in **phagocytosis**, the process of engulfing and removing harmful agents, as well as cells essential in promoting healing and developing an immune response.
2. Increased fluid dilutes harmful substances at the site of the injury.

Inspection of a scraped knee after a bike accident will show a layer of watery fluid that seeps from the wound. This **exudate** (watery fluid) that accumulates at the site of injury has a high protein and leukocyte concentration. This is a sure sign that the vessels have become more permeable and that cells active in phagocytosis are present and are ready to fend off microorganisms. Healing can then begin.

This whole process is orchestrated through the work of potent chemicals, referred to as inflammatory mediators. **Inflammatory mediators**, specifically vasoactive inflammatory mediators, facilitate the process of widening and loosening of the blood

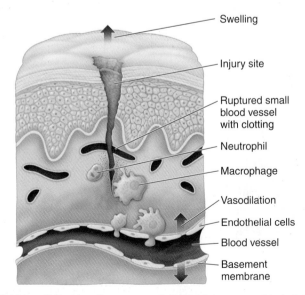

■ **Figure 3.2** Vascular response. Inflammation causes widening of endothelial cell junctions and vasodilation. (Image modified from Werner R, Benjamin BE. *A Massage Therapist's Guide to Pathology.* 3rd ed. Baltimore: Lippincott Williams & Wilkins; 2005, with permission.)

vessels at the site of injury. Inflammatory mediators are located in the blood plasma and in many cells, including platelets, mast cells, basophils, neutrophils, endothelial cells, monocytes, and macrophages. The location of inflammatory mediators is important; these substances must be constantly ready to respond to injury anywhere in the body. Figure 3.3 illustrates the major roles of the inflammatory mediators in the inflammatory process. Refer to this figure frequently as you move through this chapter.

INFLAMMATORY MEDIATORS WITHIN CELLS

As mentioned, some inflammatory mediators are formed within the blood plasma and some are formed within cells. Within cells, most of these inflammatory mediators are generated in the cell plasma membrane or are made up of proteins within the cell. Most commonly, it is white blood cells that produce and release inflammatory mediators; platelets, endothelial cells, and injured tissue cells are also potential sources. The generation and activation of inflammatory mediators is a complex process. Try not to get overwhelmed. In this section, focus on the key inflammatory cells, where they are located, examples of inflammatory mediators released from those cells, and what their role is in the inflammatory process.

Inflammatory Mediators within White Blood Cells

The **mast cell** is an important inflammatory mediator. Mast cells are leukocytes (white blood cells) that are housed throughout the connective tissues of the body and near all blood vessels. The placement of the mast cell allows for a rapid response directly at the site of injury. Mast cells are similar to having emergency first responders trained in all neighborhoods. They are right there on the scene. The mast cell is responsible for the production and immediate release of inflammatory mediators through a process of **degranulation**, the mast cell breaks apart and releases inflammatory mediators in the form of extracellular granules (grain-like particles). The **basophil**, a white blood cell that also contains granules, functions in the same manner. Examples of inflammatory mediators released by mast cells include histamine, leukotrienes, and prostaglandins.

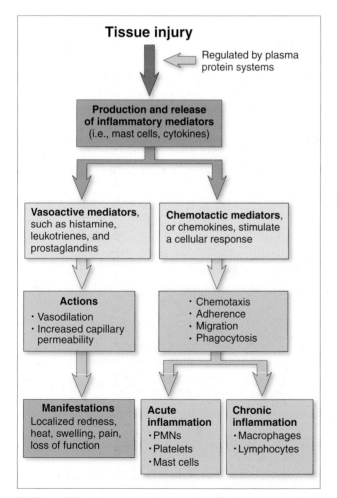

STOP *and Consider*

Where have you heard the names of the various inflammatory mediators listed above? What do you already know about these inflammatory mediators?

Signals to trigger, enhance, and discontinue the inflammatory response are also generated within other white blood cells, such as lymphocytes and monocytes/macrophages. For example, **cytokines** are more than a hundred distinct cell proteins most often found within white blood cells that have a vital role in regulating inflammation; they are active from the onset of vasodilation and increased vascular permeability to the resolution of the inflammatory response. Each of the different cytokines is released from a specific cell and serves a specific purpose. For example, cytokines released from lymphocytes are called lymphokines. Those released from monocytes or macrophages are called monokines. Other examples of cytokines include interleukins, growth factors, interferons, and chemokines. Now try not to hyperventilate

Figure 3.3 Concept map. An overview of the importance of chemical mediators in the vascular and cellular responses of inflammation. PMNs, polymorphonuclear neutrophils. (Image modified from Rubin E, Farber JL. *Pathology*. 4th ed. Philadelphia: Lippincott Williams & Wilkins; 2005, with permission.)

here. The main point is that potent inflammatory mediators are released from a variety of white blood cells in order to effectively orchestrate the inflammatory process.

Inflammatory Mediators within Platelets

Platelets are also active in generating and releasing inflammatory mediators to promote vasodilation, clotting, attraction of white blood cells, and healing of injured tissues. Serotonin is one example of an inflammatory mediator found in platelets. Serotonin causes vasodilation and increased vascular permeability, allowing cells of healing to arrive quickly to the site of injury. Histamine, also found in white blood cells, can be housed in platelets as well as functions similarly to serotonin.

Inflammatory Mediators within Endothelial or Injured Tissue Cells

Inflammatory mediators can also be released from endothelial cells or injured tissue cells. For example, **platelet-activating factor** is a complex lipid stored in cell membranes, including those of endothelial cells that line blood vessels and in many other types of cells that can become injured. Platelet-activating factor is a potent inflammatory mediator that has a key role in promoting vessel vasodilation, clotting, and attracting infection-fighting white blood cells to the site of injury.

Another example is arachidonic acid. **Arachidonic acid** is a substance, derived from the plasma membrane of an injured cell, which generates various inflammatory mediators through a complex chemical conversion. Inflammatory mediators associated with arachidonic acid include prostaglandins, lipoxins, leukotrienes, and thromboxane. These inflammatory mediators are active in the processes of vasodilation and vasoconstriction, increasing vascular permeability, bronchodilation and bronchoconstriction, and attraction of leukocytes. Corticosteroids are a highly effective group of anti-inflammatory drugs that work to block the production of arachidonic acid, thereby decreasing the inflammatory response. Corticosteroids also have a role on inhibiting the immune response, as discussed in Chapter 4.

⬤ **STOP** *and Consider*

Why would you want to block the production of arachidonic acid and inhibit the work of the inflammatory mediators?

INFLAMMATORY MEDIATORS WITHIN PLASMA

Inflammatory mediators can also circulate continuously within blood plasma. This is usually accomplished through the work of three major interrelated pathways. These pathways are responsible for the activation and deactivation of inflammatory mediators that circulate in the plasma. Table 3.1 summarizes these three pathways.

Multiple sources and pathways to induce and suppress inflammation are necessary because the inflammatory response *must occur* to heal tissues, and the inflammatory mediators are so *potent and powerful* that multiple pathways are needed to regulate these substances. Impaired activation of inflammation can lead to inadequate blood flow to the injured area. This will impair healing by limiting phagocytosis, clot formation, and repair of injured tissues. Impaired inhibition of inflammation can lead to an uncontrolled inflammatory response, the depletion of proteins needed within the three pathways (complement, clotting, and kinin). Loss of the ability to shut down the inflammatory response

Table 3.1 Continuously Circulating and Interrelated Plasma Systems That Regulate Inflammation

System	Key Characteristics
Complement	Several proteins that comprise 10–15% of plasma; produced in liver
	Triggered by the presence of microorganisms
	Once triggered, activates a cascade of inflammatory mediators
	Primary role to destroy and remove microorganisms to prevent infection through **opsonization** (making bacteria vulnerable to phagocytosis) and cell **lysis** (destruction)
Clotting	Promotes coagulation through a cascade of clotting factors
	Suppresses coagulation when clotting is complete
	Various clotting factors produce and release inflammatory mediators
Kinin	Source of highly potent vasoactive inflammatory mediators
	Amplifies the inflammatory response by triggering other inflammatory mediators

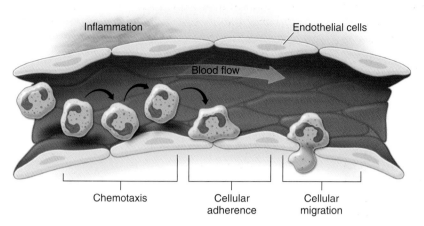

■ **Figure 3.4** Cellular response: chemotaxis, adherence, migration. (Image modified from Rubin E, Farber JL. *Pathology*. 4th ed. Philadelphia: Lippincott Williams & Wilkins; 2005, with permission.)

effectively can also lead to **autoimmunity**, a self-attack against body tissues.

To summarize, the initial steps in the inflammatory response influenced by vasoactive inflammatory mediators include:

- Tissue injury
- Blood vessel vasodilation
- Increased vascular permeability
- Activation of clotting cascade
- Continued release and circulation of vasoactive inflammatory mediators

Cellular Response

After the vessels are dilated and permeable, the cells essential for healing are needed at the injury site. As with the vascular response, the cellular response is regulated by inflammatory mediators. Three steps are needed for a successful cellular response: (1) chemotaxis; (2) cellular adherence; and (3) cellular migration (Fig. 3.4).

Chemotaxis is a process of moving certain cells to the site of injury. Specific inflammatory mediators, referred to as **chemotactic factors**, are activated, which attract specific types of cells. The neutrophil chemotactic factor attracts neutrophils. The eosinophil chemotactic factor attracts eosinophils, and so forth.

Blood cells are constantly moving through the vascular system. Attraction and binding, or cellular **adherence**, is another step essential for effective phagocytosis. Cellular adherence is regulated by:

- Inflammatory mediators; specifically, chemotactic factors released by endothelial cells
- Receptors that bind leukocytes to the surface of endothelial cells near the site of injury

Cellular migration is the third essential step in the cellular response. The cellular response depends on the ability of cells, primarily leukocytes, erythrocytes, and platelets, to migrate, or move across, endothelial cells and get to the exact site of the injury. In the process of **diapedesis**, cells can move between and through endothelial junctions. The role of the major cells activated in the cellular response is summarized in Table 3.2. Leukocyte is a global term for many different types of white blood cells, including neutrophils, monocytes, macrophages,

Research Notes

Recently, inflammatory and immune mechanisms continue to be "hot" topics in research. Several studies have attempted to link inflammatory and immune mechanisms to chronic health conditions such as Alzheimer's disease, coronary artery disease, and even diabetes mellitus. Elevations in inflammatory markers can be detected early in some diseases and sometimes even before diagnosis. The major dilemma is likened to the age-old question: "What came first, the chicken or the egg?" That is, does inflammation appear and cause the disease, or does the disease appear, and inflammation is the natural result?[1-3]

Table 3.2 Cells Active in the Cellular Response

Cell	Role
Leukocyte (white blood cell)	Phagocytosis; removal of dead tissue
Neutrophil	A type of white blood cell; earliest phagocytic responders
Macrophages	A type of white blood cell; large, long-lived phagocytes associated with a prolonged (chronic) inflammatory response; monocytes are immature macrophages
Erythrocyte (red blood cell)	Carry oxygen to tissues
Platelet	Trap harmful substances; stop bleeding; form structural origin of repair

mast cells, basophils, and T and B lymphocytes. Because there is extensive crossover of cellular activity between the inflammatory response, immune response, and the subsequent development of infection, this discussion of the cells will continue into the next two chapters and beyond.

During phagocytosis, inflammatory cells release inflammatory mediators to attract more neutrophils. The neutrophil itself also releases potent inflammatory mediators as it works to engulf and digest impaired tissue. During this aggressive process, unaffected, healthy tissue is also destroyed. Tissue destruction is minimized by the work of inhibitor proteins in the plasma-derived complement, clotting, and kinin systems.

GENERAL MANIFESTATIONS

The local manifestations of acute inflammation are often referred to as **cardinal signs**. These signs include **erythema** (redness), heat, swelling, pain, and loss of function. **Lymphadenitis**, or enlargement and inflammation of the nearby lymph nodes, can occur as a function of filtering or draining

Table 3.3 Local Manifestations of Acute Inflammation

Manifestation	Rationale
Redness (erythema)	Vasodilation; increased blood flow to the injured area
Heat	Vasodilation; increased blood flow to the injured area
Incapacitation	Loss of function is related to tissue damage from injury, pain, and swelling at the site
Pain	Increased vascular permeability and accumulation of fluid causes compression in the tissues; inflammatory mediators can also directly elicit a pain response
Exudate and edema	Extracellular fluid accumulation often in tissues because of increased vascular permeability

microorganisms. **Leukocytosis** is an elevation in white blood cells, or leukocytes, with a count usually above 10,000/mm^3. Typically, the individual has a white blood cell count of 5,000 to 10,000/mm^3. All laboratory information is approximate because variability in laboratory ranges exists among various populations and sources. Leukocytosis demonstrates the increased circulation of white blood cells to aid in healing. Plasma proteins are also increased as a result of the three plasma protein systems discussed previously. These proteins are called acute-phase reactants and can be measured through the use of laboratory tests, such as C-reactive protein (CRP). Common blood tests used to detect inflammation are presented in Table 3.4.

From the Lab

CRP and the erythrocyte sedimentation rate (ESR) are two nonspecific tests of inflammation. Elevations in either test will signify inflammation is present, but neither will identify the exact source or location of the inflammation. CRP is often the preferred test for acute inflammation. CRP signifies the presence of a specific protein triggered by plasma protein systems during the inflammatory process. The ESR (also referred to as a sed rate) is a nonspecific method of testing for inflammation. During the inflammatory process, the coagulation cascade results in increased circulating levels of fibrinogen, which causes cells to stick together. When measured in a tube in the lab, red blood cells (RBCs) exposed to the inflammatory process will fall faster and will clump together. The ESR test then measures (in mm/hr) the level of RBC stacking.[4]

harmful substances at the injury site. Local manifestations with rationales are presented in Table 3.3. These manifestations are primarily related to vasodilation and fluid accumulation in the tissues as a result of the activation of inflammatory mediators.

Systemic manifestations related to the inflammatory response include fever, leukocytosis, and a higher percentage of circulating plasma proteins. **Pyrexia**, or fever (an elevated core body temperature), is a result of inflammatory mediators acting directly on the hypothalamus. The hypothalamus is responsible for controlling body temperature. An elevated body temperature stimulates phagocytosis and can also inhibit the growth of certain

STOP *and Consider*

What does an elevation in leukocytes, ESR, or CRP tell you about the location of acute or chronic inflammation?

TREATMENT

The inflammatory response has multiple components and is often considered "overzealous," which explains the efforts of the booming pharmaceutical industry to find effective anti-inflammatory drugs. Damage to healthy surrounding tissue is a common

Table 3.4 Common Blood Tests Used to Detect Acute Inflammation

Blood Test	Reference Values	Changes with Inflammation
White blood cell count	5,000–10,000 white blood cells/mm^3	Circulating white blood cells are increased, often above 10,000/mm^3
White blood cell differential	Neutrophils 45–75% Bands (immature neutrophils) 0–5% Eosinophils 0–8% Basophils 0–3% Lymphocytes 16–46% Monocytes 4–11%	Measures proportion of each of the five types of white blood cells; the proportion of immature neutrophils (bands) is increased in comparison to other white blood cell types
Erythrocyte sedimentation rate	0–17 mm/hr for men 1–25 mm/hr for women 44–114 mm/hr in pregnancy 1–13 mm/hr for children	Detects red blood cell clumping or stacking as a result of increased fibrinogen levels; levels increase, often above 100 mm/hr for those with inflammation
C-reactive protein	Routine CRP <10 mg/L High sensitivity CRP 0.1–3.8 mg/L	>10 mg/L indicates significant inflammatory disease
Complement activity	Total complement 63–145 U/mL C3 (comprises 70% of total protein in the complement system) 80–184 mg/dL	Elevated in inflammation signifying the activation of complement; over time may decrease, indicating that complement factors are exhausted
Prothrombin time	Measured in time to coagulate, approximately 11.2–13.2 seconds	Increased prothrombin levels result in a reduced time to coagulate
Fibrinogen	175–400 mg/dL	Elevated during inflammation to promote coagulation

CRP, C-reactive protein.

occurrence in the acute inflammatory response. Therefore, the initial treatment principles for acute inflammation are to:

1. Reduce blood flow to the local area
2. Decrease swelling
3. Block the action of various inflammatory mediators
4. Decrease pain

The goal of treatment is to minimize the damage to healthy, unaffected tissue and promote rapid healing. Pharmacologic, or drug, treatments for inflammation most commonly block the action of inflammatory mediators, thereby reducing the swelling, pain, redness, and warmth typical of inflammation. Table 3.5 illustrates the actions of common pharmacologic treatments for inflammation. Nonpharmacologic treatments for inflammation initially include rest, ice, compression, and elevation. Once the initial treatment has been employed, resolution may improve with the application of warmth/heat and increased movement. As with all health conditions, optimal fluid and nutrient intake is needed to facilitate healing.

● **STOP** *and Consider*

The RICE (rest, ice, compression, elevation) protocol is employed frequently in acute injury to minimize the effects of inflammation. How does each of these components reduce inflammation?

RESOLUTION OF ACUTE INFLAMMATION

The acute inflammatory response is self-limited. Once the offending agent has been destroyed and removed, feedback systems regulated by the three plasma protein systems (clotting, complement, and kinin), along with the relevant inflammatory mediators, deactivate the inflammatory response, allowing the tissue to heal.

Table 3.5 Common Pharmacologic Agents Used to Treat Inflammation

Pharmacologic Agent	Action
Aspirin	Inhibits the conversion of arachidonic acid to prostaglandins to suppress inflammation, reduce pain, and reduce fever
Nonsteroidal anti-inflammatory drugs	Similar to aspirin; inhibits the anti-inflammatory conversion of arachidonic acid to prostaglandins (NSAIDs). Examples: ibuprofen, naproxen
Glucocorticoids	Act through several mechanisms to interrupt the inflammatory process: inhibit synthesis of chemical mediators and reduce swelling, warmth, redness, and pain; suppress infiltration of phagocytes and avert tissue damage from release of lytic (cell-destroying) enzymes; suppress lymphocyte proliferation; and reduce immune component of inflammation. Example: prednisone

NSAIDs, nonsteroidal anti-inflammatory drugs.

Module 2

Healing and Tissue Repair

Tissue repair is similar to home repair. If a home is damaged, the destroyed area needs to be sealed off to prevent further exposure to the external environment. Then, a process can begin to clear the debris, rebuild the walls and roof, and restore the interior working contents of the home, such as the electrical system, appliances, or heating system. Likewise, the goal of tissue healing and repair is to cover the wound, clear the debris, and restore the structural and functional integrity of the injured area. This process is often divided into three phases: the inflammatory phase, the proliferative phase, and the remodeling phase. Within these phases, structural supports must be rebuilt and functional cells and tissues regenerated or replaced (Fig. 3.5).

The construction workers of tissue repair fit into the following categories:

- Clotting (coagulation) factors to stop bleeding and form a fibrin clot
- Inflammatory mediators to promote chemotaxis to the affected area
- Proteinases (enzymes) to degrade dead tissue
- Proteinase inhibitors to prevent healthy tissue breakdown
- Matrix, or structural, proteins to rebuild architectural supports
- Molecule receptors to attract cells needed to form a structural matrix
- Adhesion molecules to provide "stickiness" to these cells
- Growth factors to promote regeneration of new cells and tissues

◢ Covering the Wound

Inflammatory mediators released from platelets and other cells constrict blood vessels and form a clot at the site. A protective scab is formed from dried blood and exudate. This protective clot and subsequent scab is also called a **thrombus**. The role of the thrombus is to form a physical barrier to prevent additional harmful substances from entering the wound. This covering also prevents the loss of plasma. Epithelial (skin) cells regenerate under the thrombus. Once re-epithelialization is complete, enzymes degrade the scab.

⬤ STOP *and Consider*

Why is it not a good idea to pick off a scab before a wound has healed?

CLEARING THE DEBRIS

Chemical mediators activate neutrophils to move into the injured area and begin the work of healing. The inflammatory response activates neutrophils and later macrophages to engulf, digest, and remove harmful substances and debris. The process of healing cannot begin until the necrotic cells and tissues are removed.

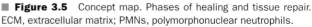
■ **Figure 3.5**   Concept map. Phases of healing and tissue repair. ECM, extracellular matrix; PMNs, polymorphonuclear neutrophils.

Restoring Structural Integrity

Restoring structural integrity depends on the delicate balance of tissue destruction and construction. Tissue lysis, or breakdown and removal, is accomplished through the work of enzymes that are needed to rid the body of the damaged tissue. Growth factors and matrix proteins are responsible for rebuilding the **extracellular matrix** (ECM), the layers of architectural structures that support the cells.

Extracellular matrices include the basement membrane and connective tissue layers. The basement membrane serves to:

1. Provide a supportive architectural structure
2. Support **re-epithelialization**, or the movement of epithelial cells to form a covering over the wound
3. Store growth factors
4. Restore neuromuscular function
5. Support the development of **parenchymal** tissues; that is, those tissues made up of cells with a specific function (such as neurons, myocardial cells, and epithelial cells)

The basement membrane is reproduced by endothelial, epithelial, muscle, adipose (fat), and Schwann (nerve fiber) cells. The basement membrane must be restored before re-epithelialization can occur. Extensive damage to the basement membrane is a hindrance to re-epithelialization because the basement membrane must be replaced first.

Another structural extracellular matrix is connective tissue (Fig. 3.6). The connective tissue layer is composed primarily of collagen, elastin, and glycoproteins. This layer is also referred to as stromal or interstitial tissue. The connective tissue layer provides storage of proteins, an exchange medium between proteins and other cells, and architectural support and physical protection from trauma by resisting stretching or compressing of tissues. Cells such as fibroblasts, adipose cells, endothelial cells, osteocytes, and chondrocytes stimulate the replacement of connective tissue.

Fibroblasts are important cells that produce and replace the connective tissue layer. Fibroblasts are stimulated by macrophages. The fibroblast moves into the area to support the constructive phase of wound healing. Fibroblasts actively manufacture and secrete **collagen**. Collagen helps to fill in the gaps left after the removal of damaged tissues. Excess collagen production leads to tissue fibrosis and can result in scarring at the site of injury.

The connective tissue layer is also composed of elastin and glycoproteins. **Elastin** allows stretching and

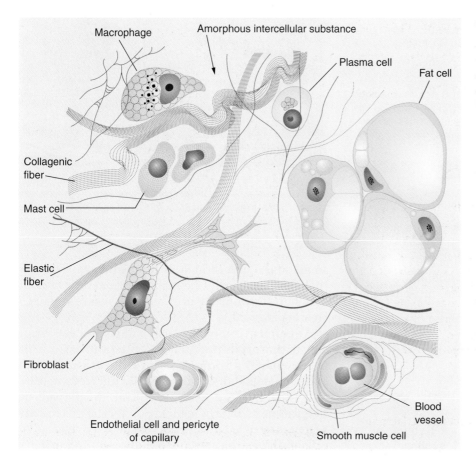

Figure 3.6 Diagram of cells that may be seen in loose connective tissue. The cells lie in the extracellular matrix that is bathed in tissue fluid that originates in capillaries. (From Cormack DH. *Ham's Histology.* 9th ed. Philadelphia: J.B. Lippincott; 1987, with permission)

recoil of tissue. Elastin is somewhat resistant to damage, but is also slow and difficult to replace. Damaged tissue is often less flexible after injury. Glycoproteins are essential within the basement membrane and connective tissue layer. **Glycoproteins** regulate cell movement across the matrix, provide a place for attachment of the cells to the matrix, and prompt the cells to function.

Basement membranes and connective tissue layers are continuously present and must be replaced to support architectural structure and tissue function. A third, temporary, extracellular matrix also forms in response to injury. This temporary matrix, called a **provisional matrix**, promotes healing by decreasing blood and fluid loss at the site and attracting and supporting fibroblasts, endothelial cells, and epidermal (skin) cells. When an injury occurs, increased vascular permeability allows proteins from the plasma to move to the site and form this provisional protective layer.

Macrophage activity converts this provisional matrix into **granulation tissue** (Fig. 3.7). Granulation tissue is connective tissue characterized by extensive macrophages and fibroblasts, and the promotion of **angiogenesis**, or the generation of new blood vessels, at the site. The generation of blood vessels, particularly capillaries, at the site is needed for oxygen/carbon dioxide exchange and to provide other nutrients to the newly developing tissue. Granulation tissue is most noted for the presence of an extensive network of capillaries. As the wound heals, granulation tissue loses the excessive capillary network and retains only that needed to support the final connective tissue matrix. The provisional matrix and specialized granulation tissue are no longer needed and are reabsorbed once the wound is healed and the final connective tissue matrix is in place.

Restoring Functional Integrity

A major goal in healing is to restore the functional integrity of parenchymal tissues. Parenchymal tissues are those that perform a specific body function, such as neuronal (brain) tissue, epithelial (skin) tissue, cardiac myocyte (heart) tissue, or hepatocyte (liver) tissue. Without restoring functional integrity, even minor injuries would become problematic. Restoring functional integrity can be accomplished by one of the three processes:

1. Resolution
2. Regeneration
3. Replacement

Resolution is healing in response to mild injury with minimal disruption to cells, such as with a

Figure 3.7 **A:** Crush injury to thigh. **B:** The patient was treated and developed an excellent granulation base. **C:** The wound was closed with a skin graft. (From Bucholz RW, Heckman JD. *Rockwood & Green's Fractures in Adults.* 5th ed. Philadelphia: Lippincott Williams & Wilkins; 2001, with permission.)

small superficial scratch or mild sunburn. The epithelial cells basically slough and regenerate without incident. Resolution is like "business as usual." Healing is rapid.

Regeneration of parenchymal tissues can occur only in those cells that undergo mitotic division. This is accomplished through (1) **proliferation** (growth and reproduction), (2) **differentiation** (cells mature and become more specialized), or (3) **diapedesis** (migration of nearby cells). Some cells constantly regenerate through mitosis, particularly epithelial cells of the skin, gastrointestinal tract, and urinary

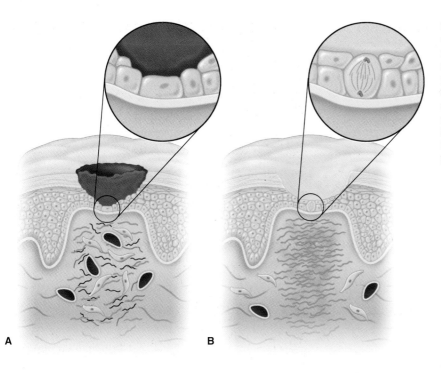

A   B

■ **Figure 3.8** Regeneration and migration of epidermal cells. **A:** The migration of epidermal cells, sustained by the mitotic activity of neighboring cells, fills the wound gap and displaces the scab. **B:** The gap created by the wound has been repaired. The mitotic activity of the epidermal cells will restore the epidermal thickness. (Image modified from Rubin E, Farber JL. *Pathology*. 4th ed. Philadelphia: Lippincott Williams & Wilkins; 2005, with permission.)

tract, and blood cells in the bone marrow. These cells are often referred to as **labile cells**. The skin is a common tissue that requires regeneration after injury. Basal epithelial cells (the bottom, or the deepest, layer) are re-established through mitosis in a process called re-epithelialization. Once this continuous basal layer is re-established, the cells mature and are shed off and regenerated every few days. A prerequisite for epithelial cell replacement is the presence of the basement membrane. In the process of re-epithelialization, the skin cells at the periphery of the wound undergo mitosis and migrate inward until the process is complete (Fig. 3.8). Multiple substances, including growth factors, adhesion molecules, and receptor molecules, direct this activity.

Other cells stop regenerating when growth is complete but can resume regeneration if injured. These cells are referred to as **stable cells**. Hepatocytes in the liver are one example. Similar to epithelial cell regeneration, an intact extracellular matrix is needed to support cell division. The liver has tremendous capacity to regenerate with the support of the matrix.

Replacement through the production of scar tissue occurs in extensive wounds and when regeneration is not possible (Fig. 3.9). **Permanent cells**, such as neurons, cardiac myocytes, and the lens of the eye, do not undergo mitosis and are unable to regenerate. When permanent cells are damaged, the functional tissue is replaced with connective tissue. For example, if neuronal tissue of the brain is destroyed by a brain tumor, the neurons do not regenerate, and the damaged area of the brain does not function as it did prior to the injury. Connective

tissue, or scar tissue, can also replace labile or stable cells if the injury and subsequent damage is extensive. For example, in a severe burn that covers a large area of the body, connective scar tissue will replace the epithelial tissues of the skin. The scar tissue fills in the gap but does not function as the parenchymal tissue.

Conditions That Promote Wound Healing

Wound healing involves multiple variables. Promotion of wound healing depends primarily on adequacy of the vascular and cellular inflammatory responses, reformation of the extracellular matrix (including collagen deposition), and regeneration of those cells capable of mitosis.

These processes are enhanced and supported by an adequate dietary intake of proteins, carbohydrates, fats, vitamins, and minerals. The most beneficial of these nutrients are proteins and vitamins, particularly vitamins A and C. Proteins are needed during every phase of repair, including extracellular matrix regeneration and angiogenesis. Vitamins A and C are needed for re-epithelialization and collagen synthesis. Further review of nutritional needs and altered nutrition is discussed in Chapter 14. Adequate blood flow is also needed to transport inflammatory cells and products of healing to the injured site and to oxygenate cells and tissues. Perfusion is discussed in depth in Chapter 14.

Necrotic (dead) myocardial muscle cells

Mixture of fibrocytes and leukocytes

A

Fibrosis

New capillaries (angioneogenesis)

Scar of dense fibrous tissue

B

Normal, undamaged myocardial muscle cells

— Inflammation
— Fibrocyte migration
— Angioneogenesis

— Fibrocyte proliferation
▢ Granulation tissue
⋯ Collagen accumulation (scar development)

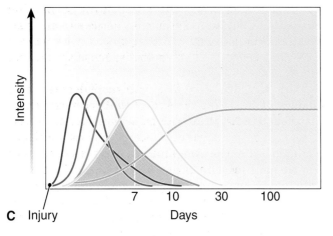

C   Injury   Days

Figure 3.9 Granulation tissue in a healing myocardial infarct ("heart attack"). **A:** Ten days after infarct, some dead muscle cells remain; others have been replaced by a mixture of inflammatory cells, edema, fibrous tissue, and new blood vessels (granulation tissue). **B:** Healed myocardial infarct, months or years old. Dead muscle cells (which cannot regenerate) have been removed and replaced by dense scar tissue. Nearby are normal, undamaged cardiac muscle cells. **C:** Process timeline. After injury and inflammation, fibrocytes migrate into the wound and begin proliferating as inflammation fades. New blood vessels sprout and form a rich fibrovascular mix called granulation tissue, which fades as collagen deposited by fibrocytes accumulates as a scar.

wound edges are those that are "lined up" or close together, such as that which occurs with a paper cut or a surgical incision. These wounds heal by **primary intention**. When healing occurs by primary intention, the wound is basically closed with all areas of the wound connecting and healing simultaneously. The risk for infection is reduced and scarring is minimal.

Larger, open, craterlike wounds must heal by **secondary intention**. These wounds heal from the bottom up. The process is much slower and more involved than the primary intention process. Healing by secondary intention results in a greater risk for infection and scarring. Figure 3.10 compares healing by primary intention with healing by secondary intention.

⬤ **STOP** *and Consider*

What did you eat and drink yesterday? What nutrients did you consume that would promote wound healing?

🔲 Healing By Intention

Wounds that are smaller with approximated wound edges will heal much more quickly and easily than wounds that are large and craterlike. Approximated

⬤ **STOP** *and Consider*

How does the concept of healing by primary or secondary intention compare to the body's three lines of defense?

A Healing by primary intention (wounds with approximated edges)

B Healing by secondary intention (wounds with separated edges)

■ **Figure 3.10** Comparison of healing by primary versus secondary intention. **A:** Healing by primary intention. **A1:** A wound with closely approximated edges and minimal tissue loss. **A2:** Such a wound requires minimal cell proliferation and neovascularization to heal. **A3:** The result is a small scar. **B:** Healing by secondary intention. **B1:** A wound in which the edges are far apart with substantial tissue loss. **B2:** This wound requires extensive cell proliferation and granulation tissue to heal. **B3:** The wound is re-epithelialized from the margins, and collagen fibers are deposited into the granulation tissue. **B4:** Granulation tissue is eventually reabsorbed and replaced by a large scar. (Image modified from Rubin E, Farber JL. *Pathology.* 4th ed. Philadelphia: Lippincott Williams & Wilkins; 2005, with permission.)

Complications of Healing and Tissue Repair

Impaired wound healing can occur at any point in the process of closing the wound, clearing the debris, and restoring structural and functional integrity. Primary factors that impact wound healing are an ineffective inflammatory response, inadequate immune response, inadequate nutritional status, and poor tissue perfusion. Common complications of wound healing include:

- Infection
- Ulceration
- Dehiscence
- Keloid development
- Adhesions

Infection (Chapter 5) refers to invasion by microorganisms. Destroying the first line of defense, along with many other factors, such as a poor inflammatory and immune response, will promote infection and ultimately impair wound healing. As mentioned, tissue healing also requires adequate **perfusion** (passage of oxygenated blood) to the site. Poor perfusion can lead to ulceration. **Ulcers** are circumscribed, open, craterlike lesion of the skin or mucous membranes. These areas are necrotic and open to further invasion by microorganisms. Ulcers are often resistant to healing because of the lack of perfusion to the site and persistent habitation by microorganisms. Ulcers are a common complication of gastritis, one of the clinical models in this chapter.

Wound **dehiscence** is a problem of deficient scar formation, in which the wound splits or bursts open, often at a suture line. Wound separation, like ulceration, opens the area to invasion by microorganisms. This is a possible complication early after surgery because of mechanical stresses put on the wound during movement or coughing. Poor development of the extracellular matrix and ineffective or inadequate collagen is often the cause of wound dehiscence later in the recovery period.

Keloid development is the opposite of dehiscence. **Keloids** are hypertrophic scars that result from excessive collagen production at the site of injury (Fig. 3.11). Keloids occur with higher frequency in those with deeply pigmented skin and tend to develop in those between the ages of 10 and 30 years of age with a familial disposition to developing keloids. Keloids are often seen only as a cosmetic problem, but these large areas of scarring represent ineffective healing at the site. Attempts at removal of the keloid often result in another keloid forming in the same location.

Adhesions are also a problem with collagen deposition. Collagen fibers can develop and form

■ **Figure 3.11**   Keloid. This woman developed a keloid as a reaction to having her earlobe pierced. (Image modified from Rubin E, Farber JL. *Pathology*. 4th ed. Philadelphia: Lippincott Williams & Wilkins; 2005, with permission.)

adhesions with injuries located in or nearby serous (watery) body cavities, such as the peritoneum (inner lining of the abdomen). **Adhesions are fibrous connections between serous cavities and nearby tissues, which do not allow the surrounding tissues to move freely.** Abdominal surgery presents an increased risk for adhesion development. The collagen fibers connect to organs within the peritoneum, such as the bowel, bladder, and ovaries. Adhesions restrict free movement of the organ and cause pain and loss of organ function.

Module 3

Chronic Inflammation

Chronic inflammation represents a persistent or recurrent state of inflammation lasting several weeks or longer. This state occurs when the acute inflammatory and immune responses are unsuccessful. Chronic inflammation can be related to an unrelenting injury, persistent infectious process, or an autoimmune condition. Autoimmunity occurs when the immune system identifies self-cells as "foreign" and attacks these cells (Chapter 4). Often, injuries or infections that cause chronic inflammation are subtle and slow-growing. Chronic inflammation differs from acute inflammation in many ways, as illustrated in Table 3.6.

Cells of Chronic Inflammation

Cellular activity is notably different between acute and chronic inflammation. The longer lasting activity of monocytes, macrophages, and lymphocytes are more prominent in chronic inflammation. Monocytes circulate in the blood to the site of injury and mature into macrophages in the tissues. As monocytes mature into macrophages, they produce **proteinases** and fibroblasts. Proteinases are enzymes that destroy elastin and other tissue components. These enzymes help to break down

dead tissue; unfortunately, these enzymes do not discriminate. Proteinase activity is responsible for ongoing tissue destruction at and surrounding the site of persistent injury. Fibroblasts are also active in chronic inflammation. Fibroblasts are responsible for collagen development, which contributes to the extensive scarring characteristic of chronic inflammation. Scarring leads to permanent loss of function and deformity of the tissue or organ.

Granuloma Formation

In some cases, chronic inflammation results in **granuloma** formation (Fig. 3.12). Granulomas are nodular inflammatory lesions that encase harmful substances. Granuloma formation is also regulated by macrophages. Granulomas typically form when the injury is too difficult to control by the usual inflammatory and

Table 3.6 Comparison of Acute and Chronic Inflammation

Characteristic	Acute Inflammation	Chronic Inflammation
Time	Resolution within a few weeks	Present for a prolonged period of time, usually greater than 6 months
Chief Phagocytic Cells	Neutrophils	Monocytes Macrophages Lymphocytes
Restoration	Minimal scarring	Marked by fibrosis, scarring, or granuloma formation

immune mechanisms, such as with foreign bodies or certain microorganisms. One classic example of a microorganism that results in granuloma formation is *Mycobacterium tuberculosis*, the bacteria responsible for tuberculosis infection (Chapter 5).

By forming granulomas, macrophages protect healthy, unaffected surrounding tissue from further damage. Macrophages adapt into **giant cells** or **epithelioid cells**. Giant cells are phagocytes that can engulf particles much larger than the typical macrophage. Epithelioid cells gather and contain smaller substances by forming a wall, or fibrotic granuloma, around the affected area. Inside the wall, macrophages are busy phagocytizing harmful substances. As a result, necrosis fills the inside of the granuloma. Gradually, the necrosis diffuses through the granuloma wall and a fibrotic capsule remains.

GENERAL MANIFESTATIONS

The general manifestations of chronic inflammation can be similar to those of acute inflammation during a flare-up of symptoms, such as redness, heat, pain, swelling, and loss of function. These symptoms may lead to scarring in the affected area or granuloma formation as discussed above. Other systemic manifestations associated with chronic inflammation may include fever, malaise, anemia, fatigue, anorexia, weight loss, or weakness. Remission of the chronic inflammation can occur in some conditions; during these times, the patient will have no symptoms.

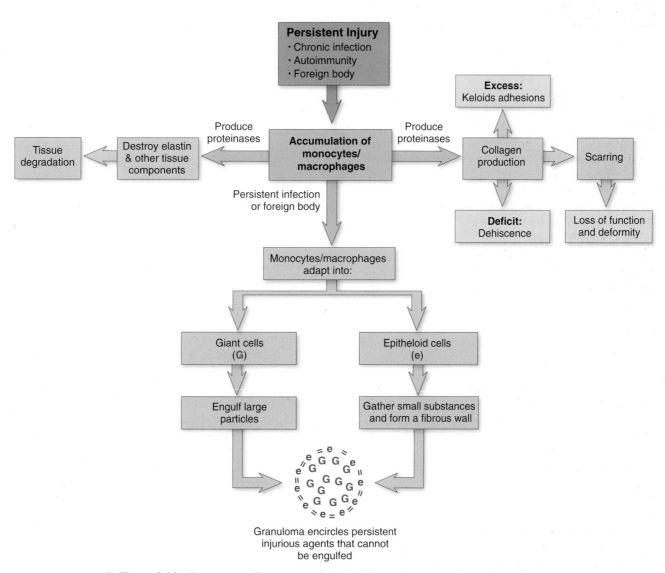

Figure 3.12   Concept map. The process of chronic inflammation leading to granuloma formation.

TREATMENT

The treatment of chronic inflammation is aimed at removing the source of injury if possible and managing symptoms. Long-term use of anti-inflammatory, analgesic, or immune-modifying drugs is often needed. Chronic infections as a source of chronic inflammation would be treated with antimicrobial drugs (Chapter 5). Nonpharmacologic treatments are important as well, such as the use of heat or cold, immobilization, dietary changes, exercise/physical therapy, and rest. Complementary therapies, such as homeopathic preparations, acupuncture, and guided imagery, should also be explored with patients and monitored for safety and effectiveness.

Module 4

Applied Pathophysiology Clinical Models

The following clinical models have been selected to aid in the understanding and application of inflammatory processes. When reading about the clinical models, visualize the process of acute versus chronic inflammation and healing and note the commonalities and unique features of each model.

Burn Injuries

Every year in the United States, burns cause 500,000 people to seek medical treatment with 4,000 of these resulting in death.[5] The most common causes include fire/flame exposure (46%), scalding (32%), hot object contact (8%), electrical burns (4%), and chemical burns (3%). The vast majority of burn injuries cause an inflammatory response in the skin and other structures of the integumentary system.

FUNCTION OF THE SKIN

The skin serves as an important barrier between the body and the external environment. It is composed of the dermis, which is a dense, irregular connective tissue, and the epidermis, a layer of epithelial tissue. The epidermis and dermis are separated by the basement membrane. The skin protects internal structures from invasion by infectious or harmful agents and mechanical damage. The skin prevents dehydration, regulates body temperature, and produces vitamin D. Understanding the vital function of the skin is important since loss of function is a critical manifestation of inflammatory processes.

BURNS

Pathophysiology

Burns can result from thermal injury, electrical injury, caustic chemical injury, radiation exposure, or inhalation of noxious fumes. In thermal injuries, the higher the temperature and increased length of heat exposure increases the severity of the burn. As temperatures exceed 45°C (113°F), proteins denature and irreversible cellular damage occurs.[6] The extent of damage from chemical injuries depends on the toxicity of the chemical, location of exposure (particularly in the eyes, respiratory tract, or gastrointestinal tract), and length of exposure. Electrical injuries follow the path of least resistance in the body; that is, along tissue, fluids, blood vessels, and nerves. Serious electrical trauma results from the electrical current passing through vital organs, nerves, and blood vessels. Electrical currents can disrupt cardiac conduction and cause immediate death.

With all burns, the injury triggers an acute inflammatory response. The extent and nature of the inflammation, along with corresponding clinical manifestations, diagnostic criteria, and treatment, primarily depend on the surface area that is affected as well as the depth of the burn injury (Fig. 3.13).

Superficial partial-thickness burns, also known as first-degree burns, damage the epidermis. Mild sunburn is one example. This radiation-induced injury triggers vasodilation of the dermal blood vessels and increased capillary permeability, causing erythema, pain, and swelling of affected areas. Superficial partial-thickness burns do not result in cell necrosis or scarring. The extracellular matrix generally remains intact, allowing uneventful healing of superficial partial-thickness burns as endothelial and epithelial cells rapidly regenerate. Healing occurs within a week.

Deep partial-thickness burns, also known as second-degree burns, damage epidermal skin layers and penetrate some dermal skin layers. Scalding with hot liquids, more severe sunburn, mild to moderate chemical burns, or flash flame exposure can lead to deep partial-thickness burns. Epidermal and dermal layers separate, fluid accumulates between these layers, and blisters form (Fig. 3.14).

Epidermis

Dermis

Subcutaneous tissue

Muscle

Superficial partial thickness (first degree)

Deep partial thickness (second degree)

Full thickness (third degree)

■ **FIGURE 3.13** Classification of burns by depth of injury. Superficial partial-thickness burns enter the epidermis. Deep partial-thickness burns penetrate the epidermis and dermal layers. Full-thickness burns penetrate all skin layers and can progress to underlying structures as well. (Asset provided by Anatomical Chart Company.)

A loss of function of the skin as the first line of defense allows microorganisms to invade the tissue. If necrosis occurs in the upper epidermal cell layers but the basal cell layer remains intact, scarring is avoided. More commonly, however, necrosis results in both epidermal and upper dermal layers. Collagen fills in the gaps left after the removal of damaged tissues. Excess collagen production often leads to tissue fibrosis and scarring at the burn site. The process of healing occurs within approximately 2 to 4 weeks.

Full-thickness burns, also known as third-degree burns, damage the epidermis and dermis and can penetrate subcutaneous layers as well. Contact with extremely hot objects, exposure to a flame, electrical exposures, and caustic chemicals are likely to result in full-thickness burns. The severity depends on the temperature or type of chemical and the length of exposure. Destruction of blood vessels is also common as heat cauterizes the vessels. The healing of full-thickness burns is challenged by extensive loss of elastin, replacement of skin cells with collagen, and invasion by microorganisms. Regeneration of epithelial cells is impaired because of the destruction of extracellular matrix. Scarring is often extensive. Loss of elasticity is evidenced by **contractures**, areas of thick, shortened, and rigid tissue.

● **STOP** and *Consider*

> Hematocrit is a laboratory test that indicates the percentage of red blood cells in a designated volume of blood. Would an individual with partial- and full-thickness burns covering 20% body surface area have a decrease or an increase in this laboratory value? What would be the impact of this change?

The loss of skin function results in multiple potential complications, particularly in severe burn injuries, defined as full-thickness burns covering greater than 20% of the adult body surface area, including:

1. Body fluid shifts that cause impaired blood circulation, edema, and dehydration
2. Microorganism invasion that leads to infection
3. Overwhelming metabolic demands that increase the risk for malnutrition
4. Problems with temperature regulation

In widespread inflammation, impaired blood circulation and cellular dehydration can result as fluids shift from cells and blood vessels into the tissues (edema). This is due to massive capillary permeability and direct damage to blood vessels at the site of the burn injury (Fig. 3.15). In patients with

■ **Figure 3.14** Deep partial-thickness (2nd degree) sunburn. Epidermal and dermal layers separate, fluid accumulates between the layers, and blisters form. (From Fleisher GR, Ludwig S, Baskin MN. *Atlas of Pediatric Emergency Medicine*. Philadelphia: Lippincott Williams & Wilkins; 2004, with permission.)

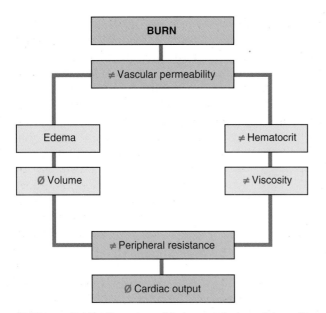

▓ **Figure 3.15** Hemodynamic changes in burn injury. (From Nettina, Sandra. *The Lippincott Manual of Nursing Practice.* 7th ed. Lippincott Williams & Wilkins; 2001, with permission.)

full-thickness burns, approximately 0.3 mL of body water per square centimeter is lost per day.[7] When full-thickness burns cover 70% of the body, extensive fluid shifts out of the blood vessels and swells into the tissues, resulting in severe hypovolemia (low fluid volume in the blood vessels).[7] The blood becomes viscous (thick), heat converts red blood cells from a concave to a spherical shape, and the flow of blood is altered. At the local site of the burn, thrombi, or clots, can develop, oxygenated blood flow is restricted, and necrosis can develop as the burned tissue becomes hypoxic. An inadequate amount of blood in the circulation leads to **shock**, a state of inadequate perfusion (oxygenated blood flow) to peripheral tissues. Poor perfusion is particularly problematic in vital organs, which require a constant flow of oxygen to survive. In partial-thickness burns, capillary permeability is restored after 24 to 48 hours and interstitial fluid shifts decrease after this time. This allows the volume of fluid in the blood vessels needed for optimal circulation. A more detailed description of altered fluid balance in the body is provided in Chapter 8. Altered perfusion and shock are further discussed in Chapter 14.

The loss of skin function as a result of burn injuries also allows for ready access for microorganisms and stresses the metabolic and reparative processes of the body. Burns covering a larger surface area pose a greater risk for the development of **sepsis**, which is a bacterial infection of the blood, and septic shock. In full-thickness burns, dead tissue and exudate convert into an **eschar**, which is a thick, coagulated crust. The eschar must be surgically removed to prevent extensive microorganism growth. Energy, protein, and oxygen use are also increased due to the extensive reparative processes required in substantial burn injuries. If these increasing needs are not met, tissue hypoxia, tissue wasting, and infection are the potential results.

Clinical Manifestations

Clinical manifestations primarily depend on the depth of the burn injury. Superficial partial-thickness burns result in erythema, warmth, pain, swelling, and loss of function of affected areas. Deep partial-thickness burns lead to blistering, along with erythema, warmth, pain, edema, and **serous exudate**, which is a clear fluid that seeps out of the tissues. Erythema, eschar formation, edema, and exudate characterize full-thickness burns. Full-thickness burns destroy nerve endings, sweat glands, and hair follicles. Destruction of nerve endings inhibits the pain response in areas where the burn has penetrated all skin layers. The individual with a full-thickness burn is not pain free, however. Areas of deep and superficial-thickness burns, like a bull's-eye, often surround full-thickness burns. Pain is notable in these surrounding tissues.

Diagnostic Criteria

Wound depths (superficial, deep partial, or full thickness) are classified according to the affected tissue layers. Surface area is also a significant variable in determining the diagnosis and treatment of a burn injury. Calculation of adult body surface area is aided using the "rule of nines" depicted in Figure 3.16. For children under 5 years, body proportions do not match that of the adult. For example, although the trunk and arms are similar in proportion to the adult, the infant's head and neck make up 18% of total body surface area, and each lower extremity accounts for 14%. Health care professionals who treat childhood burns should refer to a "modified rule of nines" appropriate for the specific age of the child.[8]

Estimation of the rule of nines, along with a determination of the thickness of the burn, allows the health professional to determine the severity of the injury and direct treatment. The American Burn Association has published criteria for distinguishing minor, moderate, and major burns (Table 3.7).[9]

Treatment

In the last 15 years, significant advances in the medical treatment for burns have greatly increased survival rates, with over half of patients surviving with burns covering 80% of the body.[10] Initial treatment for minor and moderate burns requires

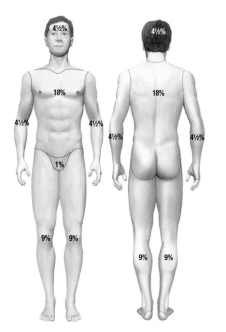

Figure 3.16 Rule of nines. Estimating the extent of burns in adults. (Asset provided by Anatomical Chart Company.)

removing the source of injury and stopping the burning process. Chemical burns should be flushed with copious amounts of water. In minor burns, the wound is cleansed with tepid (cool but not cold) water. In some cases, the wound is covered with an antimicrobial ointment and dressed with fine-mesh gauze. Dressings are usually changed every 1 to 2 days. Frequent (daily) dressing changes aid in **debridement**, which is a process of mechanically removing debris, including necrotic tissue, from the wound. Analgesics can be used to treat pain.

Moderate and major burns require emergency medical attention. Also, burns larger than the palm of the hand or those that involve the face, hands, feet, or genital areas require specialized intervention in a burn treatment center. Treatment for moderate and major burns, as with other emergencies, focuses on the airway, breathing, and circulation. Once these are stabilized, administration of intravenous fluids is instituted to replace water and sodium losses. Administering fluids helps to restore the circulating blood volume and improves perfusion of vital organs. Because metabolic demands increase significantly with the stress of a burn injury, nutrition support in the form of increased calories and protein is needed. Analgesics and antibiotics are also used to treat pain and infection. Protective isolation measures are often instituted to protect the patient from contact with microorganisms as much as possible.

Wound management for major burns involves removing necrotic tissue, closing the wound, and preventing infection. Hydrotherapy, which involves soaking in a tub or showering once or twice per day, is used to cleanse the wound by removing dead tissue and exudate. Full-thickness burns are unable to undergo re-epithelialization and require surgical excision and grafting to close the wound. Skin grafting is a process of using self or donor tissue to cover and protect the exposed area. This transplanted epithelial tissue supports cellular regeneration, decreases invasion by microorganisms, and minimizes scarring. Long-term rehabilitation (tertiary prevention) involves prevention of complications such as scar formation, contractures, deformity, and chronic pain. Treatment may also involve psychosocial support because those with burn injuries may experience depression or other psychologic sequelae.

Arthritis

Arthritis is a generic term for degeneration or inflammation of the joints and refers to a group of diseases of varying pathogenesis. Inflammatory arthritis is usually a result of chronic infections, autoimmune conditions, or other chronic irritants in the joint capsule. Rheumatoid arthritis (RA), a systemic autoimmune disease leading to chronic inflammation of synovial tissue, is the selected clinical model.

FUNCTION OF SYNOVIAL JOINTS

The primary function of joints is skeletal stability and mobility. Synovial joints, particularly those in the knees, wrists, hands, fingers, and feet, are

Table 3.7 American Burn Association (ABA) Burn Severity Grading Scale

	Minor[a]	Moderate	Major
Partial-Thickness	<10% TBSA	10–20% TBSA	>20% TBSA
Full-Thickness			ALL
Treatment	Usually treated at home	Admission to hospital; may require specialized burn center treatment	Admission to specialized burn center

[a]Minor burns exclude any burn involving the face, hands, feet, and perineum; also exclude electrical burns, inhalation injuries, or other trauma.

TBSA, total body surface area.

Source: American Burn Association. Hospital and prehospital resources for optimal care of patients with burn injury: guidelines for development and operation of burn centers. *J Burn Care Rehabil*. 1990;11:98–104.

Pilletteri A. *Maternal and Child Nursing Care*. 4th ed. Philadelphia: Lippincott Williams & Wilkins; 2003.

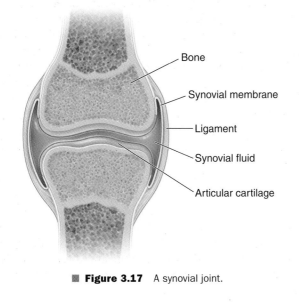

- Bone
- Synovial membrane
- Ligament
- Synovial fluid
- Articular cartilage

■ **Figure 3.17** A synovial joint.

From the Lab

Rheumatoid factor (RF), a substance that can be found in the blood, synovial fluid, and synovial membranes, signifies that antibodies (IgM, IgG, or IgA) are acting against other antibodies (mainly IgG). RF is present in the vast majority of patients that have RA and can also be found in a variety of other conditions. The presence of RF in RA often signifies more severe disease.

highly mobile and common targets for inflammation (Fig. 3.17). Synovial joints are also highly vascular. The two-layer synovial membrane lines the joint capsule. One layer is composed of connective tissue, elastin, adipocytes, fibroblasts, macrophages, and mast cells. The second layer is a row of synovial cells, which are capable of phagocytosis and secreting synovial fluid. Synovial fluid nourishes, cushions, and protects the joint from microorganisms. Synovial cells are labile cells, which can quickly regenerate.

Between the bone and synovial membrane is cartilage. Cartilage is composed of chondrocytes, collagen, water, and protein glycans. Collagen forms an extracellular matrix, which attaches bone to the cartilage. Cartilage is needed to distribute body weight and to decrease joint friction. Cartilage must be replaced by collagen if damaged; chondrocytes do not regenerate.

RHEUMATOID ARTHRITIS

RA is a systemic autoimmune disease characterized by chronic inflammation and hyperplasia of the synovial membranes with increased synovial exudate, leading to swelling and thickening of the synovial membranes, joint erosion, and pain. The onset

of disease occurs typically between the ages of 36 and 50 years of age. RA affects 0.8% of adults worldwide. Females are affected three times more often than males.[11]

Pathophysiology

Although the exact cause of RA is unknown, the etiology is likely a combination of:

- Genetic susceptibility
- An immune triggering event
- The subsequent development of autoimmunity against synovial cells

The triggering injury in RA that leads to inflammation is difficult to pinpoint and is often never determined. Despite the lack of an identifiable trigger, autoimmunity plays a key role. CD4+ helper T cells have been implicated as activating the inflammatory response along with the release of cytokines. Lymphocytes and plasma cells then form antibodies in the synovial membrane and cartilage. The antibodies are formed against specific antigens. The antibodies actually see other antibodies within the body as foreign "antigens" (see From the Lab).

In RA, the antigens and antibodies form complexes called immune complexes. These immune complexes are found in the synovium of most individuals diagnosed with RA. These antigen–antibody complexes trigger the complement system thereby stimulating an exaggerated inflammatory response.

The inflammatory response is marked by excess production and release of inflammatory mediators. These inflammatory mediators act on the vasculature of the joints to cause increased vasodilation and capillary permeability. The joint becomes erythematous, warm, swollen, painful, and difficult to move. Exudate accumulates in the synovium. Neutrophils and macrophages move into the site to defend against harmful substances. This process, while necessary, also promotes the production of destructive tissue enzymes. Synovial cells adapt by rapidly regenerating. The synovium, after the initial bout of inflammation, is altered and causes the following changes:

1. Mild edema
2. Accumulation of the cells of chronic inflammation (macrophages, plasma cells, and lymphocytes)
3. Acceleration of angiogenesis
4. Accumulation of fibrin
5. Synovial cells continue to undergo reactive hyperplasia

These initial synovial changes usually demonstrate minimal damage to the joints.

Exacerbations of the disease progressively damage affected joints through pannus formation, cartilage erosion, fibrosis, and joint fixation and deformity (Fig. 3.18). **Pannus** is granulation tissue that forms over the inflamed synovium and cartilage as a result of accelerated angiogenesis. Pannus is filled with synovial cells, which undergo hyperplasia and migrate, along with the pannus, over the cartilage. The pannus and synovial cells are joined by mast cells, lymphocytes, and macrophage giant cells. These cells further exacerbate inflammation and tissue destruction. Pannus separates the cartilage from synovium, thereby depriving the cartilage of nutrients. The pannus also produces enzymes that break down the cartilage and can erode the adjacent bone as well. These erosions are irreversible. Fibroblasts work to form and replace the connective tissue layer by producing and secreting collagen. Collagen fills in the gaps that remain after tissue damage. As a result, fibrosis forms in the joint capsule. Fibrosis impairs joint mobility and can result in a debilitating fixation of the joint, a condition termed **ankylosis**. Limited joint movement decreases the workload of surrounding muscle tissue, leading to muscle tissue atrophy. Inflammatory cells can also irritate surrounding muscle tissue, resulting in muscle spasms.

Clinical Manifestations

The severity of RA can range from mild to debilitating. Involvement is characteristically symmetric

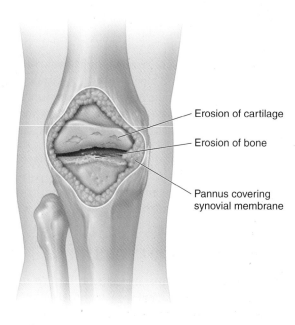

■ **Figure 3.18** Effects of rheumatoid arthritis.

and can involve any number of joints, producing erythema, pain, swelling, warmth, and decreased mobility. Malalignment or deviation of symmetrical joints is a common clinical manifestation of long-standing RA (Fig. 3.19). Malalignment is caused by a combination of cartilage and bone erosion, fibrosis, ankylosis, muscle spasms, and muscle atrophy. Pain and stiffness are often most notable upon rising in the morning and after periods of immobility.

Common systemic manifestations during disease exacerbations are low-grade fever, fatigue, anorexia, weight loss, and weakness. Chronic pain can also lead to isolation and depression. Manifestations of long-standing RA can also be found outside of the joint capsule. Granulomas, called nodules, can form on blood vessels throughout the body. Vasculitis, an inflammatory condition involving small and medium-sized arteries, may also occur in those with long-standing disease.

Diagnostic Criteria

No definitive test exists to diagnose RA. Diagnosis is based on history and physical examination (during which stiffness and pain in symmetrical joints are demonstrated), and it may involve several diagnostic tests. Test results that increase the likelihood of RA as the diagnosis include:

1. An elevated serum ESR level
2. An elevated serum CRP level
3. The presence of RF significant for antibodies against IgG
4. A positive antinuclear antibody (ANA) assay indicating suspected autoimmune disease
5. The presence of inflammatory products in a synovial joint fluid analysis
6. Visualization with a radiograph demonstrating joint damage

RA presents a diagnostic challenge because multiple autoantibodies are known to be associated with this disease. Many of these tests are nonspecific and indicate the presence of an inflammatory or autoimmune process but do not directly point to RA as the cause. Each test also has a risk of false-positive (positive result without the disease) or false-negative (negative result with the disease) results. RF appears to have the greatest advantage in diagnosing early RA compared with multiple other autoantibody tests. It is unlikely that a single antigen is involved in the development of RA.[12] The diagnostic challenge can lead to frustration for the patient and health care professional and may lead to a delay in treatment.

Treatment

Treatment of RA involves a careful balance of pharmacologic and nonpharmacologic treatment

A

B

■ **Figure 3.19** Deviation of joints in rheumatoid arthritis, as shown in a radiograph **(A)** and a photograph **(B)**. (Image A reprinted with permission from Harris JH Jr, Harris WH, Novelline RA. *The Radiology of Emergency Medicine*. 3rd ed. Baltimore: Williams & Wilkins; 1993:440. Image B reprinted with permission from Smeltzer SC, Bare BG. *Textbook of Medical-Surgical Nursing*. 10th ed. Philadelphia: Lippincott Williams & Wilkins; 2003, with permission.)

strategies. Medications employed include anti-inflammatory drugs, immunosuppressive drugs, and medications that otherwise induce remission. Nonpharmacologic strategies involve the balance of activity and rest, physical therapy exercises to promote joint mobility, and the use of splints and

Research Notes

The traditional view of chronic inflammation leading predictably to destruction of the joint in RA has been viewed recently by researchers as too simplistic. Research has shown that the relationship between disease activity and subsequent damage is not perfectly correlated whereas many patients with active disease may not show progressive damage. The pathophysiology of RA has been proposed by some to involve two distinct processes: synovial inflammation and synovial hyperplasia. Treatment measures must therefore be aggressive and target both processes, including the subclinical inflammation that goes undetected in many patients and is responsible for much of the tissue and bone destruction characteristic of RA.[13]

other devices that allow the joints to rest and help to prevent deformities. Heat or cold therapy can be helpful. In some cases, synovectomy or total joint replacement surgery may be needed to reduce pain and deformity.

Gastritis

Gastritis refers to inflammation of the lining of the stomach, or gastric mucosa, thereby impairing gastric function. Gastritis can be both acute and chronic.

FUNCTION OF THE STOMACH

The stomach functions as an organ of protection, digestion, and absorption, primarily absorbing water and alcohol. Stomach acid forms a first line of defense by destroying many types of microorganisms and other harmful substances on contact. During the digestive process, foods and liquids are mixed with gastric secretions, comprised of mucus, acid, enzymes, hormones, and intrinsic factor (IF). Secretion of these substances is accomplished through the work of gastric glands lined by specialized epithelial cells (Fig. 3.20).

Epithelial cells form a tight connection. This connection is an important source of protection from the corrosive effects of gastric acid. Prostaglandins also play a key role in maintaining the integrity of the gastric mucosa through the stimulation of a protective mucus barrier.

● STOP *and Consider*

Explain how anti-inflammatory drugs that inhibit prostaglandins can cause or further exacerbate gastritis.

The surface mucus barrier is highly vascular and dependent upon a rich blood supply to support gastric function. Restriction or loss of perfusion to this layer can be a cause of gastritis. For example, altered perfusion can occur in the case of shock when blood is shunted to vital organs and not to the stomach, causing the protective mucus barrier to form ulcers and perforate.

ACUTE GASTRITIS

Acute gastritis refers to inflammation in the gastric mucosa most often caused by the ingestion of irritants such as aspirin,

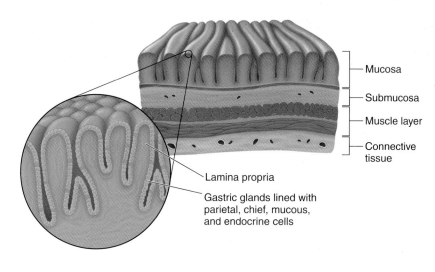

Mucosa

Submucosa

Muscle layer

Connective tissue

Lamina propria

Gastric glands lined with parietal, chief, mucous, and endocrine cells

alcohol, or certain microorganisms. Acute gastritis typically occurs over a short period and is considered reversible when the causative agent is removed. Although gastritis is often associated with having too much stomach acid, the role of gastric acid hypersecretion is unclear.

Pathophysiology

The gastric mucosa is accustomed to and functions best in the acidic environment of the stomach. Exposure to gastric irritants inhibits the production of gastric mucosa and makes the mucosa more vulnerable to acidic stomach contents. This leads to an acute inflammatory response ranging from mild erythema to erosion and gastric perforation (Fig. 3.21). Epithelial cells become necrotic. The underlying gastric tissue is eroded. Hemorrhaging often occurs. Gastric acid is allowed to escape the confines of the

gastric mucosa and corrode nearby tissues. Perforation may occur in severe cases.

Clinical Manifestations

Clinical manifestations are dependent upon the severity and range from mild to severe abdominal pain, which can be accompanied by indigestion (heartburn), loss of appetite, nausea, vomiting, and hiccups. Hematemesis, or vomiting blood, can occur. Anemia may result from mild gastric hemorrhage. Severe hemorrhage and perforation are quickly followed by shock and this is a medical emergency (Chapter 14).

Diagnostic Criteria

The history often reveals aspirin or other nonsteroidal anti-inflammatory drug use, excessive alcohol intake, recent contaminated food intake, or conditions causing ischemia of the gastric mucosa. The physical examination may reveal abdominal tenderness. Direct visualization of the stomach with an endoscope is needed to visualize ulcers in the mucosa and a stool analysis may show occult blood in the fecal material. Hemoglobin or hematocrit levels provide information about anemia.

Treatment

Treatment begins with removal of the gastric irritant. Medications are then needed temporarily to buffer gastric acid and/or decrease gastric acid production. The healing of gastritis and gastric ulceration depends on regeneration of the epithelial cells that line the gastric mucosa. Most acute gastritis improves rapidly when the irritant is removed and treatment is initiated.

Perforating Ulcer

Penetration of wall creating a passage for gastric acids, other fluids and air to enter adjacent spaces of the body

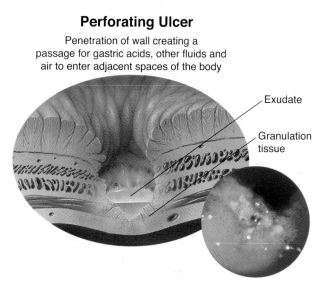

Exudate

Granulation tissue

■ **Figure 3.21** Gastric perforation as a result of acute gastritis.

CHRONIC GASTRITIS: *Helicobacter Pylori* INFECTION

Chronic gastritis is related to an unrelenting injury, such as with chronic infection or autoimmunity. Chronic gastritis due to *H. pylori* is an example caused by chronic infection. *H. pylori* infection is most prevalent in Asia and in developing countries with poor sanitation. Worldwide, an estimated 50% of the population is infected.[14]

Pathophysiology

H. pylori are gram-negative protobacteria that are passed from person to person through infected saliva and stool. The microorganism is ingested and multiplies on the epithelial surface cells and mucus barrier. *H. pylori* produce enzymes that neutralize gastric acid and the microorganism is able to survive. The microorganisms then produce toxins that can destroy the mucosal barrier (Fig. 3.22).

In response to the microorganism-induced injury, inflammatory mediators trigger an intense inflammatory response. Phagocytes work to engulf, destroy, and remove these aggressive microorganisms. Neutrophils migrate to the lamina propria and gastric epithelium to phagocytize the bacteria. As the infection becomes chronic, macrophages and T and B lymphocytes move in an attempt to rid the body of the offending bacteria. *H. pylori* tends to remain contained within the mucosal barrier and surface epithelial cells and, unlike acute gastritis, there are no erosions of the gastric mucosa. Instead, epithelial cells and mucosal glands atrophy. Eventually, the chronic inflammatory response wanes. The mucosal lining of the stomach remains thin, and the gastric acid production and secretion is impaired.

Clinical Manifestations

Dyspepsia, a vague epigastric discomfort associated with nausea and heartburn, is a possible clinical manifestation. Some patients may experience a loss of appetite or vomiting. Most infected people, however, are asymptomatic carriers.

Diagnostic Criteria

Diagnosis of chronic gastritis caused by *H. pylori* infection is accomplished through direct endoscopic visualization and biopsy of gastric tissue. A breath test can be used to measure the presence of an enzyme given off when the bacterium converts urea to carbon dioxide in the lungs. Protein antibodies against *H. pylori* may also be detected in the blood, indicating past or present infection with the bacteria.

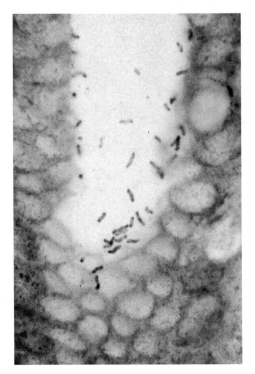

■ **Figure 3.22** Infective gastritis. *H. pylori* appears as small curved rods on the surface of the gastric mucosa. (From Rubin E, Farber JL. *Pathology*. 3rd ed. Philadelphia: Lippincott-Raven; 1999:687, with permission.)

Treatment

Because *H. pylori* are buried deep in the stomach mucosa, multiple antibiotics are needed to treat this infection along with proton pump inhibitors or bismuth, which have antimicrobial properties and raise gastric pH. Over time, certain strains of *H. pylori* can lead to chronic ulcers and gastric cancer.

CHRONIC GASTRITIS: AUTOIMMUNE

Chronic gastritis can also result from autoimmune processes. Although rarer than other forms of chronic gastritis, antibodies are produced against gastric parietal cells or IF.

Pathophysiology

Parietal cells secrete hydrochloric acid. When antibodies are formed against parietal cells, gastric acid secretion is impaired. IF is needed for intestinal absorption of B_{12}. When antibodies are formed against IF, absorption of B_{12} is impaired. B_{12} is a critical vitamin that promotes DNA synthesis in red blood cells. Impaired DNA synthesis in red blood cells leads to a marked decrease in red blood cells and low hemoglobin levels. This condition is known as pernicious anemia (Chapter 15). Chronic inflammation related to autoimmunity allows T cells to infiltrate the gastric mucosa, destroying epithelial cells and causing gastric atrophy.

Clinical Manifestations

Autoimmune gastritis can be asymptomatic. The presence of pernicious anemia may be the first clue that chronic gastritis is present. Manifestations of anemia include weakness, light-headedness, pale mucous membranes, and fatigue. Clinical manifestations can also include dyspepsia, vague abdominal pain, nausea, vomiting, and anorexia.

Diagnostic Criteria

Diagnosis of autoimmune gastritis can be determined only with histologic examination of the gastric mucosa. Several biopsy samples are obtained and analyzed for atrophic changes in the cells. Antiparietal or anti-IF antibodies may present in a blood sample, which indicate an autoimmune process against the parietal cells or IF. Because autoimmunity against IF impairs B_{12} absorption, a low B_{12} level will be noted in the blood.

Treatment

Treatment is aimed at blocking the autoimmune attack against the parietal cells. The administration of B_{12} intramuscular injections monthly is needed to facilitate absorption of this important vitamin. Similar to *H. pylori*, autoimmune gastritis can lead to gastric cancer.

Inflammatory Bowel Disease

Inflammatory bowel disease (IBD) refers to chronic inflammatory processes most commonly in the small and large intestine, but it can occur anywhere along the gastrointestinal tract from the mouth to the anus. The most common forms of IBD include Crohn disease and ulcerative colitis.

The incidence of IBD is the highest in developed countries where persons in colder climates and urban areas have an increased risk.[15] The American Jewish population has a four to five times greater prevalence than in other groups. Among those of European descent in the United States, the prevalence of ulcerative colitis is estimated at 116 per 100,000 people and this is slightly increased at 133 per 100,000 people for Crohn disease. The risk appears similar for African Americans but is lower for Asian Americans and Hispanic Americans. Males and females are equally affected.[15]

Figure 3.23 Wall of small intestine.

FUNCTION OF THE SMALL INTESTINE

The small intestine is composed of several layers (Fig. 3.23). From inner to outer, these layers consist of the mucosa, submucosa, muscularis, and serosa. The innermost mucosal tissue is composed of three sublayers: mucous columnar epithelium, lamina propria (connective tissue), and the thin muscularis layer. The mucous epithelium layer lines the villi, which provide a large surface area. These villi are lined with columnar cells, which secrete mucus, enzymes, and hormones. The submucosa is a thick connective tissue layer that houses nerves, small glands, and blood vessels.

The primary functions of the small intestine are digestion and absorption. Enzymes secreted by villi promote digestion. Vitamins, minerals, fats, carbohydrates, proteins, water, and electrolytes, such as sodium and potassium, are absorbed through columnar epithelium of the intestinal mucosa. The lamina propria houses infection-fighting macrophages, plasma cells, and lymphocytes. Replacement of columnar epithelial cells is rapid, primarily because of the presence of the crypts of Lieberkühn. These pitlike depressions store cells that can quickly differentiate into replacement cells. The rate of production and differentiation of epithelial cells is increased with injury, thereby promoting healing and repair.

CROHN DISEASE

Crohn disease is selected as a clinical model to demonstrate chronic inflammatory process in the small intestine. It is recurrent and characterized by a granulomatous inflammatory process. Although Crohn disease can be found anywhere along the gastrointestinal tract, the small intestine and ascending colon, particularly the submucosal layers, are most often affected (Fig. 3.24).

Pathophysiology

The exact cause of Crohn disease is unknown. Consistent with many other chronic inflammatory conditions, autoimmunity and genetic etiologies have been suggested. Family history does play a role: those with a family history of bowel inflammation are more likely to develop Crohn disease. Environmental factors, such as smoking, diet, or microorganisms, may trigger the condition as well. As with all conditions, Crohn disease has varying levels of disease severity.

As mentioned, chronic inflammation occurs in patchy segments (called "skip lesion") of the intestine and penetrates all layers of those segments. Between affected areas of intestine is unaffected, noninflamed bowel tissue. Inflammation begins in the mucosa and submucosa. Increased permeability and vascularity contributes to edema and fibrosis. Macrophages, plasma cells, and lymphocytes are released in response to inflammatory mediators. Granulomas develop to wall off affected areas.

As the affected bowel segments become further inflamed, interior surfaces thicken due to excessive edema, fibrosis, and granuloma formation (Fig. 3.25). The thickening of the bowel can lead to total bowel obstruction. Ingested food is unable to move through the digestive tract, which is a life-threatening emergency. Although thickening and granuloma formation is most characteristic of Crohn disease, ulcers can form in the intestinal mucosa. These ulcers can become deep and penetrate through bowel layers, forming a fistula. A **fistula** is an abnormal track or passage that forms between two segments of bowel or other epithelial tissue. At the base of a fistula, an **abscess**, or a pocket of purulent (containing pus) exudate, is likely to develop. External surfaces can also be affected by the chronic inflammatory response. Outer surfaces can stick to other sections of bowel and form adhesions further limiting bowel function.

Destruction of the mucosa and submucosa leads to damage to the villi and crypts. This damage impairs absorptive and epithelial regenerative

functions within the affected areas. Malnutrition from the inability to properly absorb nutrients further exacerbates problems with healing. The most severe complication is massive infection and shock from total bowel obstruction and perforation.

Clinical Manifestations

Clinical manifestations are related to rapid stool transit time, intestinal edema and fibrosis, and loss of absorptive function that results from bowel inflammation during periods of exacerbation. Symptoms depend upon the location of the affected areas. Abdominal pain, intermittant nonbloody diarrhea, malnutrition, and **occult**, or hidden, blood in the stool are possible clinical manifestations. Nonbloody diarrhea often indicates greater involvement in the submucosal layer as compared to the mucosal layers. If the colon mucosal layer is involved, diarrhea may contain mucus, blood, or pus. Abdominal pain is often relieved with defecation. Systemic manifestations are also common with Crohn disease and can include fever, weight loss, and fatigue. Anemia is often present when there is chronic blood loss through the gastrointestinal tract.

Diagnostic Criteria

Diagnosis of Crohn disease is based on the patient history, physical examination, and diagnostic tests. Direct visualization with an endoscope (sigmoidoscopy) or

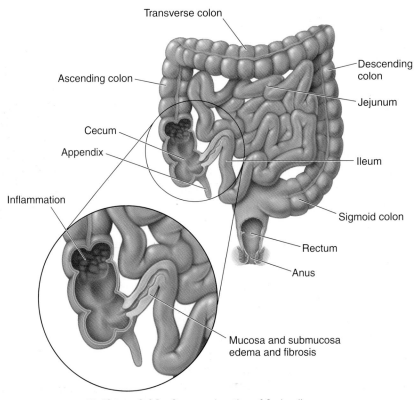

Figure 3.24 Common location of Crohn disease.

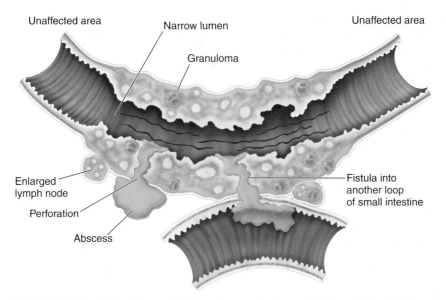

Figure 3.25 Major features of Crohn disease. (Image modified from Rubin E, Farber JL. *Pathology*. 4th ed. Philadelphia: Lippincott Williams & Wilkins; 2005, with permission.)

with radiographs show a cobblestone pattern to the mucosa with alternating affected and unaffected areas of inflammation. Complications, such as abscesses or fistulas, can also be detected through radiographs or CT scan. Stool cultures may be needed to rule out infectious processes.

Treatment

Treatment is symptomatic. Medications that suppress the inflammatory and immune responses are most often used. Dietary changes are required and foods that irritate the bowel, such as spicy foods, should be avoided. Individuals with Crohn disease need a diet high in calories and protein, and low in fat and fiber during exacerbations. Surgical intervention may be needed to remove damaged bowel or to repair fistulas. Those with Crohn disease are at increased risk of small intestine and colorectal cancer.

FUNCTION OF THE LARGE INTESTINE

The anatomy of the large intestine is similar to the small intestine with the notable absence of villi in the large intestine. Columnar epithelial cells and mucus-secreting cells make up the mucosa of the large intestine. The major function of the large intestine is to absorb water and electrolytes.

ULCERATIVE COLITIS

Ulcerative colitis is selected as a chronic inflammatory condition of the colon. Ulcerative colitis is found exclusively in the large intestine and does not affect other areas of the gastrointestinal tract (Fig. 3.26). It most often affects the mucosal layer but can extend into the submucosa.

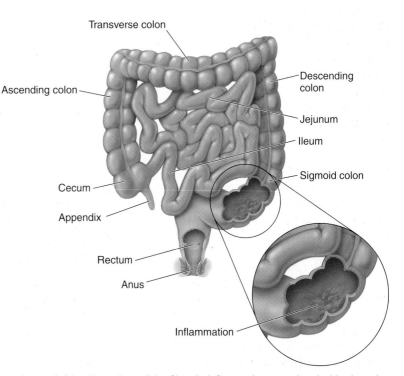

Figure 3.26 Ulcerative colitis. Chronic inflammation associated with ulcerative colitis is found exclusively in the large intestine.

Figure 3.27 Ulcerative colitis. Prominent erythema and ulceration of the colon begin in the ascending colon and are most severe in the rectosigmoid area. (From Ruben E, Farber JL. *Pathology.* 3rd ed. Philadelphia: Lippincott-Raven; 1999:731, with permission.)

Pathophysiology

The exact cause of ulcerative colitis is not known. Autoimmunity has been implicated because antibodies to epithelial cells in the colon have been found in some individuals with ulcerative colitis. Ulcerative colitis typically begins in the distal region of the rectum and extends up the descending colon. The area of inflammation often remains on the surface of the mucosa and is continuous; ulcerative colitis does not skip any areas of the colon along the way (Fig. 3.27).

With ulcerative colitis, inflammation invades the superficial mucosa and causes **friability**, a state where tissue readily bleeds. The mucosa becomes erythematous and granular. Hemorrhagic lesions in the crypts of Lieberkühn, highly characteristic of ulcerative colitis, can form into abscesses. Extensive exudate is present early in the process, and necrosis and ulceration are common. Inflammatory processes promote the development of pseudopolyps. Over time, epithelial cells of the mucosa begin to atrophy. Metaplasia can occur. Those with long-standing ulcerative colitis demonstrate a higher risk for colorectal cancer than those with Crohn disease. Other potential complications include obstruction, perforation, and massive hemorrhage. Table 3.8 and Figure 3.28 compare pathophysiologic differences with Crohn disease and ulcerative colitis.

Clinical Manifestations

Clinical manifestations are related to large intestine irritability and friability. Diarrhea, often with rectal bleed-ing, is the most common clinical manifestation. Abdominal pain, fever, weakness, fatigue, and anemia can also occur. Functional losses with ulcerative colitis are related to the extent of inflammation; impaired water and electrolyte absorption are notable with extensive disease.

Diagnostic Criteria

Ulcerative colitis is diagnosed through endoscopy, which shows mucosal erythema. Radiographs can detect colonic dilation, ulcers, perforation, or obstruction. Severity is based on the number of bowel movements with rectal bleeding and the presence of systemic manifestations:[16]

- Mild = fewer than four bowel movements per day; no systemic manifestations
- Moderate = greater than four bowel movements per day; no systemic manifestations
- Severe = greater than four bowel movements per day with systemic manifestations and low blood albumin (protein) levels

Treatment

Treatment is symptomatic. Anti-inflammatory, antidiarrheal, and immunosuppressive medications are sometimes used. A healthy diet and adequate fluid intake are recommended. Avoidance of certain foods, such as milk, caffeine, or spicy foods may be recommended. Surgery may be needed if medical therapies are ineffective, or if perforation or obstruction occurs.

Summary

- Inflammation is required for tissue healing and occurs in response to tissue injury.
- Inflammatory mediators, under the direction of the three plasma protein systems, regulate the inflammatory response.

Table 3.8 Comparison of Crohn Disease and Ulcerative Colitis

	Crohn Disease	Ulcerative Colitis
Location	Small intestine and ascending colon	Descending colon
Pattern	Skip lesions	Continuous
Depth	Primarily submucosal	Primarily mucosal
Diarrhea	Watery	Bloody
Abdominal Pain	Yes	Yes
Bowel Obstruction	Common	Uncommon
Cancer Risk	Increased	Higher risk than with Crohns

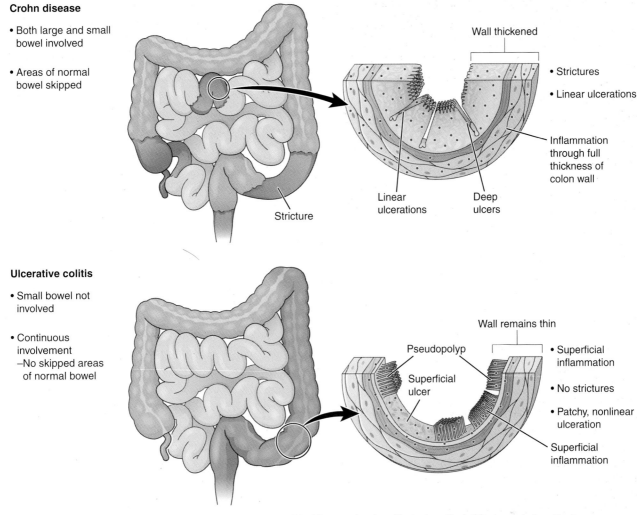

Crohn disease

- Both large and small bowel involved

- Areas of normal bowel skipped

Stricture

Wall thickened

- Strictures
- Linear ulcerations

Inflammation through full thickness of colon wall

Linear ulcerations

Deep ulcers

Ulcerative colitis

- Small bowel not involved

- Continuous involvement
  –No skipped areas of normal bowel

Wall remains thin

Pseudopolyp

Superficial ulcer

- Superficial inflammation
- No strictures
- Patchy, nonlinear ulceration

Superficial inflammation

Figure 3.28 Crohn disease and ulcerative colitis. The two drawings illustrate critical differences in how the two diseases affect the gastrointestinal tract.

- Inflammatory mediators elicit vascular and cellular responses characterized by vasodilation, increased capillary permeability, chemotaxis, cellular adherence, and cellular migration.
- Phagocytic cells (neutrophils and later macrophages) taxi to the site to engulf and destroy harmful substances.
- Removal of the injury will direct resolution of the acute inflammatory response.
- Tissue healing is a multistep process that involves covering the wound, clearing the debris, and restoring structural and functional integrity.
- The results of the inflammatory response are to either repair, regenerate, or replace damaged tissue.
- Persistent injury, such as with chronic infection or autoimmune conditions, results in chronic inflammation.
- Chronic inflammation differs from acute inflammation in the types of prominent cells and in the tissue repair process. Macrophages and fibroblasts

are much more prominent, resulting in increased tissue destruction, fibrosis, scarring, and granuloma formation.
- Chronic inflammatory outcomes contribute to poor wound healing. Other complications of wound healing include infection, ulcers, wound dehiscence, keloid formation, and adhesions.

Case Study 3.1

A friend has disclosed that she has been having problems with heartburn. She has been told that she has gastroesophageal reflux disease (GERD) in which stomach acid backs up into the esophagus. Think about which clinical model is most related to this process. From your reading related to cellular injury and adaptations, as well as to inflammation, answer the following questions:

1. *What anatomic problem would most likely lead to gastroesophageal reflux?*
2. *What is the injury in gastroesophageal reflux?*
3. *What would the acute inflammatory response look like?*
4. *Why might this condition become a chronic problem?*
5. *What pathophysiologic changes would most likely occur with chronic gastroesophageal reflux?*
6. *What would you expect for clinical manifestations?*
7. *What diagnostic tests might be used?*
8. *What treatment measures would you anticipate?*

Log on to the Internet, using the search words "gastroesophageal reflux." Search for relevant journal articles or Web sites that detail this condition, and confirm your predictions.

Case Study 3.2

Jason is a long-distance runner. He is in the clinic today complaining of heel pain and tightness along the back of this foot and ankle. He has been recently running indoors on the treadmill as the weather has been too cold to run outside. He is diagnosed with achilles tendonitis. From your reading related to cellular injury and adaptations as well as to inflammation, answer the following questions:

1. *What anatomic problem most likely leads to tendonitis?*
2. *What is the injury in tendonitis?*
3. *What would the acute inflammatory response look like?*
4. *Why might this condition become a chronic problem?*
5. *What pathophysiologic changes would most likely occur with tendonitis?*
6. *What would you expect for clinical manifestations?*
7. *What diagnostic tests might be used?*
8. *What treatment measures would you anticipate?*

Log on to the Internet, using the search words "tendonitis." Search for relevant journal articles or Web sites that detail this condition, and confirm your predictions.

Practice Exam Questions

1. You get a paper cut and experience pain at the site. This response is related to:
   a. Increased perfusion at the site
   b. Increased exudate and chemical mediators at the site
   c. Bacteria that have entered the wound
   d. Vasoconstriction at the site

2. Inflammation is ultimately needed to:
   a. Increase inflammatory mediators at the site to vasoconstrict the area
   b. Increase platelets at the site for clotting
   c. Restore functional cells
   d. Prepare the site for healing

3. A wound is 6 cm × 6 cm × 4 cm. A wound with these dimensions needs to heal through:
   a. Secondary intention
   b. Primary intention
   c. Tertiary intention
   d. Scar tissue formation

4. A major difference between the acute and chronic inflammatory response is that in chronic inflammation:
   a. Inflammatory mediators are released
   b. Neutrophils are much more prominent
   c. Granulomas form around certain invaders
   d. Granulation tissue is present

5. Which is not a local manifestation of acute inflammation?
   a. Edema
   b. Redness
   c. Loss of function
   d. Leukocytosis

6. Depth of injury is important to determine with burns. You are in the sun too long without sunscreen and develop redness and blistering on your face, chest, and back. What depth of burn did you experience?
   a. Superficial partial-thickness burn
   b. Deep partial-thickness burn
   c. Full-thickness burn
   d. Dermal-thickness burn

7. The hospitalized burn patient wants to know why you need to remove his dressings every day. It is painful and he wants to avoid uncovering

his burn injury. You explain that removing the dressings promotes:
a. Debridement
b. Infection
c. Skin function
d. Drying the exudate

8. What is the one definitive test to diagnose rheumatoid arthritis?
a. A positive rheumatoid factor (RF)
b. An elevated erythrocyte sedimentation rate (ESR)
c. A positive antinuclear antibody (ANA)
d. One test is not definitive

9. Which of the following is the most common cause of acute gastritis?
a. Poor gastric perfusion
b. Too much stomach acid

c. Ingestion of aspirin, alcohol, or other chemicals
d. *H. pylori* infection

10. Why is Crohn disease more likely to cause intestinal obstruction than ulcerative colitis?
a. Crohn disease is located in the small intestine
b. Crohn disease causes granulomas to form in the submucosal layer
c. Crohn disease causes abdominal pain and watery diarrhea
d. Crohn disease is exacerbated by certain foods, such as spicy foods

Discussion and Application

1. What did I know about inflammation and tissue repair prior to today?

2. What body processes are affected by inflammation? What are the expected functions of those processes? How does inflammation impact those processes?

3. What are the potential etiologies for inflammation? How does inflammation develop?

4. Who is most at risk for developing inflammation? How can inflammation be prevented?

5. What are the human differences that affect the etiology, risk, or course of inflammation?

6. What clinical manifestations are expected during inflammation?

7. What special diagnostic tests are useful in determining the diagnosis and course of inflammation?

8. What are the goals of care for individuals with inflammation?

9. How does the concept of inflammation build on what I have learned in the previous chapters and in previous courses?

10. How can I use what I have learned?

RESOURCES

American Burn Association Web site:
http://www.ameriburn.org/
E-medicine Web site:
http://emedicine.medscape.com/
Inflammatory Bowel Disease tutorial Web site:
http://medlib.med.utah.edu/WebPath/TUTORIAL/IBD/IBD.html

REFERENCES

1. vanExel E, deCraen A, Remarque E, et al. Interaction of atherosclerosis and inflammation in elderly subjects with poor cognitive function. *Neurology.* 2003;61:1695–1701.
2. Yaffe K, Lindquist K, Penninx B, et al. Inflammatory markers and cognition in well-functioning African-American and white elders. *Neurology.* 2003;61:76–80.
3. Christensen D. Inflammatory ideas: new thoughts about causes of diabetes. *Sci News.* 2003;162:136–138.
4. Corbett J. *Laboratory Tests and Diagnostic Procedures with Nursing Diagnoses.* Upper Saddle River, NJ: Prentice Hall; 2004.
5. American Burn Association. 2007 Burn incident fact sheet. Available at: http://www.ameriburn.org/resources_factsheet.php. Accessed April 7, 2009.
6. Wong D. *Whaley & Wong's Nursing Care of Infants and Children.* 6th ed. St. Louis, MO: Mosby; 1999.
7. Rubin E, Gorstein F, Rubin R, et al. *Rubin's Pathology: Clinicopathologic Foundations of Medicine.* 4th ed. Baltimore: Lippincott Williams & Wilkins; 2005.
8. Helvig E. Pediatric burn injuries. *AACN Clin Issues.* 1993;4:433–442.
9. American Burn Association. Hospital and prehospital resources for optimal care of patients with burn injury: guidelines for development and operation of burn centers. *J Burn Care Rehabil.* 1990;11:98-104.

10. Saffle J. Predicting outcomes of burns. *N Engl J Med*. 1998;338: 387–388.

11. Gabriel S. The epidemiology of rheumatoid arthritis. *Rheum Dis Clin North Am*. 2001;27:269–281.

12. Goldbach-Mansky R, Lee J, McCoy A, et al. Rheumatoid arthritis associated autoantibodies in patients with synovitis of recent onset. *Arthritis Res*. 2000;2:236–243.

13. Boers M. Pathophysiology of rheumatoid arthritis: split or lump? *Arthritis Rheum*. 2008;58:2925–2927.

14. Sepulveda A, Dore M, Bazzoli F. Chronic gastritis. 2007. Available at: http://emedicine.medscape.com/article/176156-overview. Accessed April 7, 2009.

15. Rowe W. Inflammatory bowel disease. 2008. Available at: http://emedicine.medscape.com/article/179037-overview. Accessed April 7, 2009.

16. Khan A, Sheen A, McDonald S, et al. Ulcerative colitis. 2009. Available at: http://emedicine.medscape.com/article/375166-overview. Accessed April 7, 2009.

Chapter 4

Altered Immunity

LEARNING OBJECTIVES

1. Define and use the key terms listed in this chapter.
2. Describe the function of the cellular components (lymphocytes, macrophages, and antigen-presenting cells) in adaptive immune defense process.
3. Differentiate between the innate and adaptive immune responses.
4. Define the processes of primary and secondary antibody responses in the development of immunity.
5. Outline the similarities and differences between the types of T lymphocytes active in cell-mediated immunity.
6. Predict the potential alterations in immune responses resulting from dysfunction in the immunoglobulins IgA, IgD, IgE, IgG, and IgM.
7. Compare and contrast the process of altering immune function associated with host defense failure, hypersensitivity, autoimmunity, and alloimmunity.
8. Recognize the interactions between cell-mediated and humoral immune responses necessary for mounting an effective immune response.
9. Apply concepts of altered immune function to select clinical models.

INTRODUCTION

People live in a world in which there is a constant risk of harmful substances entering their bodies. Even when asleep, the body's defenses are protecting against overwhelming infection. These defenses are provided by the coordination of the many components that make up the immune system. The first line of defense, the skin and mucous membranes, and the second line of defense, the inflammatory response, were reviewed in detail in Chapter 3. The innate immune response is rapid and nonspecific, involving inflammatory response processes. The adaptive immune response, the third line of defense, allows the body to seek out and destroy new and old foreign invaders and is the focus of the discussion here in Chapter 4. The adaptive immune response is targeted and specific, involving two primary processes: cell-mediated immunity and humoral immunity.

This chapter provides a brief review of normal function, followed by the pathophysiology of alterations in immune function. Examples of conditions with pathogenesis resulting from altered immunity will highlight the application of concepts of altered immune responses. Developing an understanding of these responses will help to translate the signs and symptoms of disease states that result from maladaptive immune responses. Application of these concepts will form the basis for diagnosis, prevention, and treatment of a variety of conditions associated with altered immunity.

Module 1

Review of Immune Function

The process by which the body recognizes foreign substances and neutralizes them to prevent damage is known as **immunity**. Adaptive immune defense is characterized by:

- Specificity: the immune cells seek out and destroy targeted foreign invaders
- Memory: the immune cells produce substances that remember and more easily destroy return offenders

Immunology is the study of the structure and function of the immune system as well as the phenomena of immunity, induced sensitivity, and allergy. The immune system response, referred to as adaptive immunity, is stimulated when specialized cells come in contact with an **antigen**, a substance that induces a state of sensitivity or an immune response. Typically, the antigen is foreign and recognized as "nonself," prompting an immune response that spares "self" body cells. The adaptive immune response is initiated by two main components: the type of antigen presented to the cells and the type of cells to which the antigen is presented. The processes of cell-mediated and humoral immunity work together in the destruction of specifically targeted cells. The adaptive immune response involves central and peripheral immune structures, as well as primary and accessory cellular components in the development of specific immune responses, summarized in Table 4.1. The cells and organs of the body work in exquisite harmony to protect the body against bacteria, parasites, viruses, and allergens in well-defined processes.

Cellular Components of Immunity

Many of the cell types involved in immune response were first introduced in Chapter 3 because some of the same cells are involved in the inflammatory response. The initial, rapid response to foreign invaders is known as the innate immune response, a nonspecific response associated with inflammation.

The cellular components involved in innate immunity are also important in adaptive immunity as they are able to process the foreign antigens through phagocytosis and then present them to the cells involved in adaptive immunity. This step is essential for the recognition of foreign antigens by adaptive immunity cells. Cellular components of immune defense are illustrated in Figure 4.1.

IMMUNE CELL ORIGIN

The immune cells of adaptive immunity have a common origin in the pluripotent hematopoietic stem cells. Originating in the bone marrow, the pluripotent hematopoietic stem cells produce two precursor cell types: the **lymphoid progenitor** and the **myeloid progenitor**. Natural killer (NK) cells, T lymphocytes and B lymphocytes, are derived from the lymphoid progenitor cells. The myeloid progenitor cells produce other types of cells through the granulocyte/macrophage progenitor. These cells include the monocytes, dendritic cells, granulocytes, and mast cells.

Lymphoid Progenitor Cells

White blood cells (WBCs), also known as leukocytes, are the basic functional units of the immune system. Lymphocytes account for 25 to 35% of the leukocytes circulating in the blood, although 99% of lymphocytes are located in the lymph fluid. Three major categories of WBCs are derived from the lymphoid progenitor cells and play an essential role in immune function. These cell types include:

1. T lymphocytes
2. B lymphocytes
3. Natural killer cells

Table 4.1 Function of Immune Defense Components

Component	Location and Function
Central Immune Structures	*Immune Cell Production and Maturation*
Bone marrow	Production of lymphocytes
	Maturation of B lymphocytes
Thymus	Gland located in the mediastinum
	Differentiation and maturation of lymphocytes
Peripheral Immune Structures	*Process Antigen and Promote Association with Mature Immune Cells*
Lymph nodes	Rounded mass of lymphatic tissue
	Spread out along lymphatic vessels
	Contain many lymphocytes, which filter the lymphatic fluid
Spleen	Organ that produces lymphocytes
Lymphoid mucosal tissue (tonsils, Peyer's patches, appendix)	Site of lymphocyte aggregation
Primary Cellular Components	
T lymphocytes	Matured in thymus
	Essential in adaptive cell-mediated immunity
	Destruction of cellular antigens
	Promote antibody production by B lymphocytes
	Account for 60% of blood lymphocytes
B lymphocytes	Matured in bone marrow
	Essential in mediating adaptive humoral immunity
	Production of antibodies/immunoglobins
	Account for 10–20% of blood lymphocytes
Accessory Cellular Components	
Macrophage	Essential in mediating innate immunity
Neutrophil	Bind invading microbes to cell surface receptors
Dendritic cells	Process and present antigen to T and B lymphocytes, stimulating adaptive immune response
	Phagocytosis to prevent colonization, entry, and spread of microbes

The **T lymphocytes** mature and fully differentiate in the *thymus*. T lymphocytes require contact with an antigen that signals the T lymphocytes to proliferate and differentiate into the following classifications of cells:

- **Cytotoxic T lymphocytes**: direct destruction of antigen carrying cells
- **Helper T lymphocytes**: enhance humoral and cell-mediated responses of the immune system
- **Suppressor T lymphocytes**: inhibit humoral and cell-mediated responses

The cytotoxic T lymphocyte attacks cells infected with viruses while helper T lymphocyte activates other cells needed for an appropriate immune response. Suppressor T lymphocytes provide a balance, limiting immune responses. Each T lymphocyte has a unique receptor, or **T-cell receptor**

(TCR), which is able to bind to antigens, promoting a specific immune response.

B lymphocytes develop in the *bone marrow*. B lymphocytes migrate from the bone marrow to the peripheral lymphoid tissues where they become activated after contact with an antigen. Binding of the antigen with the B lymphocyte stimulates differentiation of B lymphocytes into antibody-secreting plasma cells. The B lymphocytes recognize specific antigens due to the **B-cell receptor** (BCR) bound to the cell membrane of the B lymphocytes. The uniqueness of antigen–BCR binding contributes to the specificity of the adaptive immune response. After antigen–BCR binding, the B lymphocytes differentiate into plasma cells, which proliferate and begin to produce and secrete large quanities of antibodies that target the specific antigen bound to the BCR. Antibodies are released from the membranes of plasma cells. The secreted

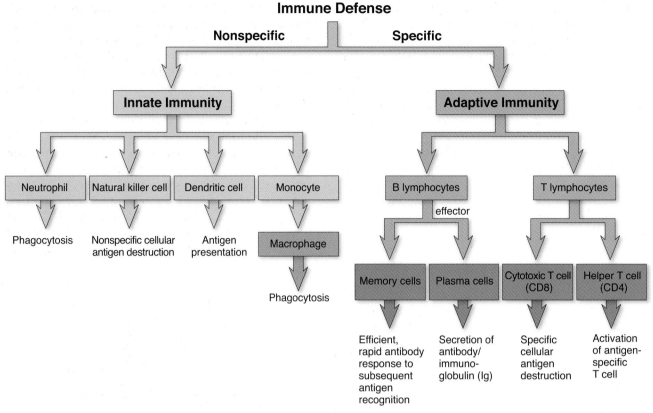

Figure 4.1   Concept map. Cellular components involved in immune defense.

antibody is known as **immunoglobulin (Ig)**. The main classes of immunoglobulins include IgA, IgG, IgM, IgD, and IgE (Table 4.2). These antibodies are designed to detect and bind to *specific* antigens, each playing a different role in the immune response.

Natural killer cells are large, granular lymphocytes. NK cells differ from T cells and B cells in that they are not antigen specific, similar to other cells

active in innate immunity. NK cells circulate until they come in contact with cells they can recognize as a threat, such as infected cells or tumor cells; they then attack and kill these cells.

Myeloid Progenitor Cells

Myeloid progenitor cells produce granulocytes and monocytes, which are leukocytes essential to

Table 4.2 Primary Role of Immunoglobulin Classes

Immunoglobulin	% of Total	Characteristics
IgA	15	Concentrated in bodily secretions such as breastmilk, tears, and saliva
		Protection of mucous membrane lined structures
IgG	75	Most common circulating antibody
		Produced in primary and secondary immune responses
		Activates complement
		Antibody activity against toxins, viruses, and bacteria
		Passive immunity in newborns via placental transfer
IgM	10	First immunoglobulin to proliferate in immune response
		Bound to B lymphocytes
		Activates complement
IgD	0.2	Bound to and activates B cells
IgE	0.004	Bound to mast cells in skin and mucous membranes
		Stimulates mast cell release of histamine in allergic immune response, leading to inflammation

immune function. Granulocytes, named for the cytoplasmic granules common to all types, are phagocytic cells. Monocytes are also phagocytic cells, able to engulf larger quantities of debris than granulocytes.

The **granulocytes**, also known as polymorphonuclear (PMN) leukocytes, include neutrophils, eosinophils, and basophils. Although these cells do not live long, their production can be dramatically increased when stimulated. **Neutrophils** are present in the greatest number and are most important in the rapid response to bacterial infection. Neutrophils are phagocytes that are the first responders in the inflammatory response. **Eosinophils** offer the greatest protection against parasites, whereas **basophils** complement the actions of mast cells, important in the establishment of allergic reactions.

Monocytes are large, mononuclear leukocytes representing 3 to 7% of the total number of circulating leukocytes.[1] Circulating monocytes become activated when in contact with an antigen, prompting differentiation into **macrophages** and movement out of the circulation into the tissues. The antigen carrying cell is injested by the macrophage where it undergoes phagocytosis. During the processing of the antigen, macrophages display antigen markers on the cell surface where they can be recognized by the receptors on T and B lymphocytes. Macrophages are known by different cell names that are determined by the location of tissues where they reside. These cell types include:

- Histiocytes (loose connective tissue)
- Microglial cells (brain)
- Kupffer cells (liver)

Dendritic cells are critical to the processing and display of antigens to T lymphocytes. Mature dendritic cells take up antigens when they are encountered in the circulation. **Langerhans' cells**, immature dendritic cells in the skin, carry surface receptors for immunoglobulin and complement, important in the immune response.

Lymphatics

The lymphatic system is composed of central and peripheral organs and is important in the establishment of the immune response. Lymphocytes are produced and differentiated in the central organs, bone marrow, and thymus. The **peripheral organs** serve as sites for maintenance of the lymphocytes and are the organs in which immune responses are often initiated. These organs include the spleen, lymph nodes, and other lymphoid mucosal tissue, such as tonsils and the appendix. The **lymphatic system** circulates the

lymphocytes in lymph fluid. **Lymph fluid** is a filtration product of extracellular fluid from tissues and is returned to blood. **Lymph nodes** are joined segments of lymphatic vessels. The vessels of the lymphatic system work in concert with the blood vessels to promote an effective immune response (Fig. 4.2).

The lymphatic system traps antigen captured by cells of the immune system. This process allows the antigen to be presented to immune cells and stimulates the immune response. The lymph also serves to maintain signals to the **naive lymphocytes**, or those that have not yet encountered an antigen, enabling them to survive. The absence of such a signal results in apoptosis, or programmed death of cells, as discussed in Chapter 2. This

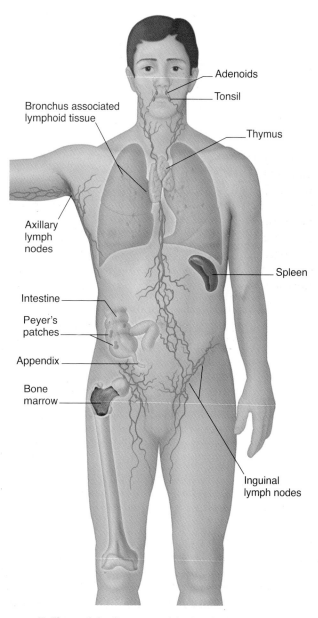

Figure 4.2 Structures of the lymphatic system.

process is essential to the regulation of the number and type of circulating lymphocytes.

STOP *and Consider*

When increased lymphocyte production is stimulated, the additional cells travel to the lymph nodes. How could you determine if this was occurring with a physical examination? What signs and symptoms might a person have if this occurs?

IMMUNE PROCESSES

The immune response is vital to an individual's survival. As a result, the immune system involves processes that are both redundant and complementary to one another. The two distinct and specialized processes of immunity are adaptive immunity and innate immunity. **Innate immunity** is the first responder to insult. This immune response is rapid and can be initiated by many different pathogens without requiring prior exposure. **Adaptive immunity**, humoral and cell-mediated, occurs over a lifetime, promoting the body's ability to adapt to the threat of reinfection.

INNATE IMMUNITY

Macrophages, neutrophils, and dendritic cells are the primary cell types involved in innate immunity. The cells of the innate immune system are the rapid responders to organisms that pose a threat of infection. In addition, these cells work in harmony with the adaptive immune system to initiate and direct continued protection from infection. The functions of the innate immune system include:

- Prevention of microbe colonization
- Prevention of microbe entry
- Prevention of microbe spread

The first exposure to a microorganism initiates an immune response through the detection of foreign antigens, as discussed in Chapter 3. An inflammatory response is then initiated. The receptors on the surface of macrophages recognize components common to bacterial, viral, fungal, and parasitic organisms. The inflammatory response initiates the phagocytic process and stimulates the release of chemical mediators with specific purposes. This rapid, early response of the innate immune system is critical to the defense against infection, and it may be adequate to control infection without further action.

Dendritic cells located in the tissues are primarily responsible for presenting the antigen and phagocytosis, which is stimulated in the same manner as macrophages and neutrophils. Dendritic cells are especially important in recognizing hidden antigens. Certain pathogens conceal themselves in envelopes but can be shown to lymphocytes after ingestion by dendritic cells. For this reason, mature dendritic cells are also known as **antigen-presenting cells**. They assist in the recognition of particles that are not part of the individual, or are **nonself**. The innate immune system initiates the activity of the adaptive immune system by this process of recognition of nonself.

ADAPTIVE IMMUNITY

B and T lymphocytes and dendritic cells are the primary cell types involved in adaptive immunity. The adaptive immune system is stimulated by phagocytosis and activation of antigen-presenting cells (APCs). Key properties of the adaptive immune system include:

- Specificity: targeted response to a distinct antigen
- Diversity: recognition of a wide variety of antigens
- Memory: rapid and robust response to previously recognized antigens
- Self and nonself recognition: ability to distinguish between antigens on body cells and foreign antigens

Adaptive immunity is characterized by a slower response to the introduction of microorganisms than that of the innate immune system. When an organism is reintroduced, immune memory leads to a more rapid and intense immune response. Immunity can be acquired in different ways:

- Active
  - Development of antibodies in response to an antigen
  - Achieved through actually having a specific disease or vaccine immunization against a particular disease
- Passive
  - Immunity transfer from host to recipient
  - Achieved via mother to infant transfer via placenta or breastmilk or injection with high concentrations of antibody, such as immune gamma globulin

The adaptive immune system, including humoral and cell-mediated immunity, provides essential defense against specific antigens.

Humoral Immunity

Antibodies, essential components of adaptive immunity, were first identified in the plasma, or humor as it was once known. The term **humoral immunity** refers to adaptive immunity-involving antibodies. **Antibodies** are immunoglobulins that react with an antigen in a specific way. Immunoglobulins are composed of two regions. The **constant region** forms the base of the Y-shaped antibody and is the most stable component. The two **variable regions** are structured to allow binding to specific antigens. IgG is the most abundant class of immunoglobulin. Due to its size and shape, IgG is able to enter body tissues from body fluids. IgG is the only immunoglobulin that is able to cross the placenta, providing passive immunity to the developing fetus. IgA provides passive immunity from mother to newborn through breastmilk, transferring essential immune defense prior to the development of an adequate immune response in the infant. IgM is the initial circulating antibody produced in response to antigen challenge and the first to be produced by the newborn. Located on the B lymphocyte cell membrane, IgD is involved in the binding of antigen and stimulation of differentiation of B lymphocytes into plasma cells. IgE on the cell surfaces of mast cells and basophils leads to cellular degranulation upon antigen binding, triggering the release of chemical mediators involved with inflammation and allergies.

Each B lymphocyte carries a single, specific receptor that recognizes a unique antigen pattern. When an antigen is recognized by the BCR, B lymphocyte activation is initiated, causing proliferation and differentiation of targeted B lymphocytes into **effector cells** (plasma cells that secrete antibodies). The process of activation and differentiation of naive lymphocytes into effector cells takes approximately 4 to 5 days. Most of these effector cells undergo apoptosis (programmed cell death) after the end of their lifespan, although some continue to exist after the antigen is eliminated. These remaining cells are then known as **memory cells**, an important component of **immunologic memory**. These memory cells respond much more rapidly when re-exposed to the same antigen, dramatically shortening and intensifying the immunologic response (Fig. 4.3). This process is accomplished through the secretion of higher levels of antibodies and those that bind with higher affinity to the antigens.

Clones of the B lymphocytes carrying cell surface receptors for specific antigens (**clonal selection**) respond by differentiating into plasma cells capable of secreting large quantities of single specificity antibody (**clonal expansion**), the result of antigen occupying the specific BCR (Fig. 4.4). In this way, the humoral immune response can generate a defense that recognizes and targets distinct antigens in a specific manner.

Figure 4.3 Primary and secondary antibody responses. The level of antibodies in the primary and secondary responses to a specific antigen. (Image from Premkumar K. *The Massage Connection: Anatomy and Physiology*. Baltimore: Lippincott Williams & Wilkins; 2004, with permission.)

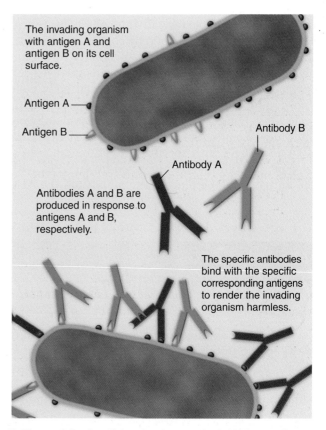

Figure 4.4 Specificity of antigen–antibody binding. Antibodies bind with specific antigens, stimulating clonal expansion, the proliferation of antigen-specific lymphocytes capable of mounting an immune response.

Antibodies protect cells from pathogens in three major ways:

1. The binding of the antigen to the antibody, which prevents the antigen from infecting cells (**neutralization**). The antigen–antibody complex is removed by agglutination (clumping together) or precipitation (falling out of solution).
2. The promotion of phagocytosis and destruction of the pathogen through the phagocyte's ability to recognize the constant region of the antibody that is bound to or coating the antigen (**opsonization**).
3. The activation of complement, which supplements that of the innate system, further enhancing the actions of the antibodies.

Cell-Mediated Immunity

Cytotoxic T lymphocytes are the primary immune cells involved in **cell-mediated immunity**, a component of the adaptive immune response. Cell-mediated immunity results in the recognition and the destruction of cells carrying nonself antigens. Cytotoxic T lymphocytes detect pathogens inside the cell where they cannot be recognized by antibodies. Cells infected with viruses displayed on the cell surface are recognized by cytotoxic T lymphocytes. The cytotoxic T lymphocytes kill the cells before viral replication is complete, thereby controlling the further spread of infection. The specificity of T lymphocyte recognition of foreign antigens involves cell surface markers on APCs and infected body cells known as major histocompatibility complex (MHC) molecules, lymphocyte identification by membrane molecules known as **clusters of differentiation** (CD) and TCRs with specific antigen binding sites. In short, the antigen is processed by an APC, with the antigen epitope placed onto a MHC on the APC surface. T lymphocytes recognize and bind processed antigens with a specific TCR, leading to death of the affected cell.

T lymphocytes display membrane surface molecules, known as CD, contributing to cell specificity. CD molecules determine specific functions and responses of T-cell subtypes. The molecule CD8 is expressed on the surface of cytotoxic T lymphocytes (**CD8 T lymphocytes**). Helper T lymphocytes express CD4 on their surfaces and are known as **CD4 T lymphocytes**. Helper T lymphocytes provide a regulatory function, enhancing the responses of other types of T lymphocytes.

Two classes of CD4 T lymphocytes are responsible for different roles in immune defense. One subset, T_H1 cells, is particularly important in the control of bacterial intracellular infection. T_H1 cells activate macrophages, secrete chemokines, and cytokines to attract macrophages, promote fusion of lysosomes with vesicles containing bacteria, and stimulate phagocytosis. T_H2 cells, the second subset of CD4 T lymphocytes, activate B cells to produce antibodies.

Targets are recognized by T lymphocytes through TCR detection of antigens displayed by MHC molecules. MHC molecules are important in the recognition of the body's "self" antigens from foreign "nonself" antigens. MHC molecules are also known as **human leukocyte antigens (HLAs)**. Two subsets of MHC molecule, MHC class I and MHC class II, trap an antigen within the cell and then transport it to the cell surface, where it can be displayed to T lymphocytes. The **MHC class I molecule** is found on nucleated body cells and is recognized by the CD8 cytotoxic T lymphocytes. The **MHC class II molecule** is found on APCs and is recognized by the CD4 helper T lymphocytes (T_H1 or T_H2). A summary of the steps involved in activation of the adaptive immune system is depicted in Figure 4.5.

Module 2

Process of Altering Immune Function

Daily defense against infection requires interplay between the immune system processes. Failure of even one component in the immune system can result in catastrophic consequences, presenting a significant risk for disease and death. Altered immunity can result from:

- Failure of host defense mechanisms: the impaired ability to mount an immune defense
- Hypersensitivity: inappropriate excessive immune responses

- Autoimmunity: inappropriate response to "self"
- Alloimmunity: reactions directed at tissue antigens from other individuals of the same species

Host Defense Failure

Failure of the **host** (the person on which the pathogen lives) to defend against infection occurs in a variety of ways. Pathogens can trick the immune

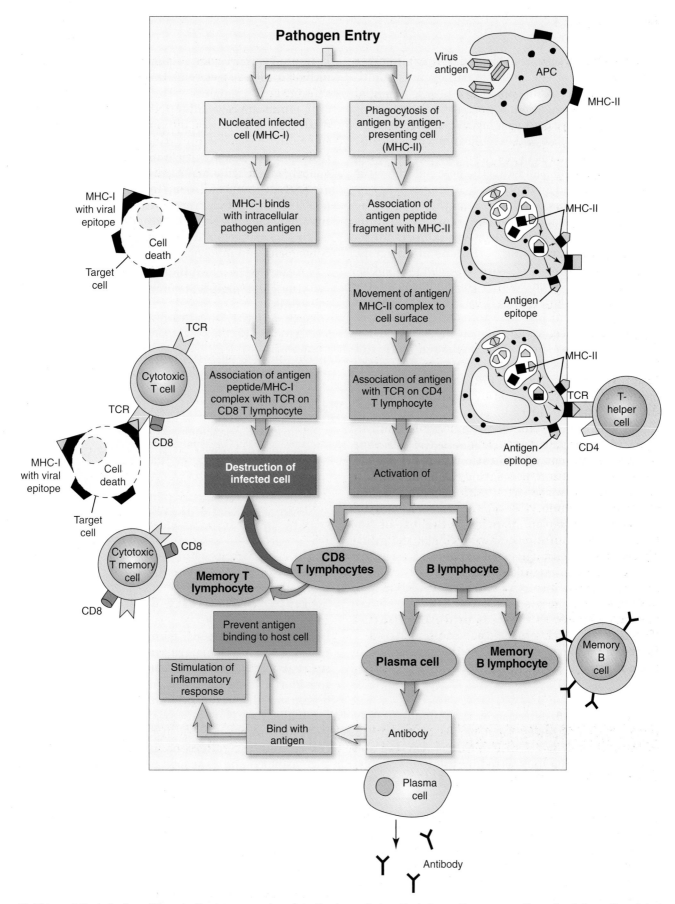

Figure 4.5 Activation of the adaptive immune system. Adaptive immunity is activated on pathogen recognition, stimulating cell-mediated and humoral immunity. Cell-mediated immunity is activated when the major histocompatibility complex (MHC) I–antigen complex binds to the T-cell receptor (TCR) on cytotoxic (CD8) T lymphocytes. Humoral immunity is activated on the association of the MHCII/antigen complex with the TCR on helper (CD4) T lymphocytes. B lymphocyte effector plasma cells produce antigen-specific antibodies that prevent antigen binding to the host cell and stimulate the inflammatory response.

system, evading the normal signal that stimulates a defense response. The ability of pathogens to multiply in the host cell and spread to others is essential to continued propagation. A "successful" pathogen is one that grows without alerting the immune system to mount a response and is replicated without causing immediate harm to the host. For example, if a virus is too vigorous and kills the host cell, the virus will not be able to multiply.

One of the most effective methods used by pathogens to evade detection from the immune system is called **antigenic variation**. Many pathogens have multiple variations of antigens, making recognition by T and B lymphocytes potentially difficult. Even though the body may have been previously infected by one variant of the pathogen and was able to mount an effective immune response, a variation in the same pathogen will appear new. The pathogen may not be recognized and therefore does not stimulate the immune "memory." Antigenic variation explains the potential of reinfection by a pathogen with a slightly different antigenic epitope. Variations in antigens can also occur because of genetic mutations. Mutated antigens are genetically different enough to prevent identification as a previously recognized pathogen, preventing the mounting of a rapid antibody response. Health concerns resulting from antigenic variation occur each year as influenza (flu) season approaches. Because of frequent genetic mutations, new strains of the influenza virus develop that are capable of escaping detection by the immune system.

STOP *and Consider*

People can suffer from the same illness, such as a cold, many times. What is a possible explanation for this?

Viruses can evade detection by the immune system by going into **latency**, or a period of inactivity. When a virus is latent, it is not being replicated and therefore remains undetected by the immune system. This characteristic is further discussed in Chapter 5.

Some pathogens resist destruction by using the immune system. Pathogens that use the cells of the immune system as host cells may prevent their own destruction. This is the case with *Mycobacterium tuberculosis*, in which the pathogen escapes destruction by the lysosome, which instead protects the pathogen. However, some pathogens can stimulate a strong immune response, which then promotes suppression of the immune system. This is sometimes seen after infection with the virus that causes measles.

Immunosuppression resulting from inhibition or incapacitation of even one immune component has significant consequences. The most significant form of immunosuppression is that caused by **immunodeficiency**. Primary immunodeficiency is often caused by a genetic mutation, impairing immune responsiveness. Primary immunodeficiency is frequently identified when recurrent, severe infections are seen in young children. Table 4.3 describes common forms of primary immunodeficiency. Immunodeficiency that is a result of another disease is known as secondary immunodeficiency. These deficiencies can involve:

- Defective humoral function
- Deficient phagocyte numbers and functional ability
- Altered T lymphocyte signaling
- Altered cytokine production and function

The absence of an adequate immune response may lead to overwhelming infection.

STOP *and Consider*

Some immunodeficiency diseases primarily affect one cell type. What part of the immune defense would be affected if the number of neutrophils was decreased? What would occur with a decrease in the number of macrophages? What would occur with a decrease in the number of plasma cells?

Hypersensitivity

Disorders that result from excessive immune responses to allergens are known as hypersensitivity reactions. **Allergens** are antigens commonly considered to be harmless, unlike the pathogenic organisms discussed previously. The response to these allergens is inappropriate, ranging in severity from mild to severe, and it can be potentially life threatening. The allergens may be environmental, such as pollen, dust, or food products (e.g., nuts), or they may be certain proteins or components found in drugs. In other words, potential allergens are things encountered as a daily part of life.

Allergic reactions to insect stings, primarily honeybees, yellow jackets, hornets, wasps, and fireants, cause cutaneous reactions (swelling, itching, redness) with the potential for severe systemic reaction. The location of insects causing allergic reactions varies throughout the regions of the United States, with yellow jackets prominent in the northern region, wasps in the southwest, and fireants in the southeast. Food allergies affect both children

Table 4.3 Primary Immunodeficiencies

Condition	Immune Deficit	Immune Manifestation
X-linked agammaglobulinemia (Bruton disease)	B cell • Absent to few B cells	No antibody production
Common variable immune deficiency (CVID) (hypogammaglobulinemia)	Normal B-cell number, but impaired function • Low levels of gamma globulins • Low levels of IgA	Common form of primary immunodeficiency Variable in manifestations
Selective IgA deficiency	B cell • Low levels of IgA	Common form of primary immunodeficiency (1:300) Mild presentation Frequent and unusual infections May not be diagnosed until third or fourth decade
Severe combined immunedeficiency	T and B cell • Complete lack of immune defense	Most rare (1:500,000) multiple forms associated with decreased NK cells, circulating T cells, and serum Ig
DiGeorge anomaly	T cell • Underdeveloped thymus • Decrease in circulating T cells	Frequent infections diagnosed soon after birth
X-linked hyper-IgM syndrome	B cell • Absent IgA, high IgM • T cells impaired communication for Ig type switching to B cells	Neutropenia, opportunistic infections GI and liver dysfunction
Wiskott–Aldrich syndrome	T and B cell • Progressive disease in T cells • Decreased IgM	Lymphoma Eczema Autoimmune disease
Ataxia-telangiectasia	T and B cell • Decreased IgA, IgG • Decreased circulating T cells • Immature thymus	Malignancies of the lymphoid tissues X-ray sensitivity
Chronic granulomatous disease	• Impaired phagocytosis • Inability to produce compounds for oxygen transport	Recurrent, severe bacterial and fungal infections

GI, gastrointestinal; NK, natural killer.

and adults, with incidence declining with age. In children, more than 90% of food allergies are due to milk, eggs, wheat, soy, peanuts, and tree nuts. Among adults, peanuts, tree nuts, fish, and shellfish are the most common culprits. Drug allergies account for >5% of all hospital admissions.[1] Allergies to penicillin are commonly reported, although only a minority of individuals indicating a penicillin allergy have a positive skin test documenting an IgE response to the drug. If a true allergy to penicillin is documented, other similar drugs (i.e., penicillin, ampicillin, and amoxicillin) should be avoided as well, such as the cephalosporin class drugs. These drugs contain a common structure, the beta lactam ring, that can stimulate the allergic response. Hypersensitivity disorders are classified based on four major types of reactions, described in Table 4.4.

Symptoms of allergy result from tissue injury and can vary depending on the route and the "dose" of the allergen exposure. Allergen exposure can occur through inhalation, ingestion, injection, or physical

Table 4.4 Types of Hypersensitivity Reactions

Category	Etiology	Activated Immune Cells	Injury
Type I, immediate hypersensitivity reaction	IgE mediated	Helper T (T_H2) Mast cells Basophils	Allergic reaction: local (atopic) inflammation; systemic (anaphylactic) life threatening
Type II, antibody-mediated reaction	IgG or IgM mediated	Macrophage	Reaction against normal "self" antigens; opsonization and lysis of cells
Type III, immune complex-mediated reaction	IgG and IgM mediated	Complement Neutrophils	Deposition of insoluble antigen–antibody complex
Type IV, cell-mediated hypersensitivity reaction	T-cell mediated	CD8 T lymphocytes CD4 T_H1 lymphocytes	Inflammatory response leading to cell lysis

contact. Symptoms can be local (itching and irritation at the point of contact) or systemic (difficulty breathing and oxygenating, as occurs in asthma or anaphylaxis).

 Research Notes

Immunotherapy for the treatment of hypersensitivity reactions resulting from insect stings has been used to improve prognosis. While effective in reducing the manifestations of type I hypersensitivity responses, venom immunotherapy (VIT) is also associated with adverse systemic effects. In a recent clinical trial, the use of purified and nonpurified formulations of VIT and the association with adverse systemic effects was investigated. The use of purified VIT extract reduced the incidence of severe local and systemic reactions, providing evidence of improvement in treatment options in individuals with hypersensitivity to insect stings.[2]

Special testing to determine specific allergens capable of stimulating hypersensitivity reactions can be completed. Several methods may be used, including:

- Scratch skin test
  - A small amount of a suspected allergen is placed on the skin, followed by scratching or pricking the skin, introducing the allergen to the skin surface. An allergen is identified when a local hypersensitivity reaction occurs
- Intradermal skin test
  - The allergen is injected under the skin, followed by observation of a local hypersensitivity reaction.
- Skin patch test
  - The allergen is placed in a liquid solution on a pad secured to skin, followed by observation of a local hypersensitivity reaction in 24 to 72 hours.
- Measurement of serum IgG

  - Hypersensitivity reaction is determined by the amount of specific IgE antibodies in the blood.
- Elimination diet
  - Suspected food allergens are eliminated, followed by reintroduction and observation of hypersensitivity reaction.

Allergy testing involves exposure of an individual to a potential allergen. Severe reactions can result, requiring testing to be completed under close medical supervision. Allergy testing is an effective method to determine specific allergenic substances. This information can be used to inform individuals of substances to avoid, if possible, and to prevent and treat hypersensitivity reactions.

TYPE I OR IMMEDIATE HYPERSENSITIVITY REACTION

Immediate hypersensitivity reactions are also known as IgE-mediated hypersensitivity responses to antigen challenges. Initial exposure to an allergen in a vulnerable individual stimulates the production of **IgE**, an immunoglobulin important in the development of protective immunity. Allergy is most often caused by inhaled allergens taken in at low doses. These small, dry allergens dissolve and become soluble when they come in contact with mucous membranes. Dendritic cells are activated by these allergens. Dendritic cells then travel to the lymph nodes where they present the allergens to naive T lymphocytes, promoting their differentiation into T$_H$2 cells. Specific chemical signals can cause B lymphocytes to produce IgE antibodies in place of other types of antibodies. IgE produced by the plasma cells within inflamed tissue binds with high affinity to receptors on mast cells and basophils. When IgE encounters and binds an allergen, mast cells and basophils degranulate, release chemical mediators and cause injury to cells, producing the symptoms associated with allergy. Lipid products from cell membranes, including leukotrienes and prostaglandins, are also released in this process. Repeated exposure to the same allergen produces a IgE-mediated hypersensitivity response that is responsible for a range of symptoms, some of which can be life threatening. Type I hypersensitivity reaction is an example of a pathophysiologic exaggeration of a defensive immune response (Fig. 4.6).

Immediate hypersensitivity reactions are initiated within minutes of allergen exposure. Some hypersensitivity reactions, including asthma, are known to have symptoms associated with two separate response stages. The symptoms associated with stage one are related to mast cell degranulation followed by the release of chemical mediators. They include vasodilation and nonvascular smooth muscle contraction that last approximately 1 hour. The second stage follows in approximately 2 to 8 hours and results in symptoms associated with the lipid mediators released from the plasma membrane of degranulated cells. These symptoms are similar to those in stage one but last longer. In addition, recruitment of eosinophils and leukocytes results in an inflammatory response in the affected tissues.

Not everyone develops hypersensitivity reactions after allergen exposure. People who develop symptoms after exposure to a wide number of commonly encountered allergens are described as **atopic**, which means that IgE responses are stimulated from exposure to these typically benign substances. Many allergies are familial, meaning they are genetic tendencies that are passed on from one generation to another. Avoidance of potential allergens may prevent the development of atopy, especially early in development.

Systemic manifestations of type I immediate hypersensitivity reactions are potentially life threatening. **Anaphylaxis** represents an extremely serious response to type I immediate hypersensitivity reaction. It is characterized by edema and vasodilation and leads to hypotension. Anaphylaxis is discussed in detail in Module 4: Clinical Models.

TYPE II OR ANTIBODY-MEDIATED REACTIONS

Antibody-mediated reactions are the result of mistaken identity. Usually harmless substances are identified as harmful; an immune response is mounted that results in cell damage. The reaction in type II hypersensitivity is tissue specific, usually involving destruction of a target cell by antibody binding to antigen on the cell surface. Cell destruction and tissue damage often result from harm inflicted by macrophage phagocytosis and complement-mediated effects. This is a direct response resulting from an antigen–antibody reaction.

Responses of these types are seen in certain drug reactions, blood transfusion reactions, Graves disease, and hemolytic disease of the newborn. Often, the affected cells include blood cells. When the antibody binds to the antigen on the cell, the cell is lysed and destroyed. This results in disease related to the loss of these cells and includes anemia (decreased red blood cells [RBCs]), thrombocytopenia (decreased platelets), and leukopenia (decreased WBCs). Symptoms are related to the degree of loss of these blood cell types (Fig. 4.7).

Treatment for this type of reaction involves removal of the antigen causing the reaction. When a drug is

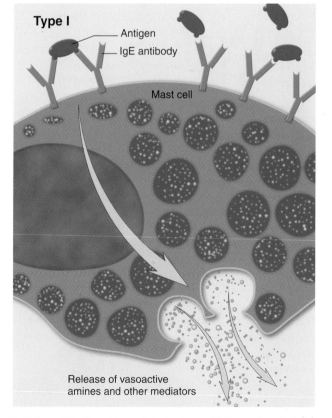

Figure 4.6 Type I immediate hypersensitivity reaction. Antigen–IgE antibody binding induces release of chemical mediators from mast cells.

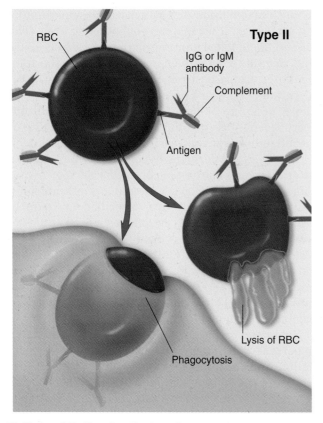

■ Figure 4.7 Type II antibody-mediated hypersensitivity reaction. Cell-bound antigen binds to IgG or IgM antibodies leading to a cytotoxic reaction. RBC, red blood cell.

involved, the administration of the drug is halted to prevent further immune-mediated cellular damage. Avoidance of the antigen is recommended to prevent subsequent, increasingly serious reactions. This drug information is requested and marked prominently on medical records to prevent inadvertent administration in the future. When a patient's treatment involves blood replacement with transfusion, a lab procedure called blood typing and cross matching is done on recipients to allow matching with donor blood. If a reaction occurs inadvertently during transfusion, the administration of blood is immediately halted. A similar condition known as Rh isoimmunization, or hemolytic disease of the newborn, is covered in greater detail in the clinical model section of this chapter.

TYPE III OR IMMUNE COMPLEX-MEDIATED REACTION

Cellular and tissue damage caused by type III reactions are the indirect result of complement activation stimulated by the deposition of insoluble antigen–antibody complexes. Immune complex activation of complement results in widespread damage from several mechanisms. Altered blood flow, vascular permeability, and the response of inflammatory cells result

in damage to blood vessels and organs, including kidney glomeruli, small blood vessels in the skin, and the synovial lining of joints. The deposition of antigen–antibody complexes triggers the inflammatory immune response of complement activation and the recruitment of inflammatory cells (Fig. 4.8). This response was originally seen in individuals who received horse antisera, once used as a treatment for tetanus. These individuals developed a condition referred to as **serum sickness** and responded with local symptoms of itching and rash at the injection site as well as systemic symptoms of edema and fever approximately 7 days after antisera injection. These symptoms resulted from antigen–antibody complex deposition in blood vessels and tissue, prompting complement activation and an inflammatory response.

When the location of this complex-mediated immune response is in the skin, the resulting area of localized tissue necrosis is referred to as an **Arthus reaction**. Although the initial exposure results in symptoms that resolve with time, subsequent exposure can cause a more serious response, sometimes resulting in death. Conditions most commonly associated with this response include the

■ Figure 4.8 Type III immune complex-mediated reaction. Type III reactions are the result of the formation and deposition of immune complexes in tissues, causing acute inflammation polymorphonuclear neutrophil (PMN).

autoimmune diseases of systemic lupus erythematosus (SLE) and rheumatoid arthritis (as discussed in Chapter 3). The administration of certain drugs, including antilymphocyte globulin (an immunosuppressive agent used in transplant patients) and streptokinase (thrombolytic agent used with patients having a myocardial infarction), can also stimulate this response.

TYPE IV OR CELL-MEDIATED HYPERSENSITIVITY REACTION

The heightened immune responses in type IV reactions are caused by T lymphocyte mediated reactions rather than antigen–antibody reactions. Two types of these reactions are distinguished by different mechanisms and associated response times. They include direct cell-mediated cytotoxicity and delayed type hypersensitivity reactions.

In **direct cell-mediated toxicity**, damage occurs in cells and tissues as a direct response to CD8 cytotoxic T lymphocyte destruction of cells with recognized antigens. CD8 cytotoxic T lymphocytes attack all infected cells with recognized antigens, whether the antigen is harmful or not. This response can actually be more harmful than the damage inflicted by the pathogen, as in the case of some forms of hepatitis, in which liver damage is primarily caused by the cell-mediated toxicity rather than by the virus itself.

Delayed hypersensitivity reactions are mediated by antigen-specific T lymphocyte. T lymphocyte responds to antigens presented to them as described in the earlier discussion of their normal role in immune response. Often, these responses occur on the skin and are mediated by APCs and CD4 helper T lymphocytes of the T_H1 type. Antigens more likely to cause this reaction are small, can penetrate the skin, and can stimulate itching. These antigens react with "self" proteins and create complexes that can bind to MHC molecules seen as foreign by T lymphocytes, stimulating an immune response (Fig. 4.9).

The two phases of delayed hypersensitivity reaction are sensitization and elicitation. The **sensitization phase** begins when the antigen crosses the skin, the first line of defense. Antigens are taken up by Langerhans' cells and transported to the lymph nodes. Once in the lymph nodes, Langerhans cells develop into mature dendritic cells, which are able to present antigens to helper T lymphocytes and activate them. Memory cells are produced and become localized in the dermis.

During the **elicitation phase**, the memory T lymphocytes in the dermis are stimulated by a subsequent exposure to the specific antigen. Cytokines and chemokines are released, stimulating the attrac-

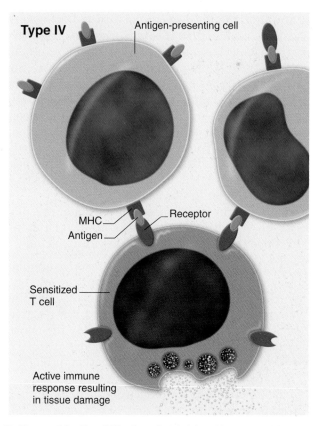

■ **Figure 4.9** Type IV T-cell mediated delayed hypersensitivity reaction. Type IV reactions occur 1 to 3 days after antigen exposure, resulting in erythema and itching. MHC, major histocompatibility complex.

tion of macrophages and additional T lymphocytes to the area. This results in a visible local reaction at the site of antigen entry. Blood vessel permeability is increased, leading to swelling. The T cell–mediated response takes between 24 and 72 hours. This condition is often referred to as contact dermatitis. It can also be initiated by the injection of an antigen to determine an individual's prior exposure to *M. tuberculosis*, commonly referred to as a tuberculin or Mantoux test. Reactions from poison ivy are also the result of type IV hypersensitivity reactions.

Autoimmunity

One of the critical functions of the immune system is to distinguish "self" from "nonself." When this recognition fails or is not controlled, severe **autoimmune** (directed at an individual's own tissues) disease can develop. The two major ways in which this occurs are by specific recognition of "self" antigens and by overzealous responses to chronic infection. The acute autoimmune response can convert to a chronic response if the involved antigen is not adequately cleared or if a positive feedback loop develops in response to the inflammatory process, as described in Chapter 3.

Autoimmune disease can be directed at specific organs, as seen in type II hypersensitivity reactions, or it can have a systemic or whole body effect, as seen in type III hypersensitivity reactions. For example, in Graves disease, the organ affected is the thyroid gland, and antibodies are specifically directed against the thyroid itself (Fig. 4.10). In contrast, SLE is characterized by antibodies formed against proteins found in cells throughout the body, causing systemic disease. We will discuss the specific pathology related to autoimmunity seen in SLE in Module 4, later in this chapter.

Failure in the development of self-tolerance may occur at various steps of immune development. Situations that can trigger autoimmunity include:

* Inadequate elimination of self-reactive lymphocytes in central lymphoid tissues
* Altered **lymphocyte ignorance** (converting lymphocytes from nonresponsive to self-reactive)
* Stimuli, such as infection, overriding the nonresponsive nature of naive T lymphocytes
* Impaired T lymphocyte inactivation (prolonged or irreversible)
* Failure to recognize antigen due to MHC–antigen complex interaction
* Release of antigens sequestered during development
* Close resemblance between foreign and self-antigen, also known as **molecular mimicry**
* Inappropriate activation of T-cell receptors by superantigens

A **familial tendency**, or propagation of autoimmunity among family members, is a common trait in autoimmune disease. Both genetic predisposition and environmental factors appear to promote the development of disease. Although a few types of autoimmune diseases are caused by an alteration in a single gene, most involve many genes (most of which are unknown), making identifying a responsible target and determining an effective treatment difficult. Drugs and chemical toxins can also precipitate the development of autoimmunity, although the exact mechanism involved is unclear.

Although difficult, treatment and prevention of autoimmunity continue to be areas of intense interest. The development of newer techniques and increased knowledge of the science of immunology have been instrumental in promoting recent advances to develop effective clinical treatments. The study of T-cell-mediated responses has uncovered the existence of suppressor cells, also known as **regulatory T cells**. These cells, as their name implies, are able to suppress autoreactive lymphocytes and regulate the immune response. Isolation of these specialized T lymphocytes and the administration of them to individuals are future potential therapeutic strategies for those diagnosed with autoimmune disease.

Alloimmunity

Alloimmunity occurs when an immune response is stimulated in response to the presence of cells from another individual of the same species. Alloimmunity can occur after allograft (transplantation of body tissues) or allotransfusion (transfusion of body fluids, such as blood or plasma).

GRAFT REJECTION

Grafts (unattached tissues or organs used for implantation) are commonly used in the treatment of disease. The acceptance of grafted tissue donated from one individual to another depends on the matching of MHC molecules. MHC molecules are **polymorphic** (occurring in more than one form) and **polygenic** (containing several MHC class I and II genes). These two characteristics make matching the MHC molecules challenging. The likelihood of a match increases when both donor and recipient are related, but even then matching is not guaranteed. Grafts from different sites on the same person (**autograft**) or from genetically identical individuals/monozygotic twins (**syngeneic**) are fully accepted; however, a graft between unrelated individuals (**allograft**) is often rejected after 10 to 13 days without drugs to control immune response.

STOP *and Consider*

Why is there less chance of rejection when a transplant occurs between identical twins? Is the chance of rejection the same if the twins are fraternal (not identical)?

Adaptive immune responses mediated by T lymphocytes (CD4 and CD8) are responsible for rejection of grafted tissue due to the recognition of **alloantigens** (proteins that vary between individuals) as foreign. When APCs from the donor leave the graft site and travel via the lymphatic system, host T lymphocytes are activated. These activated T lymphocytes travel back to the graft and attack the alloantigens, destroying the grafted tissue.

The presence of **alloantibodies** (antibodies produced against alloantigens) can contribute to the rapid rejection of grafts, known as **hyperacute graft rejection**. These antibodies recognize and attack antigens on endothelial cells lining blood vessels, stimulating both the complement and clotting cascades. Vessels become **occluded**, or blocked,

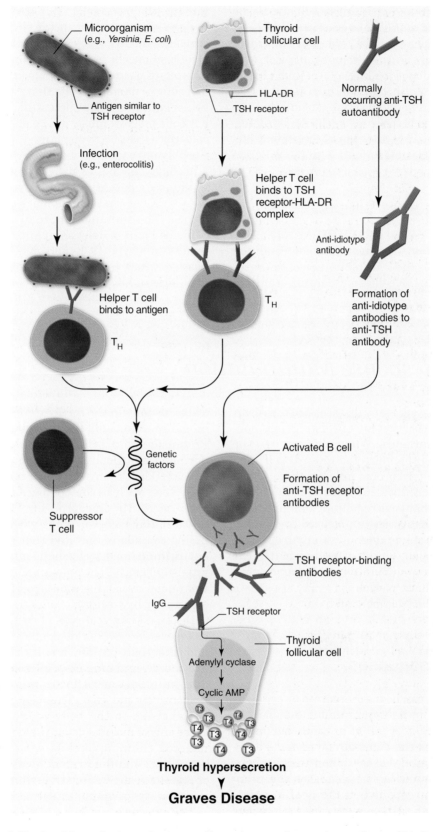

Thyroid hypersecretion

Graves Disease

■ Figure 4.10 Possible mechanisms of organ-specific autoimmune disease: Graves disease. This figure depicts three possible pathways by which B cells are activated to produce anti-TSH receptor antibodies. These antibodies stimulate thyroid cells to secrete T3 and T4. Indirect pathways shown to the left and middle involve activation of helper T cells along with genetic factors that inhibit suppressor T cells. The pathway on the right shows antibodies against anti-TSH antibodies cross-reacting with the TSH receptor. HLA-DR, human leukocyte antigen-D related. (Modified from Rubin E, Farber JL. *Pathology*. 4th ed. Philadelphia: Lippincott Williams & Wilkins; 2005.)

preventing perfusion and resulting in cell and tissue death to the affected site. This is often seen in **blood transfusion**, the most common form of tissue transplant. The antibodies in the recipient interact with antigens from the donor leading to systemic effects, because blood type antibodies can bind to all tissue types. This issue can be avoided by ensuring that the recipient's blood type is the same as the donor (determined by **blood typing**) and that the recipient has no antibodies that are able to react with the WBCs of the donor (determined by **cross matching**).

GRAFT VERSUS HOST DISEASE

Graft versus host disease (GVHD) presents a contrast to graft rejection. The most common condition resulting in GVHD is the transplantation of **hematopoietic stem cells**, or cells that can differentiate into healthy blood cells. This treatment is often used to fight bone marrow cancers such as leukemia or to cure immunodeficiencies. Transplantation of hematopoietic stem cells can result in an individual's ability to produce normal, healthy blood cells in place of the deficient or damaged cells that result in disease. For transplantation to be successful, the diseased recipient bone marrow must first be destroyed. Donor stem cells may then be transplanted. GVHD occurs when the T lymphocytes of the donor recognize the recipient's body as being different or foreign. Donor-immunocompetent T lymphocytes (CD4 and CD8) detect antigens in the recipient's tissue and mount an attack. The immunocompromised recipient tissue cannot mount a defense against the attack, which results in a type IV hypersensitivity reaction. This disease, which can be fatal, is characterized by rash, diarrhea, and liver disease.

Module 3

Immune Response Manipulation

As previously discussed, many diseases are the result of an immune response that fails to distinguish "nonself" from "self" antigens. When this occurs, the immune response is then directed toward "self" and serves as the basis for chronic inflammation, which leads to cellular alterations and injury. As the understanding of the mechanisms regulating immune function grows, these discoveries can be used to manipulate the immune system favorably. Many treatment strategies are based on interference with the responses seen in autoimmunity and hypersensitivity. Exploitation of these mechanisms may also play a significant role in the treatment of disease.

◢ Treatment of Maladaptive Immune Responses

Immune responses can be inappropriate or exaggerated as is the case in allergy, autoimmune disease, and tissue rejection. Control of unwanted immune responses decreases the signs and symptoms associated with illness and disease. Suppression of the immune system, which also suppresses the inappropriate immune response, is the goal of treatment. This general response carries with it the risks associated with immunosuppression, particularly the increased risk of opportunistic infection (see Chapter 5).

A number of classes of drugs are used to regulate immune responses, and each target a particular mechanism. The first class is anti-inflammatory drugs, usually in the corticosteroid family. One of the most common of these drugs is prednisone. Prednisone is a synthetic analog of **cortisol**, the hormone synthesized in the adrenal cortex (see Chapter 11). Prednisone has a body-wide effect typically seen with hormones because almost all body cells carry the receptor for cortisol. When the intracellular receptor binds with prednisone, a signaling cascade is initiated that regulates the **transcription** (transfer of genetic information) of a large number of genes. The amount of prednisone taken for treatment translates into blood levels much higher, or **supraphysiologic**, compared with that found with the normal secretion of cortisol. This causes an exaggerated cellular response with both beneficial and potentially harmful results. The beneficial effects are the desired outcomes of treatment and include anti-inflammatory effects as a result of immune response suppression. The adverse effects are wide-ranging due to the body-wide responses induced; these effects include elevated blood sugar, loss of bone mineral, thinning of skin, weight gain, altered fat deposition, and fluid retention. A delicate balance to create the desired effect and minimize adverse effects is necessary for optimal treatment outcome.

● STOP *and Consider*

The adrenal gland stops producing cortisol during prednisone treatment. Why does this happen? What are the special considerations made when prednisone treatment is no longer needed?

A second class of drugs commonly employed in regulation of immune response is cytotoxic drugs. Commonly used drugs in this family include methotrexate, azathioprine, mycophenolate, and cyclophosphamide. A common mechanism among these drugs includes interference with DNA synthesis in dividing cells. Rapidly dividing cells are most sensitive to the effects of this mechanism and include the cells of the bone marrow (lymphocytes, RBCs, and platelets), the cells lining mucosal membranes of the gastrointestinal tract, the cells of a developing fetus, and hair follicle cells. The proposed target in this method of treatment is dividing lymphocytes, with the desired outcome of decreased immune function. As a result of the nonspecific nature of the drugs, their use is associated with significant adverse effects. High doses of these toxic drugs are used when the treatment goal is elimination of all dividing lymphocytes. These patients then require bone marrow transplant to resume production of necessary blood cells. Lower doses, commonly accompanied by anti-inflammatory drugs, are used to manage unwanted immune responses.

Bacterial and fungal derivative drugs are a third class of drugs used to regulate immune function. These drugs alter signal transduction pathways in T lymphocytes, reducing inflammation by alteration of the reproductive cell cycle. Commonly used drugs in this family include cyclosporine A, tacrolimus, and rapamycin. Predominantly used in transplant patients, these drugs prevent tissue rejection by binding to a group of intracellular proteins. These proteins then form complexes that alter signal transduction pathways used in the proliferation of T lymphocytes and the clonal expansion of activated T lymphocytes. Because each of these drugs has a specifically targeted mechanism of action in the signal pathway, they are often used in combination. Another class of drugs target cytokine activity, limiting immune responses. These drugs are designed to interfere with the binding of the cytokine tumor necrosis factor-alpha (TNF-α) to its receptor, reducing inflammation. Interferons also reduce inflammation and are used in the treatment of the autoimmune condition multiple sclerosis (Chapter 9).

Ideally, drugs specifically targeting the mechanism of chronic inflammation resulting from inappropriate immune responses will be developed. The optimal treatment effect of regulating inappropriate immune responses and maintaining functional responses is the objective in the management of related diseases. The use of this biologic therapy is ongoing clinically to specify targets in the signal transduction pathway.

Immune Response in Disease Management

Using the body's own immune system to attack pathologic cells is another mechanism by which the immune system can be exploited to achieve a positive outcome. Cancer, a disease resulting from uncontrolled proliferation of a single transformed cell, is a central target for this type of strategy. Pathophysiologic processes associated with cancer are discussed in detail in Chapter 7. Development of a drug that can promote the ability of the immune system to distinguish normal cells from transformed cancer cells would be a useful treatment strategy. The desired outcome is the recognition and destruction of cancer cells while avoiding the destruction of normal cells, thereby preserving immune function and minimizing adverse effects.

Immune Response in the Prevention of Disease

Vaccines work by stimulating immunity through exposure to an antigen. This immune response is designed to reactivate quickly when re-exposure to the antigen occurs, the result of immunologic memory. Early vaccination technique was attempted to prevent smallpox by using a small amount of actual pathogen to stimulate immunity. However, the safety of this technique was not ensured—some people actually contracted the illness and died. Later, the use of vaccines made from pathogen analogs derived from other species was effective in stimulating immunity and was a much safer alternative. For vaccines to be effective, the following requirements must be met:

- Vaccines must be safe and must avoid the development of actual disease.
- Vaccines must protect against illness caused by live pathogens.
- Vaccines must provide long-lasting protection.
- Vaccines must stimulate antibody production and T-cell-mediated immunity.
- Vaccines must be accessible and affordable.
- Vaccines must have minimal side effects.

Modern vaccination techniques include the use of **attenuated** (reduced ability to cause disease) or killed organisms. In some cases, **conjugated vaccines,** which promote activation of more than one cell type, are necessary to stimulate an adequate immune response to a specific pathogen.

The use of adjuvants, or substances that increase immune response to antigens, is sometimes necessary for stimulation of protective immune responses.

● **STOP** *and* **Consider**

Many vaccines are available to protect against common diseases and conditions. What are some reasons why people do not get immunized?

Module 4

Clinical Models

The following clinical models have been selected to illustrate the concepts of altered immunity. As you read the descriptions that follow, think about the concepts of altered immune function as they apply to the specific conditions to help understand and apply these concepts to the models.

▨ Immune Maladaptation: AIDS

AIDS is a condition representative of altered host defense. It is a secondary immunodeficiency caused by infection with the **human immunodeficiency virus (HIV)**. HIV is an enveloped retrovirus that infects CD4 helper T lymphocytes, dendritic cells, and macrophages. Symptoms of the primary infection include vague flulike complaints associated with the activation of CD8 cytotoxic T lymphocytes and CD4 T_H1 lymphocytes. Initially, this response works to control infection by killing HIV-infected cells, followed by antibody production against the virus. Symptoms resolve during the early period, although viral replication continues. The hallmark of AIDS is the loss of cell-mediated and humoral immunity due to the loss of CD4 T_H1 lymphocytes.

The continent of Africa has been particularly affected by the HIV epidemic. According to UNAIDS, a joint United Nations and World Health Organization program on HIV/AIDS, people living in Sub-Saharan Africa accounted for 32% of all new HIV infections and AIDS-related deaths worldwide.[3] In the United States, there are 1.2 million individuals living with HIV, with males representing 74% of cases among adolescents and adults.[4] Among young adults aged 20 to 24 in the United States., almost 10,000 men and women were living with AIDS at the end of 2006.[5] In North America, AIDS continues to disproportionately affect African Americans and Aboriginal people in the United States and Canada, respectively.[6]

PATHOPHYSIOLOGY

HIV is transmitted by sexual contact, blood contamination, and perinatally between individuals.

Infection with HIV occurs across mucosal surfaces covered with stratified squamous epithelium, including the vagina, cervix, and anus. Dendritic cells bind HIV and transport it to the lymphoid tissues where it encounters the CD4 helper T lymphocytes. When the virus enters the host cell, the viral RNA is transcribed into complementary DNA, which is then integrated into the host cell, stimulating replication of this provirus. The virus undergoes rapid replication, associated with the generation of many viral mutations. These mutations are numerous and can occur within a day, promoting the development of antigenic variation. Viral drug resistance develops rapidly, requiring the use of combination therapy.

CLINICAL MANIFESTATIONS

As the disease progresses, the CD4 helper T lymphocyte number gradually declines, promoting significant immunosuppression. The loss of CD4 T lymphocytes is caused by the killing of infected cells by viruses, the apoptosis (programmed cell death) of infected cells, and the killing of CD4 helper T lymphocytes by CD8 cytotoxic T lymphocytes. Cell-mediated immunity is lost when the CD4 helper T lymphocyte level is too low, contributing to the risk of opportunistic infection. Resistance is lost to many common pathogens, including the fungi *Candida*. Activation of latent viruses may occur, promoting symptoms and disease. Pneumonia, especially the type caused by *Pneumocystis jiroveci* pneumonia (formerly *carinii*), is a common opportunistic infection. Kaposi's sarcoma, a tumor of endothelial cells, is also a common finding in patients with AIDS. Figure 4.11 shows many of the conditions experienced by patients with immunosuppression due to AIDS. These conditions are normally controlled or prevented by CD4 helper T lymphocyte stimulated cell-mediated immunity, lost when CD4 host T lymphocyte numbers are significantly decreased.

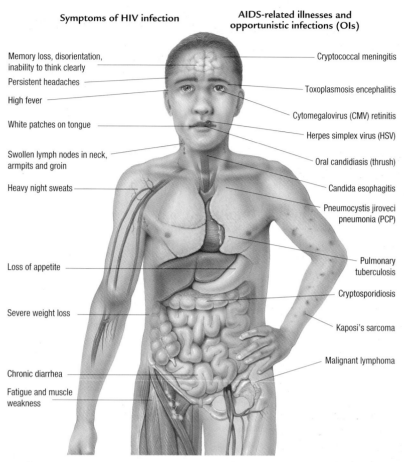

Symptoms of HIV infection

AIDS-related illnesses and
opportunistic infections (OIs)

Memory loss, disorientation,
inability to think clearly

Persistent headaches

High fever

White patches on tongue

Swollen lymph nodes in neck,
armpits and groin

Heavy night sweats

Loss of appetite

Severe weight loss

Chronic diarrhea

Fatigue and muscle
weakness

Cryptococcal meningitis

Toxoplasmosis encephalitis

Cytomegalovirus (CMV) retinitis

Herpes simplex virus (HSV)

Oral candidiasis (thrush)

Candida esophagitis

Pneumocystis jiroveci
pneumonia (PCP)

Pulmonary
tuberculosis

Cryptosporidiosis

Kaposi's sarcoma

Malignant lymphoma

■ **Figure 4.11** Manifestations of HIV infection and AIDS. (Asset provided by Anatomical Chart Company.)

● **STOP** *and Consider*

Why are immunosuppressed patients at greater risk for cancer?

DIAGNOSTIC CRITERIA

The criteria used in the diagnosis of HIV infection are often based on initial screening tests that identify antibodies to the virus. Recommendations for HIV screening from the Centers for Disease Control and Prevention (CDC) include routine initial screening in individuals aged 13 to 64. Annual repeat screening is advised for all those at high risk for HIV infection.[6] Individuals at risk for infection (i.e., intravenous drug users, individuals exposed to blood products, men who have sex with men, and the women who have sex with these individuals) should be screened for the presence of antibodies to HIV. It takes most people about 3 months from time of exposure to develop antibodies to HIV. This occurrence is known as **seroconversion**. People are usually asymptomatic at this time and can unknowingly infect others with the virus.

Progression of the disease from HIV infection to the diagnosis of AIDS is based on laboratory criteria and on signs and symptoms of immunosuppression. Early symptoms of infection include **lymphadenopathy** (swelling or enlargement of the lymph nodes). Later complications related to immunosuppression include infection with candidiasis, cytomegalovirus, mycobacterium, toxoplasmosis, *P. jiroveci* pneumonia, movement disorders, dementia, non-Hodgkin lymphoma, or Kaposi's sarcoma of the skin and mucous membranes. The CDC established three clinical categories based on symptoms.[7] Category designations and examples of associated symptoms include:

- Clinical category A
  - ▪ asymptomatic
- Clinical category B
  - ▪ Symptomatic conditions complicating the course of someone with HIV infection that are not of adequate severity to be AIDS—defining
    - ▪ Oropharyngeal/vulvovaginal candidiasis
    - ▪ Cervical dysplasia
    - ▪ Herpes zoster (shingles)
- Clinical category C
  - ▪ Severe symptoms consistent with the diagnosis of AIDS
    - ▪ Recurrent bacterial pneumonia

- Kaposi sarcoma
- Candidiasis of the bronchi, trachea, lungs, esophagus
- Cervical carcinoma
- Wasting syndrome
  - Involuntary loss of >10% body weight
  - Fever
  - Chronic diarrhea or weakness

At this time, the diagnosis of AIDS can be made based on symptoms included in clinical category C. In addition to clinical findings, laboratory determination of CD4 T lymphocyte counts is used in AIDS diagnosis. Laboratory diagnostic criteria are determined by the number of CD4 helper T cells. CD4 cell counts less than 200 cells/μL (or 14% CD4 cells) meet the criteria for the definition of AIDS. Worsening disease and immune status is correlated with a progressively decreased number of CD4 helper T lymphocytes.

TREATMENT

Recommended treatment of HIV is the use of antiretroviral agents. The goals of antiretroviral therapy include:

- Maximal and long-lasting viral load suppression
- Restoration or preservation of immune function
- Reduction in morbidity and mortality related to HIV

From the Lab

Diagnosis of HIV infection is made by the detection of the presence of HIV antibodies. A screening test known as enzyme linked immunoassay (EIA) detects the HIV antibody. Body fluid samples (saliva, blood, or urine) are tested. A positive screening test is not diagnostic of HIV infection and requires a confirmatory test. Often, a test called Western blot is used that detects antibodies to specific HIV antigens or proteins. Other tests that can confirm HIV infection include isolation of antibodies from tissues and tests that detect the HIV antigen. The amount of HIV in the blood can be determined by a test for viral load. The competency of the immune system can be determined by measurement of the CD4 T lymphocyte cell count.

Because of the ability of the HIV retrovirus to evade the immune system by mutating into different forms, resistance to drug therapy develops rapidly if only one or two drugs are used. Highly active antiretroviral therapy (HAART) is the treatment strategy designed to delay disease progression by suppressing viral replication and addressing the issues of increasing drug resistance.[8] Drugs used in HAART target viral replication processes. These drugs can be categorized into classes known as nucleoside and nucleotide analog reverse transcriptase inhibitors; nonnucleotide reverse transcriptase inhibitors, protease inhibitors, entry inhibitors, and integrase inhibitors. Although the use of HAART has increased effectiveness over monotherapy or combined two-drug therapy, significant barriers contribute to failed treatment regimens. To increase the patient's willingness and ability to use these drugs, ongoing counseling and assistance with problem areas are critical to successful treatment. More information about specific strategies can be found in the guidelines for counseling by the CDC listed in the resource section at the end of this chapter.

● STOP *and Consider*

What special considerations must a person with AIDS take to limit illness caused by immunosuppression? What considerations must others make to protect a person with AIDS?

▨ Immune Maladaptation: Anaphylactic Reaction

This clinical model represents a systemic response to a type I hypersensitivity reaction. Anaphylaxis can occur from exposure to drugs, environmental compounds, insect venom or stings, or food products that stimulate an exaggerated immune response. Re-exposure to an allergen is responsible for triggering this IgE-mediated event. The induced systemic response produces a hypersensitivity reaction affecting many organ systems, which is potentially fatal without treatment.

PATHOPHYSIOLOGY

Exposure to an allergen in an individual previously sensitized by that allergen stimulates the classic allergic hypersensitivity response of degranulation of mast cells and basophils. The IgE bound to receptors on these cells induces the release of chemical mediators when binding with the allergen occurs (Fig. 4.12). The reaction occurs locally but is spread beyond the site of allergen entry by the bloodstream. Vascular smooth muscle dilates, bronchial smooth muscle constricts, and vascular permeability increases, accounting for the clinical manifestations seen in this condition. These effects are potentially fatal without intervention and supportive care.

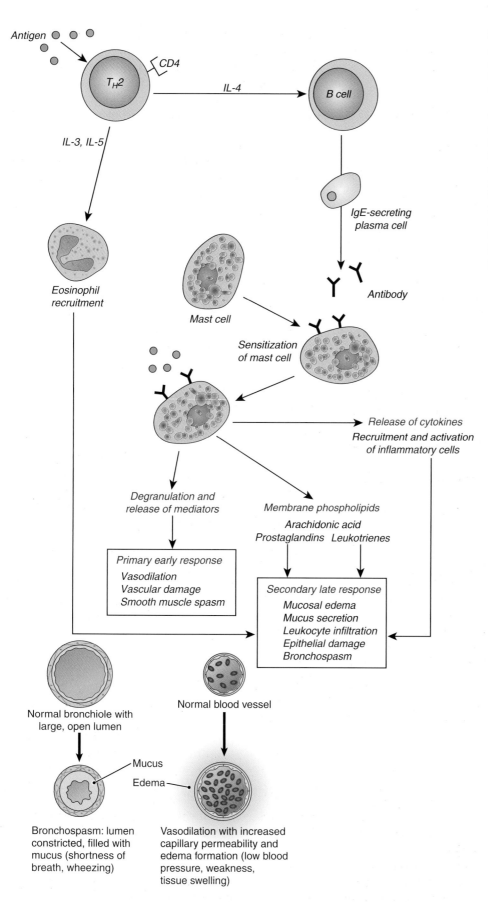

■ **Figure 4.12** IgE-mediated response in anaphylactic reaction. Allergen triggers B lymphocyte differentiation into IgE-secreting plasma cell, stimulated by an activated type II helper T lymphocyte (T_H2). IgE attaches to the mast cell. When the allergen reappears, it binds to the mast cell-bound IgE and triggers mast cell degranulation, releasing chemical mediators that stimulate primary early response manifestations. Secondary late response manifestations are the result of lipid mediators released from phospholipids in the destructed cell membrane and recruitment of eosinophils by T_H2 lymphocytes.

CLINICAL MANIFESTATIONS

The clinical manifestations stimulated by anaphylactic reaction are determined by the amount of antigen-specific IgE present, the dose of the antigen, and the route of antigen transmission. A biphasic (two-phase) response results from the release of chemical mediators, including histamine, prostaglandins and leukotrienes (bronchoconstriction), and cytokines (increased IgE production and inflammation). The initial response occurs within minutes to a few hours and includes severe **bronchospasm** (contraction of the smooth muscle in the bronchi and bronchioles of the lungs, decreasing airway size and making it difficult to breathe), skin flushing, **urticaria** (itching), and **angioedema** (sudden subcutaneous edema). The first phase is a response to short-acting chemical mediators, and the second phase of this reaction is caused by longer-acting substances occurring approximately 4 hours after the first phase reaction. During the second phase, severe bronchospasm recurs and is often accompanied by severe hypotension and edema. Immediate evaluation and treatment of these manifestations must be instituted due to the emergency nature of anaphylaxis. Severe reactions can result in anoxia and death.

⬤ STOP *and Consider*

Why don't all people stung by insects develop systemic symptoms of anaphylaxis?

DIAGNOSTIC CRITERIA

Diagnosis is based on symptoms and history. People on multiple drugs and people suffering from insect sting, atopy, or food allergy are especially susceptible. Testing to determine the responsible antigen can be done to educate the patient about specific allergens to avoid or to provide the basis of future treatment. Prognosis is based on the severity of symptoms and the time it takes to provide treatment for acute symptoms.

TREATMENT

Initial treatment is designed to treat symptoms and limit inflammation. Immediate administration of epinephrine to relax bronchial smooth muscle, reform endothelial tight cell junctions in blood vessels, and control cardiovascular effects is the first line of treatment. Inhaled bronchodilators may also assist in the treatment of bronchospasm. Antihistamines may help reduce the symptoms stimulated by histamine release, such as itching and increased vessel permeability. Fluids may be provided to restore intravascular volume. If the initial treatment is delayed, the prognosis worsens. The symptoms associated with the second phase are much more difficult to treat and may require intubation and mechanical ventilation to provide oxygenation.

Long-term treatments include desensitization and signaling pathway blockade of effectors. The goal of desensitization is to:

1. Switch the IgE response to an IgG response
2. Bind the allergen and prevent stimulation of IgE-mediated responses by skin injection of allergen in progressively larger doses
3. Change the helper T lymphocyte effectors from T_H2 to T_H1 cells to downregulate the IgE response

Blockade of signaling pathways of mediators stimulating hypersensitivity responses, including cytokines, is another potential long-term treatment.

▨ Immune Maladaptation: Systemic Lupus Erythematosus

SLE is an example of a type III hypersensitivity reaction. SLE is considered an autoimmune disease and features responses from both the innate and humoral immune systems. The chronic nature of this disease is a result of persistent antigen-promoting complex deposition and inflammation. Autoantibodies are targeted against the self-antigenic components of the cell membrane (antiphospholipid), cytoplasm (anticytoplasmic), and cell nucleus (antinuclear), including the DNA. Binding of antigen with these antibodies stimulates activation of the complement system and accumulation of immune complexes. The location of these complexes and the organs that are involved determine the symptoms of the disease (Fig. 4.13). Because the involved antigens are present in all of the cells, SLE is a chronic, systemic disease that can potentially damage a wide range of cell types and locations.

PATHOPHYSIOLOGY

The exact events that stimulate the development of SLE are not fully known. A genetic or familial tendency combined with hormonal and environmental influences seems to make a person more susceptible to developing the disease (Fig. 4.14). SLE, most commonly found in women, tends to run a course with exacerbations (disease flare ups) and **quiescence** (decreased symptoms). The MHC and HLA

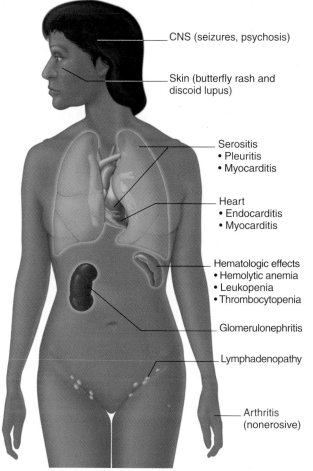

Figure 4.13 Complications of systemic lupus erythematosus. CNS, central nervous system.

CNS (seizures, psychosis)

Skin (butterfly rash and discoid lupus)

Serositis
• Pleuritis
• Myocarditis

Heart
• Endocarditis
• Myocarditis

Hematologic effects
• Hemolytic anemia
• Leukopenia
• Thrombocytopenia

Glomerulonephritis

Lymphadenopathy

Arthritis (nonerosive)

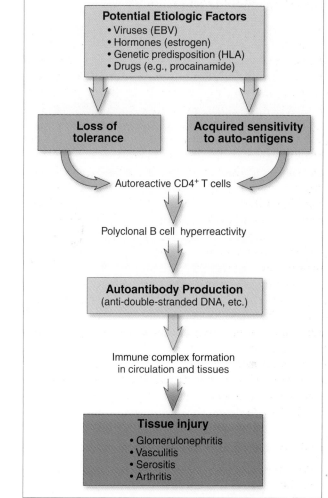

Figure 4.14 Pathogenesis of systemic lupus erythematosus. EBV, Epstein–Barr virus; HLA, human leukocyte antigen. (Image from Rubin E, Farber JL. *Pathology*. 4th ed. Philadelphia: Lippincott Williams & Wilkins; 2005, with permission.)

systems appear to be involved in the development of autoimmune activity, triggered by an unknown event, perhaps infection or another pathologic process. A breakdown in self-tolerance results in the stimulation of APCs, the evasion of normal immune response by molecular mimicry, or the alteration of antigens that make them unable to be recognized as "self." The ability to remove cells that recognize "self" by apoptosis is altered. The result is the activation of the B lymphocytes to develop autoantibodies and cytotoxic T lymphocytes, which then promote inflammation and complex deposition in susceptible organs of the body, causing permanent organ damage.

CLINICAL MANIFESTATIONS

Clinical signs and symptoms develop in the organs affected by the pathology associated with SLE. Organs most commonly affected include the skin, kidney, and musculoskeletal system. In addition, people diagnosed with lupus may develop neurologic,

pulmonary, and cardiac disease. Typical manifestations in SLE include:

• Joint pain and swelling
• Skin rashes
• Fatigue
• Pericardial effusion (swelling around the heart)
• Pleural effusion (swelling around the lungs)

These systemic clinical manifestations contribute to the diagnosis of the disease and can also provide valuable information about the activity of the disease and effectiveness of treatment strategies.

DIAGNOSTIC CRITERIA

Diagnosis of SLE is determined by a combination of subjective symptoms, objective physical findings, and laboratory values. Criteria to be used in classifying SLE patients for inclusion in clinical and research studies have been established by the American

■ **Figure 4.15** Malar (butterfly) rash in systemic lupus erythematosus. (Image from Goodheart HP. *Goodheart's Photoguide of Common Skin Disorders.* 2nd ed. Philadelphia: Lippincott Williams & Wilkins; 2003, with permission.)

College of Rheumatology (ACR).[9] Although not intended for diagnostic purposes, these criteria are often used for that purpose. Eleven criteria are outlined by the ACR, four of which must be present to obtain a diagnosis of SLE. These criteria include:

1. Rash over cheeks (**malar**) (Fig. 4.15)
2. Red, raised, **discoid** (round) rash, sometimes with scaling or plugged follicles
3. Sensitivity to the sun resulting in rash (**photosensitivity**)
4. **Ulcers**, or open areas, in the mouth or nasopharynx
5. Arthritis, associated with tenderness, swelling, or fluid buildup (as seen in rheumatoid arthritis [RA]) in at least two peripheral joints
6. **Pleuritis** (inflammation of the lining of the lungs or pleural cavity) or **pericarditis** (inflammation of the lining of the heart)
7. **Proteinuria** (protein in the urine) greater than 5 g/dL or +3 on a dip stick, or **cellular casts** (compacted collection of protein, cells, and debris that are formed in kidney tubules) suggesting renal involvement
8. Seizures or psychosis, suggesting neurologic involvement

9. Anemia, leukopenia, or **thrombocytopenia** (abnormally low number of platelets), suggesting hematologic involvement
10. Lab values including anti-DNA antibody, anti-Sm (antibody to Smith nuclear antigen), or a false-positive test for syphilis
11. Abnormal antinuclear antibody

The criteria reinforce the importance of looking at the entire person, rather than just a lab test, to identify the disease and illness accurately. The entire clinical picture is necessary to provide proper treatment and care for a specialized condition.

TREATMENT

Treatment for SLE varies among individuals. Considerations for treatment include clinical manifestations, duration of desired treatment, and toleration of associated side effects. Early treatment is essential to minimize morbidity and mortality, although this must be balanced with the significant risk of adverse effects from the treatments themselves, including the development of atherosclerotic heart disease, osteoporosis, hypertension, diabetes, infection, and even death (Table 4.5).

Table 4.5 Treatment Options for Systemic Lupus Erythematosus

Drug	Desired Effect	Adverse Effect
Salicylates	Anti-inflammatory	GI bleeding and upset
NSAIDs	Anti-inflammatory	GI bleeding and upset
Glucocorticoids	Anti-inflammatory	Hypertension Hyperglycemia Hyperlipidemia Hypokalemia Osteoporosis Infection Fluid retention Weight gain
Hydroxychloroquine	Immunosuppression	Macular damage Photosensitivity Rash
Azathioprine	Immunosuppression	Myelosuppression (anemia, thrombocytopenia) Hepatotoxicity
Cyclophosphamide	Immunosuppression	Myelosuppression Malignancy Infection Cystitis Infertility
Methotrexate	Immunosuppression	Myelosuppression Hepatotoxicity Pulmonary disease

GI, gastrointestinal; NSAIDs, nonsteroidal anti-inflammatory drugs.

Initially, pharmacologic management may involve nonsteroidal anti-inflammatory drugs (NSAIDs), although ultimately it often involves the use of corticosteroids for symptom control and anti-inflammatory effects. The disease is often managed with other drugs designed to delay the progress and resulting damage, including disease-modifying antirheumatoid drugs (DMARD) as are used in RA. The antimalarial drug Plaquenil may be used to slow disease progress. In more aggressive cases, immunosuppressant drugs including cyclophosphamide, azathioprine, and mycophenolate may be necessary. Providing appropriate drug treatment to prevent damage while simultaneously decreasing potentially damaging side effects is difficult and often requires care planned by a rheumatologist who specializes in these types of conditions.

From the Lab

Lab tests used to diagnose SLE are designed to detect the antibodies directed against cell components in the cytoplasm and nucleus. These include antinuclear antibodies and extractable nuclear antigens, a group of several cellular proteins and antibodies that include antibodies to Smith antigen (anti-Sm). Once SLE is diagnosed, laboratory tests used to evaluate disease activity and prognosis include measurement of anti-double-stranded DNA (anti-dsDNA; detecting antibodies against DNA) and complement (C3 and C4). Future work in determining more specific and sensitive biomarkers of SLE includes evaluation of the products of complement activation and inhibition, cytokines (including the interleukins and TNF-α), circulating immune complexes, measurement of the number of abnormal T-cell types by cell surface marker (i.e., CD4, CD8), and markers of B-cell activation.

Research Notes

Currently, a great deal of research is being conducted that focuses on the development of a pharmacologic treatment for SLE that is both effective and has minimal side effects. Increasingly, refined approaches are being investigated to achieve maximum benefit and improve treatment outcome. A treatment approach in individuals with significant renal involvement based on histologic characteristics has the potential to reduce drug dosage and duration of use. In lupus nephritis, the site of accumulation of immunoglobulins in the renal glomeruli, the specificity of the immunoglobulins to antigens and the inflammation induced upon antigen–antibody complex deposition are factors that may be used to determine optimal therapy for this serious manifestation of SLE.[10]

Immune Maladaptation: Rh Isoimmunization

This clinical model represents a type II cytotoxic antibody-mediated reaction. Rh isoimmunization is a direct antigen–antibody hypersensitivity reaction between a mother and her fetus. The damage that results from this reaction includes cell destruction of the antigen target, which are the fetal RBCs. This condition, known as **hemolytic** (destruction of blood cells) disease of the fetus and newborn, is a result of this blood cell destruction.

PATHOPHYSIOLOGY

Hemolytic disease of the fetus and newborn is caused by maternal alloantibodies, which target paternally inherited antigens. Many antigens can be targeted in this disease, but the antigen usually involved is D(Rho), one of the primary antigens responsible for the determination of Rh-positive blood type. If a person is D antigen positive, he or she is identified as being Rh positive; a person without the D antigen is known as Rh negative.

A fetus often has a different R factor from the mother. This does not usually cause any immune response because each has a separate circulation not designed to mix. Maternal blood circulates through the maternal portion of the **placenta,** a specialized organ sustaining the fetus, by providing oxygenation, nutrition, endocrine, and excretion functions. The chorionic villi contain fetal capillaries that allow exchange of substances between mother and fetus across a membrane, without the actual mixing of maternal and fetal circulations. Most substances in the maternal and fetal circulations, with the exception of high molecular weight compounds, can cross the placental membrane using a variety of transport mechanisms. These transport mechanisms include passive diffusion, facilitated diffusion, and active transport. If the mother has not had prior exposure to the D antigen and therefore no production of antibodies against it, the mother is unable to stimulate an immune response to an antigen it cannot recognize in the separate fetal circulation.

If fetal blood enters the maternal circulation unintentionally, fetal D antigen on the fetal RBCs can pass into the maternal blood supply. In a D antigen naive Rh-negative individual, the D antigen is recognized as foreign, stimulating an antibody response against the antigen. Though IgG has the ability to cross the placenta to reach the target of the D antigen on RBCs in the fetal circulation, the

■ **Figure 4.16**   Maternal sensitization. (From Nath J. *Using Medical Terminology: A Practical Approach.* Baltimore: Lippincott Williams & Wilkins; 2006, with permission.)

response of maternal primary antibody production is slow and therefore does not severely affect the fetus. Once antibodies are produced, the mother is then "sensitized" against the antigen and is able to mount a rapid, robust immune response if the antigen presents itself to the maternal system in the future due to immunologic memory.

If the Rh-negative mother becomes pregnant again with an Rh-positive fetus, maternal anti-D IgG will cross the placenta into the fetal circulation. Maternal anti-D IgG will recognize and target the D antigen-bearing fetal RBCs for destruction. The memory cells, a component of the humoral immunologic memory response, respond rapidly and are able to produce increased levels of antibodies with a higher affinity to the fetal D antigen. The transplacental passage of maternal antibody (IgG) into the fetus results in RBC destruction and the condition known as hemolytic anemia (Fig. 4.16).

CLINICAL MANIFESTATIONS

Fetuses suffering from Rh isoimmunization are at increased risk for the development of anemia, hydrops (accumulation of edema), and death. Severe hemolysis of fetal RBCs can be worsened by increased erythropoiesis, resulting in the production of large numbers of immature nucleated erythro-

cytes, known as erythroblastosis fetalis. Destruction of RBCs allows the release of cellular components, some of which can produce additional pathology. One of the components of the breakdown of hemoglobin in RBCs is bilirubin. Bilirubin, in its unconjugated form, is lipid soluble, a characteristic that prevents excretion of this potentially toxic substance. After birth, infants may have a newborn course complicated by kernicterus (unconjugated bilirubin deposits in the basal ganglia of the brain), lethargy, hearing loss, cerebral palsy, and learning problems.

● **STOP** *and Consider*

Is an Rh-positive mother at risk of becoming sensitized to her Rh-negative fetus? Why or why not?

DIAGNOSTIC CRITERIA

Identification of a mother at risk for sensitization and those who are sensitized is completed as a component of routine prenatal care. Maternal blood is screened to determine whether the mother is Rh positive or negative as the initial step in identifying risk. In addition, a screen for antibodies to the D antigen is completed to identify whether the mother is already sensitized.

Fetal blood type and Rh are not determined in routine pregnancies because that would require an invasive procedure with more risk than benefit. In a sensitized mother, the high-risk nature of the pregnancy requires careful screening of fetal status during growth in the uterus. Detection of the fetal RBC antigen can be determined by performing an **amniocentesis** (insertion of a needle into the uterine cavity to obtain a sample of amniotic fluid) and by using the technique of genotyping. If the fetus is also Rh negative, no further testing needs to be done because the fetus does not carry D antigen and therefore is unable to stimulate the maternal memory cells to initiate an immune response. A noninvasive method of determining fetal Rh status is to measure circulating fetal DNA in the maternal plasma.

In an Rh-positive fetus, measurements of amniotic components, including bilirubin, provide an indirect measure of hemolysis and anemia. Amniocentesis may be required several times during the pregnancy, or serially, to determine disease severity and progression. A noninvasive procedure may be used to reliably quantify fetal anemia and guide treatment decisions. Measurements of fetal middle cerebral artery peak systolic velocity (MCA PSV) using ultrasound can also provide information about fetal heart rate, tissue oxygenation, or blood **viscosity** (concentration) to detect fetal anemia.

TREATMENT

When hemolysis of fetal RBCs occurs, fetal oxygenation is decreased because of the decreased hemoglobin available to transport oxygen to cells and tissues. One of the primary treatments of a fetus with severe anemia is to provide healthy RBCs in exchange for hemolyzed RBCs, using an in utero exchange transfusion. The need for transfusion is based on the determinations by amniocentesis or MCA PSV, as described previously. The transfusion procedure, completed under ultrasound guidance, uses the fetal umbilical cord arteries and vein to add healthy cells and remove damaged cells. The risks associated with this potentially dangerous procedure include infection, pregnancy loss, premature labor, or rupture of membranes, worsening isoimmunization and decreased fetal heart rate. The transfusion procedure may also need to be completed in a serial manner, depending

From the Lab

Maternal antibodies to the fetal D antigen can be detected in the serum using an indirect Coombs test to determine whether the mother is sensitized. For sensitization to be prevented after maternal exposure to fetal D antigen, an adequate dosage of RhIg must be given. The standard prenatal dose is 500 and 1500 IU at the time of delivery. If there is an increased risk of an excessive maternal exposure to fetal cells (i.e., after blunt trauma), testing to quantify the number of fetal cells present in the maternal circulation, the Kleihauer–Betke test, can be completed to assure adequate dosing of RhIg.

Research Notes

RhIg has drastically reduced the number of women who become sensitized to the D fetal antigen. As a result, sensitization to other antigens in the Rh system (anti-FYa, anti-c, anti-E, and anti-K) is now getting more attention. No specialized treatments exist to prevent other forms of Rh sensitization. RhIg is often the treatment of choice in the protection against sensitization and has proven to be an effective strategy.[12]

on the progress of fetal disease. Once a mother is sensitized against the fetal D antigen, there are no procedures to desensitize her. The focus of managing disease in the fetus is the primary intervention.

The development of prevention strategies has reduced the rate of sensitization in at-risk mothers. This is accomplished by providing the Rh-negative mother with Rh immunoglobin (RhIg) when there is a risk of maternal exposure to fetal RBCs. Initiated in 1968, RhIg was administered to Rh-negative mothers by injection within 72 hours of delivering an Rh-positive fetus, when the risk of maternal and fetal circulations mixing is high. The RhIg binds to D antigen on fetal cells circulating in the maternal circulation, providing a protective coating around the cells and preventing detection by the maternal immune system and subsequent anti-D antibody production.

Current prevention strategies include provision of RhIg administration to Rh-negative nonsensitized mothers during pregnancy at times when the likelihood of combined circulations is the greatest and the fetal Rh factor is unknown. RhIg can be administered during invasive procedures, such as amniocentesis, upon early termination of pregnancy (as in the cases of abortion and ectopic pregnancy), following physical trauma and at 28 weeks' gestation to provide protection from inadvertent antigen exposure. RhIG continues to be administered to Rh-negative mothers within 72 hours of delivery if the newborn is Rh positive. The optimal dosage and administration regimen of RhIg continues to be reevaluated to maximize effectiveness and safety.[11]

Summary

- The cellular components of the immune response work together to mount the third line of defense against invasion of pathogens.
- Innate and adaptive (cell-mediated and humoral) immune responses combine to provide protection against infection and illness.
- T lymphocytes proliferate and differentiate into cytotoxic or helper T cells when presented with an antigen, leading to cell-mediated immunity.
- B lymphocytes produce and secrete antibodies, each capable of detecting specific antigens, leading to humoral immunity.
- Granulocytes respond quickly and broadly to infectious agents.
- The lymphatic system traps antigens captured by cells of the immune system, allowing the antigen to be presented to antibody.
- Molecules known as MHC or HLA display antigens to T cells, stimulating the immune response.
- Receptors on T and B lymphocytes recognize unique antigen and antigen-MHC complexes in a specific manner resulting in targeted destruction of antigen-bearing cells.
- Altered immune function may be caused by inability to mount an immune defense, exaggerated immune responses, inappropriate immune responses to "self," and immune response directed toward transplanted tissues.
- Maladaptations in immune response, either exaggerated or impaired, contribute to acute and chronic disease.
- Immunosuppression is the result of a primary or secondary immunodeficiency.
- Hypersensitivity responses are mediated by IgE, antigen–antibody, immune–complex or cytotoxic reactions.
- Autoimmunity is the failure to distinguish "self" from "nonself," leading to an immune response against an individual's own tissues.
- Alloimmunity results from an immune response directed against the tissues of another individual of the same species, often seen in transplantation.
- Protection of immune function and the manipulation of the immune system to prevent disease are exciting prospects that will significantly decrease morbidity and mortality resulting from many chronic diseases in the United States and throughout the world.

Case Study 4.1

C.J., a 19-year-old white female, has a history of hay fever, which seems to get worse during the summer months. After a weekend camping trip, she developed difficulty breathing and needed to seek care for these symptoms, diagnosed as an exacerbation of asthma. Think about which clinical model is most related to this process. From your reading related to inflammation and immune function, answer the following questions:

1. What anatomic problem would most likely lead to difficulty breathing as a consequence of allergy and asthma?
2. What is the injury in asthma?
3. How would the immune system respond?
4. Why is this a chronic problem?
5. What pathophysiologic changes would most likely occur with chronic asthma and allergy?
6. What would you expect for clinical manifestations?
7. What diagnostic tests might be used?
8. What treatment measures would you anticipate?

Log onto the Internet. Search for a relevant journal article or Web site that details asthma with an allergic component to confirm your predictions.

Case Study 4.2

A.L., a 25-year-old Native American female, is pregnant with her second child. She was exposed to a child with chicken pox at a recent family event. A.L. has not had chicken pox, and she has not been immunized. Her 4-year-old son was immunized (initial and booster) against the varicella virus that causes chicken pox. From your reading related to immunity, answer the following questions:

1. What is A.L.'s risk for infection with the varicella virus?
2. Explain A.L.'s son's risk for infection with the varicella virus.
3. Discuss the risk for A.L.'s unborn child for infection with varicella.
4. Discuss prevention and treatment strategies that can be used to prevent varicella infection in each of these individuals.
5. What strategies should be used to protect other household family members?
6. Identify whether prevention strategies for A.L., her son, and fetus stimulate passive or active immune responses.
7. How can it be determined if an individual has immunity to varicella?

Log onto the Internet. Search for a relevant journal article or Web site that details varicella infection prevention during pregnancy and childhood and special considerations in immune responses in these groups to confirm your predictions.

Practice Exam Questions

1. During flu season, you get exposed to the influenza virus. Which component of your immune system will be the first to respond to this foreign pathogen?
   a. Innate
   b. Adaptive
   c. Humoral
   d. T-cell mediated

2. The following season, you are concerned about getting the flu again. Which of the following statements is true?
   a. You continue to be at risk because nothing can protect you from reinfection.
   b. Vaccination for prevalent strains of influenza virus can provide improved protection against the disease.
   c. Premedication with immunosuppressants will provide protection against infection.
   d. Because you have had the flu once, you will be protected from getting it again.

3. Immune suppression in AIDS is related to:
   a. Decreased platelet count
   b. Decreased red blood cell count
   c. Decreased lymphocyte count
   d. Elevated lymphocyte count

4. Which of the following conditions represents pathologic responses caused by immunologic memory?
   a. Common cold
   b. Anaphylaxis
   c. Shingles
   d. Strep throat

5. The pathology related to systemic lupus erythematosus is due to:
   a. Neutrophil activation
   b. Delayed immunity
   c. Immunosuppression
   d. Immune complex deposition

6. Immunodeficiency is the result of:
   a. Failure of host defense mechanisms
   b. Hypersensitive immune responses
   c. Inappropriate immune response to self
   d. Immune response stimulated by antigens from other individuals

7. A hypersensitivity reaction resulting from a yellow jacket sting is an example of:
   a. Type I, immediate hypersensitivity reaction
   b. Type II, antibody-mediated reaction
   c. Type III, immune complex reaction
   d. Type IV, cell-mediated reaction

8. A hypersensitivity reaction resulting from complement activation due to insoluble antigen–antibody deposition is an example of:
   a. Type I, immediate hypersensitivity reaction
   b. Type II, antibody-mediated reaction
   c. Type III, immune complex reaction
   d. Type IV, cell-mediated reaction

9. Autoimmunity may be triggered by which one of the following?
   a. Elimination of self-reactive lymphocytes in central lymphoid tissues
   b. Persistent lymphocyte ignorance
   c. Impaired T-cell activation
   d. Close resemblance between foreign and self-antigen

10. Treatment of an altered immune response with corticosteroids is associated with which one of the following adverse effects?
    a. Decreased blood sugar
    b. Loss of bone mineral
    c. Thickening of skin
    d. Weight loss

11. The transfer of secretory IgA from mother to infant during breast feeding is an example of
    a. Hypersensitivity reaction
    b. Active immunity
    c. Passive immunity
    d. Alloimmunity

12. Which of the following is true regarding cytotoxic T lymphocytes?
    a. Recognize the MHC class I–antigen complex
    b. Recognize the MHC class II–antigen complex
    c. Carry the CD4 marker
    d. Present antigen to B lymphocytes for antibody production

13. Which of the following are considered antigen-presenting cells?
    a. Dendritic cells
    b. Eosinophils
    c. B lymphocytes
    d. T lymphocytes

14. Which of the following markers identifies a nucleated body cell?
    a. CD4
    b. BCR
    c. MHC I
    d. MHC II

15. Which of the following is true regarding pharmacologic treatment for AIDS?

    a. Drugs are used to target increased red blood cell number
    b. Drugs are used to target increased white blood cell number
    c. Drugs are used to increase host DNA replication
    d. Drugs are used to inhibit HIV replication

Discussion and Application

1. What did I know about basic alterations in immunity before today?

2. What body processes are affected by altered immune function? How does immunity impact those processes?

3. What are the potential etiologies for altered immune function? How do alterations in immune function develop?

4. Who is most at risk for developing altered immunity? How can these alterations be prevented?

5. What are the human differences that affect the etiology, risk, or course of altered immunity?

6. What clinical manifestations are expected in the course of altered immunity?

7. What special diagnostic tests are useful in determining the diagnosis and course of illness due to altered immune function?

8. What are the goals of care for individuals with altered immunity?

9. How does the concept of altered immunity build on what I have learned in the previous chapter and in the previous courses?

10. How can I use what I have learned?

RESOURCES

The American College of Rheumatology:
http://www.rheumatology.org/index.asp?aud=mem
This site is a resource for information about autoimmune disorders.

Immune Deficiency Foundation:
http://www.primaryimmune.org/
Learn more about primary immune deficiency.

National Institute of Allergy and Infectious Disease (NIAID):
http://www3.niaid.nih.gov/
Find out more about general immune function.

REFERENCES

1. National Institute of Allergy and Infectious Diseases, National Institutes of Health. Current trends in allergic reactions: a multidisciplinary approach to patient management. *Clinician.* 2003;21(3):1-19.
2. Bilò MB, Severino M, Cilia M, et al. The VISYT trial: venom immunotherapy safety and tolerability with purified vs nonpurified extracts. *Ann Allergy Asthma Immunol.* 2009;1(102):57–61.
3. UNAIDS, World Health Organization. *Sub Saharan Africa AIDS Epidemic Update Regional Summary.* Switzerland: UNAIDS; 2007. Retrieved at http://data.unaids.org/pub/Report/2008/JC1526_epibriefs_subsaharanafrica_en.pdf on September 13, 2009.
4. UNAIDS, World Health Organization. *North America, Western and Central Europe AIDS Epidemic Update Regional Summary.* Switzerland: UNAIDS; 2007. Retrieved at http://data.unaids.org/pub/Report/2008/JC1526_epibriefs_subsaharanafrica_en.pdf on September 13, 2009.
5. Gavin L, MacKay AP, Harrier S, et al. Sexual and reproductive health of persons aged 10-24 years – United States, 2002-2007. *Morb Mortal Wkly Rep.* 2009;58(SS06):1–58.
6. Branson BN, Hansfield HH, Lampe MA. Revised recommendations for HIV testing of adults, adolescents, and pregnant women in health care settings. *Morb Mortal Wkly Rep.* 2006;55(RR14):1–17.
7. Centers for Disease Control and Prevention. 1993 Revised classification system for HIV infection and expanded surveillance case definition for AIDS among adolescents and adults. *Morb Mortal Wkly Rep.* 1992;41(RR-17):1–23.
8. Panel on Antiretroviral Guidelines for Adult and Adolescents. Guidelines for the use of antiretroviral agents in HIV-infected adults and adolescents. Department of Health and Human Services, November 3, 2008; 1–139. Available at: http://www.aidsinfo.nih.gov/contentfiles/adultandadolescentGL.pdf. Accessed on September 13, 2009.
9. American College of Rheumatology Ad Hoc Committee on Systemic Lupus Erythematosus Guidelines. Guidelines for referral and management for systemic lupus erythematosus in adults. *Arthritis Rheum.* 1999;9(42):1788–1796.
10. Molino C, Fabbian F, Longhini C. Clinical approach to lupus nephritis: recent advances. *Eur J Intern Med.* 2009;5(20):447–453.
11. Pilgrim H, Lloyd-Jones M, Rees A. Routine antenatal anti-D prophylaxis for Rh-D negative women: a systematic review and economic evaluation. *Health Technol Assess.* 2009;10(13):1–126.
12. Gottvall T, Filbey D. Alloimmunization in pregnancy during the years 1992-2005 in the central west region of Sweden. *Acta Obstet Gynecol Scand.* 2008;8(87):843–848.

Chapter 5

Infection

LEARNING OBJECTIVES

1. Define and use the key terms listed in this chapter.
2. Relate the development of infection to breaks in the three lines of defense.
3. Identify the ways in which microbes can become pathogens to human host cells.
4. Differentiate between the basic types of microbes.
5. Determine measures to break the chain of infection at each link.
6. Identify the phases of acute infection.
7. Discuss the potential complications of acute infection.
8. Distinguish common clinical manifestations related to infection.
9. Identify laboratory and diagnostic tests relevant to infection.
10. Discuss treatment modalities effective against various types of infection.
11. Apply concepts of infection to the clinical models in this chapter.

INTRODUCTION

How many infections have you had in your lifetime? There have probably been too many to count! Infection is a state of cellular, tissue, and sometimes even organ destruction resulting from invasion by microorganisms. Multiple sites throughout the body contain specialized defense mechanisms to protect against microbe invasion (Fig. 5.1). Immune mechanisms (Chapter 4) also play a critical role in guarding against microorganism invasion and maintaining homeostasis. Unfortunately, with infection, harmful microorganisms have penetrated the three lines of defense, including these specialized defense mechanisms, and have caused disease.

Even with the advent of new antibiotics and vaccinations, infectious disease remains a health care challenge. The overuse or incomplete use of antimicrobial drugs has led to multiple drug-resistant microbes. Globalization has promoted the rapid spread of harmful microbes around the world. Importation and mass distribution of perishable food items has also contributed to infectious disease spread. A thorough understanding of infection is therefore critical to your work in the health professions.

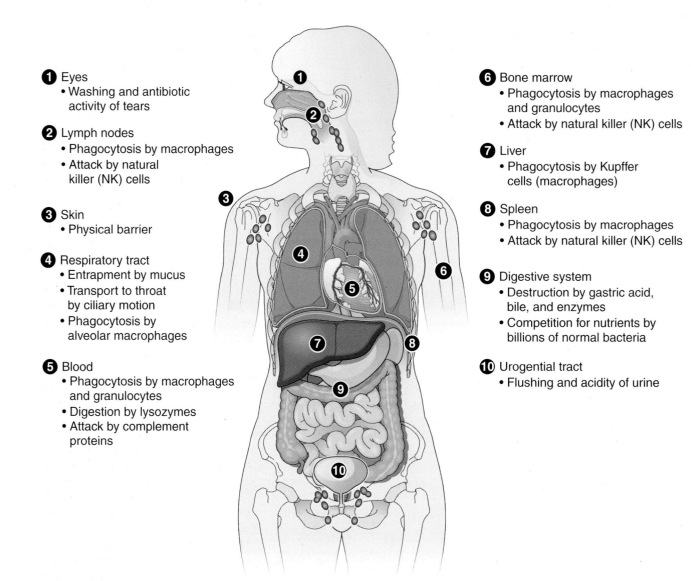

1 Eyes
 • Washing and antibiotic
   activity of tears

2 Lymph nodes
 • Phagocytosis by macrophages
 • Attack by natural
   killer (NK) cells

3 Skin
 • Physical barrier

4 Respiratory tract
 • Entrapment by mucus
 • Transport to throat
   by ciliary motion
 • Phagocytosis by
   alveolar macrophages

5 Blood
 • Phagocytosis by macrophages
   and granulocytes
 • Digestion by lysozymes
 • Attack by complement
   proteins

6 Bone marrow
 • Phagocytosis by macrophages
   and granulocytes
 • Attack by natural killer (NK) cells

7 Liver
 • Phagocytosis by Kupffer
   cells (macrophages)

8 Spleen
 • Phagocytosis by macrophages
 • Attack by natural killer (NK) cells

9 Digestive system
 • Destruction by gastric acid,
   bile, and enzymes
 • Competition for nutrients by
   billions of normal bacteria

10 Urogentical tract
 • Flushing and acidity of urine

▥ **Figure 5.1**   Nonimmune antimicrobial protective mechanisms. The numbered areas show the functions of various organs and systems that defend against bacteria and other microbes.

Module 1

Microbes

Microbes, including bacteria, viruses, fungi, and protozoa, are everywhere in the human environment. **Resident flora** are microorganisms that live on or within the body in nonsterile areas, such as the skin, mucous membranes, bowel, rectum, or vagina, without causing harm. Inflammatory and immune attacks are generally not waged against these inhabitants as long as the skin and mucosa remain intact. Resident flora compete with disease-producing microorganisms to protect the body against certain infections and to provide a type of natural immunity.

A delicate balance of homeostasis is needed because often more than one type of resident flora can be found in nonsterile areas. Destroying one type of resident flora can allow overproliferation of another competing type. For example, if a person experiences a bacterial infection and is prescribed an antibiotic, the antibiotic may also destroy the helpful resident bacteria living in nonsterile areas of the body. The resident fungi no longer have to compete with the destroyed resident bacteria. The fungi overproliferate, resulting in a fungal infection.

This example helps to explain why vaginal yeast (fungal) infections are common in women who are on antibiotics.

Pathogens

A **pathogen** is a disease-producing microbe. To cause disease in humans, a pathogen must be capable of binding to specific receptors on the human host cell. If the microorganism is not able to bind to the receptors, the host cell remains unaffected. This explains why some microorganisms found in the environment are not harmful to humans. Receptors also provide clues to the types of cells to which the pathogen will attach. For example, influenza virus attaches only to receptors in respiratory tract epithelial cells. The basic local clinical manifestations (i.e., cough, nasal congestion, and sore throat) reflect respiratory epithelial cell necrosis elicited by the pathogen. Receptor binding offers some clues to the racial and geographic differences in human infection. For example, some African American individuals lack receptors for the microorganism that causes malaria and are therefore not susceptible to this infection.[1]

Once receptor attachment has been established, the mechanism by which the pathogen causes disease in the human host cell includes one or more of the following:

1. Direct destruction of the host cell by the pathogen
2. Interference with the host cell's metabolic function
3. Exposing the host cell to toxins produced by the pathogen

The **pathogenicity**, or qualities that promote the production of disease, involves multiple factors, including the pathogen's potency, invasiveness, ability to evade the immune system, speed of replication, production of toxins, adherence to the human host cell, and degree of tissue damage that is elicited. The following factors affect the variability with which the pathogen is able to elicit disease.

- **Virulence** is the potency of the pathogen indicated by the ratio of the number of cases of disease in a population compared with the number of people exposed to the microorganism. A more virulent microorganism is one that causes severe disease in a large proportion of those exposed to the microorganism.
- **Infectivity** is the proportion of exposures needed to cause infection in an individual based on the pathogen's ability to enter, survive in, and multiply in the host. Virulence and infectivity are related. A more infective organism is one that takes one exposure, takes hold, multiplies, and causes disease in the host.
- **Toxigenicity** is the ability of the pathogen to produce harmful toxins that increase host cell and tissue damage.
- **Antigenicity** is the level to which a pathogen is viewed by the host immune system as foreign. A more antigenic pathogen elicits a more prominent immune response. Those with low antigenicity can readily elude immune mechanisms and continue to survive in the host.
- **Antigenic variability** is a process of eluding the human host defenses and is often a result of altering the antigens present within or on the surface of the microorganism. This means that many infectious microorganisms can escape human host defenses through slight genetic variations unrecognized by the host. These mutations are responsible for much of the infectious disease burden throughout the world.
- **Pathogenic defense mechanisms** are the ways in which many pathogens have developed ways to avoid destruction by the host, such as through thick protective capsules, which prevent phagocytosis.
- **Coinfection** is a phenomenon of hosting two or more pathogens simultaneously. Certain pathogens, such as those that cause chlamydia and gonorrhea, are more likely to be transmitted and to coexist in the host. Coinfection presents a greater challenge to the immune system.
- **Superinfection** is when an infection arises in addition to one that is already present. Superinfection often results from compromised host defenses and overproliferation of resident flora.

TYPES OF PATHOGENS

Basic types of microorganisms that can cause disease include bacteria, viruses, fungi, and protozoa. Understanding the distinctive quality of each microorganism can provide clues to the transmission and spread of infectious disease.

Some microorganisms live and reproduce independently of the host. Other microorganisms are considered parasites. **Obligate parasites** require the host for metabolism and reproduction. **Facultative parasites** may live on the host but can also survive independently. Helminths (worms) are capable of eliciting disease in humans. They are not considered microorganisms but rather are a highly diverse group of multicellular parasites. Helminth eggs can be found in contaminated food, water, or soil, as well as within infected insects. Once infected, the helminth matures within the host and can grow to be quite large.

Flagellum
Capsule
Cell wall
Cell membrane
Nucleoid
Cytoplasm

B

■ **Figure 5.2**   Bacterial cell **(A)** scanning electron microscopy; basic structure of bacteria **(B)**.

Bacteria

Bacteria are single-celled microorganisms (Fig. 5.2). Most can reproduce outside of host cells. Bacteria that require oxygen for growth are called **aerobic**; those that do not are called **anaerobic**. Oxygen requirements dictate where the bacteria can best survive. Anaerobic bacteria survive best in deep tis-

sues of the body where oxygen supply is limited. This type is difficult to treat because antimicrobial drugs often travel within the vascular system to affect local tissues. Deeper tissues are much more difficult to penetrate. Some bacteria can survive in both aerobic and anaerobic environments.

Bacteria are often referred to by their shape: cocci (spheres), bacilli (rods), and spirochetes (spirals). They contain an indiscrete nucleus, a cytoplasm, and an outer cell membrane. The "indiscrete" nucleus does not have a nuclear membrane and is therefore not separate from the cytoplasm. Like the nucleus, the cytoplasm is also different from human cells. The cytoplasm of bacteria is referred to as **cytosol**. Cytosol contains extensive ribosomes, proteins, and carbohydrates but does not contain mitochondria, endoplasmic reticulum, or other membranous components.

The innermost cell membrane, also called the cell envelope, has multiple functions:

● Formation of a barrier surrounding the bacterial cell
● Protein and DNA synthesis
● Cell division

Most bacteria also include a rigid cell wall that surrounds this inner membrane. The cell wall provides shape and structure. Because human cells do not have a cell wall, antibiotic treatment is commonly aimed at inhibiting synthesis of the bacterial cell wall during bacterial replication. Therefore, the bacteria are destroyed and the human host cell is unharmed. Some bacteria can also have a capsule covering this cell wall. Bacteria with a capsule more easily adhere to host cells. The capsule is also highly resistant to phagocytosis. The variability of each type of cell envelope, cell wall, and capsule is important in the pathogenicity of the bacteria and will often direct treatment decisions.

From the Lab

Laboratory tests are important in differentiating the specific types of bacteria that are causing the infection. The goal is to "match the bug to the drug;" that is, aiming treatment at the specific bacteria without harming the host cells or resident flora. Cultures can be obtained and the bacteria grown and identified. This usually takes 3 days or more. Two other important clues that allow more rapid identification of bacteria characteristics are the Gram stain and tests for coagulation. Bacterial cell walls, when exposed to a Gram stain in the lab, become either dark blue or red (when counterstained). Bacterial cell walls that preserve the stain and turn dark blue are considered Gram-positive. Examples of gram-positive bacteria include *Staphylococcus aureus*, *Streptococcus pneumoniae*, and *Clostridium difficile*. Those that do not retain the dark blue color and instead turn red when another stain is applied are considered gram-negative. Examples of gram-negative bacteria include *Neisseria gonorrhoeae*, *Helicobactor pylori*, and *Escherichia coli*. Coagulase tests differentiate potentially pathogenic staphylococcus species from other gram-positive cocci. Staphylococcal bacteria that cause coagulation (clotting) in the blood are more resistant to phagocytosis or antibody destruction. A coagulase-positive test indicates a pathogenic strain of staphylococcal bacteria that should be treated aggressively.

STOP *and Consider*

What aspects of bacterial activity would be effective targets for pharmacologic treatment?

The damage caused by bacteria can result from bacterial structural properties and exotoxin release. Structural properties critical to the pathogenicity of bacteria include

● Independent survival: Bacteria can survive outside the human host and can infect and reinfect if not destroyed.

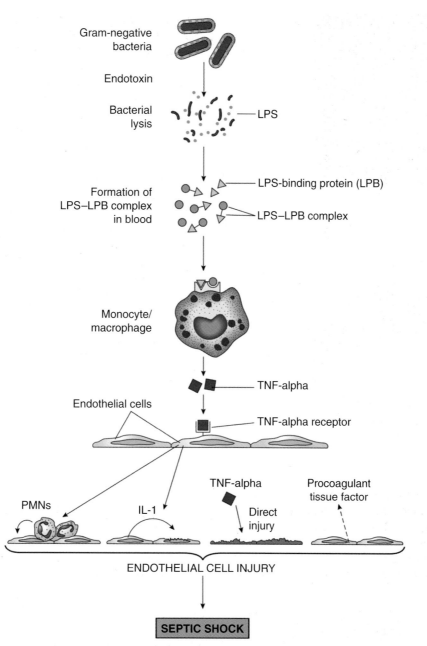

Figure 5.3 Pathogenesis of endothelial cell injury in endotoxic shock. In sepsis caused by gram-negative bacteria, the lysis of the organisms releases endotoxin into the circulation in the form of lipopolysaccharide (LPS), where it binds to the LPS-binding protein (LBP). The LPS–LPB complex binds to monocytes/macrophages, which are stimulated to secrete substantial quantities of tumor necrosis factor-alpha (TNF-alpha), a potent inflammatory mediator. TNF-alpha mediates septic shock by causing endothelial cell injury by a number of mechanisms: (1) direct cytotoxicity; (2) enhancing the adherence of polymorphonuclear leukocytes; (3) stimulating the release of interleukin-1 (IL-1), a cytokine that injures endothelial cells; and (4) promoting the expression of procoagulant tissue factor, thereby leading to thrombosis and local ischemia.

- Stimulation of an inflammatory response: Bacteria stimulate an inflammatory and immune response that will destroy surrounding host tissues in an effort to rid the body of the invader.
- Bacterial capsule: Encapsulated bacteria are adherent and highly resistant to phagocytosis.
- Endotoxin: The presence of endotoxin in the gram-negative bacterial cell envelope activates the plasma protein systems (Chapter 3). **Endotoxin**

is a complex of phospholipid–polysaccharide molecules that form the structural component of the gram-negative cell wall. Endotoxin causes inflammatory mediators to be released, leading to a massive inflammatory response (Fig. 5.3). This in turn can result in a state of septic shock accompanied by severe diarrhea, fever, and leukocytosis. When inducing fever, these endotoxin-containing bacteria are referred to as **pyogenic** bacteria.

Pathogenic Bacteria

Neisseria meningitidis

Types of infection:
• Meningitis

Streptococcus pyogenes

• Septicemia
• Myositis
• Necrotizing fascitis

Streptococcus pneumoniae

• Pneumonia
• Meningitis
• Otitis media

Staphylococcus aureus

• Endocarditis
• Cellulitis
• Pneumonia
• Osteomyelitis
• Septicemia

Escherichia coli

• Urogenital tract infection
• Diarrhea

Salmonella typhi

• Enterocolitis
• Bacteremia
• Typhoid
• Localized infections

Pseudomonas aeruginosa

• Urinary infection
• Wound infection

Sites of Infection

Key

A—Brain
B—Lung
C—Heart
D—Liver
E—Stomach
F—Large intestine
G—Small intestine
H—Bladder

■ **Figure 5.4**   Sites of bacterial infection for each type of pathogenic bacteria. (Asset provided by Anatomical Chart Company.)

- Endospores: Some bacteria can produce spores that survive in a latent state that is resistant to environmental extremes and lack of nutrients. When the environment is more conducive to replication, the bacteria will emerge from the spore state, multiply, and may cause infection in a susceptible host.

Many bacteria are also capable of producing toxins, called **exotoxins**, and enzymes, which result in host cell dysfunction or lysis. Exotoxins are potent substances, often bacterial-derived proteins, released into the surrounding tissues that cause local or systemic injury to the host. The target tissue can be in the brain and spinal cord (neurotoxic), the gastrointestinal (GI) tract (enterotoxic), the liver (hepatotoxic), the blood (hemotoxic), and so forth. Figure 5.4 depicts examples of pathogenic bacteria and the sites of infection for each type.

Viruses

Viruses are considered obligate intracellular parasites. This means that viruses cannot replicate outside of the host cell. The virus binds to specific receptors on the host cell and then moves into the host cell. Once inside the host cell, the virus converts the host cellular metabolism to nucleic acids and proteins that are encoded and controlled by the virus. Viruses have the ability to either directly kill the cell or modify certain cellular functions, such as protein synthesis. Viruses can cause cells to proliferate rapidly and randomly, causing tumors to form in the body (Chapter 7). The cell ultimately loses its ability to function. The virus next releases particles outside of the cell, called **virions**, which can enter and infect other nearby cells (Fig. 5.5).

Initially, viruses evade many defense mechanisms by hiding within host cells. As the virus moves from cell to cell, the immune response is activated. Viral infections are often severe enough to spark a strong, eradicating immune response. This exaggerated immune response allows neutralization of the virus and resolution of the infection. The infected host cells are eliminated and the virus can no longer replicate. In this regard, many viruses, such as those associated with the common cold, are considered self-limiting; that is, the infection ceases after a definite period.

Some viruses are sustained for longer periods in the host. If the initial, acute infection does not provoke a strong viral-eradicating immune response, the individual is more likely to host a chronic viral infection. Other factors that support chronic infection with a virus include

1. The size of the virus that is inoculated into the body
2. The process of viral replication
3. The viral genotype
4. Host susceptibility

For example, in an immunocompetent healthy adult, hepatitis B becomes a chronic infection in 10% of cases. This same virus, when spread to a fetus from an infected mother, becomes chronic in 90% of newborns.[3] The major difference between the two scenarios is the immaturity of the newborn's immune system, allowing the virus to continue to replicate.

Also characteristic of chronic viral infections is a period of **latency**, or dormancy. During this period, the virus is integrating itself into the host cell's genetic material. The virus will reside in a host cell and cause minimal or no loss of functional capabilities for that cell. The virus demonstrates low antigenicity, although cellular mitosis continues and new cells that contain viral material are generated. Immunocompromise, including that induced by physical and emotional stress, provides a medium for active viral replication. Active viral replication can be triggered weeks to years after the initial inoculation with the virus. This process results in host cell death. Cell death leads to recognizable signs and symptoms of disease. A common example of a latent virus is herpes simplex virus, which causes cold sores. The virus remains dormant. Replication is triggered by immunocompromise (often stress related). The local clinical manifestations characteristic of herpes simplex infection (e.g., itching, blistering, and erythema) then become apparent. These local necrotic cells are removed from the body by inflammatory/immune mechanisms; however, other cells containing viral material remain and can cause active disease again at another point.

Another example of latency is a disease condition caused by herpes zoster virus. The original infection with herpes zoster virus causes varicella, or chicken pox. During the initial battle, some of the viral particles leave the skin blisters from the chicken pox and move into the nervous system. When the varicella virus reactivates, often years later, the virus moves back down the long nerve fibers from the sen-

Research Notes

Prions, protein particles that lack DNA or RNA, have been found to cause infectious disease in humans. Prion diseases are implicated in such conditions as Creutzfeldt-Jakob disease and bovine spongiform encephalopathy, also known as mad cow disease. Interestingly, prion diseases are not known to elicit a notable immune response by the host, and the mechanism by which they destroy brain tissue is poorly understood. It is known, however, that animal prion diseases pose a significant public health risk with recent reports of secondary person-to-person spread.[2]

■ **Figure 5.5** Consequences of viral infection in host cells. **A:** Cell lysis. **B:** Continuous release of budding viral particles. **C:** Latency. **D:** Tumor formation. (Image modified from Porth CM. *Pathophysiology: Concepts of Altered Health States.* 7th ed. Philadelphia: Lippincott Williams & Wilkins; 2004, with permission.)

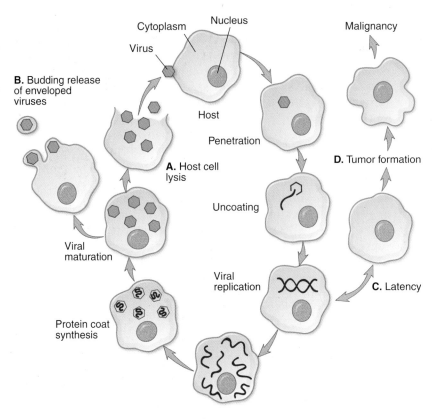

sory cell bodies to the skin, causing severe pain along these nerves. Blisters are often present as well. This disease recurrence is known as shingles. Examples of other select viral diseases are listed in Table 5.1.

● **STOP** *and* **Consider**

Why are antiviral drugs difficult to develop and use effectively?

Rickettsiae, Mycoplasmas, and Chlamydiae

Rickettsiae, mycoplasmas, and chlamydiae are unique pathogens that have characteristics of both bacteria and viruses. Rickettsiae, like viruses, are obligate intracellular parasites that cannot replicate outside the host. However, rickettsiae are also gram-negative bacteria that are capable of producing energy. Rickettsiae target human endothelial cells of the blood vessels and capillaries. Mycoplasmas lack a cell

Table 5.1 Select Viruses and Related Disease Conditions

Virus	Transmission	Disease Condition	Clinical Manifestations
Respiratory syncytial virus (RSV)	Respiratory droplets	Lower respiratory tract infection in young children	Fever, runny nose, cough, wheezing
Paramyxovirus	Respiratory droplets	Measles	Fever, runny nose, cough, rash
Rotavirus	Primarily fecal–oral	Gastroenteritis	Severe, watery diarrhea; vomiting
Coxsackievirus	Direct contact with stool or infected secretions	Hand–foot–mouth disease	Fever, sores in the mouth, rash with blisters, especially on hands and feet
Human parvovirus B19	Respiratory droplets	Fifth disease	Mild rash with "slapped cheek" appearance on face, fever, malaise
Adenovirus	Respiratory droplets or fecal–oral	Common cold with respiratory droplets, gastroenteritis with fecal–oral transmission	Common cold: runny nose, sore throat, fever, malaise; gastroenteritis: diarrhea, vomiting
Rhinovirus	Respiratory droplets	Common cold	Fever, runny nose, sore throat, body aches, malaise
Coronavirus	Respiratory droplets	Severe acute respiratory syndrome (SARS)	High fever, headache, body aches, cough, pneumonia, diarrhea

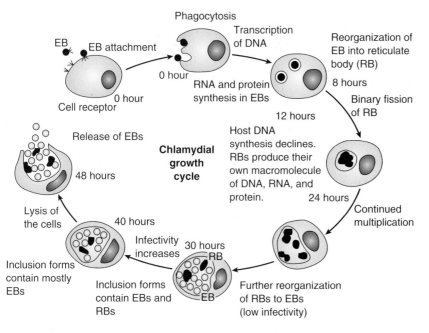

Phagocytosis

EB   EB attachment

Transcription of DNA

Reorganization of EB into reticulate body (RB)

0 hour   RNA and protein synthesis in EBs

8 hours

Cell receptor   0 hour

Binary fission of RB

12 hours

Chlamydial growth cycle

Release of EBs

48 hours

Host DNA synthesis declines. RBs produce their own macromolecule of DNA, RNA, and protein.   24 hours

Lysis of the cells

40 hours

Continued multiplication

Infectivity increases   30 hours

Inclusion forms contain mostly EBs

RB

Inclusion forms contain EBs and RBs

EB

Further reorganization of RBs to EBs (low infectivity)

Figure 5.6 Chlamydial growth cycle. EB, elementary body; RB, reticulate body (From Thompson SE, Washington AE. Epidemiology of sexually transmitted *Chlamydia trachomatis* infections. *Epidemiol Rev.* 1983;5:96–123, with permission.)

wall and survive on the surface of host cells, but they do not enter the host cell for replication. Chlamydiae reproduce through binary fission yet are obligate intracellular parasites (Fig. 5.6). These pathogens use the host metabolism to reproduce. The life cycle of chlamydiae has the following distinct phases:

1. The metabolically inactive elemental body enters the body, attaches to, and internalizes the host cell.
2. The elemental body becomes metabolically active and transforms into a reticulate body, which takes over the host cell.
3. The chlamydiae are then capable of replication.
4. Each replicated pathogen goes through the life cycle, causing epithelial cell necrosis.

Fungi

Fungi are relatively large organisms compared to bacteria and viruses. They have a nuclear membrane, cytoplasm, and organelles. Unicellular forms are called **yeasts**; multicellular forms are called **molds** (Fig. 5.7). Yeasts reproduce by budding and form an elongated chain, called **pseudohyphae**. Mold colonies have tubules that branch to form **hyphae**; clusters of hyphae form **mycelium**. Some fungi can grow as either yeasts or molds. Superficial or deep-tissue invasion occurs when pseudohyphae or hyphae multiply. This invasion results in inflammatory and immune responses. Infections with fungi are referred to as **mycoses** or mycotic infections.

Fungi are common resident microbes. These organisms frequently inhabit the skin surface or mucous membranes and are kept at bay by intact integument, inflammatory, and immune cells. Resident bacteria also compete with and regulate

growth of resident fungi. As previously mentioned, reduction of resident bacteria, often via antibiotics, disturbs this balance and allows fungal overgrowth.

Fungal infections can also be opportunistic. **Opportunistic pathogens** are those that cause

Yeasts   Hyphae

Mycelium   Pseudohyphae

Figure 5.7 Basic structure of fungi. Molds grow as branching hyphae, forming a mycelium. Yeasts multiply by budding and form elongated pseudohyphae. (Asset provided by Anatomical Chart Company.)

disease only in a host with a compromised immune system. Patients with fungal invasion of tissues are frequently immunocompromised, such as persons with AIDS (Chapter 4). One of the most common opportunistic yeast infections involves *Candida*. Yeast grows well in warm, moist, dark environments; common sites for superficial candidal epithelial cell infection include those with skin–skin contact, such as beneath the breasts in women, the diaper area in infants, and the perineum, between toes, nail beds, and oral mucosa in susceptible individuals. **Maceration**, a softening and breaking down of these tissues, is often related to excessive moisture and is required for candidal infections to gain a foothold. Deep-tissue infections, such as those found in the lungs, kidney, and heart, are life threatening and are found almost exclusively in immunocompromised persons.

Clinical manifestations of superficial *Candida* cutaneous invasion include skin redness, itching, and burning at the site. In oral candidiasis, lesions are white and resemble cottage cheese attached to an erythematous oral cavity; these lesions bleed easily and can be painful if scraped (Fig. 5.8). Vulvovaginal candidiasis also produces redness, itching, and burning at the site along with a thick, white, vaginal discharge.

Protozoa

Protozoa are unicellular, complex microorganisms. They are characterized by an irregular or fluctuant

Figure 5.8 Oral candidiasis. These curdlike lesions can be easily removed with gauze. (Image from Goodheart HP. *Goodheart's Photoguide of Common Skin Disorders*. 2nd ed. Philadelphia: Lippincott Williams & Wilkins; 2003, with permission.)

shape without a cell wall, and many are motile. Transmission can occur through sexual contact, contaminated food or water, or a **vector**, which carries the protozoa, such as by an insect or other arthropod. Some protozoa are parasites and some are capable of living independently of the host. Those that are parasites compete for and deprive host cells of nutrition, causing tissue destruction.

Module 2

Communicable Disease

Communicable diseases are those that are spread from person to person, often through contact with infected blood and body fluids. Although all communicable diseases are infectious, not all infectious diseases are communicable. Communicable diseases are infections caused by microorganisms that live and reproduce in a human host.

STOP *and Consider*

What sources of infection would not be considered communicable?

The chain of infection is a useful organization for recognizing the factors inherent in the transmission and spread of communicable disease (Fig. 5.9). The

infectious agent link refers to the pathogens described above. Infection control measures seek to break one or more of these links. For example, breaking the chain of infection at the level of the pathogen requires sterilization of the environment to remove all pathogens from contact with the human cell. Sterilization is performed using physical or chemical agents, heat being the most important. An **autoclave** is a device that uses steam heat at high pressures to sterilize objects.

Reservoir

The reservoir is the "holding tank" for the microorganism. The reservoir could include an infected person, an animal, or the environment, such as pond

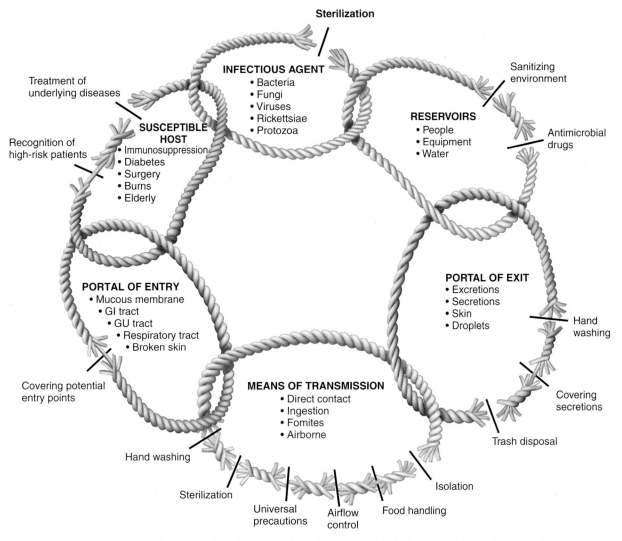

Sterilization

INFECTIOUS AGENT
• Bacteria
• Fungi
• Viruses
• Rickettsiae
• Protozoa

Treatment of underlying diseases

SUSCEPTIBLE HOST
• Immunosuppression
• Diabetes
• Surgery
• Burns
• Elderly

Recognition of high-risk patients

Sanitizing environment

RESERVOIRS
• People
• Equipment
• Water

Antimicrobial drugs

PORTAL OF ENTRY
• Mucous membrane
• GI tract
• GU tract
• Respiratory tract
• Broken skin

Covering potential entry points

PORTAL OF EXIT
• Excretions
• Secretions
• Skin
• Droplets

Hand washing

Covering secretions

Trash disposal

MEANS OF TRANSMISSION
• Direct contact
• Ingestion
• Fomites
• Airborne

Hand washing

Sterilization

Universal precautions

Airflow control

Food handling

Isolation

Figure 5.9 Chain of infection. Sources of infection are depicted along with interventions used to break the chain of infection at each link. GI, gastrointestinal; GU, genitourinary. (Image modified from Smeltzer SC, Bare BG. *Texbook of Medical-Surgical Nursing*. 10th ed. Philadelphia: Lippincott Williams & Wilkins; 2003, with permission.)

water. Breaking the chain at the level of the reservoir includes providing antimicrobial drugs to the carrier or taking action to destroy the presence of the microorganism in the environment.

Portal of Exit

The portal of exit represents the passage by which the microorganism leaves the reservoir. In human hosts, common portals of exit include the respiratory tract, GI tract, skin, mucous membranes, placenta, and blood. If you have a respiratory infection, wearing a mask or otherwise covering your mouth and nose during sneezing will help to block the portal of exit.

Mode of Transmission

All infection will occur through some form of contact with a pathogen. This contact can be direct or indirect. The mode of transmission refers to the mechanism of transference from the reservoir to the portal of entry. The modes of transmission include

• **Direct contact**. As a mode of transmission, direct contact implies physically touching or otherwise coming in contact with the reservoir. Examples of direct contact transmission include touching the blood or body fluids of an infected person, kissing, or sexual intercourse. This mode can also involve close contact by touching another person or a surface in the environment that is holding the pathogen.

- **Droplet transmission**. Larger respiratory particles, produced by sneezing, coughing, or talking, can pass through the air from the reservoir to the host. For droplet transmission to occur, the host must be within 3 feet of the reservoir. The heavy droplet particles drop to the ground beyond this distance. Most respiratory illnesses are spread through droplet transmission.
- **Airborne transmission**. Smaller respiratory particles can remain suspended in the air and are subject to airborne transmission. The particles can remain in the area of the reservoir for an extended period. Infection can be transmitted to a person who enters this area and breathes the air. Tuberculosis and varicella (chicken pox) are examples of respiratory diseases spread through airborne transmission.
- **Vector transmission**. A **vector** is a vehicle that harbors the pathogen and carries it to the host. Biological vectors are those that support the life cycle of the pathogen. Arthropods, such as mites, ticks, and spiders, and insects, are examples of biologic vectors. Mechanical vectors are not essential to the life cycle of the pathogen and can include dogs, mosquitoes, and even food.

Universal precautions are a standard of health care that recognizes all blood and body fluid as potentially infected. Universal precautions dictate that health care providers wear gloves when having *any* contact with blood and body fluids. Masks and protective eyewear are also recommended if splattering of blood or body fluids is anticipated. Additional precautions are implemented depending on the mode of transmission.

STOP *and Consider*

How can you break the chain of infection at each of the different modes of transmission?

Portal of Entry

The portal of entry refers to the access point for the microorganism into the **host**, or the individual who is exposed to and contracts the infection. The most common locations for microorganisms to enter the body include through the mucous membranes, eyes, respiratory tract, genitourinary tract, gastrointestincal tract, or placenta.

Loss of physical (skin) and chemical barriers can also provide access to the portal of entry. Breaking the chain of infection at the level of the portal of entry involves covering and protecting potential entry points. Examples include wearing gloves, mask, protective eyewear, and condoms. Each of these measures prevents entry of the microorganism into host tissues.

Host Factors

When host lines of defense are compromised and microbes gain access to vulnerable areas, infection can result. Factors that increase host susceptibility to experiencing infection are primarily related to impaired host defense mechanisms (problems with skin/mucous membranes, inflammation, and/or immunity). Immunosuppression is often related to poor nutrition, the extremes of age, concurrent chronic illness, and severe stress. Coinfection and superinfection impact the load placed on the host immune defenses and can further complicate infectious processes.

Module 3

Acute Infection and Complications

Acute infection in both communicable and noncommunicable infectious diseases progresses along five distinct phases (Fig. 5.10):

1. **Exposure**. Exposure is contact with the pathogen through any of the modes of transmission described above.
2. **Incubation**. The incubation phase extends from exposure to the onset of any signs or symptoms. During the incubation period, the individual often has no idea that he or she has been exposed to, or will develop, the illness.

With communicable disease, it is often during this incubation period that transmission of microorganisms to others is greatest. For example, chicken pox has an incubation period of 7 to 21 days from exposure to recognizable signs and symptoms.

3. **Prodrome**. The prodromal phase involves the onset of vague, nonspecific signs and symptoms, including fatigue, low-grade fever, nausea, weakness, and generalized muscle aches. This phase is often described as feeling

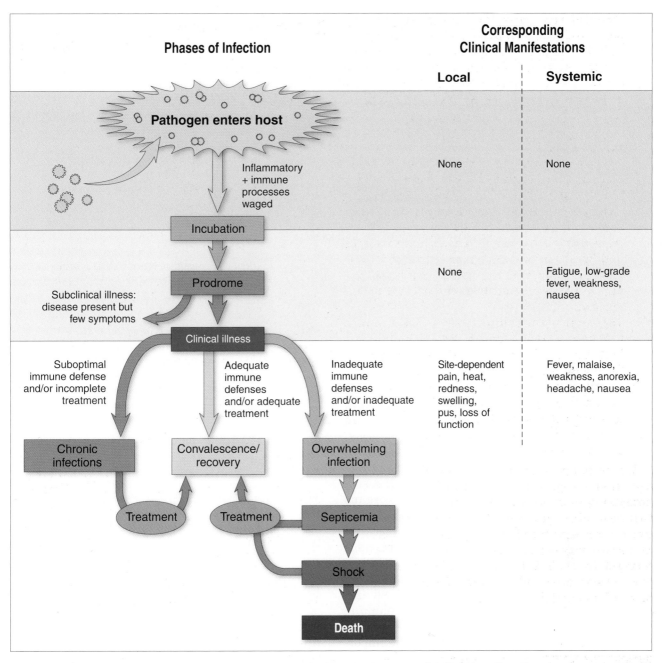

Phases of Infection

Corresponding Clinical Manifestations

	Local	Systemic
Pathogen enters host / Inflammatory + immune processes waged / **Incubation**	None	None
Prodrome	None	Fatigue, low-grade fever, weakness, nausea
Clinical illness	Site-dependent pain, heat, redness, swelling, pus, loss of function	Fever, malaise, weakness, anorexia, headache, nausea

Subclinical illness: disease present but few symptoms

Suboptimal immune defense and/or incomplete treatment

Adequate immune defenses and/or adequate treatment

Inadequate immune defenses and/or inadequate treatment

Chronic infections — Treatment

Convalescence/ recovery — Treatment

Overwhelming infection — Septicemia — Shock — **Death**

■ **Figure 5.10** Concept map. Phases of infection and corresponding clinical manifestations.

"under the weather." The specific signs and symptoms related to the disease have not yet emerged.

4. **Acute clinical illness**. The clinical illness phase represents the manifestation of signs and symptoms specific to the disease. Often, the accurate medical diagnosis is applied more confidently during this time. In many cases, the immune response peaks or treatment is initiated and the body is able to overcome the pathogen.

5. **Convalescence**. The convalescent phase extends from waning clinical manifestations to

full recovery from the disease. Fatigue is a common concern during this time of recovery.

Complications of Infection

Acute infection can result in two major complications: septicemia and chronic infection. **Septicemia** occurs when microorganisms gain access to the blood and circulate throughout the body. When septicemia is caused by bacteria, the term **bacteremia** is often used. The development of overwhelming systemic infection is based on the degree of microorganism

Table 5.2 Common Laboratory and Diagnostic Tests to Detect Infection

Test	Purpose	Interpretation
White blood cell count	A nonspecific test that examines an increase or decrease in white blood cells to assist in determining the presence of inflammatory or infectious process	**Leukocytosis**: elevation in white blood cells, which may indicate an infectious process, often bacterial in origin **Leukopenia**: decrease in white blood cells, which may indicate a viral infection or a problem with suppression of white blood cell production
Serum antibody levels	A specific blood test that detects the presence of certain antibodies against pathogens	Presence of specific antibodies indicates an exposure to the antigen at some point
Cultures	Identifies presence and density of microorganisms that grow in a specific medium over a period of time (usually 3 days or so); sample extracted from body tissues (including blood) or exudates	Positive test indicates the microorganism is present
Sensitivities	Identifies which antimicrobial drugs would be most effective for a specific pathogen	If the microorganism is sensitive to a certain antibiotic, that is the recommended treatment

pathogenicity and immunocompromise in the host. Once pathogens enter the blood and gain access to all perfused tissues, the infection can result in septic shock and become life threatening. **Septic shock** is a process of systemic vasodilation due to severe infection, often with gram-negative bacteria (the endotoxin component). Massive vasodilation leads to poor perfusion of vital organs (Chapter 14).

Chronic infection is defined as an infection that lasts for several weeks to years. The mechanism for eliciting a chronic viral infection was discussed earlier in the chapter. Chronic bacterial infection can result when pathogens are not fully destroyed as a result of a suboptimal inflammatory or immune response or incomplete antibiotic treatment. Patients need to be clearly informed of the importance of taking an entire course of an antibiotic to prevent this complication. The pathophysiologic processes and outcomes are the same as with chronic inflammation, which is described in depth in Chapter 3.

Clinical Manifestations

Infection with a microorganism triggers the inflammatory and immune responses. Clinical manifestations are consistent with these responses. Acute local infection is usually manifested by pain, heat, redness, swelling, lymph node enlargement and tenderness, and site-dependent loss of function. The presence of exudate is common and can be **purulent**, or containing pus. Systemic manifestations

include fever, malaise, weakness, anorexia, headache, and nausea.

Laboratory and Diagnostic Tests

The diagnosis of infection is based on a thorough history and physical examination along with the performance of relevant laboratory and diagnostic tests. Common laboratory and diagnostic tests are summarized in Table 5.2.

Treatment Modalities

Antimicrobial drugs are often used to treat infection. Antimicrobials function to destroy pathogens or to decrease the growth of the offending microorganisms. The major mechanisms of action are to alter the cellular structure of the microorganism or to disable enzymes produced by pathogens. Antibacterial drugs can inhibit synthesis of the bacteria cell wall, damage the cytoplasmic membrane, and disable nucleic acid metabolism or protein synthesis. Antifungals function by binding to the fungal cell membrane, increasing permeability, and reducing viability of the fungal cells. Because bacteria do not contain the same components as fungal cells, antifungal medications are not active against bacteria. Antiviral treatment has been met with limited success because viral growth employs the host cell. Therefore, destruction of the virus can significantly damage host cells as well. Symptomatic treatment, such as fluids, rest, and analgesics, is often recommended with all infections.

Module 4

Clinical Models

The following clinical models have been selected to aid in the application of knowledge related to infection. When reading through the clinical models, differentiate between the types of pathogen, acute or chronic features of the disease, and the roles of inflammatory and immune responses.

Influenza

Influenza is a viral infection of the epithelial cells of the airway. The virus is transmitted via respiratory droplets from another infected person or contaminated surface. Three different types of influenza viruses (A, B, or C) can cause influenza disease; each of these types also has several strains, or subtypes.

PATHOPHYSIOLOGY

The respiratory epithelial cells are armed with cilia, mucus, and antibodies. The influenza virus enters the respiratory tract, attaches to the surface epithelial cells, impairs cilia, mucus, and antibodies, moves into the cells, and replicates. The virus causes these epithelial cells to die, resulting in necrosis and sloughing of the dead cells. In many cases, influenza results in an uncomplicated upper respiratory infection or can progress to viral pneumonia. In more severe cases, viral infection in the lung tissue can lead to bacterial pneumonia, impaired ventilation and diffusion (Chapter 13), and even death. Young children (under 2 years of age), adults 65 years of age and older, pregnant women, and individuals with chronic cardiopulmonary, renal, metabolic, or immunodeficient conditions are predisposed to greater morbidity and mortality when infected with influenza.

Influenza viruses are well adapted to escape host defenses and gradually change genetic composition during replication in the human host cell in a process called **reassortment**. This process results in viral offspring with altered antigenic properties. These minor genetic modifications result in ongoing host susceptibility to the influenza virus. The development of vaccines is adjusted yearly to take into account these shifts.

CLINICAL MANIFESTATIONS

The clinical manifestations of influenza are based on the inflammatory response and cell necrosis in the respiratory tract and include cough, sore throat, nasal congestion and drainage, and shortness of breath. Systemic signs of inflammation are also common and include chills, fever, body aches, weakness, and malaise.

DIAGNOSTIC CRITERIA

Diagnosis is based on a health history significant for the clinical manifestations described previously. Influenza is a clinical diagnostic challenge because many symptoms resemble that of the common cold. However, influenza is more likely to have an abrupt onset, severe body aches, fever, anorexia, headache, malaise, and a dry cough. During influenza outbreaks, rapid viral assays are available to identify type A and B viruses. These tests of nasopharyngeal secretions are quick (10 to 20 minutes) but do demonstrate a 30% false-positive or false-negative error rate.[6]

TREATMENT

Influenza is highly contagious and epidemics are common worldwide. Because this infection is viral, treatment is usually symptomatic and focuses on hydration, adequate nutrition, and control of body aches with analgesics. Aspirin use should be avoided in children to prevent the development of Reye syndrome. Antiviral drugs may help reduce the duration of disease if they are started early in the course of infection. Prevention and infection avoidance is an important strategy. Vaccines are developed annually to prevent infection of susceptible individuals.

Research Notes

Epidemiologists are concerned with tracking the movement of influenza viruses worldwide to predict the most effective vaccine strategy. Selection of the most appropriate vaccine combination is based on antigenic analyses of recently isolated influenza viruses, epidemiologic data, and postvaccination serologic studies in humans. The Food and Drug Administration's Vaccines and Related Biological Products Advisory Committee (VRBPAC) makes a final vaccine recommendation for the United States based on these data.[4,5]

Hepatitis

Hepatitis is inflammation of the liver and can have numerous causes, the most notable being viral infection. Hepatitis can also result from alcohol abuse or ingestion of other toxic substances that damage the liver.

The Function of the Liver

The major roles of the liver include

- Secretion of bile
- Metabolism of bilirubin
- Blood storage
- Synthesis of clotting factors
- Metabolism of nutrients
- Metabolic detoxification
- Storage of minerals and vitamins

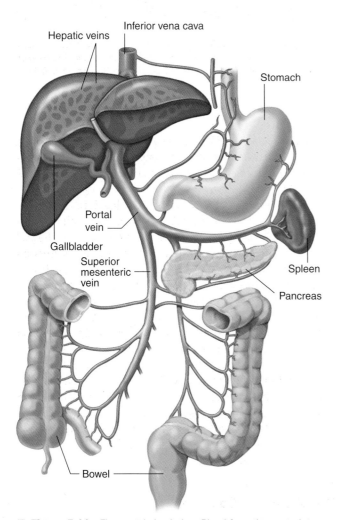

■ **Figure 5.11**   The portal circulation. Blood from the gastrointestinal tract, spleen, and pancreas travels to the liver via the portal vein before moving into the vena cava for return to the heart.

The liver has a major impact on health status and multiple important functions, but it also has excellent regenerative and restorative capabilities. Injury to the liver often affects the blood vessels, lymphatics, and nerves, which are concentrated in the outer coating of the liver, called the Glisson capsule. When inflamed or enlarged, the Glisson capsule causes right upper-quadrant pain.

The liver has an active role in venous blood return for the circulatory system. Deoxygenated blood from the GI tract, spleen, and pancreas travels to the liver by way of the portal vein before moving on to the vena cava and heart. This blood bypass is called **portal circulation** (Fig. 5.11). Obstruction of portal circulation from liver damage causes backup of blood flow to the GI tract, spleen, and pancreas.

Within the capsule are hepatocytes, the functional cells of the liver that are capable of regeneration. Hepatocytes are responsible for secretion of bile. Bile contains bile salts, cholesterol, bilirubin, electrolytes, and water. Bile is needed for fat emulsification and absorption. Damage to hepatocytes therefore inhibits bile production and can affect fat absorption. The liver converts fats (primarily triglycerides) to glycerol and free fatty acids to provide energy to the cells. Glucose is another source of energy affected by liver disease, which causes blood glucose fluctuations (Chapter 18). The liver is capable of releasing glucose during hypoglycemia, converting amino acids and glycerol to glucose if needed, and taking up glucose from the blood during hyperglycemia.

Blood volume and pressure regulation is also aided by the work of the liver in producing plasma proteins. The role of plasma proteins in regulating plasma oncotic pressure is further discussed in Chapter 8.

The liver plays a critical role in detoxification. The liver alters toxic substances, such as alcohol, medications, and even hormones, and helps remove these substances from the body. Damage to the liver from excess amounts of toxins or from other sources will affect the levels of toxic substances circulating in the body. Patients with liver disease must be cautious about taking medications that are metabolized in the liver because these may continue to circulate at high levels without being inactivated and removed.

Not to be confused with bile production, bilirubin metabolism is another major role of the liver. Recall that bile contains bilirubin. Bilirubin results from the destruction of aged red blood cells. The liver is responsible for breaking down and removing these dying red blood cells. The aged red blood cells are engulfed and destroyed by phagocytes housed in the liver called **Kupffer cells**. Small capillaries perfuse the liver and are lined with Kupffer cells. Kupffer cells are phagocytes that readily engulf harmful substances. This helps to explain why bacterial and other foreign invaders in the liver are less likely to cause disease than viral microorganisms. When damage to the liver occurs, bilirubin is allowed to circulate freely. Bilirubin is responsible for the yellow-tinged skin color and sclera of the eyes (**jaundice**) in individuals with liver disease (Fig. 5.12). Similarly, the obstruction of bile flow can result in jaundice. The presence of liver disease marked by jaundice is often referred to as the **icteric phase**. Newborns often experience some degree of physiologic (expected) jaundice due to liver immaturity. In newborns, this physiologic jaundice typically resolves spontaneously within a week.

Kupffer cells separate hemoglobin into heme and globin. The globin is degraded into amino acids. The amino acids are then used again to form new protein. The iron cleaved from the heme component can be stored in the liver or used by the bone marrow for **erythropoiesis**, which is the formation of new red blood cells. In patients with protein and iron malnourishment, deficiencies are even more striking when liver disease is present. The liver also produces clotting factors, making those with liver disease more prone to bleeding and bruising.

■ **Figure 5.12** Jaundice marked by the presence of a yellow sclera. (Image from Bickley LS, Szilagyi P. *Bates' Guide to Physical Examination and History Taking*. 8th ed. Philadelphia: Lippincott Williams & Wilkins; 2003, with permission.)

Viral Hepatitis

Viral hepatitis refers to inflammation of the liver caused by viral infection. The hepatitis viruses (A, B, C, D, and E) are often implicated in this disease. These are referred to as HAV, HBV, and so forth. Table 5.3 details the route of transmission, incubation, and other characteristics of the major hepatitis viruses. Other viruses, including herpes simplex virus, Epstein-Barr virus, and even Ebola virus, can also cause liver inflammation.

PATHOPHYSIOLOGY

The major routes of transmission for the hepatitis viruses include fecal–oral contact or contact with infected blood and body fluids. Fecal–oral transmission is a problem of hand contact with infected feces in which the virus is transmitted to another when encountering the oral mucosa. For example, if a food preparation worker does not thoroughly wash his or her hands after toileting, he or she can transmit the virus to restaurant patrons who consume the handled food. Contact with blood and body fluids, as

with hepatitis B, C, and D, are of particular concern for health care workers who are at high risk of contracting these infections because of frequent contact with blood and body fluids.

Once infected, hepatitis can lead to acute or chronic disease. Hepatitis B can also exist in an asymptomatic carrier state. In general, fecal–oral transmission leads to acute hepatitis, whereas transmission by blood and body fluids results in chronic disease. The level of damage in acute viral hepatitis can vary from death of a few hepatocytes to massive hepatic necrosis. An inflammatory response is waged and the local Kupffer cells help remove necrotic cells. Affected hepatocytes regenerate. Regeneration generally begins within 48 hours of hepatocyte necrosis. With severe infection, **fulminant hepatitis**, which is hepatic failure from severe acute hepatitis, can occur. Obstruction can occur in the blood vessels that perfuse the liver, resulting in tissue hypoxia. Bile flow can also become obstructed.

● **STOP** *and Consider*

What is the role of bile and why is obstruction of bile flow problematic?

Table 5.3 Characteristics of Hepatitis Viruses

	Transmission	Incubation	Carrier State	Chronic	Vaccine	Diagnosis
Hepatitis A	Fecal–oral from another infected person; contaminated food and water supplies	1–2 months	No	No	Yes	Blood detection of anti-HAV
Hepatitis B	Contact with infected blood and body fluids; infected mother to fetus	2–3 months	Yes	Yes	Yes	Blood detection of HBsAg
Hepatitis C	Contact with infected blood	2–3 months	Yes	Yes	No	Blood detection of anti-HCV
Hepatitis D	Contact with infected blood and body fluids; infected mother to fetus; *must* have HBsAg to be infected with hepatitis D (coinfection or superinfection)	2–3 months	Yes	Yes	No	Blood detection of anti-HDV
Hepatitis E	Fecal–oral from another infected person	1–2 months	No	No	No	Blood detection of anti-HEV

Likewise, chronic hepatitis can range from minimal damage to widespread hepatocyte necrosis, fibrosis, diffuse scarring, and cirrhosis. Chronic hepatitis is represented by impaired liver function for more than 6 months. The liver is infiltrated with macrophages and lymphocytes. Patients with chronic hepatitis also carry an increased risk of developing hepatocellular carcinoma related to persistent cell injury.

Cirrhosis is an end-stage liver disease marked by interference of blood flow to the liver and widespread hepatocyte damage. Interference of blood flow to the liver (1) exacerbates hypoxia of the hepatocytes and results in further cell death; (2) causes blood and bile to back up into the liver resulting in further injury and inflammation; and (3) obstructs blood flow from portal circulation. Liver failure and death may result.

STOP *and Consider*

Compare fulminant hepatitis and cirrhosis to general infection complications: septicemia and chronic infection.

CLINICAL MANIFESTATIONS

All types of viral hepatitis can cause acute, icteric illness. Three phases, similar to the general phases of infection, characterize acute hepatitis infection:

1. **Prodrome**: A period of fatigue, anorexia, malaise, headache, and low-grade fever. The prodrome usually lasts about 2 weeks.
2. **Icterus**: Marked by the onset of jaundice, dark urine, and clay-colored stools 2 weeks after exposure to the virus. This phase corresponds to the clinical illness phase discussed previously and lasts approximately 2 to 6 weeks. The liver is enlarged and tender.
3. **Recovery**: Marked by the resolution of jaundice around 8 weeks after the initial exposure to the virus. Signs and symptoms improve with the exception of the liver, which remains enlarged and tender for an additional 1 to 4 weeks.

A careful glance at Figure 5.13 will reveal the connection between pathophysiologic processes and clinical manifestations of liver failure.

DIAGNOSTIC CRITERIA

Diagnosis is often based on detection of viral antibodies, such as anti-HAV, anti-HCV, anti-HDV, and anti-HEV, in the blood of the infected person. The core of the hepatitis B virus contains two antigens: the core antigen (HBcAg) and the e antigen (HBeAg). Since there are three possible clinical courses for hepatitis B—complete recovery, asymptomatic carrier state, or chronic infection—the health professional must look at the corresponding antigen and antibody levels. Antibodies to the hepatitis B core antigen (IgM anti-HBc) are required for the diagnosis of acute hepatitis B infection.[7] Cells infected with hepatitis B virus also present surface antigens on the outer coating. The hepatitis B surface antigen (HBsAg) may be present in acute infection or in those who are chronic asymptomatic carriers. Other findings that may aid in diagnosis and prognosis include the detection of bilirubin in the urine, elevated serum bilirubin levels (more than 30 mg/dL indicates more severe disease), and prolonged clotting time (a grave finding that indicates impaired liver function).[7]

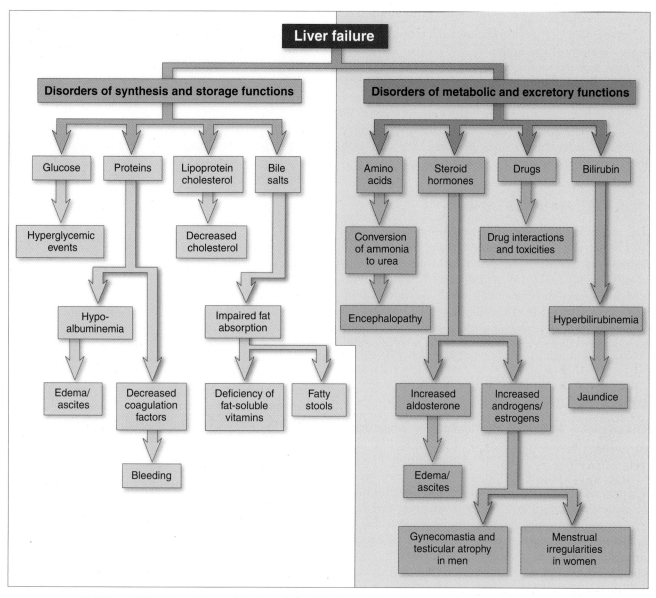

Figure 5.13 Concept map. Alterations in liver function and manifestations of liver failure. (Image modified from Porth CM. *Pathophysiology: Concepts of Altered Health States*. 7th ed. Philadelphia: Lippincott Williams & Wilkins; 2004, with permission.)

TREATMENT

Hepatitis A and hepatitis B can be prevented through vaccination. Treatment of acute viral hepatitis, as with other viral infections, is symptomatic. Fluids, rest, and analgesics are recommended, particularly during the icteric phase of illness. Avoidance of strenuous physical activity or contact sports is often recommended because of liver enlargement. Because bile helps with fat emulsification and absorption and because bile production may be impaired during liver disease, a low-fat diet is recommended. Antiviral medications may be used in chronic viral hepatitis to decrease viral replication. Avoidance of transmission to others is critical through careful hand washing, avoidance of contact with infected fecal material, and avoidance of contact with blood and body fluids where appropriate.

Urinary Tract Infection

Urinary tract infections (UTIs) are **ascending**; that is, microorganisms enter at the distal urethra and move up toward the bladder. The bacteria attach to the urinary tract epithelium, resulting in an acute inflammatory response.

PATHOPHYSIOLOGY

Escherichia coli is the most common microorganism implicated in UTI. *E. coli* is an aerobic, gram-negative bacterium and is resident flora in the GI tract. When gaining access into the urinary tract (which is a sterile area of the body), *E. coli* causes infection. Women are particularly vulnerable due to a short urethra and close proximity between the urethra and the anus. Mechanical obstruction of the urinary tract, such as with renal calculi (kidney stones) or an enlarged prostate, and introduction of urinary catheters into the urethra and bladder can also increase the likelihood of developing a UTI.

CLINICAL MANIFESTATIONS

The tissues in the urinary tract become edematous and hyperemic, which results in **dysuria** (pain with urination), urinary **urgency** (the need to immediately urinate), and urinary frequency. Tissue destruction in the urinary tract may result in **hematuria**, or blood in the urine. The inflammatory response to these bacteria produces a purulent exudate, which can be detected as cloudy urine with a microscopic increase in leukocytes.

DIAGNOSTIC CRITERIA

Diagnosis is based on the history of presenting symptoms along with physical examination and diagnostic tests. Physical examination may demonstrate suprapubic tenderness with palpation. Urinalysis and urine culture are required and must be obtained using a midstream or catheterized sample using the appropriate technique. **Pyuria**, or purulent exudate (pus) in the urine, found by performing the leukocyte esterase dip test, increases the likelihood of bacterial infection. The definition of UTI is based on a urine culture noting greater than 1,000 colonies of a single organism per milliliter. Imaging studies may be needed if urinary obstruction is suspected.

TREATMENT

The process of urination does assist in "flushing" out much of the bacteria that attempt to ascend the urethra. For this reason, increasing fluid intake is important for patients with UTI. Drug therapy with an antibiotic effective against gram-negative aerobic bacteria, such as *E. coli*, is the primary treatment intervention. Patients with diabetes mellitus, immunosuppression, or urinary tract obstruction, or patients who are pregnant, are more likely to develop complications with a UTI and must be aggressively treated with a prolonged course of antibiotics.[8] If UTI is untreated, the bacteria can continue to ascend into the kidneys and result in **pyelonephritis**, an acute kidney infection. Chronic infections in the urinary tract and kidneys can also occur. Chronic pyelonephritis is associated with scarring and impaired renal function.

Tinea

Tinea is a group of fungal skin diseases that occur in various locations, including the feet (tinea pedis), nails (tinea unguium), scalp (tinea capitis), groin (tinea cruris), and skin (tinea corporis and tinea versicolor). Fungal infections of the skin, hair, and nails are also called **dermatophyte** infections and are considered minor but extremely common.

PATHOPHYSIOLOGY

The major mode of transmission is direct contact with another person or surface reservoir. Risk factors for the development of dermatophyte infections include exposure to moist conditions, genetic predisposition, immunocompromise, and sharing of hygiene facilities (such as public showers) with infected persons. The dermatophyte attaches to and produces thickening of keratinized cells. The infection often remains localized. Complications include bacterial superinfection or generalized invasive dermatophyte infection.

CLINICAL MANIFESTATIONS

Clinical manifestations vary depending on the location of infection. All forms result in changes in the skin, hair, or nails. Tinea corporis is known as "ringworm" because the infection spreads circumferentially like an erythematous bull's-eye (Fig. 5.14A). Tinea versicolor presents as patches of hypopigmentation on the skin of the trunk and extremities. Tinea capitis results in hair loss or breakage at the site of infection. Tinea pedis is notable for scaling, fissuring, and maceration, most often between or around the toes. Tinea cruris ("jock itch") is characterized by erythematous lesions that have central clearing and raised borders. Tinea unguium affects the nails and leads to thickened, discolored (white, yellow, brown, or black), dystrophic changes and nail plate separation from the nail bed (Fig. 5.14B). Most forms of tinea can also cause pruritus (itching).

DIAGNOSTIC CRITERIA

The diagnosis of tinea is based on physical examination and laboratory studies, including direct microscopic examination of infected skin, nail, or hair, fungal cultures, and wood light examination. Hyphae on skin or nails and spores within or around

Figure 5.14 Tinea. **A:** Tinea corporis (ringworm). (Image provided by Stedman's.) **B:** Tinea unguium. (Image from Goodheart HP. *Goodheart's Photoguide of Common Skin Disorders*. 2nd ed. Philadelphia: Lippincott Williams & Wilkins; 2003, with permission.)

the hair shaft can be detected with microscopic examination. Wood light is a procedure of moving a portable ultraviolet light over the site of infection and noting a bright yellow-green or dull green fluorescence (i.e., glowing). This procedure is used primarily for tinea capitis.

TREATMENT

Fungal infections are treated with topical or oral antifungal agents. Treatment with topical therapy for dermatophyte infections of the skin commonly extends from 2 to 8 weeks. Topical therapy is ineffective for treating tinea in the hair and nails. These types require prolonged oral antifungal therapy. Prevention measures are also critical to avoid recurrence of infections. Practicing proper hygiene and avoiding contact with suspicious lesions on others can deter infection.

Bacterial Meningitis

Meningitis is inflammation of the membranes (meninges) of the brain and spinal cord (Fig. 5.15). The meninges are comprised of the dura mater, arachnoid, and pia mater. These tissue layers cover and protect the brain and spinal cord. Meningitis commonly results from infection with bacteria or viruses. Worldwide, the rates of meningococcal disease are highest in infants. Adolescents, young adults, and the elderly are also at risk. The epidemic prevalence of meningitis is 100 to 800 per 100,000 population. This rate is more than 2,000 cases per 100,000 in the "meningitis belt" (a lateral stretch across the bulge of the continent from Ethiopia to Senegal) of sub-Saharan Africa.[9]

PATHOPHYSIOLOGY

The most common bacterial cause of meningitis is *Neisseria menigitidis*, an aerobic, gram-negative bacterium. There are at least 13 different *N. menigitidis* subtypes, which are exclusively responsible for lethal epidemic meningitis.[10] Viral meningitis is often referred to as aseptic meningitis. It is generally less severe than bacterial meningitis and often resolves without specific treatment. Fungi can result in meningitis in individuals who are immunocompromised. Table 5.4 compares the different types of meningitis.

The mode of transmission for meningitis is respiratory droplets passed from an infected person to the host. The microorganism enters the respiratory tract and attaches to epithelial cells. Inflammatory and immune responses are waged. Immunoglobulins in the respiratory mucosa can provide protective immunity against the microorganisms. However, in some cases, the bacteria move through the mucosa and get into the central nervous system or the blood. The mechanism for entry into the blood and central nervous system is often unknown.

In the central nervous system, the bacteria multiply along the meninges and in the cerebral spinal fluid (CSF). The rapid proliferation of bacteria is related to few antibodies, complement components, and white blood cells in the CSF. The inflammatory response causes the brain tissues to become edematous (swollen) and hyperemic (filled with blood). The infectious process is perpetuated by the replication of bacteria (along with the influx of inflammatory cells) and increased capillary permeability. Exudate accumulates throughout the CSF, causing damage to cranial nerves, obstruction of CSF pathways, obstruction of blood flow to brain tissue, and reduced

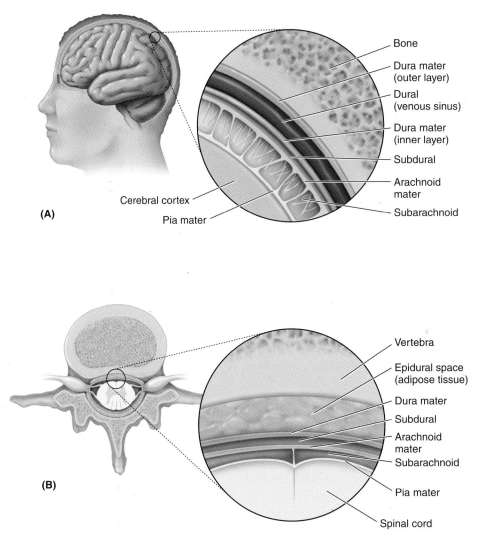

(A)

- Bone
- Dura mater (outer layer)
- Dural (venous sinus)
- Dura mater (inner layer)
- Subdural
- Arachnoid mater
- Subarachnoid

Cerebral cortex

Pia mater

(B)

- Vertebra
- Epidural space (adipose tissue)
- Dura mater
- Subdural
- Arachnoid mater
- Subarachnoid
- Pia mater

Spinal cord

■ **Figure 5.15**   Meninges of the **(A)** brain and **(B)** spinal cord. (Images from Nath J. *Using Medical Terminology: A Practical Approach*. Baltimore: Lippincott Williams & Wilkins; 2006, with permission.)

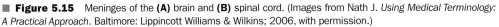

Table 5.4 Comparison of the Types of Meningitis

	Bacterial	Viral	Fungal
Common pathogens	*S. pneumoniae, N. meningitidis,* and *H. influenzae* (in those unimmunized)	Aseptic; variety of viral agents including enteroviruses, herpesviruses, HIV	Opportunistic fungi
Onset	Rapid (less than 24 hours)	1–7 days	>7 days
Severity of symptoms	Severe	Mild to moderate	Often mild
Predominant cells	Neutrophils	Lymphocytes	Lymphocytes
Changes in intracranial pressure	Increased	Normal or slightly increased	May be increased
CSF Gram stain	Positive bacteria	Negative	Negative
Glucose in CSF	Decreased	Normal	Decreased
Treatment	Antibiotics	Symptomatic, supportive	Antifungals

CSF, cerebral spinal fluid.

oxygen to the brain. Meningitis can result in septicemia. Septicemia damages endothelial cells of the vessels. Massive, systemic inflammation can then lead to septic shock.

CLINICAL MANIFESTATIONS

Acute bacterial meningitis is noted for a rapid and severe onset of symptoms (often within less than 24 hours). Irritation of the meninges results in the characteristic clinical manifestations: severe headache, light sensitivity (**photophobia**), and a hyperextended stiff neck (**nuchal rigidity**). The increase in intracranial pressure (ICP) from brain edema and resultant hypoxia (low oxygen) in the brain leads to decreased alertness, loss of consciousness, changes in mental status, vomiting, and seizures (Chapter 9). Systemic manifestations include fever, leukocytosis, and anorexia.

DIAGNOSTIC CRITERIA

The diagnosis of meningitis is often made through history and physical examination, blood and CSF analysis, and cultures. Kernig and Brudzinski signs are two common physical examination tests performed to determine the presence of meningeal irritation. Meningeal irritation is related to the influx of chemical mediators, inflammatory cells, and exudate into the CSF and meningeal tissues. To elicit meningeal pain using the **Kernig sign**, the patient is placed supine with the knees bent and hips flexed. The practitioner lifts and extends one knee upward. The Kernig sign is considered positive if moving the leg upward stretches the irritated meninges and elicits pain. Similarly, with the **Brudzinski sign**, the patient is supine. The practitioner quickly flexes the neck to the chest. Again, this activity stretches the irritated meninges at the neck. A positive Brudzinski sign occurs when the patient protects the irritated meninges by involuntarily flexing the hips and knees.

TREATMENT

Treatment involves intravenous antibiotics, corticosteroids, fluids, and other methods to decrease inflammation, maintain adequate blood pressure,

and maintain vital organ perfusion. Treatment should be started early in the disease to avoid septicemia and septic shock. The mortality rate is 50% to 90% for patients who are not diagnosed until after the onset of severe neurologic impairment.[11] Appropriate antibiotic treatment of most common types of bacterial meningitis should reduce the risk of dying from meningitis to below 15%. However, even with early recognition and treatment, the mortality risk is higher among the elderly. Treatment is also indicated for close household contacts who may have been exposed to *N. meningitidis*. Hospitalization may require respiratory isolation until the patient has been on antibiotics for at least 24 hours to prevent bacterial spread to other patients.

Immunization is an important step in preventing bacterial meningitis in all populations. Vaccination for *Haemophilus influenzae* is part of the recommended vaccine schedule for children. In October 1997, the American College Health Association recommended that all college students consider vaccination against meningococcal disease. College students are at particular risk due to close living quarters. One vaccine protects against four strains of *N. meningitidis* and would deter the onset of disease in this population.[11]

Summary

- Exposure to a microorganism elicits the inflammatory and immune responses. Infection results from inadequacies of the three lines of defense and represents a state of tissue destruction resulting from invasion by microorganisms.

- The chain of infection is a useful organization for recognizing the factors inherent in the transmission and spread of communicable disease. The links in the chain include the pathogen, portal of entry, reservoir, portal of exit, mode of transmission, and host. Infection control measures seek to break one or more of these links.
- Microorganisms that cause infection are called pathogens. The pathogenicity, or qualities that promote the production of disease, involves multiple factors, including the pathogen's potency, invasiveness, ability to evade the immune system, speed of replication, production of toxins, adherence to the human host cell, and degree of tissue damage that is elicited.
- Bacteria, viruses, fungi, and protozoa are common types of pathogens. Understanding the distinctive quality of each can provide clues to transmission and spread of each pathogen.
- Major modes of transmission include direct contact, droplet, airborne, and vector transmission. Hand washing is a critical step in preventing the spread of infection by direct contact. Universal precautions are a standard of health care that recognizes all blood and body fluid as potentially infected. Universal precautions dictate that health care providers wear gloves when having *any* contact with blood and body fluids. Masks and protective eyewear are also recommended if splattering of blood or body fluids is anticipated.
- Phases of an acute infection include exposure, incubation, prodrome, clinical illness, and convalescence. Clinical symptoms are dictated by the cells that are damaged by the invading microorganism.
- Complications of acute infection include septicemia and chronic infection with loss of function in the affected tissues.

Case Study 5.1

You are the parent of a 6-month-old child who is fussy and is tugging on her ears. You take her to the clinic and are told that she has otitis media, a middle ear infection. From your reading and experience regarding infectious processes, answer the following questions:

1. *Outline the process that is most likely occurring in this child's body.*
2. *What anatomic differences in a child would predispose to this type of infection?*

3. *What are the probable sources of this infection?*
4. *What would you expect for local and systemic clinical manifestations?*
5. *What diagnostic tests could be used? How could you differentiate between viral or bacterial pathogens?*
6. *What treatment measures would you anticipate?*
7. *What would be the potential complications?*

Log on to the Internet. Search for a relevant journal article or Web site that details otitis media and confirm your predictions.

Case Study 5.2

Jamie is a 48-year-old black woman who comes into the emergency department complaining of painful swelling, drainage, and redness over the past 5 days in the left hand. She spends a lot of time outdoors working in her garden and said she had a "pretty nasty" mosquito bite on the top of that hand before the swelling started. After 3 days of increased swelling and redness she went to her doctor and received an oral antibiotic and was told it was probably a mild infection from the insect bite. Now, she presents because her hand is increasingly painful, tight, and the drainage has worsened. She noticed that she had a fever this morning of 102.9°F. Laboratory test results today show a WBC count of 18,500. After intravenous antibiotic treatment and hospitalization the wound culture is found to be positive for methicillin-resistant *Staphylococcus aureus* (MRSA). From your reading and experience regarding infectious processes, answer the following questions:

1. *Outline the process that is most likely occurring in Jamie's body.*
2. *What is the probable source of this infection?*
3. *What would you expect for local and systemic clinical manifestations?*
4. *What diagnostic tests were used or could be used? How could you differentiate between viral or bacterial pathogens?*
5. *What additional treatment measures would you anticipate? How is MRSA treated differently than nonresistant pathogens?*
6. *What would be the potential complications?*

Log on to the Internet. Search for a relevant journal article or Web site that details MRSA and confirm your predictions.

Practice Exam Questions

1. You are looking to break the chain of infection by washing your hands frequently as you provide care for patients. Which of the following links in the chain will be broken by this activity?
   a. Reservoir
   b. Host
   c. Portal of entry
   d. Mode of transmission

2. Which of the following may make a person more susceptible to getting an infection?
   a. Age between 6 and 46 years
   b. Experiencing a surgery that is healing by primary intention
   c. Final exams week
   d. A functioning immune system

3. The feeling that "something is not quite right" is considered which stage in infection?
   a. Point of infection with pathogen
   b. Incubation
   c. Prodrome
   d. Acute symptoms

4. Which of the following clinical manifestations is not typically found with inflammation but is more characteristic of a bacterial infection?
   a. Purulent exudate
   b. Redness and swelling at the site
   c. Lymphadenopathy
   d. Fever

5. A white blood cell differential shows an increase in the number of monocytes and macrophages in the blood. This typically means that
   a. This is a new infection
   b. This is a chronic infection
   c. This is a viral infection
   d. The differential provides no useful information

6. Given the mode of transmission for influenza, how would you break the chain of infection and prevent spread?
   a. Administer antibiotics as directed
   b. Wash hands after toileting
   c. Disinfect table surfaces in the room
   d. Wear a mask

7. What aspects of bacterial activity would be effective targets for pharmacologic treatment?
   a. hepatitis B surface antigen (HBsAg)
   b. hepatitis B core antigen (HBcAg)
   c. Prothrombin time (PTT)
   d. There is no way to distinguish the different forms of hepatitis B

8. What is the most likely complication of an untreated UTI?
   a. Glomerulonephritis
   b. Pyelonephritis
   c. Fulminant UTI
   d. Urethritis

9. Treatment for tinea unguium must include
   a. Oral antifungals
   b. Topical antifungals
   c. Both topical and oral antifungals
   d. Nail removal and topical antifungals

10. Which of the following scenarios is most likely in the CSF of a patient with bacterial meningitis?
    a. CSF has high neutrophil count and high protein count
    b. CSF has high neutrophil count and low protein count
    c. CSF has high glucose level and high red blood cell count
    d. CSF has high lymphocyte count and low red blood cell count

Discussion and Application

1. What did I know about infection prior to today?

2. What body processes are affected by infection? What are the expected functions of those processes? How does infection affect those processes?

3. What are the potential etiologies for infection? How does infection develop?

4. Who is most at risk for developing an infection? How can infection be prevented?

5. What are the human differences that affect the etiology, risk, or course of infection?

6. What clinical manifestations are expected in the course of infection?

7. What special diagnostic tests are useful in determining the diagnosis and course of infection?

8. What are the goals of care for individuals with infection?

9. How does the concept of infection build on what I have learned in the previous chapters and in previous courses?

10. How can I use what I have learned?

RESOURCES

The World Health Organization (WHO) provides valuable information about the global infectious disease threat. The organization Web site can be accessed at:
http://www.who.int/.
An excellent review of the WHO strategy for containment of antimicrobial resistance can be found at www.who.int/drugresistance/en/.

The Centers for Disease Control and Prevention (CDC) provides a wealth of information on infectious disease prevention and spread. The Web site can be accessed at:
http://www.cdc.gov/.

The National Institute of Health provides research-based information related to allergy and infectious disease at:
http://www.niaid.nih.gov.

REFERENCES

1. Pouniotis D, Proudfoot O, Minigo G, et al. Malaria parasite interactions with the human host. *J Postgrad Med*. 2004;50(1):30–34.
2. Belay E, Schonberger L. The public health impact of prion diseases. *Annu Rev Public Health*. 2005;26:191–212.
3. Berzofsky J, Ahlers J, Janik J, et al. Process of new vaccine strategies against chronic viral infections. *J Clin Invest*. 2004;114:450–462.
4. Centers for Disease Control. Vaccines and preventable disease 2009. Available at: http://www.cdc.gov/vaccines/vpd-vac/default.htm. Accessed April 23, 2009.
5. Smith D, Lapedes A, deJong J, et al. Mapping the antigenic and genetic evolution of influenza virus. *Science*. 2004;305:371–376.
6. Montalto N. An office-based approach to influenza: clinical diagnosis and laboratory testing. *Am Fam Physician*. 2003;67(1):111–118.
7. Sjogren M. Serologic diagnosis of viral hepatitis. *Gastroenterol Clin North Am*. 1994;23:457–477.
8. Miller L, Tang A. Treatment of uncomplicated urinary tract infections in an era of increasing antimicrobials resistance. *Mayo Clin Proc*. 2004;79:1048–1054.
9. World Health Organization. Meningococcal disease 2009. Available at: http://www.who.int/ith/updates/2009_03_20/en/index.html. Accessed April 23, 2009.
10. Lepow M, Hughes P. Meningococcal immunology. *Immunol Allergy Clin North Am*. 2003;23:769–786.
11. Schuchat A, Robinson K, Wenger J. Bacterial meningitis in the United States in 1995. Active surveillance team. *N Engl J Med*. 1997;337:970–976.
12. Kyne L, Hamel M, Polavaram R, et al. Health care costs and mortality associated with nosocomial diarrhea due to *Clostridium difficile*. *Clin Infect Dis*. 2004;34:346–353.

Chapter 6

Genetic and Developmental Disorders

LEARNING OBJECTIVES

1. Define and use the key terms listed in this chapter.
2. Identify the implications of alteration in the structure and function of genes and chromosomes.
3. Describe inheritance patterns in single gene disorders and chromosomal disorders.
4. Compare and contrast the inheritance patterns of multifactorial and altered chromosomal disorders.
5. Discuss the influence of gene–environment interactions on developmental disorders and adult-onset development of disease.
6. Analyze the biologic, social, and ethical implications of genetic screening.
7. Apply concepts of alterations in genetics and development to clinical models.

INTRODUCTION

How do you feel today? How will you feel a week from now? How about a month or year from today? Although you probably do not think that far ahead, the story of your future health and risk of disease can be told by your genetic makeup. The study of genetics is the study of **heredity**, the passage of characteristics from parent to offspring. Your story is but one chapter in your family's book of heredity. Your health has been influenced by the genetic contributions of your parents and the contributions from all of the generations before them. Your genes will contribute to future chapters when passed on to your children. The road map of your life's journey toward health is designed by the genes that make you who you are. Your genetic makeup can sometimes lead directly to disease or can just point you in that direction, which can be changed by other things that you encounter along the way. An understanding of the genetic influences of health and disease provides the basis for the application of these concepts to the promotion of health and the prevention of disease.

Module 1

Review of Genetic Processes

Chapter 2 introduced the basic components of the genetic system in the discussion of cellular structure. This chapter expands on the genetic components of the cell and introduces other influences that are important in genetic regulation of health and disease. The nucleus houses the genetic components essential to life processes. The organization of these components will be presented in an ordered fashion to provide an overview of both structure and function. The processes of transcription and translation of genes and the replication of chromosomes will be highlighted as the basis for improved application to genetic and developmental alterations discussed in the modules that follow this review.

 DNA

Deoxyribonucleic acid (DNA) is a type of nucleic acid that contains a sugar (deoxyribose). DNA is usually found in the cell nucleus and mitochondria. DNA is responsible for the storage of genetic information. It is made up of four nitrogenous bases, including the **purines**, adenine (A) and guanine (G), and the **pyrimidines**, cytosine (C) and thymine (T). DNA is usually double stranded, with two single strands linked by the purine/pyrimidine combinations of A–T and C–G, also known as **base pairs**. These linked combinations bring the two single strands together in a double helix structure, connected by phosphate bonds. These products combine in specific ways, forming genes and chromosomes.

Genes

Genes are small functional hereditary units located on a specific site of a chromosome. Made up of pieces of DNA, most genes contain the information, or **genetic code**, for making a specific protein. Genes vary in size, and associated DNA nitrogenous base pairs total anywhere between several hundred to 1 million. Genes occur in pairs in somatic (body) cells and singly in gametes such as ova and sperm,

consistent with the chromosome makeup of those same cell types.

The four nitrogenous bases (adenine, guanine, cytosine, and thymine) that are the foundations for DNA base pairs and are also important in the formation of the genetic code. The sequence of three of these bases forms a **codon** (nucleotide triplet), a fundamental triplet code necessary for protein synthesis. The basic compounds produced by these codons are **amino acids**. Twenty different types of amino acids combine to form the basis of human proteins, produced by **ribonucleic acid (RNA)** as a result of reading the genetic code. Redundancy is built into this process, allowing production of a single amino acid from more than one combination of triplet nitrogenous bases in most cases (Table 6.1). The base pairs in RNA are similar to those described for DNA, with the exception that T is substituted by uracil (U) in the genetic code, resulting in purine/pyrimidine combinations of A–U and C–G (Fig. 6.1). RNA delivers DNA's genetic message to the cytoplasm of a cell where proteins are made. The process of protein production by genes is complex. A brief

Table 6.1 Amino Acids and Their Genetic Codes

Amino Acid	Symbol	Codons
Alanine	Ala	GCA, GCC, GCG, GCU
Cysteine	Cys	UGC, UGU
Aspartic acid	Asp	GAC, GAU
Glutamic acid	Glu	GAA, GAG
Phenylalanine	Phe	UUC, UUU
Glycine	Gly	GGA, GGC, GGG, GGU
Histidine	His	CAC, CAU
Isoleucine	Ile	AUA, AUC, AUU
Lysine	Lys	AAA, AAG
Leucine	Leu	UUA, UUG, CUA, CUC, CUG, CUU
Methionine	Met	AUG
Asparagine	Asn	AAC, AAU
Proline	Pro	CCA, CCC, CCG, CCU
Glutamine	Gln	CAA, CAG
Arginine	Arg	AGA, AGG, CGA, CGC, CGG, CGU
Serine	Ser	AGC, AGU, UCA, UCC, UCG, UCU
Threonine	Thr	ACA, ACC, ACG, ACU
Valine	Val	GUA, GUC, GUG, GUU
Tryptophan	Trp	UGG
Tyrosine	Tyr	UAC, UAU

Cytosine

Guanine

Adenine

Uracil

Nitrogenous
bases

RNA
Ribonucleic
acid

Nitrogenous bases

Base pair

Sugar
phosphate
backbone

DNA
Deoxyribonucleic
acid

Cytosine

Guanine

Adenine

Thymine

Nitrogenous
bases

Figure 6.1 Base pairs in RNA and DNA. Uracil is the nitrogenous base in RNA, corresponding with the thymine base in DNA. Note the single helix structure of RNA in contrast to the double helix structure of DNA.

The process of making a protein from a gene is highly complex and sometimes difficult to understand. One way to think of this process in a more simplified way is to consider the basic steps of transcribing and translating a gene with something more familiar, like reading. The nucleus is like the library. It contains the complete complement of genetic materials as the library has a full range of books needed to satisfy any reader. Within the nucleus are the chromosomes that contain genes. The genes are located along specific areas of each numbered chromosome. This is like the books arranged in the library by the Dewey Decimal or Library of Congress Classification systems so that what is sought can be easily found. Within each section of books are those that are arranged by topic or subject matter. This is similar to the arrangement of the organization of exons and introns along genes that serve to provide the code and regulation for the transcription of the DNA nucleotide bases. The mRNA reads the series of DNA nucleotide bases and *transcribes* them into complementary RNA nucleotide bases, a process similar to identifying the letters in a word. Each letter is taken so that pieces of words or syllables are formed, like the process of sounding out each part of a word in the process of reading. This process is similar to taking the transcribed mRNA nucleotide bases and *translating* them into the nucleotide triplet, or codon. The nucleotide bases that make up each codon are translated by the tRNA, complementing those transcribed by the mRNA. Next, each syllable comes together to make a word. The tRNA moves the nucleotide triplet out of the nucleus to the ribosomes where each triplet is made into the corresponding amino acid. The amino acids combine in particular ways to form polypeptide chains, similar to how words form sentences. Finally, polypeptide chains combine to form large proteins of various sizes in the way that sentences come together to form paragraphs, chapters, and whole books.

overview is presented in Figure 6.2 to help apply this information to health and disease.

Three types of RNA are involved in the process of protein production. **Messenger RNA (mRNA)** provides a template for protein synthesis depending on a codon sequence that is based on that of the complementary strand of DNA (cDNA). Through the process of **alternative splicing**, certain pieces of the RNA called **exons** are retained, and other segments, **introns**, are excised. The genetic code directs the specific splice location, allowing for a large variety of mRNA molecules to be transcribed from a single gene. **Transfer RNA (tRNA)** delivers these products into the cell (Fig. 6.2). Each tRNA recognizes and binds a specific amino acid, which it then transfers to organelles called ribosomes. Ribosomes are formed by a combination of **ribosomal RNA (rRNA)** produced in the nucleolus and nuclear ribosomal proteins. These ribosomes are transported from the nucleus to the cytoplasm where many attach to the endoplasmic reticulum, associate with mRNA, and begin protein synthesis, also known as **translation** of the genetic code.

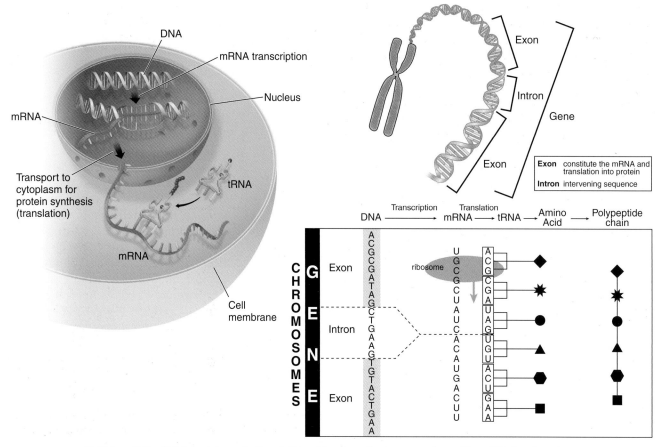

Figure 6.2 RNA in protein production. In the cell nucleus, the gene exon is read by mRNA, forming a template based on the DNA nucleotide bases for transcription of the genetic code. The message is transported to the cytoplasm, where it is transferred by tRNA to ribosomes on the endoplasmic reticulum producing amino acids. Translation of the genetic code begins the process of protein synthesis.

Chromosomes

Chromosomes are composed of double-stranded DNA containing threadlike sections of genes, most commonly found in the cell nucleus (Fig. 6.3). During cell division, chromosomes reproduce their physical and chemical structures, passing on genetic information. The process of cell division and creation of new cells is a result of the processes of **mitosis** and **meiosis**. In mitosis, the chromosomes in the nuclei of somatic cells go through a series of phases (prophase, prometaphase, metaphase, anaphase, and telophase) resulting in the creation of daughter cells with the same chromosome number and genetic makeup as the original somatic cell. The somatic cells of the body each contain chromosome pairs, also known as chromatids, linked by a **centromere**. The end of each chromatid is comprised of DNA segments known as telomeres. DNA is wound around spool-like protein cores known as histones. Each human somatic body cell contains 23 pairs of chromosomes, or a total of 46, also known as the **diploid** number of chromosomes. Of the total number of chromosomes, 44 are **autosomes** (chromosomes

Figure 6.3 Nuclear chromosomes. Chromosomes are comprised of two chromatids joined by a centromere. Chromosomes contain compacted DNA with an individual's unique genetic information.

other than a sex chromosome) and 2 are **sex chromosomes**. The two sex chromosomes, known as X and Y, are the genetic determinants of the sex of an individual. Females possess two X chromosomes and males one X and one Y.

Gametes (ova and sperm) contain only one of the chromosome pairs, known as the **haploid** number of chromosomes. Germ cells (ova and sperm) are produced through a process known as meiosis. In meiosis, one cell produces four cells, each with half the number of chromosomes, known as gametocytes. When sperm divide, four spermatids result. When ova divide, three polar bodies and only one ovum are produced. These cell numbers reflect their roles in reproduction. The combination of ova and sperm genetic material at the time of conception results in a cell with the diploid number of chromosomes. In this way, each parent contributes one chromosome; therefore, children get half of their chromosomes from their mothers and half from their fathers.

Chromosomal Replication

Each of the DNA strands of the double helix is important in replication of genetic information, but only one forms the template for **transcription**, or the transfer of the genetic code from one type of nucleic acid to another. The other strand serves as a complement to the strand used in transcription. Before cellular reproduction, the two DNA strands separate from the helix, and each forms new strands made up of matching base pairs next to each original strand. The result is four strands, doubles of each of the two original strands (Fig. 6.4). When the cell divides by the process of mitosis, these duplicated molecules are separated and placed in a daughter cell, each with a double

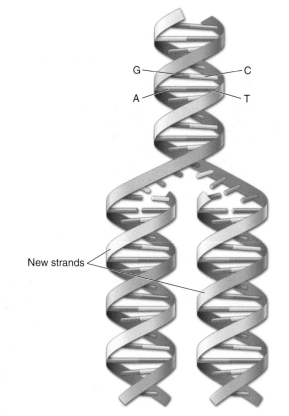

Figure 6.4 Genetic replication. The DNA strands in the double helix replicate to form two identical double helices to be placed in the daughter cells when the cell divides.

strand formed by the transcription strand and its complement.

STOP *and Consider*

What would happen to protein synthesis if the gene didn't turn on? If one of the nucleotide bases was substituted for another? If one extra nucleotide base was added to an exon?

Module 2

Inheritance of Genetic Disorders

Since the 1850s, when Gregor Mendel began the first work on the study of genetics in his experiments with garden peas, much has been learned about human genetics and the way traits are passed on from one generation to the next. Although none of the genetic concepts was known at the time, Mendel recognized the presence of factors that controlled the physical features of plants. He also realized that some of these "factors" had more influence, or were more dominant,

than others. Mendel determined laws of genetic traits, described by the following categories:

* Autosomal dominant
* Autosomal recessive
* Sex-linked dominant
* Sex-linked recessive

The discovery of the double helix structure of DNA by Watson and Crick in 1953 was followed by other discoveries that greatly improved our understanding of genetics.

Study of the human genome, or the full DNA sequence, is known as **genomics**. Genomics reflects not just the study of single genes but the functions and interactions of all the genes in the genome, including interactions between genes and with genes and the environment. An international research project, the Human Genome Project, was started in 1990 with goals to map each human gene and to completely sequence human DNA. After completion of the project in 2003, work continues to analyze the tremendous amount of data generated by this project. The identification of the location of specific genes on chromosomes provides an opportunity for scientists to pinpoint the cause of genetic disease and is the basis for current and future strategies to prevent or treat genetic defects. The interactions between genes and the environment provide the basis for application in other areas of study including nutrigenomics (the effect of nutrients on health through nutrient–genome interactions) and pharmacogenomics (interactions between drugs and the genome that affect the efficacy or toxicity in the human response).

It may be possible to improve health by understanding the mechanisms of disease contributing to complex conditions such as hypertension, diabetes, and asthma through the study of the human genome.[1] Instead of targeting specific individuals for screening of genetic information to predict disease, genetic screening in the future will be done on entire populations, allowing the identification of risk groups to determine susceptibility to disease.[2]

Identification of individuals with risks for specific conditions provides an opportunity to intervene and initiate strategies to prevent the development of disease before it begins. Newborn screening is an example of this type of screening and has been in place since the 1960s. All states require newborns to be screened for certain genetic disorders, although not all states have the same requirements. Recommendations from the March of Dimes include testing for 29 different genetic disorders with known treatments, and an additional 25 secondary target disorders without any known effective treatment. Some of the most commonly tested newborn diseases are included in Table 6.2.

Transmission and Expression of Genetic Traits

Traits are transmitted to each generation by the gametes: the ova and the sperm. Each parent contributes one set of chromosomes, ensuring that each off-

Table 6.2 Common Newborn Screening Tests

Disease	Pathology	Newborns Affected	Consequences If Left Untreated	Treatment
Phenylketonuria (PKU)	Inability to break down the amino acid, phenylalanine	1 in 14,000	Brain damage and mental retardation	Avoid foods with phenylalanine
Hypothyroidism	Thyroid hormone deficiency	1 in 3,000	Retards growth and brain development	Replacement of thyroid hormone
Galactosemia	Inability to convert the sugar galactose into glucose for energy	1 in 50,000	Death, blindness, and mental retardation	Avoid foods with galactose
Sickle cell anemia	Inherited blood disease causing abnormal shape and function in RBCs	1 in 400 African American	Infection, pain, organ damage, and death	Early identification and treatment of symptoms and prevention of infection and triggers
Congenital adrenal hyperplasia (CAH)	Group of disorders from deficiencies in hormones	1 in 19,000	**Altered genital development, kidney function,** and death	Replacement of missing hormones
Biotinidase deficiency	Deficiency of biotinidase, an enzyme that recycles biotin, a B vitamin	1 in 60,000	Frequent infections, hearing loss, mental retardation, and death	Replacement with additional biotin
Maple syrup urine disease	Inability to break down the essential amino acids leucine, valine, and isoleucine	1 in 230,000	Mental retardation, seizure, and death	Diet low in leucine, valine, and isoleucine
Homocystinuria	Inability to break down the amino acid methionine	1 in 340,000	Growth problems, developmental delay, and mental retardation	Vitamin B_6 therapy
Medium-chain acyl-CoA dehydrogenase **deficiency**	Inability to use fat for energy	1 in 20,000	Sudden infant death and mental retardation	Steady food intake and avoidance of fasting

spring has two genes at each locus, or location on the chromosome, when these chromosomes combine. The combination of the ova and sperm at the time of conception determines the genetic makeup of an individual, or the **genotype**. The genotype of a person is not always apparent or visible. A person's **phenotype** refers to the traits that are apparent or observable. Examples of these kinds of traits include gender, blood type, and eye or hair color. Genes may have many forms, such as those determining hair or eye color, that determine offspring traits, due to **alleles** (a series of two or more different genes occupying the same location on a specific chromosome). Other traits, known as **polygenic**, result from the interaction of several genes and are influenced by environmental factors. The transmission of genetic traits is specific for the trait and can be a complex process.

Many diseases result from damage to genes or chromosomes. These defects can be the result of spontaneous damage (de novo), environmental insult, or they can be an inheritable defect. Errors in DNA duplication can occur and result in genetic **mutations**. These mutations become permanent structural alterations in DNA. They are often resolved by DNA repair mechanisms, which prevent serious harm. However, when these repair mechanisms fail, the damaged genetic material can be passed on. The effects of mutations can be variable, ranging from no effect at all, to change in the expression of a trait or the function of a cell. Occasionally, a **somatic mutation** (not inheritable) can result in a **polymorphism** (gene occurring in more than one form). This common DNA variation can occur among individuals and have no impact on health (e.g., having one brown eye and one blue eye). Other mutations result in permanent change in genetic material, forming the basis of disease. In some cases, mutations affecting the control of cellular proliferation can result in cancer, which is discussed in Chapter 7. The transmission of genetic mutation is affected by the **expressivity** of the mutation, or the way the gene is expressed in the phenotype, which can range from mild to severe. **Penetrance**, the ability of a gene to express a mutation, can also influence the effects of genetic mutations. Obviously, many variables influence the complexity of the transmission of genetic traits.

Inheritance of Single Gene Disorders

Some traits are passed on by the transmission of a single gene and are known as **single gene traits**.

When people have identical alleles on each chromosome, they are **homozygous** for that gene. If they have two different alleles on each chromosome, they are **heterozygous** for that gene. Inheritance of single gene traits follows a **Mendelian pattern** of predictable trait transmission based on autosomal dominant or recessive genotypes. On autosomal chromosomes, some alleles have more influence than others. **Dominant** forms of a gene are more likely to be expressed in a person. **Recessive** genes are less influential, requiring homozygous alleles to be expressed. A dominant allele, when combined with a recessive allele, may prevent the phenotypic expression of the recessive gene, although both alleles comprise the genotype. An example of the application of this concept is a person who is heterozygous for the alleles that contribute to eye color. That person may have a dominant allele for brown eyes and a recessive allele for blue eyes in his or her genotype but express the trait of brown eyes in his or her phenotype due to the imbalance in the influence of the two alleles. A person must be homozygous for a recessive gene in order for it to be expressed in the phenotype. Therefore, for a person to express the recessive trait of blue eyes, he or she must be homozygous for the allele for blue eyes (Fig. 6.5).

The sex chromosomes, X and Y, determine gender at conception. X chromosomes are much larger than Y and carry much more genetic material. Females have two copies of the X chromosome (XX), whereas males have one copy of X and one of Y (XY). The X chromosome is inherited from both parents in the female but only from the mother in the male. Traits passed on by sex chromosomes are known as **sex-linked**. These traits are most often recessive and are linked to the X chromosome. While females possess two copies of the X chromosome, one becomes inactivated, leading to variable expression patterns of X-linked genes. In males, the genes are inherited on the single copy of the X chromosome. Males are usually affected by this recessive disorder because they have only one X chromosome. Females are usually carriers because they have two copies of the X chromosome.

From the Lab

Newborn screening is done using a variety of different types of tests. One of the oldest tests is the Guthrie bacterial inhibition assay, initially developed to identify infants with the metabolic disorder phenylketonuria (PKU). The use of tandem mass spectrometry allows for the identification of a wide array of amino acid, fatty acid, and organic acid metabolic disorders from a sample of dried blood on filter paper.[3] DNA testing of newborns for such diseases as cystic fibrosis can be done to get an early diagnosis and to initiate treatment for optimal wellness.

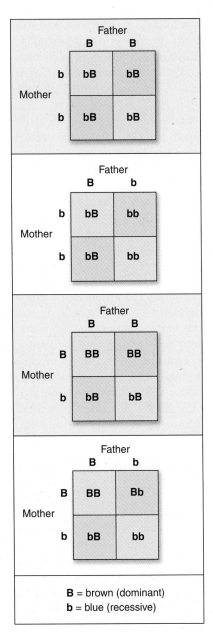

B = brown (dominant)
b = blue (recessive)

Figure 6.5 Eye color inheritance. Brown eye color will result if any of the combinations contains the dominant allele (BB, bB, Bb). Blue eyes will result from a combination of the recessive alleles (bb).

GENETIC MUTATIONS

Inheritable single gene mutations follow the Mendelian pattern of inheritance in a clearly identifiable and predictable manner. Single gene disorders occur at a specific, single site on the strand of DNA as a result of the following:

- Deletion
- Duplication
- Inversion
- Insertion
- Translocation

These mutations are caused by the change of a base pair that leads to an error in the transcription of a single codon, which in turn leads to the abnormal formation of proteins (Fig. 6.6). The resulting alteration in cellular function leads to the manifestation of disease. Specific mechanisms of genetic alterations can now be considered as causative factors of damage in autosomal and sex-linked gene errors. Table 6.3 describes the patterns of inheritance in single gene disorders.

Autosomal Dominant Disorders

Most hereditary disorders involve the genes on autosomes because there are more of these types of chromosomes (22 pairs) than sex chromosomes (1 pair). Because the genetic mutations occur on autosomes, the resulting disorders affect males and females equally (Fig. 6.7). If one parent is heterozygous for the autosomal dominant disorder, each child has a 50% chance of inheriting the damaged gene. In offspring who inherit the damaged allele, the dominant nature of the gene is likely to lead to disease, even when the offspring is heterozygous for the allele. Examples of diseases having this type of autosomal dominant inheritance pattern include Huntington disease (HD) (described in detail in Clinical Models), Marfan syndrome, and osteogenesis imperfecta.

Autosomal Recessive Disorders

Autosomal recessive inheritance patterns result in a different pattern of disease expression than the autosomal dominant disorders (Fig. 6.8). Because of the recessive nature of the genes involved, a child must be homozygous for the mutated gene to express the disease. This means that both parents must have at least one copy of the damaged gene for the disease to be passed on to their children. The mutated recessive

Research Notes

Prostate cancer is the most common cancer among American men (usually over 65 years old), causing more than 40,000 deaths. It is estimated that approximately 181 of 100,000 African American men will be diagnosed with prostate cancer this year, with 54 of those dying from the disease. This disease appears to run in families, leading to investigation into the genetic link to the disease by scientists at the National Human Genome Research Institute (NHGRI). These scientists have identified the location of a gene, called *HPC-1*, that is associated with increased risk of prostate cancer.[4]

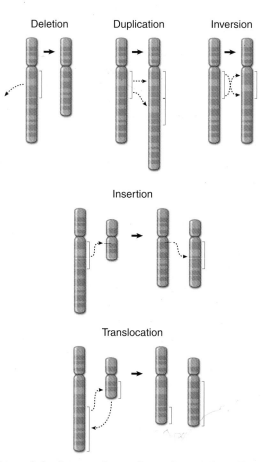

Figure 6.6 Common forms of genetic mutations. The alterations in cellular function caused by genetic mutation lead to the manifestation of disease.

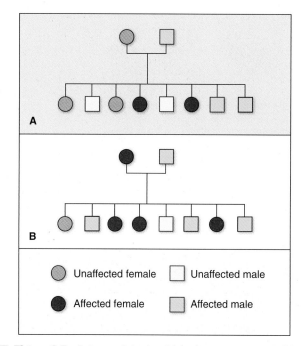

Figure 6.7 Autosomal dominant inheritance patterns. **A:** When only one parent is heterozygous for the dominant diseased gene, the child has a 50% chance of having the disease and a 50% chance of being unaffected. **B:** When both parents are heterozygous for the diseased gene, the child has only a 25% chance of being unaffected and a 75% chance of having the disease.

gene may be present in their genotype but not in their phenotype. In other words, they may be unaware that they have the mutated gene because they do not have the disease. Individuals who are heterozygous for a recessive gene mutation are known as **carriers**.

If both parents are carriers, their child has a 25% chance of expressing the disorder. If only one parent is a carrier, the child has an equal chance of being a carrier (50%) or be completely unaffected (50%). If both parents are homozygous for the gene and have the disease, all of their children will also have the disease by inheriting both damaged alleles from their parents. When one parent is homozygous for the gene mutation and has the disease and the other does not carry the recessive gene mutation, all of their children will be carriers with the ability to pass on the mutated gene. Autosomal recessive disorders appear more frequently within specific populations, where the likelihood of carriers is greater. Examples of autosomal recessive disorders are cystic fibrosis, Tay–Sachs disease, thalassemia, and sickle cell disease (described further under Clinical Models).

Table 6.3 Patterns of Inheritance in Single Gene Disorders

Inheritance Pattern	Allele Configuration	Transmission	Expression	Carrier	Noncarrier
Autosomal dominant disorders	Heterozygous	One heterozygous parent	50%	0%	50%
Autosomal recessive disorders	Homozygous	One homozygous and one noncarrier parent	None	100%	0%
		Two heterozygous parents	25%	50%	25%
Sex-linked disorders	Paternal X link	Transmitted to daughters only	0%	100%	0%
	Maternal X link	Transmitted to daughters and sons	50% sons	50% daughters	50% sons 50% daughters
Mitochondrial gene disorders	Maternal link	Transmitted to daughters and sons	Variable	Variable	Variable

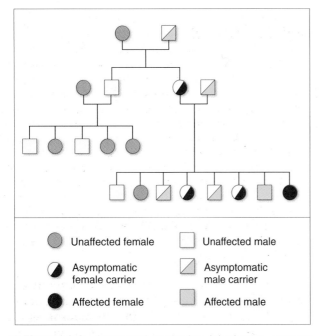

■ Figure 6.8 Autosomal recessive inheritance patterns. Recessive genes are expressed in the phenotype when the child is homozygous for the disease gene. If the inherited genotype is heterozygous, the child is a carrier of the disease gene and has the ability to continue this inheritance pattern. When one parent is a carrier, the children have a 50% chance of being a carrier themselves. If both parents are carriers, 25% of the children will be unaffected, 25% will be affected, and 50% will become carriers of the disease gene.

Sex-Linked Disorders

Mutations of genes located on the sex chromosomes, X or Y, are called sex-linked disorders. Many of these disorders are linked to genes on the X chromosome, or X-linked, and are usually recessive. For this reason, there is a gender difference in expression of X-linked disorders. Because females have two copies of the X chromosome, they are usually carriers of disease. Males have only one copy of the X chromosome and therefore are more likely to express the genetic disorder. Y-linked diseases result from the inheritance of a gene mutation on the Y chromosome from the father and are less common than X-linked disorders.

Sex-linked disorders are inherited based on which parent has the gene mutation. When the father carries the defective gene on the X chromosome, all daughters will be carriers and sons will be unaffected (Fig. 6.9A). When the mother is a carrier and passes the defective gene to her child, her daughters will have a 50% chance of being a carrier and her sons will have a 50% chance of being affected (Fig. 6.9B). Hemophilia and X-linked severe combined immunodeficiency (XSCID), often referred to as "bubble boy disease," are examples of X-linked disorders, with females carrying the defect and only males expressing the disease.

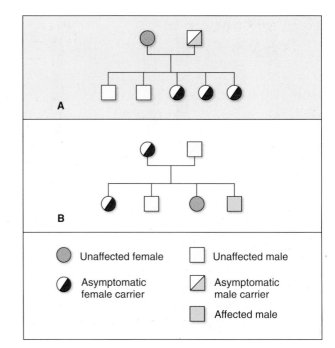

■ Figure 6.9 Sex-linked inheritance patterns. **A:** Carrier status is limited to female children and males are unaffected when the damaged gene is inherited from the father. **B:** Expression of recessive X-linked traits occurs only in males when the defective gene is inherited from the mother.

Mitochondrial Gene Disorders

The pattern of mitochondrial gene transmission is different from the transmission of nuclear genes. Although most genes can be found in the cell nucleus, several dozen genes can be found in the mitochondria. The functions of these genes are associated with the overall function of mitochondria and are often related to energy production. Sperm do not carry a significant number of mitochondrial genes; therefore, men do not pass mitochondrial gene disorders on to their offspring. Most mitochondrial genes are passed on through the maternal gametes (ova), which are dense with mitochondrial genes. For this reason, mitochondrial genes are transmitted only through female or maternal lines, in a **matrilineal** inheritance pattern.

Leigh syndrome is a condition involving mitochondrial DNA (mtDNA). Manifestations usually occur in the first year of life and include hypotonia, spasticity, peripheral neuropathy, encephalopathy, ataxia, and vision and hearing loss. Manifestations of mitochondrial gene disorders are variable because of the heteroplasmic features of these disorders. **Heteroplasmy** refers to the random distribution of mitochondria to daughter cells during embryonic cell division, leading to a variable distribution of mutant mitochondrial genes in tissues of an individual and between related individuals. Manifestations are revealed when the mutant mitochondria reach a critical level, or threshold.

Inheritance of Polygenic Disorders

Polygenic inheritance involves multiple alleles at different loci affecting phenotype. The expression of disease often involves a complex interaction of multiple factors that impact the interaction between genes and environment. Environmental influences modulate the phenotypic expression of a trait in multifactorial inheritance. An example of this type of inheritance is the height of an individual. Height is influenced by the combination of genes inherited from both parents, but it can also be influenced by environmental factors, including nutrition and hormones.

Certain environmental conditions must be present for expression of a genetic trait that leads to disease. Factors that can increase expression of disease include chemicals (alcohol, tobacco, drugs, and hormones), nutrition, and altitude. Clinical manifestations of multifactorial disorders may be seen at birth and include such disorders as cleft lip/palate, clubfoot, and neural tube defects (NTDs), including anencephaly and spina bifida (discussed in more detail in Clinical Models). Other multifactorial disorders are not expressed until the person ages, including hypertension, coronary artery disease, diabetes, and many cancers.

STOP *and Consider*

The process of genetic selection is based on reproductive practices that result in offspring with desired traits. These practices are in use today in the animal industry, where animals are bred for desired qualities such as increased milk production in dairy cows or desired characteristics in show dogs. Food products are genetically manipulated to have traits of disease resistance. What are the health implications of genetic selection in humans? What are the social and ethical implications?

Inheritance of Chromosomal Alterations

Chromosomal alterations may result from the loss, addition, or rearrangement of genetic material. Chromosomal alterations can be detected by assessing an individual's karyotype, or chromo-

Research Notes

Human genome mapping and improved technology identifying DNA patterns have stimulated applications of the gleaned information in areas beyond human health. These include the use of DNA as evidence in identifying criminals. First used in 1983, DNA evidence has been used to convict individuals of crimes and to exonerate innocent individuals.[6,7] This practice is commonly referred to as "DNA fingerprinting." Current DNA technology uses **short tandem repeats (STRs)**, lengths of DNA stretches that are unique to an individual. STRs from suspect individuals are compared with national databases for rapid and accurate identification. In addition, mtDNA provides information about maternal lineage, and Y-specific STRs provide evidence for paternal lineage. These techniques are most often used in historical identification, such as the determination of lineage of the Russian royal family, the Romanovs. These techniques were especially useful in identifying the remains of victims of the World Trade Center disaster, leading to positive identification of more than 1,500 individuals.

somal complement. A **karyotype** is a picture of arranged, paired, like chromosomes in order of largest to smallest (Fig. 6.10). Chromosomes are matched by centromere location and banding pattern (see From the Lab on page 136).

ALTERATIONS IN CHROMOSOMAL NUMBER

Chromosomes separate during mitosis and meiosis in a process known as disjunction. When chromosomes fail to separate, the result is **nondisjunction** (Fig. 6.11). Nondisjunction results in an unequal number of chromosomes between cells. The timing of nondisjunction determines the number of

■ **Figure 6.10** Karyotype. The karyotype shows the 23 pairs of chromosomes from a man. Notice the size of the Y chromosome compared with the X chromosome. (Image from Bear MF, Connors B, Paradiso M. *Neuroscience: Exploring the Brain*. Baltimore: Lippincott Williams & Wilkins; 2006, with permission.)

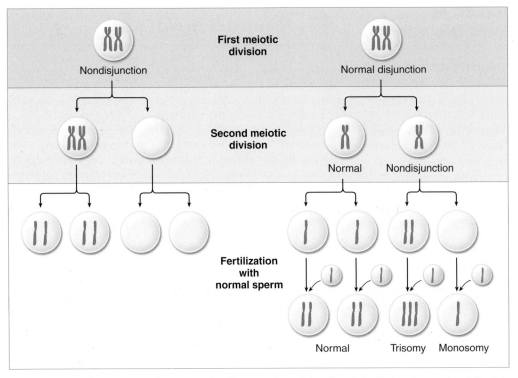

Figure 6.11 Chromosomal nondisjunction. Process of nondisjunction at the first and second meiotic divisions of the ovum and fertilization with normal sperm. (Image modified from Pillitteri A. *Maternal and Child Nursing*. 4th ed. Philadelphia: Lippincott Williams & Wilkins; 2003, with permission.)

cells involved. If it occurs soon after conception, it may affect all of the resulting cells. If it happens later, some cells will be affected and others will be normal. The term **mosaicism** refers to the combination of cells with the regular chromosome number and those with an altered number of chromosomes; the effects are determined by the ratio. The risk of nondisjunction increases with parental age.

Monosomy occurs when nondisjunction results in cells with one copy of a chromosome instead of two. If this occurs in autosomes, this defect is not compatible with life. Although monosomy in the sex chromosome is compatible with life, significant physical and mental defects result. An example of a condition that results from monosomy of the sex chromosome includes Turner syndrome (TS), described in more detail under Clinical Models.

Trisomy refers to the presence of three copies of a chromosome in a cell. The viability of the individual is determined based on which specific chromosome is affected. If a large chromosome is affected, trisomy is incompatible with life because large chromosomes contain a great deal of genetic material. When trisomy occurs in chromosome 21, the condition known as Down syndrome results. Children born with Down syndrome have characteristic facial features, small stature, physical defects, and neurologic involvement. The clinical manifestations for a person with Down syndrome can be modified by the degree of mosaicism (see Clinical Model: Down Syndrome).

From the Lab

Chromosomal abnormalities can be determined by examining the number and structure of chromosomes through evaluation of the karyotype. The first step in evaluating a person's karyotype is obtaining a cell sample. Cells are prepared and chromosomes removed during mitosis, at which time they can best be seen under a microscope. The chromosomes are attached to a slide and stained with a special dye called Giemsa. A striped, or banded, appearance results from the dye staining of regions rich in adenine and thymine base pairs. A picture of the chromosomes is then taken and the single chromosomes are matched with their pairs and arranged from largest to smallest. There are three criteria for matching chromosomes: size, Giemsa banding pattern, and centromere position.

ALTERATIONS IN CHROMOSOMAL STRUCTURE

Translocation occurs when a large segment of DNA breaks from one chromosome and reattaches to a different chromosome, often occurring during meiosis. If the translocation is balanced, this abnormal arrangement does not affect the individual because he or she still retains the same amount of genetic material. It can seriously affect any offspring who inherits the defective chromosome, as the genetic complement inherited on the altered chromosome will result in either missing or excessive genes in the offspring.

Epigenetic Inheritance

Epigenetic is defined as "around the genome." Epigenetic modifications are caused by environmental and metabolic agents that stimulate chemical modifications of genes. The chemical modifications mostly include histone acetylation and DNA methylation. The epigenetic modifications change the expression of the gene without causing genetic mutation. The change in gene expression induced by epigenetic modification may persist even after removal of the initiating agent and has the potential to be passed to offspring. Epigenetic modifications of gene expression are heritable, with the potential to influence the health of future generations.

Genomic imprinting is the mechanism that controls expression of genes based on parental origin. Genomic imprinting is an epigenetic phenomenon resulting in regulation of the expression of gene activity without alteration of genetic structure. The process of genetic imprinting is usually the result of DNA methylation, preventing transcription of the gene. Genomic imprinting occurs when both maternal and paternal alleles are present, with only one allele expressed and the other

allele inactive. Approximately 20 known genes are affected by imprinting, causing different diseases based on whether they were inherited from the mother or the father. For example, diseases inherited from the mother (maternal) include myotonic muscular dystrophy (MMD) and fragile X syndrome (FXS) (see description in Clinical Models). Those inherited from the father (paternal) include Wilms tumor, osteosarcoma, bilateral retinoblastoma, and embryonal rhabdomyosarcoma—forms of cancer resulting from inactivation of the tumor suppressor gene. Two classic conditions that illustrate the influence of imprinting on expression of genetic disorders include PWS and AS (see From the Lab below).

From the Lab

Prader-Willi syndrome (PWS) and Angelman syndrome (AS) are two separate diseases caused by changes in an identical region of DNA on the long arm (q) of chromosome 15. These diseases are the result of genomic imprinting expressed by differences in DNA modification by methylation and are determined by inheritance of the abnormality from either the mother or the father. When the methylated gene is inherited from the mother, the defect is expressed as AS. When this same defect is inherited from the father, it is expressed as PWS. A lab test to determine the methylation-induced changes in the affected region of the chromosome is available to assist in the diagnosis and differentiation of these diseases. This test is called methylation-specific polymerase chain reaction (MSPCR).[5]

Research Notes

Environmental factors that may contribute to disease in adulthood can be linked to events that occur during fetal development. Many adult diseases have been linked to a fetal environment that impairs growth of the developing fetus. The study of the fetal origins of disease suggests that the fetus whose intrauterine growth is restricted may be programmed to develop diseases, including hypertension, diabetes, and breast cancer. It may be that all of these individuals are born susceptible to these diseases, and therefore the expression of disease is determined by environmental influences.[8,9]

Module 3

Developmental Disorders

Developmental disorders are usually the result of environmental influences that alter gene function, contributing to the expression of altered structure or function of the affected tissue or organ system. Developmental disorders occur after conception and therefore are not inherited.

Congenital Disorders

Developmental disorders can be the result of chemicals, hormones, drugs, pathogens, or other environmental factors that cause congenital disorders in the

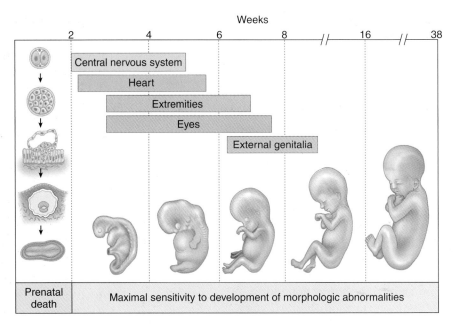

■ **Figure 6.12** Critical periods of vulnerability. Pre-embryologic (weeks 0 to 2) exposure to teratogenic insult is often incompatible with life. The embryologic period (3 to 8 weeks) represents the most vulnerable period of teratogenic damage. During the fetal period (9 weeks to delivery), risk for teratogenic insult remains, especially for tissues of the neurologic system. (Image modified from Rubin E, Farber JL. *Pathology.* 4th ed. Philadelphia: Lippincott Williams & Wilkins; 2005, with permission.)

developing child. The result of gene–environment interactions that occur during fetal development, congenital disorders are linked to events that occur at critical points in development. Factors may include the intrauterine and nutritional environments that impair appropriate anatomic and physiologic development of the embryo and fetus. Environmental influences may also be the result of a pathogen challenge prior to the fetus' ability to mount an adequate immune response. Exposure to drugs and toxins in the maternal system may also result in errors in morphogenesis, or the appropriate structure of organs and tissues. The period of intrauterine embryonic and fetal development is characterized by the dynamic processes of cellular proliferation and differentiation, increasing vulnerability to environmental insults that lead to altered function across the life span.

The risk of damage to a developing child is greatest during the embryologic period (weeks 3 through 8 of gestation). During this time, **organogenesis** (development of organ systems) is occurring. If damage occurs during this period, the organ systems most susceptible at the time of exposure are specifically affected. Damage prior to this time, the pre-embryologic period, may interfere with implantation or may be so significant that the pregnancy ends in spontaneous abortion. The fetal period begins during gestational week 9 and continues through the end of pregnancy (Fig. 6.12). Environmental insult during the fetal period has the potential to alter developing organ systems based on the timing of the challenge.

Substances that cause damage to developing embryos or fetuses are known as **teratogens**. Many substances that enter the mother's system are able to cross the placenta and enter the fetal circulation. If teratogen exposure is serious and occurs very early in the pregnancy, it can cause damage incompatible with life, resulting in spontaneous abortion or miscarriage. Damage later in fetal life is usually seen in specific organs, which were actively developing at the time of exposure. Teratogens can take many forms, including pathogens, drugs, alcohol, and environmental chemicals.

It is difficult to predict the effects of teratogen exposure because the effects are influenced by many variables. For example, it is known that maternal alcohol consumption during pregnancy is the sole causative factor identified for the development of **fetal alcohol syndrome (FAS)**. FAS is a condition characterized by significant mental handicap, growth deficit, and physical disability. The damage in FAS is linked to the amount and timing of alcohol exposure to the developing fetus. Not all babies exposed to alcohol develop FAS, suggesting the influence of environmental factors and varying susceptibility. Maternal abstinence from alcohol during pregnancy would result in the elimination of FAS, the leading cause of mental retardation in the United States.

Maternal infection during pregnancy can also result in congenital disorders in the fetus. The group of diseases described by the acronym known as TORCH is known to cause damage to the fetus if exposure occurs. These diseases are as follows:

- *T*oxoplasmosis
- *O*ther (hepatitis)
- *R*ubella

- *Cytomegalovirus*
- *Herpes*

Many pathogens in addition to those described in the TORCH group have teratogenic effects and are often manifested by fetal loss, multiple fetal malformations, and neurologic involvement. Examples of common conditionsinclude varicella (chicken pox) and parvovirus (fifth disease).

The presence or absence of agents in the environment can pose a risk for the development of genetic defects. An example of an environmental insult that can cause genetic damage is ionizing radiation. Radiation exposure to the fetus can cause genetic mutations. DNA repair mechanisms exist for this specific type of damage. If these repair mechanisms fail or if the damage is too great for adequate repair, permanent damage to DNA may result, leading to defects. There is no evidence that the radiation exposure delivered during diagnostic procedures causes damage, but women who are pregnant are cautioned to avoid radiographs unless absolutely necessary.

Maternal nutrient deficiency is linked to the development of **congenital defects**. Maternal folic acid deficiency is known to be a risk factor for the development of NTDs, including anencephaly and spina bifida. Adequate maternal intake of folic acid prior to pregnancy is associated with a reduction in the occurrence of NTDs. Since 1998, foods have been fortified with folic acid, resulting in the prevention of NTDs by 50% in the United States.[10] There has been a call for a similar strategy internationally, where dietary recommendations alone are not adequate to reduce the incidence of NTDs.[11]

Developmental Origins of Adult Disease

Observations from the "Barker Hypothesis" during the 1980s demonstrated the link between low infant birth weight and future development of heart disease, suggesting that undernutrition during pregnancy permanently changed fetal structure, function, and metabolism, programming the fetus for future development of disease.[12] Current evidence implicates epigenetic modifications triggered by the adverse intrauterine environment during fetal development as

the likely etiology of genetic predisposition to disease. As in other conditions with complex etiologies involving gene–environment interactions, the predisposition to adult disease due to fetal intrauterine adaptations requires an environmental trigger for expression of disease.[13]

The developing fetus is dependent on the maternal system for the delivery of oxygen and nutrients and the removal of wastes. The placenta is the interface between the maternal and fetal systems, playing an important role in support of fetal growth and development. The placenta has a significant endocrine function, providing hormones that support fetal and maternal adaptations needed for an optimal pregnancy outcome. Reduced maternal blood flow and variations in constituents in the maternal blood create an adverse intrauterine environment contributing to fetal adaptations that promote survival in utero, but may be mismatched with the environmental conditions of postnatal life.

Maternal nutritional status is central to the promotion of fetal development. Variations in maternal nutritional status including obesity, macronutrient and micronutrient excesses and deficiencies are associated with future development of obesity, diabetes, and heart disease.[14] Alterations in maternal hormonal status may stimulate fetal adaptations that may predispose to future development of disease. Examples of maternal hormonal conditions that have been linked to future disease include stress due to alteration in stress hormone delivery to the fetus and deficiency in maternal prohormone vitamin D levels. Impaired nutrition and stress are some of the challenges in the extrauterine environment that may provide the trigger for expression of disease, including hypertension, obesity, and diabetes.

Research Notes

Many adult-onset disorders can be predicted by genetic testing. Individuals should be counseled on the issues related to the knowledge that they have a predisposition to develop a disease. Identification of gene mutations that lead to disease may prevent a person from obtaining adequate insurance coverage for medical care. In addition, it is important to share this information with other family members who may also be at risk. Ethically, individuals should be encouraged to share their diagnosis of a genetic disorder, which the medical providers cannot themselves disclose to others because of patient confidentiality.[15] It is important to share knowledge of hereditary genetic disease with family members for them to make informed decisions about their future reproduction and health.

Module **4**

Management of Genetic and Developmental Disorders

Unlike other pathologic alterations that present with symptoms restricted to one particular organ system, the clinical manifestations of developmental and genetic disorders are specific to the affected tissues and organ systems at the time of insult. Even among individuals with similar genetic alterations, manifestations are influenced by penetrance and expressivity. Clinical manifestations of specific syndromes are presented in the clinical models in this chapter that represent a variety of developmental, genetic, and chromosomal pathologies. General methods of identification and management of alterations in genetics and development are discussed in the next section.

Screening and Diagnosis

Screening and diagnosis can be completed in an individual across the life span. Individuals may request genetic screening when family history indicates a heritable genetic risk. Genetic screening may be done in order to determine treatment decisions when faced with a diagnosis associated with known genetic risk. Individuals during the child-bearing years may consider genetic screening to determine the probability of genetic risk in offspring based on cues in maternal and paternal history or factors such as parental age. In all cases, the decision to pursue genetic screening has emotional, ethical, and economic implications.

PRENATAL SCREENING AND DIAGNOSIS

Ideally, counseling on the inheritance of genetic risk is completed prior to conception. Genetic risk can be determined when a complete family and pregnancy history is obtained. Maternal age (older than 35 years) or the family history of genetic disorders represents some of the most common reasons for seeking prenatal diagnosis. The decision to undergo screening may be made when a woman has had repetitive (three or more) spontaneous abortions, which suggests the potential for a chromosomal abnormality. Individuals who present with manifestations classically linked to single gene alterations or clinical subjective and objective findings that form a syndrome may undergo genetic screening to identify a defect and determine whether the defect can be passed on to offspring.

The goal of prenatal diagnosis is to determine recognizable chromosomal or genetic defects in the growing fetus. Initially, screening techniques can be used to determine genetic risk. Screening of maternal serum may be completed to identify NTDs or Down syndrome. Ultrasound is used to screen for abnormalities in the physical structure of the fetus. Although these techniques suggest risk, they are not diagnostic. Screening tests that suggest genetic abnormalities are usually followed by diagnostic testing. Cell samples of fetal origin must be used to diagnose fetal abnormalities. Fetal cells can be obtained from the chorionic villi, which contain cells of trophoblastic origin and therefore are fetal. The amniotic fluid that surrounds the fetus is another source of fetal genetic material and can also be used to identify genetic disorders. Finally, percutaneous blood sampling can be used to examine fetal cells obtained from a sample of fetal blood from the umbilical cord.

When the risk of transmission of a genetic defect is identified, prenatal counseling should include the option of preimplantation genetic diagnosis. **Preimplantation genetic diagnosis** is an alternative to prenatal diagnosis, and it allows for identification of abnormalities before implantation. Preimplantation genetic diagnosis requires the use of in vitro fertilization, embryo culture, and biopsy of the **blastomere** (early embryo). This procedure is costly and invasive, and its use is restricted to those individuals with identified risks, including single gene defects, X-linked disorders, **aneuploidy** (abnormal chromosome number), and those with balanced translocation.[16] Balanced translocation refers to the exchange of entire chromosome segments between two different chromosomes. Individuals with balanced translocations have the appropriate amount of genetic material, so they appear phenotypically normal. However, these individuals are carriers of this chromosomal anomaly and are able to pass one of the altered chromosomes, producing an unbalanced chromosomal complement in the offspring.

A thorough family history is often the first step toward a genetic diagnosis. Review of generational information is important in the determination of trends. This information is often depicted graphically as a pedigree, tracing genetic disorders through generations. Pedigrees are helpful in the tracking of inheritable single gene, chromosomal, and multifactorial disorders. A karyotype helps determine the presence of chromosomal abnormalities. When using a karyotype to identify chromosomal abnormalities as a cause for repeated abortion, cell samples from both parents are needed. Prenatal counseling of families with genetic disorders involves providing information to support decisions about pregnancy outcome and determining support services needed for the best possible outcome.

POSTNATAL SCREENING AND DIAGNOSIS

In the newborn period, screening for the most common genetic conditions results in earlier identification and treatment of many disorders. Learning more about genetics increases the ability to identify genetic causes of many diseases, including cancer, Parkinson disease, and Alzheimer disease. Although not all individuals with these diseases have a readily identifiable genetic mutation, many who have a family history of the disease have a genetic link. Once the gene responsible for the disease is identified, individuals at risk can be screened for the particular mutation. Disorders are discovered by determining the sequencing of DNA and identifying variations consistent with mutations that result in disease.

Genetic screening of carriers and affected individuals may provide predictive, preventive, and personalized medical care. The trend of the future is to use population-based screening to predict risk for adult-onset disorders in different ethnic and cultural groups. Knowledge of the molecular basis of disease is progressing faster than our grasp on the ethical and social implications of that knowledge. Complex implications related to the nature of patient relationships, antidiscrimination laws, and legal rules related to medical care and public health are challenges that need to be determined.[17]

● **STOP** *and* **Consider**

What are some instances in which identifying genetic information can be harmful?

▨ Treatment Strategies

Treatment of genetic disorders is disease specific. When anatomic anomalies exist, surgical correction is often implemented. If the disease results in deficiency of a particular enzyme, replacement of the missing protein is instituted, if possible. Treatment of disorders is unique to the genetic deficit and is primarily geared toward alleviation of the associated clinical manifestations.

Counseling individuals and families with genetic alterations must include communication of implications of the defect and the risk of reoccurrence. Counseling can occur in families when a risk of having children with genetic defects exists or when an affected child is born. It is important to understand the effects of the genetic condition on the individual as well as the family. A complete explanation of diagnostic strategies necessary to help the family identify risk is important. Discussion of genetic risk with families must be presented in a manner that is understood by the patients and that meets individual patient and family needs. The following are some of the strategies used:

1. Assess literacy level of the individual and family.
2. Ask for interpretation of information about testing procedures and possible outcomes.
3. Provide information about rates of risk in both positive and negative terms.
4. Promote ability to make informed decisions.

Module 5

Clinical Models

The following clinical models have been selected to illustrate the concepts of alterations in genetics and development. As you read the descriptions that follow, think about the processes of altering genetic traits as they apply to the specific conditions to help in the understanding and application of these concepts. Figure 6.13 provides a summary of genetic alterations in human disease.

▨ Autosomal Dominant Genetic Disorder: Huntington Disease

HD is a neurologic disorder caused by degeneration of the basal ganglia and cortical regions of the brain. HD affects approximately 5 of 100,000 predominantly White males and females of northern European ancestry.[18] A parent with HD has a 50%

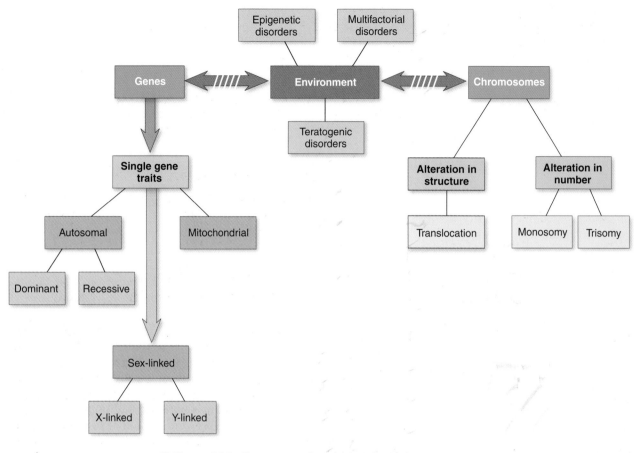

■ Figure 6.13   Concept map. Genetic alterations in human disease.

chance of passing the condition on to each child due to the autosomal dominant transmission of this condition. All individuals who inherit the mutated gene will eventually develop the clinical manifestations of this fatal condition. Manifestations usually appear by the mid-40s and include impaired function of movement, emotion, and cognitition. There is no known cure for this condition.

PATHOPHYSIOLOGY

HD is a progressive, autosomal dominant disorder caused by a defect in the *huntingtin* gene on chromosome 4. The gene defect results in a triplet cytosine–adenine–guanine (CAG) expansion mutation, with an increased number of mutations associated with earlier onset of the clinical manifestations of the disease. The genetic mutation generates a code for the abnormal huntingtin protein, which then accumulates to toxic levels and destroys nerve cells, resulting in atrophy in the brain. A fragment of the huntingtin protein produced by caspase (an enzyme that breaks down protein) may also be involved in the pathology associated with HD. Mitochondrial dysfunction contributing to oxidative damage and excitotoxicity is also being investigated as a molecular mechanism underlying the damage of HD.

🔬 *From the Lab*

Screening for HD can be accomplished by analyzing DNA from a blood sample to determine if the genetic mutation is present. CAG repeats are counted, with the number of repeats considered in diagnosis. CAG repeats of 28 or fewer do not indicate HD. Individuals with CAG repeats greater than 40 are diagnosed with HD. Because of the serious nature of the diagnosis and lack of an available cure, the decision to test for the defect is a difficult one.

CLINICAL MANIFESTATIONS

Individuals with HD suffer from involuntary movements, cognitive impairment, and emotional disturbance. Early psychological manifestations include personality changes, loss of memory, antisocial and impulsive behaviors, and emotional lability. Altered motor function in the early stage of disease manifestation includes restlessness and fidget-like activity, representing early signs of **dyskinesia** (difficulty in performing voluntary movements). The progressive nature of the condition leads to immobility, severe loss of cognitive function, intellectual deterioration, delusions, and paranoia.

DIAGNOSTIC CRITERIA

Diagnosis of HD is based on a complete family and personal medical history and physical examination. Mental, cognitive, and emotional evaluation may provide indications of early signs of disease, especially when coupled with early signs of movement disorders. Genetic testing can definitively diagnose HD, revealing the associated mutation on the *huntingtin* gene. Blood samples from the affected individual, as well as a close family member, can precisely diagnose HD. In symptomatic individuals, computed tomography (CT), magnetic resonance imaging (MRI), or positron emission tomography (PET) scans can be done to detect the characteristic brain anomalies associated with HD, including shrinkage of the basal ganglia components, caudate nuclei and putamen, and enlargement of the ventricles of the brain.

Individuals with a family history of HD have the option of genetic testing prior to onset of symptoms; this is known as presymptomatic testing. Counseling should be provided before presymptomatic testing considering the profound impact a diagnosis of HD can have on an individual and the family.

TREATMENT

There is currently no cure for this condition. Research into potential treatment options has identified new pathways to preserving brain function and preventing disease. Scientists have discovered a substance known as a histone deacetylase (HDAC) activity inhibitor, which was found to prevent cell death in an animal model.[19] The use of stem cells to stimulate growth of new neurons is also a potential future treatment.[20] Investigation into pharmacotherapy to treat or cure HD has shown promise for the use of caspase inhibitors and cannabinoids.[21] Glutamate receptor antagonists, which counter the pathology believed to be caused by excitotoxicity, have been found to slow disease progression.[22] Clinical trials will provide data on patients that will ultimately determine the effectiveness of these treatments.

Research Notes

A group of researchers studied residents from an endemic population of people afflicted with HD in Venezuela. A model was developed that determined the variables contributing to age of onset of symptoms. Variables accounting for age of onset included number of repetitive triplets in the huntingtin gene as the primary determinant (72%), although other genes and environmental factors, including poverty and nutrition, explained the remaining variation.[23]

STOP *and Consider*

What are the risks and benefits of testing for HD? Are there reasons why a person would not want testing?

Autosomal Recessive Disorder: Sickle Cell Anemia

Sickle cell anemia is a disease that affects red blood cells (RBCs). **Hemoglobin A (HbA)** (adult) in the RBCs is replaced by another form of hemoglobin, *hemoglobin S* (sickled). Following an autosomal recessive inheritance pattern, sickle cell anemia is transmitted from parent to child. Sickle cell anemia is commonly found in individuals of African ancestry. In the United States, 9% of African Americans have sickle cell trait and 1 in 600 have sickle cell anemia.[24] As a result of improved screening, treatment, and education, life expectancy is increasing.[25,26] Median survival for individuals was 14 years in 1973. Recently, median survival has increased to 42 years for males and 48 years for females.[27]

PATHOPHYSIOLOGY

Sickle cell anemia is the result of a single gene mutation that follows Mendelian inheritance patterns. RBCs contain HbA, or adult hemoglobin. HbS is an abnormal type of hemoglobin found in people with sickle cell anemia. RBCs with HbA are soft, round, and pliable enough to circulate through the small blood vessels in the microcirculation. HbS changes the phenotype of RBCs, making them stiff and distorted. RBC life span is reduced from approximately 120 days to 16 days when RBCs carry HbS, further contributing to symptoms of anemia and increased demand to produce additional RBCs. The form of hemoglobin produced is determined by the two beta-globin genes (bS) located on chromosome 11. The defect in sickle cell anemia is a point mutation, in which the amino acid valine is substituted for glutamine on the β-chain of hemoglobin of RBCs. The phenotypic expression of this genetic mutation in an individual who is homozygous for the sickle bS is sickle cell anemia.

■ Figure 6.14 Red blood cells in sickle cell anemia. When red blood cells are exposed to conditions of low oxygen tension, it results in the sickle shape of the cells. (Asset provided by Anatomical Chart Company.)

From the Lab

Hemoglobin electrophoresis is used to identify specific forms of hemoglobin. This test is completed on a blood sample drawn from a person suspected or known to have sickle cell anemia. An electric charge is passed through a solution of hemoglobin. Hemoglobin varieties move to specific distances through the solution, based on composition. A person with sickle cell disease will have a predominance of HbS.

When exposed to conditions of low oxygen tension, the hemoglobin's shape is distorted into a sickled shape, known as **hemoglobin S (HbS)** (Fig. 6.14). The irregularly shaped hemoglobin causes damage to the endothelial cells that line blood vessels and to the RBCs themselves. Trapping of the RBCs in the spleen causes **hemolysis**, or breakdown of RBCs, resulting in anemia. The altered shapes of the RBCs cause difficulty in their passage through small blood vessels, resulting in decreased oxygenation. Pain related to ischemia results and can develop into necrosis and organ failure if left untreated.

As expected in autosomal recessive disorders, the genetic mutation associated with sickle cell anemia is recessive. For individuals to have the disease phenotype, their genotype must be homozygous for the defective allele. An individual who is heterozygous for the genetic mutation is a carrier and is considered to have **sickle cell trait**.

CLINICAL MANIFESTATIONS

Clinical manifestations are related to the proportion of HbS in the circulation. Certain conditions, including infection and hypoxia, are known to stim- ulate increased production of HbS, leading to sickle cell crisis.

Hemolysis, shortened red cell life, and splenic trapping result in breakdown of RBCs, releasing contents into the circulation. The two clinical manifestations of sickle cell crisis—jaundice and anemia—result. Jaundice results from the release of **bilirubin**, a yellow, lipid-soluble by-product of hemoglobin, as a result of RBC damage. The loss of RBCs results in anemia, making it difficult to oxygenate tissues adequately. This, combined with the blockade of small vessels by the sickled RBCs, further adds to the problems of tissue oxygenation. Tissue ischemia often results, promoting the development of pain, another classic clinical manifestation of sickle cell crisis. Because of the varied sites of tissue ischemia, the location of pain can occur in the chest, extremities, or abdomen. Stroke and priapism (painful, prolonged erection) can also result. Organ damage to the spleen, kidneys, and liver can result from sickle cell crisis, contributing to significant morbidity and mortality. Splenic damage can contribute to decreased immune defense, increasing the risk of overwhelming infection. In children, infection and stroke are common manifestations of sickle cell anemia.[26] Microvascular occlusion may lead to necrosis and cell death.

DIAGNOSTIC CRITERIA

Early identification of individuals with sickle cell anemia is vital to decreased morbidity and mortality. Prenatal and newborn screening for sickle cell disease has improved treatment of complications, particularly for infection in the newborn period when the risk is highest. Laboratory testing for sickle cell disease includes:

- Hemoglobin electrophoresis (see From the Lab below)
  - Identifies hemoglobin types (HbA, HbS)
  - Differentiates homozygosity from heterozygosity by proportion of hemoglobin types
    - Homozygous: 80% to 90% HbS of total hemoglobin
    - Heterozygous: 35% to 40% HbS of total hemoglobin
- Isoelectric focusing
  - Method used to separate proteins based on their isoelectric point, based on the pH when the protein net charge is zero
  - Adjunct in determination of hemoglobin type
- High-performance liquid chromatography (HPLC)

- ■ Method used in the identification of hemoglobin
  variants
  - ● DNA analysis

Prenatal diagnosis can be done by analysis of fetal DNA obtained from amniotic fluid. Newborn screening should be initiated in the first 6 months of life, with hemoglobin F (HbF) included in the distribution of hemoglobin types expected. Laboratory follow-up of individuals diagnosed with sickle cell anemia who are not experiencing complications includes evaluation of hemolysis and anemia with yearly complete blood counts (CBC) and urinalysis. Tests of liver (liver function tests: Aspartate [AST], alanine [ALT]) and kidney (serum creatinine and blood urea nitrogen [BUN]) function should be completed every 2 to 3 years. Retinal examinations should also be completed to determine evidence of damage or disease.

TREATMENT

Prevention of complications related to infection is important in the management of sickle cell anemia. Immunization against childhood and community illnesses, such as pneumococcal pneumonia, influenza, and meningococcal meningitis is important to protect from infection. Penicillin prophylaxis is an important intervention designed to support immune defense.

Treatment for patients with sickle cell anemia is usually symptom specific. Pain management is critical to the management of sickle cell anemia. Identification and avoidance of precipitating factors, including infection, extremes of temperature, and emotional/physical stress, are important for pain prevention. Lab evaluation of a CBC (hemoglobin, reticulocytes, white blood cells, granulocytes, and bands) can help determine anemia and infection. Severe episodes of pain often require the use of opiates. Blood transfusion addresses the anemia associated with sickle cell disease and decreases the proportion of circulating HbS by adding healthy donor RBCs with HbA. Transfusion has also been shown to decrease the risk of stroke in children. Folic acid supplementation is frequently used to prevent megaloblastic erythropoiesis.

Pharmacologic measures for the prevention of complications include the use of hydroxyurea. Hydroxyurea increases the production of HbF, preventing the formation of HbS. Hydroxyurea kills bone marrow cells, inducing an increased production of

Research Notes

Gene therapy in the treatment of sickle cell anemia represents an effective strategy in the prevention of disease-associated complications. Research is currently in the early stages, but recent studies show promise for this potential therapy. One approach reported in a recent study of gene therapy involved the manipulation of the differential expression of the globin genes, inducing preferential expression of HbF.[29] Therapy involving substitution of HbS with HbF through the transcriptional control of globin genes was studied as a potential therapy for sickle cell anemia. The focus of this study was to find the right DNA sequence to target and to test its effectiveness in promoting expression of HbF. Using an in vitro method involving cells, the researchers were able to selectively express HbF, reinforcing the importance of the continued development of this strategy as an effective treatment for sickle cell anemia.

cells with higher HbF content, promoting life span of cells and depressing production of HbS. Increases in HbF have been associated with improvement of the clinical manifestations related to sickle cell anemia. The use of nitric oxide during acute chest crisis may promote relaxation of the resistance arteries to promote perfusion to ischemic tissues. Future treatments in clinical development include the use of gene therapy and bone marrow transplantation that would not only treat the symptoms, but also would provide the potential for a cure.[28]

STOP *and Consider*

What are the risks to the fetus when the father has sickle cell anemia? What are the risks to the fetus when the mother has sickle cell anemia?

Mitochondrial Gene Disorder: MELAS

Mitochondrial encephalomyopathy, lactic acidosis, and stroke (MELAS) is mitochondrial gene disorder. Although uncommon, MELAS is considered a significant cause of strokelike manifestations in individuals less than 45 years of age.[30] Mean life span of those with the full clinical syndrome ranges from 20 to 40 years, with cardiopulmonary failure, pulmonary disease, and status epilepticus the most commonly reported causes of death. There is no gender or ethnic predilection for MELAS.[31]

PATHOPHYSIOLOGY

MELAS is a maternally inherited condition, characterized by mtDNA point mutations. The ovum is the source of mtDNA; therefore, this condition is maternally inherited. To date, eight mtDNA point mutations and one deletion mutation have been identified as genetic causes of MELAS. Most of the mutations are in genes that encode tRNA for the amino acids leucine and valine. A substitution of adenine to guanine in the gene-encoding tRNA accounts for approximately 80% of MELAS cases. Mutations may also affect **cytochrome oxidase (COX)**, an enzyme important in catalyzing oxidation–reduction mitochondrial reactions in cellular respiration. The prevailing theory on the underlying mechanism involved in MELAS is that a decrease in oxidative phosphorylation creates an imbalance between ATP production and usage, contributing to neuronal dysfunction.[30]

CLINICAL MANIFESTATIONS

The manifestations of MELAS are variable due to the heteroplasmic nature of this condition. Clinical manifestations of MELAS develop when mutant mtDNA reaches a threshold of 56% to 95%. The age of onset of clinical manifestations averages 10 years. Classic symptoms of MELAS include:

- Strokelike episodes in individuals younger than 40 years of age
- Encephalopathy, including seizures and dementia
- Lactic acidosis

Other associated manifestations include hearing loss, blindness, migraine headaches, vomiting, short stature, hemiparesis, hemiplegia, cardiomyopathy, diabetes, and myopathy.

DIAGNOSIS

Diagnosis of MELAS is based on family history and documentation of clinical manifestations, and it is confirmed with laboratory studies. Biochemical analyses can determine respiratory chain dysfunction and lactic acidosis. Muscle biopsy demonstrates the characteristic findings of myopathy in MELAS: the presence of ragged red fibers (see From the Lab, below). Common lab studies used in the diagnosis of MELAS include:

- Serum and cerebrospinal fluid levels of lactic acid and pyruvic acid
- Serum creatine kinase
- Skeletal muscle biopsy to determine activity of substances involved in cellular respiration
- Blood, skeletal muscle, or hair follicle samples for determination of mtDNA mutations

Imaging studies can be added to laboratory studies to confirm a diagnosis of MELAS. CT or MRI brain scans can detect neurologic damage related to seizure activity and stroke. PET scans can determine the cerebral metabolic rate for oxygen. Electroencephalogram (EEG) is useful in identifying neural activity indicating a seizure disorder. Cardiomyopathy can be detected with echocardiography (ultrasound determination of heart structure and function) or electrocardiography (ECG), a test that indicates the neural conduction in the heart.

TREATMENT

Currently, treatment strategies are focused on management of manifestations. Examples include the use of anticonvulsant medications directed at controlling seizure activity and cochlear implants to improve hearing. Treatment strategies in development include the use of agents that affect oxidative phosphorylation. Agents of this type include coenzyme Q, riboflavin, and creatine. Clinical trials are investigating the use of dichloroacetate, a compound that promotes the conversion of pyruvate (a by-product of carbohydrate metabolism) to acetyl-CoA instead of the usual product lactate, reducing the risk for development of lactic acidosis (further discussed in Chapter 8).

Alteration in Chromosome Number (Autosome): Down Syndrome

Trisomy that results in excess genetic material is often incompatible with life, especially when the defect involves larger chromosomes. When trisomy occurs on chromosome 18, the clinical manifestations are severe. Congenital heart defects, multiple joint contractures, spina bifida, hearing loss, underdevelopment or missing radial bone of forearm, cleft lip, birth defects of the eye, and small size at birth are the most common developmental complications of this syndrome. Among infants born with trisomy 18, median survival is estimated at 6 days.[33]

Down syndrome is named for Dr John Langdon Down, who identified the syndrome in the 1860s based on the pattern of

From the Lab

Diagnosis of mitochondrial abnormalities is often determined by biochemical assays that detect specific disease markers. The most common of these markers are COX and succinate dehydrogenase (SDH), both of which play a significant role in mitochondrial cellular respiration.[32] An increase in SDH leads to altered structure of muscle fibers, impairing muscle function. On microscopic evaluation, muscle fibers exposed to trichrome stain turn a bright red color, leading to the common term "ragged red fibers," characteristic of many mitochondrial gene disorders. Ragged red fibers may also be stained with other dyes to characterize presence of COX and SDH.

manifestations he recognized in the residents of an asylum for children with mental illness in England. The genetic basis of chromosome 21 trisomy was not identified until 1959. Down syndrome is one of the most common genetic birth defects, affecting approximately 1 in 800 to 1,000 babies of both genders. According to the National Down Syndrome Society, there are approximately 350,000 people living with Down syndrome in the United States. Life expectancy among adults with Down syndrome is about 55 years, although life span varies depending on the individual and his or her medical condition. An increase in the incidence of Down syndrome was expected due to delayed childbearing and an increased birth rate in women over 35 years.

PATHOPHYSIOLOGY

Down syndrome is a condition characterized by alteration in chromosome number. Also known as trisomy 21, children born with Down syndrome have three copies of chromosome 21. The additional chromosome can be caused by fertilization of a gamete with two copies of chromosome 21, by nondisjunction during cell division, or by translocation. When an error in cell division occurs after fertilization, the child may develop two cell lines: one with the usual chromosome complement and one with trisomy 21, known as mosaic Down syndrome.

CLINICAL MANIFESTATIONS

Children born with Down syndrome have a combination of birth defects, including mental retardation, characteristic facial features, and health problems including cardiac defects, intestinal malformations, and visual and hearing impairment. The severity of expression of these problems varies greatly among affected individuals. Increased risk of infection, thyroid problems, and leukemia are also possible sequelae of Down syndrome. Facial features characteristic of Down syndrome include eyes that slant upward, small, low-set ears that fold at the top, small mouth, flattened nose bridge, and short neck (Fig. 6.15). Short stature, short fingers, and decreased muscle

tone are also characteristic outward manifestations of Down syndrome.

When parents have a balanced translocation, they may be free of the disease phenotype but can pass on the defect, resulting in trisomy of their child. Balanced translocation in a parent is the only inheritable form of trisomy. Other mechanisms leading to trisomy 21 represent spontaneous events. The risk of trisomy as a result of nondisjunction increases with age. Maternal age over 35 years is associated with a greater risk of Down syndrome. The risk of Down syndrome increases with age, from about 1 in 1,250 for a woman at age 25, to 1 in 1,000 at age 30, 1 in 400 at age 35, and 1 in 100 at age 40. Strikingly, the risk is increased to 1:60 by age 42, further rising to 1:12 by age 49. However, it is important to note that about 75% of babies with Down syndrome are born to women who are under age 35, as younger women have far more babies.

From the Lab

Screening for Down syndrome can be done during the prenatal period. Noninvasive methods of screening may include biochemical analysis of substances in maternal blood, using the quadruple test, which includes measurement of serum alpha-fetoprotein, unconjugated estradiol, hCG, and inhibin-A during the second trimester, after 14 weeks' gestation. When the quadruple test was combined with an ultrasound evaluation of nuchal translucency and PAPP-A at 10 weeks (integrated test), this two-step evaluation was very accurate in detecting Down syndrome (see Research Notes below).[36]

Research Notes

Traditionally, determination of effective antenatal screening for Down syndrome was hindered by variations in study design, preventing generalizability of study findings to the population. In a recent large prospective study of 47,053 singleton pregnancies, testing of maternal serum and urine samples, as well as nuchal translucency, was conducted to determine reliable biomarkers of Down syndrome.[34] The false-positive rates for specific prenatal tests were as follows:

- Integrated test (nuchal translucency and pregnancy associated plasma protein-A (PAPP-A) at 11 weeks of pregnancy; alpha-fetoprotein, unconjugated estriol, free beta- or total human chorionic gonadotropin (hCG), and inhibin-A in the early second trimester): 0.9%
- Serum integrated test (nuchal translucency, free beta-hCG and PAPP-A at 11 weeks of pregnancy): 4.3%
- **Quadruple test** (alpha-fetoprotein, free beta- or total hCG, and inhibin-A): 6.2%
- Nuchal translucency at 11 weeks: 15.2%

DIAGNOSTIC CRITERIA

Screening for Down syndrome in the first trimester can be accomplished by looking for increased **nuchal translucency (NT)** or thickness of the nape of the

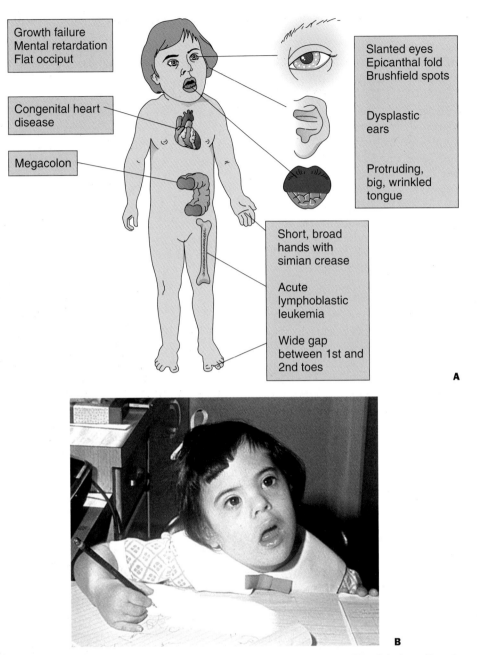

Growth failure
Mental retardation
Flat occiput

Congenital heart
disease

Megacolon

Slanted eyes
Epicanthal fold
Brushfield spots

Dysplastic
ears

Protruding,
big, wrinkled
tongue

Short, broad
hands with
simian crease

Acute
lymphoblastic
leukemia

Wide gap
between 1st and
2nd toes

A

B

■ **FIGURE 6.15** Typical clinical manifestations of a child with Down syndrome. The clinical manifestations of Down syndrome include organ system anomalies with long-term health implications (**A**) in addition to characteristic physical features (**B**). (Image modified from Rubin E, Farber JL. *Pathology*. 4th ed. Philadelphia: Lippincott Williams & Wilkins; 2005, with permission.)

neck, a common finding in fetuses with chromosomal abnormalities. Evaluation of NT uses ultrasound to measure a fluid-filled sac at the back of the fetus' neck during early pregnancy. The best time for NT testing is between 10 to 14 weeks. After that time, the fluid collected is able to drain via a more developed lymph system. Diagnostic testing requires the more invasive procedures of chorionic villus sampling and amniocentesis. These invasive procedures carry more risk and are associated with a 1% risk of pregnancy loss. More specific screening for

Down syndrome occurs during the second trimester when a pattern of anatomic anomalies can be detected by ultrasound. Some of the distinctive physical features detectable by ultrasound include:

- Short humerus
- Short femur
- Hydronephrosis
- Echogenic cardiac foci (areas in the heart, usually the left ventricle, identified as echoes or bright areas)

- Echogenic bowel (bright areas in the intestine)
- Other major anatomic defects

These findings individually may not be unusual, but when they appear in combination, the risk of Down syndrome must be addressed. When the findings from any screening tests suggest Down syndrome, further testing is offered to provide an accurate diagnosis. A limitation of some screening tests includes a high rate of "false-positive" results, meaning that the positive screening result is present in the absence of disease. Further, there is a risk of "false-negative" results, meaning the actual disease condition was not detected by the screening test, leaving families with a false assurance. Tests with high rates of "false-positive" and "false-negative" results have limited use in the identification and management of disease.

Second-trimester amniocentesis provides an opportunity to collect samples of amniotic fluid, grow fetal cells in culture, and evaluate the fetal karyotype to determine the presence of chromosomal abnormalities. Future diagnostic tests may include the genomic DNA real-time polymerase chain reaction (PCR) technique, which could serve as a reliable method for rapid prenatal diagnosis of Down syndrome.[35]

TREATMENT

Treatment in Down syndrome is focused on promotion of maximal independence and quality of life. Early intervention programs, including speech, language, and physical therapy, promote optimal function. Congenital heart disease remains the most frequent cause for early death. Treatment of cardiac or gastrointestinal complications may require surgical repair. Overall life expectancy is shorter than the general population.

Alteration in Chromosome Number (Sex Chromosome): Turner Syndrome

TS is a condition named for Dr Henry Turner, who first identified the condition in the 1930s based on the pattern of manifestations identified in his patients. The genetic basis of the syndrome was not identified for another 30 years. TS is the most common fetal monosomy, occurring with a frequency of approximately 3%. Of those fetuses affected, approximately 99% are spontaneously aborted.[37] TS occurs in 1 in 2,500 to 1 in 3,000 girls at birth, or in 25 to 55/100,000 predominantly white females. Individuals with TS have a decreased life expectancy, usually related to the associated medical complications of diabetes and heart disease.

PATHOPHYSIOLOGY

TS occurs in females when the chromosome number is altered, resulting from the loss of all or part of the sex chromosome X. Of those affected by TS, about 50% have true monosomy with only one X chromosome (45,XO), 10% have structural abnormality of the X chromosome, and remaining cases exhibit one or more additional cell lines or a mosaic karyotype.[38]

CLINICAL MANIFESTATIONS

Clinical manifestations vary based on the type of abnormality, the point in time when nondisjunction occurred, and the proportion of damaged cells in each tissue type. Manifestations common across TS include short stature and gonadal failure. Intelligence is usually normal, but girls with TS often have some learning and social problems. Other associated symptoms can be grouped into three categories:

- Skeletal abnormalities
  - Short fingers
  - Short neck
  - Cleft palate
- Soft tissue abnormalities
  - Lymphatic obstruction
  - Webbed neck
  - Low hairline
- Organ abnormalities
  - Cardiac abnormalities
  - Kidney abnormalities
  - Hearing loss

Figure 6.16 illustrates some of the physical characteristics of TS.

In addition to reproductive effects, adult women with TS may also suffer from hypothyroidism, deafness, osteoporosis, and problems related to estrogen deficiency.[39] Altered morphology of structures in the inner ear results in conductive hearing loss and otitis media.[40] Growth hormone administration promotes optimal height development. Life span in these women is decreased secondary to cardiovascular problems, including atherosclerosis.[41] Congenital malformations of the left heart, aortic rupture and

Research Notes

Individuals with TS are at increased risk of type 2 diabetes because of decreased insulin secretion.[50] Prolonged treatment with growth hormone, commonly used in TS, can also contribute to an increased risk of insulin resistance.

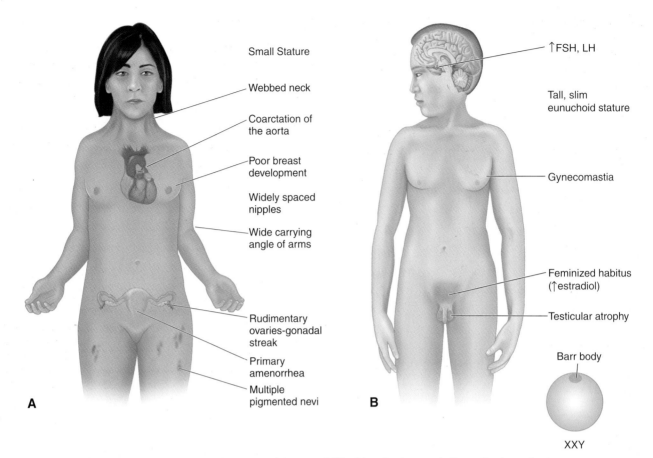

Small Stature

Webbed neck

Coarctation of the aorta

Poor breast development

Widely spaced nipples

Wide carrying angle of arms

Rudimentary ovaries-gonadal streak

Primary amenorrhea

Multiple pigmented nevi

A

↑FSH, LH

Tall, slim eunuchoid stature

Gynecomastia

Feminized habitus (↑estradiol)

Testicular atrophy

Barr body

XXY

B

■ **Figure 6.16** Clinical Manifestations of Turner and Klinefelter Syndromes. A: Turner Syndrome is characterized by physical manifestations of altered female reproductive development resulting from complete or parital monosomy of the X chromosome. B: Feminization is characteristic of Klinefelter Syndrome, due to the addition of X chromosome(s) in a phenotypic male. (Image modified from Rubin E, Farber JL. *Pathology*. 4th ed. Philadelphia: Lippincott Williams & Wilkins; 2005, with permission.)

dissection, hypertension, and ischemic heart disease are all risks for women with TS.

Klinefelter syndrome (KS) is another condition characterized by abnormal number of sex chromosomes, and it is considered a counterpart to TS. In KS, an abnormal ovum carrying an additional X chromosome (XX) is fertilized by a normal male sperm (Y). The child, with a karyotype of 46, XXY, is phenotypically male. Functionally, these individuals are infertile, with scant pubic hair, atrophic testes, and a small penis. They also have feminine features, including lack of facial hair, female hip shape, and breast development.

Clinical manifestations of Klinefelter syndrome. (Image modified from Rubin E, Farber JL. *Pathology*. 4th Ed. Philadelphia: Lippincott Williams & Wilkins, 2005.)

DIAGNOSTIC CRITERIA

Early ultrasound (14 to 16 weeks) can identify characteristics that increase suspicion of TS. These findings include a large, septated, cystic **hygroma** (cyst with a diameter larger than the biparietal diameter of the head) on the back of the neck, edema, short femur, and narrow aortic arch. Liveborn females are not routinely screened unless they present with behavioral or physical characteristics consistent with the diagnosis of TS.[42] Parents report behaviors of delayed development, feeding problems, and crying during infancy in their daughters diagnosed with TS.[43] Physical findings in the newborn period include puffy hands and feet from lymphedema, extra nuchal skin

From the Lab

Karyotyping is used to identify partially or completely missing X chromosomes, diagnostic of TS. Efforts to find a more affordable and quicker method are ongoing. Molecular detection of nonmethylated segments of the X chromosome, characteristic in TS, may be useful in screening high-risk groups.[48] MSPCR may also prove effective in diagnosing TS.[49]

from the remaining cystic hygroma, and heart defects, including hypoplastic heart and coarctation of the aorta.[38] Short stature may be the only physical characteristic in girls diagnosed in mid-childhood.

Many mosaic individuals affected with TS are not diagnosed until later in life, when gonadal failure alters reproductive development. Delayed puberty and infertility related to premature ovarian failure are common problems that lead to the identification of TS in women without other classic characteristics. Puberty and the development of adult female physical characteristics must often be induced by estrogen hormone administration.[44,45] Although ovarian follicle development in fetal life is significantly reduced, individuals who have a mosaic karyotype may have spontaneous pregnancies.[46] Repeated spontaneous miscarriage may be the characteristic leading to screening and diagnosis in these women. Women with TS often experience premature menopause.

TREATMENT

There is no specific management plan for treatment of TS. The phenotypes of individuals with TS are varied and determine screening for related health concerns and treatment of altered function. In addition to management of medical complications, assistance in socialization facilitates independent living and function. Some women require assisted reproduction techniques to achieve pregnancy, supported by hormone administration. In vitro fertilization via an oocyte donation may be needed to promote pregnancy, although these women may face increased risk of aortic rupture related to the physical stressors of pregnancy.[47]

Sex-Linked Genetic Disorder: Fragile X Syndrome

FXS is an example of a sex-linked genetic disorder that follows Mendelian inheritance patterns. As its name implies, the defect that causes the disorder is located on the X chromosome. FXS is the leading cause of inheritable mental retardation in the United States. The prevalence of FXS with the full mutation affects an estimated 1:4000 males and 1:6000 females, though it is felt that this syndrome is under-diagnosed.[51] Approximately 1:250 women are carriers of the defective gene.

PATHOPHYSIOLOGY

Located on the long arm of the X chromosome, a nucleotide mutation in the *FMR1* gene has been identified as the molecular basis of the syndrome. The unusual mutation is characterized by a variable trinucleotide repeat of the nitrogen base combination of cytosine–guanine–guanine (CGG). The number of CGG repeats within a gene determines if a person has a typical allele (less than 55 repeats), premutation (55 to 200 repeats), or a full mutation (more than 200 repeats).[52] This defect results in the impaired ability to produce the fragile X mental retardation protein (FMRP).

From the Lab

The *FMR1* gene test is specific for diagnosing FXS. Laboratory testing for FXS is done by detection of the triplet expansion region of the *FMR1* gene. The laboratory test PCR amplifies the specific alleles. After amplification, Southern blot analysis is performed to detect the expanded alleles.[53] This test has been shown to detect and measure the CGG repeat effectively, with more than 99% sensitivity and 100% specificity.

CLINICAL MANIFESTATIONS

Typical physical features associated with this genetic disorder include distinctive facial features, connective tissue problems, and macroorchidism (enlarged testicles); however, they are not specific enough to diagnose the condition. Cognitive impairment and behavioral difficulties are the distinguishing characteristics of this syndrome. As is typical in sex-linked disorders, males are affected by the disorder and females are carriers. Unlike other sex-linked disorders, the variations in the gene mutation can lead to clinical signs in female carriers. Female carriers have the clinical manifestations of mild cognitive or behavioral defects, premature ovarian failure, and a newly characterized neurodegenerative disorder: fragile X–associated tremor/ataxia syndrome (FXTAS) in more severe degrees of mutation.[52] Affected males are usually unable to live independently, whereas carrier females have learning difficulties but are able to function independently.

DIAGNOSTIC CRITERIA

Screening for the disorder is usually based on family history. The risk of recurrence is high in carrier relatives, presenting an important consideration for prenatal testing. Prenatal screening is completed using the techniques of chorionic villus sampling or amniocentesis to collect samples. Because the clini-

Research Notes

The use of gene therapy in the treatment of FXS holds promise for a potential treatment or cure. With current technology, significant challenges exist in determining the delivery of gene therapy and an effective method to target the damaged cells.[55]

cal manifestations are vague and can be associated with many other disorders, individuals with a family history of FXS should be screened for the disorder. Currently, FXS is not among the usual disorders detected by routine newborn screening.

TREATMENT

No cure currently exists for FXS. Behavioral and educational management and treatment of physical symptoms are recommended. Treatment of the behavioral problems associated with FXS is important to individual and family functioning. The use of stimulants to manage distractibility, hyperactivity, and impulsivity has been shown to be helpful. Antidepressants can help manage anxiety, obsessive–compulsive behaviors, and mood changes. Aggression may be treated with the use of antipsychotic medications. The combination of these psychopharmacologic agents for specific manifestations of FXS can contribute to enhanced individual functioning.[54]

● STOP *and Consider*

What are the benefits of early prenatal diagnosis in a child with FXS?

◢ Multifactorial Inheritance: Cardiovascular Disease

Cardiovascular disease (CVD) is the leading cause of death in the United States. Family history of CVD often reveals a predisposition to development of a variety of conditions, including atherosclerosis, hypertension, and stroke.

PATHOPHYSIOLOGY

The genetic influences in the development of cardiovascular disorders range from single gene mutations to complex interactions between genetic and environmental factors. In some of these conditions, including hypercholesterolemia, the inheritance pattern is well characterized. The mechanisms of genetic regulation in other conditions are less clear and more complex. In almost all conditions, the com-

bination of heredity and environment is critical in the development of disease in "at-risk" individuals. The genetic influences in the origin of specific cardiovascular conditions are discussed in this section to highlight the inheritance patterns and influential factors in expression of disease phenotypes.

Genetic Contributions to Atherosclerosis

A strong association exists between high levels of low-density lipoprotein (LDL) cholesterol and atherosclerotic heart disease. Genetic inheritance resulting in elevated plasma levels of LDL cholesterol demonstrates clear patterns. The mechanisms underlying inheritable hypercholesterolemia include:

1. Mutations of genes regulating uptake of cholesterol from the blood (*LDL receptor [LDLR], autosomal recessive hypercholesterolemia [ARH]* genes)
2. Binding of apolipoprotein B-100 (intermediate form of LDL) to the LDLR (APOB-100)
3. Synthesis and clearance of cholesterol (ABCG5 and ABCG8 genes)

Four specific diseases with identified single gene defects contribute to hypercholesterolemia.[56] Consequences of the genetic and metabolic impairments of these defects contribute to the inheritable conditions of familial hypercholesterolemia, ARH, familial ligand-defective APOB-100, and sitosterolemia.

Genetic Contributions to Hypertension

Hypertension (elevated blood pressure) contributes to increased risk of stroke, myocardial infarction, heart failure, and renal failure. In the general population, multiple environmental and genetic influences contribute to the development of hypertension. Existence of mutations in genes responsible for the regulation of blood pressure has been identified in families predisposed to hypertension. Single gene mutations leading to impaired renal salt handling demonstrate Mendelian inheritance patterns in affected individuals. Although these forms of hypertension are rare, improved understanding of the molecular basis of pathology contributes to the basis of treatment for elevated blood pressure. Genetic influences contributing to hypertension have not yet been fully characterized and represent complex, polygenetic influences of gene–gene and gene–environment interactions.[57]

Genetic Contributions to Cerebral Vascular Accident

Hypertension is a risk factor for cerebral vascular accident (CVA) or stroke, suggesting similar mechanisms of disease. Stroke does not develop in everyone with hypertension, suggesting the influential factor of genetic susceptibility. Single gene disorders linked to the development of hemoglobinopathies, embolic disorders, and hyperlipidemia contribute to an increased risk of stroke. An individual's risk of ischemic stroke is increased when a family history of this type of stroke exists. Two genes (*STRK1* and *STRK2*) have been associated with twice the risk of myocardial infarction and stroke.[58] In addition, mutations in genes regulating the clotting cascade have been identified. Individuals with these mutations are at increased risk for clot development leading to susceptibility to myocardial infarction, stroke, and venous thrombosis.[59]

CLINICAL MANIFESTATIONS

Clinical manifestations of CVD are discussed in detail in Chapter 14. The events preceding the clinical manifestations of CVD are initiated during embryologic/fetal development. Environmental factors can affect the fetus during pregnancy and contribute to increased cardiovascular risk. Low birth weight and length have been associated with increased risk of CVD developing later in life, which demonstrates the concept of fetal origins of disease.[9] This theory is based on the belief that insult during critical periods of fetal development may permanently alter tissue structure and function. These events may also alter genetic regulation during development, leading to a predisposition to disease.[60] Continued slow growth in childhood is associated with higher rates of coronary heart disease in adulthood.[61] The development of hypertension in offspring with restricted growth has been demonstrated in both human and animal studies.[62,63] Clinical guidelines have been developed to address these findings, recommending initiation of blood pressure measurement in children before the age of 3 years in this high-risk population.[64]

DIAGNOSTIC CRITERIA

Conditions with clearly defined genetic mutations, as in familial hypercholesterolemia, can be diagnosed using traditional genetic testing, as described previously in this chapter. Conditions resulting from multifactorial genetic influences, such as hypertension, are more difficult to identify accurately. Screening for known triggers leading to CVD, including birth history, growth patterns, family history, social habits, and past medical history, may provide identification of important indicators of risk.

TREATMENT

Studies to determine the best treatment for CVD with consideration of genetic influences, or pharmacogenomics, are the focus of current and future investigation.[65–67] Genomic considerations include pharmacokinetics, pharmacodynamics (drug targets), pathology-specific genetics, genetic physiologic regulation, and environmental–genetic interactions.[68] Environmental factors, including diet, exercise, and smoking, can influence plasma cholesterol, serving as a leading cause of hypercholesterolemia in the general population. The permissive influence of genes and environment involved in this pervasive form of the disease is poorly understood. Behavior modification can be implemented to control environmental influences, including following a low-fat diet and increasing physical activity. The genetic influences can be countered with pharmacologic use of statin (cholesterol-lowering) drugs directed at the molecular basis of disease.[69]

● **STOP** and *Consider*

What are the risk factors that can be altered to reduce CVD risk? Which ones cannot be changed?

▨ Developmental Maladaptation: Neural Tube Defects

NTDs are a group of serious birth defects involving the tissues of the nervous system (the brain and spine). These defects result from incomplete closure of the neural tube during embryonic life. The degree of neural tube closure distinguishes between the different types of defects. The most common conditions resulting from neural tube anomalies include spina bifida and anencephaly. Each of these conditions has clinical manifestations specific to the condition. The fortification of foods with folic acid is recognized as an important public health strategy in the prevention of NTDs. Pregnancies affected by spina bifida decreased from 2,490 to 1,640 annually since fortification of food with folic acid began in 1998. The number of infants born with anencephaly decreased from 1,640 to 1,380 annually during the same period. The overall risk for development of NTDs decreased by 26%, still short of the national Healthy People 2010 goal of 50% reduction.[70]

PATHOPHYSIOLOGY

NTDs are examples of developmental disorders during embryologic development. Causes that may contribute to these disorders include teratogenic or genetic insult. This defect may occur alone or in combination with other anomalies as part of a syndrome or result from a genetic or chromosomal abnormality. One of the major risks identified with the increased incidence of NTDs is maternal folic acid deficiency. There is still much to understand about the underlying biochemical and genetic mechanisms that lead to folic acid-associated NTDs.[71] Despite the currently unexplained mechanism of disease development, the recognition of folic acid as a cause of NTDs has resulted in successful efforts in prevention. In 1992, the U.S. Department of Health and Human Services, Public Health Service, and the Centers for Disease Control and Prevention issued recommendations for the use of folic acid supplementation to reduce the number of NTDs in childbearing women. Recommendations included the dietary consumption of folic acid 0.4 mg/day, or as a supplement. Because folic acid deficiency interfered with NTD development early in pregnancy, the recommendations included all childbearing-age women, including those not currently pregnant. Not all women who are folate deficient have babies with NTDs, suggesting the influence of genetic mechanisms in the development of the disease phenotype.

● **STOP** *and Consider*

Are there any risks related to fortifying foods with folic acid? Are there risks in other nonchildbearing populations (elderly, children, men) to folic acid food fortification? Is the economic cost associated with food fortification justified?

Figure 6.17 Neural tube defects. Variations in neural tube defects result from incomplete fusion of the neural tube with bone, soft tissues, or skin. (Image modified from Rubin E, Farber JL. *Pathology*. 4th ed. Philadelphia: Lippincott Williams & Wilkins; 2005, with permission.)

CLINICAL MANIFESTATIONS

The stimulus that results in incomplete neural tube closure is initiated early, often before many women even realize they are pregnant. Neural tube closure occurs between embryologic days 24 and 28, beginning cranially at the head and moving distally towards the spine. In anencephaly, the closure defect is located in the skull area, with all or part of the top of the skull and portions of the brain absent. Spina bifida is the result of a closure defect in the spine. There are three main variations of spina bifida:

1. Spina bifida occulta: incomplete closure of vertebrae without protrusion of the meninges or spinal cord
2. Meningocele: incomplete closure with protrusion of meninges and cerebrospinal fluid

3. Myelomeningocele: incomplete closure with protrusion of meninges, cerebrospinal fluid, and spinal cord/nerve roots

In most cases, anencephaly involves a significant portion of the brain, resulting in fatality. The severity of spinal bifida is determined by the involvement of the spinal nerves. Clinical manifestations can range from a dimple at the base of the spine in occulta to lower body paralysis in myelomeningocele. Variations in types of NTDs are depicted in Figure 6.17.

DIAGNOSTIC TESTING

Prenatally, when meninges are in communication with amniotic fluid, alpha-fetoprotein leaks from the cerebrospinal fluid into the amniotic fluid. This can be measured indirectly through determination of alpha-fetoprotein from a maternal blood sample (maternal serum alpha-fetoprotein [MSAFP]). A more direct measurement of alpha-fetoprotein can be obtained using amniotic fluid via amniocentesis. Anatomic anomalies may also be detected by ultrasound.

TREATMENT

Treatment in anencephaly is usually limited to supportive care and comfort. Treatment for meningocele and myelomeningocele requires surgical correction to prevent complications, but it does not alter neurologic damage.

Summary

- Alterations in genetic structure and function form the basis of many diseases.
- Components of the genetic system include genes and chromosomes.
- The double helix structure, DNA, is comprised of specific combinations of four nitrogenous bases, forming genes and chromosomes.
- The sequence of nitrogenous bases in genes produces amino acids, which combine to form proteins.
- Three types of RNA are involved in protein production and include mRNA, tRNA, and rRNA.
- The somatic cells of the body each contains 46 chromosomes: 44 autosomes and 2 sex chromosomes.
- The influence of genetics can be exerted by expression of a trait, the inheritance of a trait, or the establishment of a predisposition for disease.
- Single gene traits are inherited in an autosomal dominant, autosomal recessive, or sex-linked pattern or via a mitochondrial gene disorder.
- Syndromes caused by alterations in chromosome number or structure are associated with multiple clinical manifestations.
- Multifactorial disorders involve both genetic and environmental factors.
- Identification of risk for genetic disorders is based on family history and genetic screening.
- The combination of environment and genetics may underlie diseases that affect morbidity and mortality in the United States and throughout the world.
- As continued investigation reveals information that unlocks many genetic mysteries, the social and ethical implications of such findings must keep pace with the science.

From the Lab

MSAFP levels were measured in a large study that compared measurements before and after mandatory supplementation in the United States.[70] Consistent with the decreased incidence of NTDs, the incidence of high MSAFP values was similarly decreased by 32%, supporting the effectiveness of folic acid fortification efforts.

Research Notes

Technological advances in fetal surgery have contributed to the possibility of intrauterine closure of myelomeningocele as a preferred therapy for the future.[72] Current studies are underway to determine whether the benefits of intrauterine surgical closure are great enough to overcome the risks associated with this type of surgery.

Case Study 6.1

J.S., a 13-year-old male, has hemophilia A. He is entering middle school and wants to play intramural football. Think about a clinical model most related to this diagnosis. From your reading related to genetic disorders, answer the following questions:

1. *What is the pathology associated with hemophilia?*
2. *What are the clinical manifestations?*
3. *What are the risks of his passing hemophilia on to his future daughters? Sons?*
4. *What are the treatment options for hemophilia?*
5. *What are the risks related to treatment of hemophilia?*
6. *What should be the recommendations made in light of his request to play football?*

Log onto the Internet. Search for a relevant journal article or Web site that details hemophilia to confirm your predictions.

Case Study 6.2

William, a 2-year-old male, has a history of delayed motor milestones. He was delayed in rolling over, sitting, and standing. He began to walk at 18 months. He has a waddling gait and difficulty climbing stairs. After genetic testing, William was diagnosed with Duchenne muscular dystrophy (DMD).

1. *What is the genetic defect associated with DMD?*
2. *What are the clinical manifestations of DMD?*
3. *What are the risks of his passing DMD on to his future daughters? Sons?*
4. *What are the treatment options for DMD?*
5. *What is the life expectancy for William?*

Log onto the Internet. Search for a relevant journal article or Web site that details DMD to confirm your predictions.

Practice Exam Questions

1. A person's phenotype can be best described as:
   a. The genetic makeup of an individual
   b. Traits that are observable or apparent
   c. Traits that are inherited in a recessive pattern
   d. Traits that are inherited in a dominant pattern

2. A person's genotype can be best described as:
   a. The genetic makeup of an individual
   b. Traits that are observable or apparent
   c. Traits that are inherited in a recessive pattern
   d. Traits that are inherited in a dominant pattern

3. Which of these conditions follows a Mendelian pattern of recessive inheritance?
   a. Coronary artery disease
   b. Down syndrome
   c. Marfan syndrome
   d. Tay–Sachs disease

4. Which of these conditions follows a multifactorial pattern of inheritance?
   a. Coronary artery disease
   b. Down syndrome
   c. Marfan syndrome
   d. Tay–Sachs disease

5. Fortification of foods with folic acid has resulted in a significant reduction in the incidence of:
   a. Huntington disease
   b. Turner syndrome
   c. Neural tube defects
   d. Cleft lip and palate

6. Which of the following chromosomal abnormalities can result in an inheritable form of trisomy?
   a. Nondisjunction during meiosis
   b. Balanced translocation
   c. Insertion
   d. Deletion

7. Which one of the following hemoglobin types is produced during sickle cell crisis?
   a. HbA
   b. HbF
   c. HbG
   d. HbS

8. Mitochondrial gene disorders are transmitted to:
   a. Sons only
   b. Daughters only
   c. Both daughters and sons
   d. Neither daughters nor sons

9. Mitochondrial genes produce proteins involved in:
   a. Energy metabolism
   b. Growth
   c. Muscle development
   d. Nerve transmission

10. Which of the following is a manifestation of Down syndrome?
    a. Tall stature
    b. Testicular agenesis
    c. Gynecomastia
    d. Epicanthal eye folds

11. Which prenatal test(s) diagnose Down syndrome?
    a. Nuchal translucency
    b. Serum hCG
    c. Karyotype
    d. Serum alpha-fetoprotein

12. What is the risk of a mother with the genetic mutation that causes Fragile X syndrome passing the gene on to offspring?
    a. 100% of females affected
    b. 50% of females affected
    c. 100% of males affected
    d. 50% of males affected

13. Which of the following chromosomal anomalies is incompatible with life?
    a. Monosomy 21
    b. Trisomy 21
    c. Monosomy X
    d. Trisomy X

14. Which one of the following conditions affects females only?
    a. Klinefelter syndrome
    b. Turner syndrome
    c. Down syndrome
    d. Fragile X syndrome

15. The target of damage in Huntington disease is:
    a. Muscle tissue
    b. Skin cells
    c. Nerve tissue
    d. Connective tissue

16. Maternal serum alpha-fetoprotein (MSAFP) is a screening test for which of the following conditions?
    a. Cardiovascular disease
    b. Atherosclerosis
    c. Spinal bifida
    d. Cleft palate

Discussion and Application

1. What did I know about genetic and developmental disorders before today?

2. What are the body processes affected by genetic and developmental disorders? How do genetic and developmental disorders affect those processes?

3. What are the potential etiologies for genetic and developmental disorders? How do genetic and developmental disorders develop?

4. Who is most at risk for developing genetic and developmental disorders? How can these alterations be prevented?

5. What are the human differences that affect the etiology, risk, or course of genetic and developmental disorders?

6. What are the clinical manifestations expected in the course of genetic and developmental disorders?

7. What are the special diagnostic tests useful in determining the diagnosis and course of genetic and developmental disorders?

8. What are the goals of care for individuals with genetic and developmental disorders?

9. How does the concept of alteration in genetics build on what I have learned in the previous chapter and in the previous courses?

10. How can I use what I have learned?

RESOURCES

Fragile X Information Center:
http://www.fpg.unc.edu/~fxic

National Institute of Neurological Disorders and Stroke Huntington's Disease Information Page:
http://ninds.nih.gov/health_and_medical/disorders/huntington.htm

March of Dimes:
http://modimes.org
Find out more about newborn screening, including state-specific requirements.

National Down Syndrome Society:
http://www.ndss.org/

National Human Genome Research Institute, National Institutes of Health:
http://www.genome.gov/
Find out about genetic disorders, definitions of common genetic terms, and current genetic research.

Sickle Cell Disease Association of America:
http://www.sicklecelldisease.org/

American Heart Association. Heart Disease and Stroke Statistics—2009 Update. Dallas: American Heart Association; 2009:
http://www.americanheart.org/presenter.jhtml?identifier=3000090

REFERENCES

1. Guttmacher AE, Collins FS. Genomic medicine—a primer. *N Engl J Med.* 2002;347(19):1512–1520.
2. Khoury MJ, McCabe LL, McCabe ER. Population screening in the age of genomic medicine. *N Engl J Med.* 2003;348(1):50–58.
3. Banta-Wright SA, Steiner RD. Tandem mass spectrometry in newborn screening: a primer for neonatal and perinatal nurses. *J Perinat Neonatal Nurs.* 2004;18(1):41–58; quiz 59–60.
4. Powell IJ, Carpten J, Dunston G, et al. African-American heredity prostate cancer study: a model for genetic research. *J Natl Med Assoc.* 2001;93(12 suppl):25S–28S.
5. Buller A, Pandya A, Jackson-Cook C, et al. Validation of a multiplex methylation-sensitive PCR assay for the diagnosis of Prader-Willi and Angelman's syndromes. *Mol Diagn.* 2000;5(3):239–243.
6. Gill P. DNA as evidence—the technology of identification. *N Engl J Med.* 2005;352(26):2669–2671.
7. Rothstein MA. Genetic justice. *N Engl J Med.* 2005;352(26):2667–2678.
8. Ahlgren M, Melbye M, Wohlfahrt J, et al. Growth patterns and the risk of breast cancer in women. *N Engl J Med.* 2004;351(16):1619–1626.
9. Barker DJ, Eriksson JG, Forsen T, et al. Fetal origins of adult disease: strength of effects and biological basis. *Int J Epidemiol.* 2002;31(6):1235–1239.
10. Mills JL, Signore C. Neural tube defect rates before and after food fortification with folic acid. *Birth Defects Res Part A Clin Mol Teratol.* 2004;70(11):844–845.
11. Botto LD, Lisi A, Robert-Gnansia E, et al. International retrospective cohort study of neural tube defects in relation to folic acid recommendations: are the recommendations working? *BMJ.* 2005;330(7491):571.
12. Wadhwa PD, Buss C, Entringer S, et al. Developmental origins of health and disease: brief history of the approach and current focus on epigenetic mechanisms. *Semin Reprod Med.* 2009;27(5):358–368.
13. Swanson JM, Entringer S, Buss C, et al. Developmental origins of health and disease: environmental exposures. *Semin Reprod Med.* 2009;27(5):391–402.
14. Symonds ME, Sebert SP, Hyatt MA, et al. Nutritional programming of the metabolic syndrome. *Nat Rev Endocrinol.* 2009;5(11):604–610.
15. Offit K, Groeger E, Turner S, et al. The "duty to warn" a patient's family members about hereditary disease risks. *JAMA.* 2004;292(12):1469–1473.
16. Sampson JE, Ouhibi N, Lawce H, et al. The role for preimplantation genetic diagnosis in balanced translocation carriers. *Am J Obstet Gynecol.* 2004;190(6):1707–1711; discussion 1711–1713.
17. Clayton EW. Ethical, legal, and social implications of genomic medicine. *N Engl J Med.* 2003;349(6):562–569.
18. Anderson KE. Huntington's disease and related disorders. *Psychiatr Clin N Am.* 2005;28:275–290.
19. Hoshino M, Tagawa K, Okuda T, et al. Histone deacetylase activity is retained in primary neurons expressing mutant huntingtin protein. *J Neurochem.* 2003;87(1):257–267.
20. Lindvall O, Kokaia Z, Martinez-Serrano A. Stem cell therapy for human neurodegenerative disorders-how to make it work. *Nat Med.* 2004;10(suppl):S42–S50.
21. Aiken CT, Tobin AJ, Schweitzer ES. A cell-based screen for drugs to treat Huntington's disease. *Neurobiol Dis.* 2004;16(3):546–555.

22. Beister A, Kraus P, Kuhn W, et al. The N-methyl-D-aspartate antagonist memantine retards progression of Huntington's disease. *J Neural Transm Suppl.* 2004(68):117–122.

23. Wexler NS, Lorimer J, Porter J, et al. Venezuelan kindreds reveal that genetic and environmental factors modulate Huntington's disease age of onset. *Proc Natl Acad Sci U S A.* 2004;101(10):3498–3503.

24. Steinberg MH. Management of sickle cell disease. *N Engl J Med.* 1999;340(13):1021–1030.

25. McKerrell TD, Cohen HW, Billett HH. The older sickle cell patient. *Am J Hematol.* 2004;76(2):101–106.

26. Quinn CT, Rogers ZR, Buchanan GR. Survival of children with sickle cell disease. *Blood.* 2004;103(11):4023–4027.

27. Platt OS, Brambilla DJ, Rosse WF, et al. Mortality in sickle cell disease. Life expectancy and risk factors for early death. *N Engl J Med.* 1994;330(23):1639–1644.

28. Puthenveetil G, Malik P. Gene therapy for hemoglobinopathies: are we there yet? *Curr Hematol Rep.* 2004;3(4):298–305.

29. Graslund T, Li X, Magnenat L, et al. Exploring strategies for the design of artificial transcription factors: targeting sites proximal to known regulatory regions for the induction of gamma-globin expression and the treatment of sickle cell disease. *J Biol Chem.* 2005;280(5):3707–3714.

30. Matsumoto J, Saver JL, Brennan KC, et al. Mitochondrial encephalomyopathy with lactic acidosis and stroke (MELAS). *Rev Neurol Dis.* 2005;2(1):30–34.

31. Majamaa K, Moilanen JS, Uimonen S, et al. Epidemiology of A3243G, the mutation for mitochondrial encephalomyopathy, lactic acidosis, and strokelike episodes: prevalence of the mutation in an adult population. *Am J Hum Genet.* 1998;63(2):447–454.

32. Cao Z, Wanagat J, McKiernan SH, et al. Mitochondrial DNA deletion mutations are concomitant with ragged red regions of individual, aged muscle fibers: analysis by laser-capture microdissection. *Nucleic Acids Res.* 2001;29(21):4502–4508.

33. Brewer CM, Holloway SH, Stone DH, et al. Survival in trisomy 13 and trisomy 18 cases ascertained from population based registries. *J Med Genet.* 2002;39(e54):1–3.

34. Wald NJ, Rodeck C, Hackshaw AK, et al. SURUSS in perspective. *BJOG.* 2004;111(6):521–531.

35. Hu Y, Zheng M, Xu Z, et al. Quantitative real-time PCR technique for rapid prenatal diagnosis of Down syndrome. *Prenat Diagn.* 2004; 24(9):704–707.

36. Alfirevic Z, Neilson JP. Antenatal screening for Down's syndrome. *BMJ.* 2004;329(7470):811–812.

37. Bronshtein M, Zimmer EZ, Blazer S. A characteristic cluster of fetal sonographic markers that are predictive of fetal Turner syndrome in early pregnancy. *Am J Obstet Gynecol.* 2003;188(4):1016–1020.

38. Sybert VP, McCauley E. Turner's syndrome. *N Engl J Med.* 2004; 351(12):1227–1238.

39. Ostberg JE, Conway GS. Adulthood in women with Turner syndrome. *Horm Res.* 2003;59(5):211–221.

40. Serra A, Cocuzza S, Caruso E, et al. Audiological range in Turner's syndrome. *Int J Pediatr Otorhinolaryngol.* 2003;67(8):841–845.

41. Cooley M, Bakalov V, Bondy CA. Lipid profiles in women with 45,X vs 46,XX primary ovarian failure. *JAMA.* 2003;290(16):2127–2128.

42. Gunther DF, Eugster E, Zagar AJ, et al. Ascertainment bias in Turner syndrome: new insights from girls who were diagnosed incidentally in prenatal life. *Pediatrics.* 2004;114(3):640–644.

43. Starke MK, Albertsson W, Moller A. Parents' descriptions of development and problems associated with infants with Turner syndrome: a retrospective study. *J Paediatr Child Health.* 2003;39(4):293–298.

44. Piippo S, Lenko H, Kainulainen P, et al. Use of percutaneous estrogen gel for induction of puberty in girls with Turner syndrome. *J Clin Endocrinol Metab.* 2004;89(7):3241–3247.

45. Hanton L, Axelrod L, Bakalov V, et al. The importance of estrogen replacement in young women with Turner syndrome. *J Womens Health (Larchmt).* 2003;12(10):971–977.

46. Reynaud K, Cortvrindt R, Verlinde F, et al. Number of ovarian follicles in human fetuses with the 45,X karyotype. *Fertil Steril.* 2004;81(4):1112–1119.

47. Karnis MF, Zimon AE, Lalwani SI. Risk of death in pregnancy achieved through oocyte donation in patients with Turner syndrome: a national survey. *Fertil Steril.* 2003;80(3):498–501.

48. Longui CA, Rocha MN, Martinho LC, et al. Molecular detection of XO - Turner syndrome. *Genet Mol Res.* 2002;1(3):266–270.

49. Pena SD, Sturzeneker R. Fetal diagnosis of monosomy X (Turner syndrome) with methylation-specific PCR. *Prenat Diagn.* 2003; 23(9):769–770.

50. Bakalov VK, Cooley MM, Quon MJ, et al. Impaired insulin secretion in the Turner metabolic syndrome. *J Clin Endocrinol Metab.* 2004;89(7):3516–3520.

51. Fragile X syndrome, Centers for Disease Control. 2003. Available at: http://www.cdc.gov/ncbddd/single_gene/fragilex.htm. Accessed July 6, 2010.

52. Song FJ, Barton P, Sleightholme V, et al. Screening for fragile X syndrome: a literature review and modelling study. *Health Technol Assess.* 2003;7(16):1–106.

53. Gold B, Radu D, Balanko A, et al. Diagnosis of Fragile X syndrome by Southern blot hybridization using a chemiluminescent probe: a laboratory protocol. *Mol Diagn.* 2000;5(3):169–178.

54. Berry-Kravis E, Potanos K. Psychopharmacology in fragile X syndrome—present and future. *Ment Retard Dev Disabil Res Rev.* 2004;10(1):42–48.

55. Rattazzi MC, LaFauci G, Brown WT. Prospects for gene therapy in the fragile X syndrome. *Ment Retard Dev Disabil Res Rev.* 2004;10(1):75–81.

56. Nabel EG. Cardiovascular disease. *N Engl J Med.* 2003;349(1):60–72.

57. Naber CK, Siffert W. Genetics of human arterial hypertension. *Minerva Med.* 2004;95(5):347–356.

58. Gretarsdottir S, Thorleifsson G, Reynisdottir ST, et al. The gene encoding phosphodiesterase 4D confers risk of ischemic stroke. *Nat Genet.* 2003;35(2):131–138.

59. Ridker PM, Hennekens CH, Lindpaintner K, et al. Mutation in the gene coding for coagulation factor V and the risk of myocardial infarction, stroke, and venous thrombosis in apparently healthy men. *N Engl J Med.* 1995;332(14):912–917.

60. Drake AJ, Walker BR. The intergenerational effects of fetal programming: non-genomic mechanisms for the inheritance of low birth weight and cardiovascular risk. *J Endocrinol.* 2004;180(1):1–16.

61. Barker DJ. Fetal programming of coronary heart disease. *Trends Endocrinol Metab.* 2002;13(9):364–368.

62. Eriksson J, Forsen T, Tuomilehto J, et al. Fetal and childhood growth and hypertension in adult life. *Hypertension.* 2000;36(5):790–794.

63. Anderson CM, Lopez F, Zimmer A, et al. Placental insufficiency leads to developmental hypertension and mesenteric artery dysfunction in two generations of Sprague-Dawley rat offspring. *Biol Reprod.* 2006;74:538–544.

64. Ingelfinger JR. Pediatric antecedents of adult cardiovascular disease—awareness and intervention. *N Engl J Med.* 2004;350(21):2123–2212.

65. Cascorbi I, Paul M, Kroemer HK. Pharmacogenomics of heart failure—focus on drug disposition and action. *Cardiovasc Res.* 2004;64(1): 32–39.

66. Mellen PB, Herrington DM. Pharmacogenomics of blood pressure response to antihypertensive treatment. *J Hypertens.* 2005;23(7):1311–1325.

67. Adeyemo A, Luke A, Wu X, et al. Genetic effects on blood pressure localized to chromosomes 6 and 7. *J Hypertens.* 2005;23(7):1367–1373.

68. Siest G, Jeannesson E, Berrahmoune H, et al. Pharmacogenomics and drug response in cardiovascular disorders. *Pharmacogenomics.* 2004;5(7):779–802.

69. Engler MB. Familial hypercholesterolemia: genetic predisposition to atherosclerosis. *Medsurg Nurs.* 2004;13(4):253–257.

70. Centers for Disease Control. Spina bifida and anencephaly before and after folic acid mandate—United States, 1995–1996 and 1999–2000. *MMWR Morb Mortal Wkly Rep.* 2004;53(17):362–365.

71. Stover PJ. Physiology of folate and vitamin B12 in health and disease. *Nutr Rev.* 2004;62(6 pt 2):S3–S12; discussion S13.

72. Bruner JP, Tulipan N, Reed G, et al. Intrauterine repair of spina bifida: preoperative predictors of shunt-dependent hydrocephalus. *Am J Obstet Gynecol.* 2004;190(5):1305–1312.

Altered Cellular Proliferation and Differentiation

LEARNING OBJECTIVES

1. Define and use the key terms listed in this chapter.
2. Recognize the role of genetic mutations in the development of neoplasms.
3. Discuss major carcinogens and their role in carcinogenesis.
4. Outline characteristics of tumor cells.
5. Differentiate benign and malignant tumors.
6. Explain the mechanisms of cancer spread.
7. Classify tumors based on staging and grading criteria.
8. Identify local and systemic clinical manifestations of neoplasia.
9. Describe cancer treatment strategies.
10. Apply the principles of carcinogenesis to select clinical models.

INTRODUCTION

"You have cancer." Very little strikes more fear than those three words. Although many cancers are curable and current research continues to support prevention, early detection, and effective treatment options, cancer continues to affect millions of lives each year. For example, cancer is the second leading cause of death in the United States, second only to cardiovascular disease.[1] About 1.4 million new cancer cases are diagnosed each year in the United States, and one in four deaths is related to cancer, resulting in the death of more than 1,500 people per day.[1]

The Impact of Cancer on the Cell

Cellular **proliferation** is the generation of new, daughter cells divided from progenitor (parent) cells. Meiosis is a process of dividing germ cells resulting in ovum and sperm. Mitosis is the division and proliferation of all other nongerm cells. Cellular proliferation through mitosis occurs continuously and/or in response to needs. For example, epithelial cells of the skin constantly reproduce to replace those damaged by the external environment. These cells can increase the rate of division in times of need, such as that occurs with a wound injury. Similarly, red blood cell (RBC) proliferation replaces RBCs at the end of the cell's 120-day lifespan and also increases exponentially in the case of excessive blood loss to maintain blood volume and oxygenate tissues. A regulated balance of cell growth and death is needed to maintain homeostasis in the body. We are concerned here with the loss of regulated balance of cell division resulting in the *overproliferation* and crowding of cells.

Differentiation refers to the orderly process of cellular maturation to achieve a specific function. Regulation of proliferation and differentiation is under the control of genes, growth factors, nutrients, and stimulation from the external environment. As with proliferation, a balance of differentiated (cells with a specific function, such as RBCs) and undifferentiated (stem cells and progenitor cells) is necessary to respond to the needs of the body (Fig. 7.1).

Stem cells are highly undifferentiated units that have the potential to divide into progenitor cells, then daughter cells, which can then mature into more differentiated units with a specific function. Undifferentiated cells are valued for their flexibility and adaptability. With each step toward differentiation, the cell loses its ability to flexibly respond and adapt but gains the ability to carry out an important physiologic function. For example, with extensive blood loss, daughter cells are directed to differentiate into RBCs to replace the lost blood. Again, a balance of undifferentiated and differentiated cells is needed to maintain homeostasis. We are concerned in this chapter with the loss of differentiation, rendering the cell incapable of carrying out a designated function.

Altered Cellular Proliferation and Differentiation

At the cellular level, cancer occurs because of unrepaired gene malfunction. More specifically, cancer is caused by altering those genes that control cell

reproduction, growth, differentiation, and/or death. The cell is therefore allowed to grow uncontrollably (altered proliferation). The cell also loses its ability to carry out its specified function (altered differentiation) and does not die when expected.

CARCINOGENESIS

Carcinogenesis describes the origin and development of cancerous neoplasms. **Neoplasms** are irreversible deviant cellular developments. **Cancer** is a term used to describe highly invasive and destructive neoplasms. These are groups of cells that do not respond to orderly expected patterns of cellular proliferation and differentiation. Neoplasms can emerge from proliferating parenchymal (functional tissue and organ) or stromal (supportive structure) cells. Rapidly dividing labile cells, such as epithelial

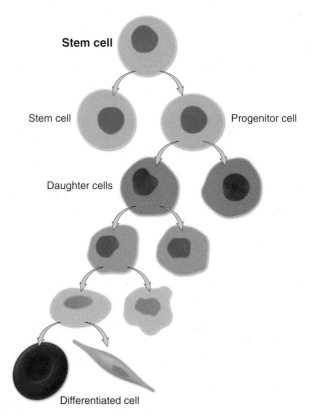

Figure 7.1 Cellular differentiation is the process by which cells become more specialized. Undifferentiated stem cells divide into like stem cells and parent (progenitor) cells, which continue to divide and further differentiate into highly specialized and functional cells. (Image modified from Porth CM. *Essentials of Pathophysiology: Concepts of Altered Health States.* Philadelphia: Lippincott Williams & Wilkins; 2003, with permission.)

cells and blood cells, are highly prone to the development of neoplasms. Permanent (undividing) cells, such as cardiac myocytes, mature neurons, and the lens of the eye, are not. The neoplastic cell ignores the genetic controls placed on cellular proliferation and differentiation.

Why a genetic defect occurs and results in cancer is often unknown. In most cases, the development of cancer is manifested through genetic mutations *after* birth. This is typically related to harmful environmental exposures, which injure the cell DNA and alter the proliferation and differentiation of cells. In a very small percentage of cases (less than 5%), cancer involves an inherited genetic defect and is therefore present *before* birth. Although relatively rare, an inherited predisposition results in an extremely high risk of developing cancer in that person's lifetime. Approximately 1% of heritable cancer syndromes are passed along germ line cells and many follow a Mendelian pattern of inheritance.[2]

Some cancer cases do not follow a clear pattern of inheritance and yet have a strong familial predisposition (i.e., cancer that "runs in families"). Assessing a family's history will reveal cancer types that have emerged in relatives over time. Familial cancers may indicate the presence of a polymorphism (occurrence of more than one form). This means that in families that develop certain types of cancer, this occurs through numerous mechanisms, such as altering the metabolism of agents that predispose to that cancer, deterring the breakdown on carcinogens, altering DNA repair, or impairing cell proliferation. Inheriting these susceptibilities does not guarantee a diagnosis of cancer. However, the risk is greatly increased.

Role of Genes

Cancer is often thought to originate from a single mutated cell, a process called **monoclonal origin**. Most of these mutations are spontaneous alterations in DNA replication or repair without an obvious cause. Given the volume of DNA replication that occurs daily, unrepaired errors in replication are not surprising. Fortunately, the majority of mutations do not affect genes that regulate cell growth and stability. Many of these mutations are of no consequence.

Three major categories of genes exist that, when altered, can lead to cancerous transformations. Typically, a combination of mutations involving more than one gene category is needed for neoplasms to develop. This mutation–transformation–neoplasia

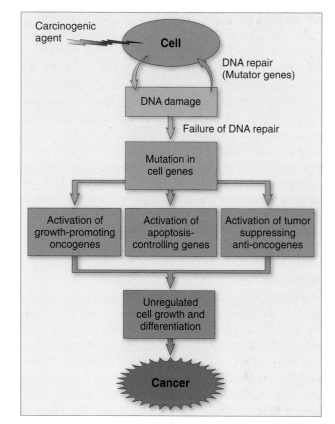

■ **Figure 7.2** Concept map. The genomic mechanisms of cancer. (Image modified from Porth CM. *Essentials of Pathophysiology: Concepts of Altered Health States.* Philadelphia: Lippincott Williams & Wilkins; 2003, with permission.)

🔬 *From the Lab*

Genetic testing may be sought by individuals newly diagnosed with cancer or those who have family members with cancer. Gene testing involves examining a person's DNA, typically taken from cells in a sample of blood, for mutations linked to that type of cancer. Specific genetic mutations have been linked to certain types of cancer, and for some cancer types, this information has been converted into a clinical test. An accurate gene test can determine if a mutation is present but does not guarantee that the disease will develop. For example, a woman with the BRCA 1 breast cancer susceptibility gene has an 80% chance of developing breast cancer by age 65. There is a 20% chance that she will not develop the disease. A woman in that same family could test negative for BRCA 1 and still acquire the disease over time at the same rate as the general population.[3] Although gene testing poses little physical discomfort or risk, the emotional and psychological consequences may be severe, particularly if there are limited prevention, early detection, or treatment interventions.

evolution is unique to each cancer type and the process often takes several years (Fig. 7.2). These categories include:

- **Mutator genes:** genes that repair mutated DNA and protect the genome
- **Oncogenes:** genes that code for proteins involved in cell growth or regulation

- **Tumor suppressor genes:** genes that prohibit overproliferation of cells and regulate apoptosis

Mutator Genes

DNA is constantly being damaged by the environment. Mutator genes repair DNA and, along with tumor suppressor genes, protect the genome. Mutator genes are highly effective and a large number of mutations in mutator genes are needed to produce cancerous neoplams. One theory proposes that cancer cells exhibit a mutator phenotype and that the mutated cells drive tumor progression. Therefore, by disabling the protective, DNA-repairing mutator genes, the environment is conducive to neoplastic development as mutations go unrepaired and the cell becomes unstable.

Oncogenes

Oncogene literally means "cancer gene." Oncogenes promote unregulated cell growth and development and can also inhibit cell death. The activation of oncogenes in germ line cells is often incompatible with life and results in spontaneous abortion. Those germ line mutations that are not lethal can develop into inheritable neoplasms. More commonly, however, activation of oncogenes is seen in the spontaneous mutation of somatic cells.

The conversion from a "normal" gene to one that induces neoplasia depends on the mutation of protooncogenes. **Protooncogenes** are important "normal" genes in the body with a vital role in regulating cell function. Protooncogenes are also considered precursor genes that, when activated, become oncogenes through one of the three ways:

1. Point mutation
2. Translocation
3. Gene amplification

A point mutation damages a single nucleotide base pair in the DNA that leads to the development of altered, unregulated proteins in somatic cells. Point mutations can arise spontaneously or from exposure to environmental influences, such as cancer-inducing chemicals or ultraviolet radiation.

Chromosomal translocations have also been implicated in the activation of oncogenes. The chromosome breaks, relocates, and unites with another chromosome. Encoded proteins become excessive and the cell deviates from expected growth, differentiation, and death cycles. Common types of cancers that result from chromosomal translocations include leukemias, lymphomas, and many solid tumors.

Gene amplification is a process of altering the chromosome by accelerating the replication of genes. Similar to translocations, this is a problem of overproducing gene products. Gene amplification is implicated in many solid tumors, including breast cancer and neuroblastoma. In many cases, the greater the gene amplification, the poorer the prognosis.

With each type of oncogene transformation, the basic mechanisms of action include:

- Encoding growth factors to stimulate cell overproliferation
- Disturbing cell surface receptors and restricting cell-to-cell communication
- Encoding proteins in the cell nucleus to alter the cell cycle, restrict apoptosis, and impact differentiation of the cell

Although oncogenes are often categorized as either viral or cellular/chromosomal, both types result in similar alterations to the cell phenotype. With viral oncogenes, the virus inserts itself into the genetic material of the host cell, replicates, and then moves on to infect other cells. During this process, the virus may capture a portion of the host cell's genetic material along with its own. The proper regulation of genes may not be possible if this occurs because the genetic repertoire of the retrovirus is limited.

The notations for oncogenes are three-letter abbreviations, such as *ras, neu,* or *myc.* The origin or location of the gene is indicated by the prefix of "v-" for virus or "c-" for cell or chromosome; additional prefixes, suffixes, and superscripts provide further delineation. For example, breast cancer has been linked to the c-*neu* oncogene and lung cancer to the c-L-*myc* gene. More than 60 human oncogenes have been identified.[2]

STOP and Consider

Why would someone with Down syndrome (trisomy 21) have an increased risk of developing leukemia?

Tumor Suppressor Genes

Tumor suppressor genes are the genes that regulate the rate at which cells divide and die. A major mechanism for regulating proliferation is to control apoptosis (programmed cell death), so that the optimal number of cells is maintained for homeostasis. When mutated, tumor suppressor genes are inactivated and the cell becomes "immortal," most likely through alteration of the cell mitochondria. This can occur in germ line or somatic cells as inherited or spontaneous mutations. The cell undergoes unrestricted proliferation, and neoplastic transformations are supported. Tumor suppressor genes can be likened to a wall or gate. When intact, growth is restricted. A mutation is like a large hole in the gate, allowing unrestricted growth of the cell.

Several tumor suppressor genes exist. Three common tumor suppressor genes that can allow neoplasias to form when mutated are the *p53* gene, retinoblastoma (*Rb*) gene, and *BCL-2* gene. The *p53* gene has been implicated as the most common mutation that leads to the development of cancer. Located on chromosome 17, this gene is deleted or mutated in three of four types of colorectal cancer and is found in many other malignancies. The *p53* gene is responsible for opposing cell division in response to cell DNA damage by delaying cell development. This delay allows time for DNA to be repaired. If the cell cannot be repaired, the *p53* gene can also force the damaged cell to undergo apoptosis. Without *p53*, cells are unresponsive to the need for repair. Cells with damaged DNA are able to reproduce and can become neoplastic.

STOP *and Consider*

What would happen to the individual who was born with a germ line mutation of p53?

The *Rb* gene is a tumor suppressor gene that, when mutated, can result in a rare childhood cancer of the retina of the eye (retinoblastoma). Just less than half of the cases are germline cell mutations; the remaining are spontaneous mutations in somatic cells. Inheritance of retinoblastoma follows a dominant pattern. The *Rb* gene has a major role in suppressing tumor proliferation. Development of other types of cancer, including osteosarcoma, breast cancer, pancreatic cancer, and lung cancer, has also been connected to inactivation of the *Rb* gene.

The *BCL-2* gene has been discovered to inhibit apoptosis. If gene *BCL-2* becomes mutated and permanently activated, the cell with the altered gene ignores all of the normal triggers to die and becomes immortal. This altered cell continues to divide by mitosis, passing along the altered gene to progeny cells. These cells accumulate and form neoplasms. *BCL-2* mutations were first found in leukocytes and are known to lead to one form of leukemia.

In summary, these gene categories (mutator, oncogene, and tumor suppressor) and other factors that promote cellular overproliferation and/or interrupt apoptosis are necessary, but not sufficient, to allow unregulated growth and to impair cell function. Mutated genes are often implicated as tumor initiators or promoters. Additional alterations in the host cell genetic material, influenced by carcinogens, are required to develop into invasive cancerous transformations.

Carcinogens

The identification of cancer-causing agents is based on epidemiological studies, experimental research, and knowledge of cellular and molecular pathology.

A **carcinogen** is a known cancer-causing agent. Carcinogens are agents that interfere with molecular pathways and can initiate or promote tumors to form in the body. Some carcinogens are considered direct because they cause modification of cell DNA and interfere with cell function. Others are considered indirect because they induce immunosuppression or chronic inflammation or act in conjunction with other carcinogens to induce DNA damage.

Certain substances or exposures are known to cause or promote cellular mutations, such as radiation, exposure to reactive oxygen species (free radicals), hormones, tobacco, infectious microorganisms, and chemicals (Fig. 7.3). Because cancer exhibits a prolonged latent period between the initiation and onset of clinical manifestations, identification of a precise carcinogen can be difficult.

Research Notes

Hill criteria are often applied to epidemiologic studies of carcinogenesis. Researchers attempt to determine whether a substance is carcinogenic based on several criteria, including the strength of the association (i.e., when exposed, how frequently the exposed get cancer), the time line, the presence of a dose–response relationship, and so on. Researchers systematically apply criteria to make logical and reasonable connections between cancer occurrences in populations and the etiology.[4]

Radiation

Ionizing radiation is both a potential cause of, and treatment for, cancer. Although radiation has many diagnostic and therapeutic applications, high-energy ionizing radiation (γ-rays, X-rays, and ultraviolet) is capable of causing genetic damage in a cell and can also kill cells directly. Radiation induces injury by producing reactive oxygen species. These unstable molecules damage the cell membrane, allowing the radiation energy to interrupt cell DNA and invoke mutations.

Labile cells are most affected by radiation exposure. Radiation treatment takes advantage of this feature with the treatment aimed at directly killing cells that are highly proliferative—most notably, cancer cells. The accumulative effect of low-dose radiation exposure is an area of extensive debate. Because all individuals are exposed to low-dose radiation over time, it is difficult to discern whether the radiation is to blame for carcinogenesis.

Ultraviolet radiation is short wavelength electromagnetic energy that, within a certain range, is also capable of inducing carcinogenesis. Sun exposure is the primary source. The risk for developing neoplasms, such as with skin cancer, from radiation exposure depends on the length of exposure, frequency of burn injuries from sun exposure, and skin tone. Similar to other types of radiation injury, the ultraviolet exposure (290 to 320 nm

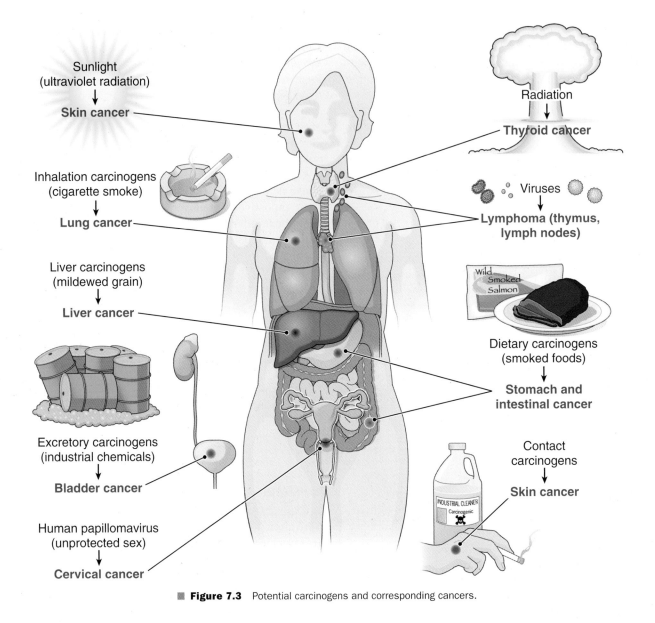

Sunlight
(ultraviolet radiation)
↓
Skin cancer

Inhalation carcinogens
(cigarette smoke)
↓
Lung cancer

Liver carcinogens
(mildewed grain)
↓
Liver cancer

Excretory carcinogens
(industrial chemicals)
↓
Bladder cancer

Human papillomavirus
(unprotected sex)
↓
Cervical cancer

Radiation
↓
Thyroid cancer

Viruses
Lymphoma (thymus, lymph nodes)

Dietary carcinogens
(smoked foods)
↓
Stomach and intestinal cancer

Contact
carcinogens
↓
Skin cancer

■ Figure 7.3 Potential carcinogens and corresponding cancers.

wavelengths) directly kills cells and can induce cellular mutation.

⬤ STOP *and Consider*

Do you think microwave ovens, electromagnetic fields, and ultrasound, as energy transmitters, would induce cellular injury?

Hormones

Hormones, like radiation, are also a cancer promoter and treatment. Some tumor cells are responsive to, or dependent on, hormones for growth. Tumors of the breast, uterus, prostate, and adrenal glands often contain receptors that are responsive to hormone levels in these tissues.

Hormones can also be considered a cancer treatment. They can be therapeutically administered to block the effects of tumor growth. For example, the

adrenal corticosteroid hormones (i.e., prednisone) can directly kill tumor cells, especially lymph cells, and can inhibit mitosis. These drugs also have potent anti-inflammatory effects. Removal of organs or tissues that secrete specific hormones in the body will also affect tumor growth. Hormones such as estrogen and testosterone can be manipulated to "starve" the tumor and prohibit further growth. Tamoxifen is a drug commonly used in breast cancer treatment. Tamoxifen blocks the action of estrogen and inhibits tumor growth in the estrogen-sensitive breast tissues.

Chemicals

Many chemicals have been implicated in carcinogenesis, such as tobacco, asbestos, benzene, insecticides, and formaldehyde. A complete list of known, probable, and possible chemical carcinogens is maintained by the American Cancer Society and is found in the reference section of this chapter.

Chemical carcinogenesis is heavily influenced by individual susceptibility, lifestyle factors (especially diet), and other environmental exposures. Predicting who will develop cancer from exposure to specific chemicals is very difficult given our frequent contact with numerous sources of varying potencies.

Chemicals lead to cancer directly without activation or indirectly. Indirectly, metabolic conversion is required to initiate or promote cancer development. Enzymes in the body are responsible for metabolizing and activating or inactivating potentially carcinogenic chemicals. These enzymes can cause the chemical to react with DNA to initiate a carcinogenic response. Genetic and environmental factors influence these enzyme levels and therefore influence chemical carcinogenesis. The basic mechanism for direct or indirect chemical carcinogenesis include the development of highly reactive species, such as free radicals, that induce cell mutation or alter cell proteins or enzymes to interfere with cell regulation.

Tobacco

Cigarette tar contains thousands of substances, many of which are carcinogenic. Approximately one in three cancer deaths in the United States can be linked to tobacco.[1] Inhaling cigarette and cigar smoke is toxic to respiratory mucosa and is known to cause lung cancer. Use of tobacco is also responsible for initiating or promoting many other types of cancer, such as laryngeal, lip, esophageal, and bladder cancer. Smoking, as with other chemical carcinogens, exhibits a dose effect; that is, the longer and heavier the smoking or tobacco use or exposure, the greater the risk for the development of neoplasms.

Microbes

Viral infections are estimated to be responsible for 15% of all human cancers. The most prevalent of these is caused by human papillomavirus (HPV) and the hepatitis viruses.[2] HPV is transmitted during sexual intercourse to the female cervix where certain strains of the virus can lead to cervical cancer. The hepatitis B or C viruses can lead to hepatocellular cancer.

Viruses vary by the mechanisms leading to neoplasia. For example, retroviruses, such as HIV, can alter genes or proteins that regulate these genes directly and also render the immune system defenseless. In the process of carcinogenesis, viral proteins are necessary to initiate, maintain, or enhance the malignant phenotype. A few bacteria, such as *Helicobacter*

pylori, are also considered carcinogenic. Chronic inflammation, a common complication of chronic infection, is known to support tumor growth.

Initiation–Promotion–Progression Theory

Carcinogenesis is a highly complex process. Multiple steps are involved in the development of neoplasms, and several theories have been suggested. One such theory proposes that an initiating event must be combined with a promoting event for cancer to develop and then progress (Fig. 7.4). This initiation–promotion–progression theory underscores the idea

From the Lab

Cultured human cells can be exposed in the laboratory setting to specific chemicals to determine whether the chemical results in a mutation in the cell. The ability to mutate these cells corresponds closely with carcinogenicity. This rapid test of mutagenicity is much preferred to waiting on epidemiologic studies, a long process of analyzing cancer deaths over time and attempting to identify the source.

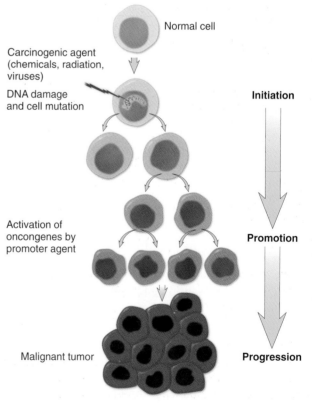

Figure 7.4 Initiation–promotion–progression theory. Initiation involves the exposure of cells to a carcinogenic agent. A promoter agent activates promotion and unregulated cell growth begins. Progression is the acquisition of independent growth of tumor cells. (Image modified from Porth CM. *Essentials of Pathophysiology: Concepts of Altered Health States*. Philadelphia: Lippincott Williams & Wilkins; 2003, with permission.)

of cofactors in cancer etiology. The **initiating event** causes a mutation in a cell. The initiating event may eventually be identified, but many times it is not. The **promoting event** is an expansion of the mutated cell's growth and reproduction. The continued growth of the cell depends on continued exposure to the promoter. A common cancer promoter is chronic inflammation. For example, chronic gastritis has been implicated in the development of gastric cancer. Other cancer promoters include hormones and chemicals in the environment. **Progression** is an extension of the promotion phase with one exception: now the cancerous growth is no longer dependent on continued exposure to the promoter. The growth now becomes autonomous. The cell is capable of functioning outside of the rules that regulate cell growth, division, and death. If either the initiating or promoting event occurs in isolation, or if the promoter occurs before the initiator, cancer does not develop.

Often, the exact initiator–promoter event is not clearly identified. Also, and perhaps most importantly, not all individuals who are exposed to a cancer-causing agent develop cancerous neoplasms. This fact highlights the complex interaction of heredity and the environment in the etiology and promotion of cancer.

Module 2

The Impact of Cancer on Tissues, Organs, and Organ Systems

Neoplasms exhibit autonomy and anaplasia. **Autonomy** refers to the unregulated proliferation of the neoplasm. **Anaplasia** refers to the loss of cell differentiation and therefore the loss of cell function. The greater the degree of anaplasia, the more aggressive, or malignant, the tumor will be. When analyzing cells under a microscope, those with greater anaplasia show wide variation in size and shape with enlarged nuclei and rapid, atypical mitosis (Fig. 7.5).

Neoplasms exhibit several other distinct characteristics:

- Loss of cell-to-cell communication, which allows further unrestricted growth of tumor cells
- Increased energy expenditure, which deprives unaffected cells of nutrients
- Increased motility and loss of cohesion/adhesion, which promotes movement to other locations
- Rapid angiogenesis, which provides extensive blood flow to the tumor cells
- Substance secretion, which alters the metabolism and degrades neighboring unaffected cells
- Present foreign antigens on the cancer cell surface, which can trigger the immune response

Proliferating cells are typically sensitive to the presence of neighboring cells. During wound healing, when cell-to-cell contact is established, the cells no longer reproduce. When this contact is lost, DNA, RNA, and proteins are triggered to synthesize new cells. Neoplastic cells are not sensitive to cell-to-cell messages. The neoplastic cells do not recognize that other cells are nearby and do not respond accordingly by decreasing the rate of reproduction. Neoplasms exhibit deviant and

■ Figure 7.5 Cellular pleomorphism. Note the irregular cell shapes and sizes and prominent nuclei.

excessive growth factors that allow rapid reproduction and angiogenesis (development of new blood vessels) to meet the extreme nutrient demands of the tumor cells. The blood flow demands of neoplastic cells deprive neighboring tissues of adequate oxygen and other nutrients, which result in tissue ischemia and necrosis. The tumor cells can also secrete enzymes that degrade the extracellular matrix and allow the tumor to move into neighboring tissues.

Cellular mutations and aberrations are seen as a type of cellular injury that is subject to destruction by the inflammatory and immune responses. The tumor cells express antigens seen as foreign to the host. Many cellular transformations are removed from the body by these active defense mechanisms and never progress to form tumors in the body. Immunodeficiency, therefore, results in a much higher risk for the development of cancer.

Paraneoplastic Syndromes

Paraneoplastic syndromes are hormonal, neurologic, hematologic, and chemical disturbances in the body, which are not directly related to invasion by the primary tumor or metastasis. Along with the local effects exerted by a growing tumor, paraneoplastic syndromes are often responsible for the range of clinical manifestations that can occur.

A significant characteristic of many neoplasms is the ability to produce and secrete ectopic hormones. **Ectopic** refers to hormone secretion from a site outside of an endocrine gland. The ectopic hormones are not under the regulatory control of the endocrine system and do not respond to the feedback mechanisms typical of that system. In some cases, substances are secreted by the tumor that mimic the hormone function and result in clinical manifestations characteristic of an oversecretion of that hormone. For example, some tumors secrete excess antidiuretic hormone. This hormone signals the body to retain water and sodium. The individual will present with widespread edema; this condition, when severe, can lead to coma and death.

Paraneoplastic syndromes also disturb neurologic function. As presented in the previous example, tumors can secrete hormones that disturb fluid and electrolyte balance, and this directly affects neurologic functioning. Tumors can also cause generalized numbness, weakness, and loss of neurologic function through several mechanisms, including promoting brain hemorrhage, promoting infection in the central nervous system (CNS), or denying the vascular supply and oxygen to neuronal tissues.

■ **Figure 7.6**   Benign versus malignant tumors. **A:** Benign tumor shows a slow-growing mass that has not yet invaded nearby tissues. **B:** Malignant tumor shows aggressive cell growth and invasion into nearby tissues and blood vessels.

Benign Versus Malignant

Tumors are classified as benign or malignant (Fig. 7.6). The terms benign and malignant refer to the tumor location and appearance related to the tissue of origin (the unaffected tissue surrounding the neoplasm). Typically, tumors that remain localized and closely resemble the tissue of origin are considered **benign**. In other words, benign tumors overproliferate but do not demonstrate a significant loss of differentiation. Benign tumors are often met with a sigh of relief; however, benign is not always equivalent to harmless. Large benign tumors can impinge on nearby structures, obstruct vital functions, and can even result in death. In some cases, benign growths, such as polyps or skin tags, are recognized as tumors but are not actually neoplastic.

Tumors that are invasive and destructive, proliferate rapidly, spread to other sites (metastasize), and do not resemble the tissue of origin are considered **malignant**. Malignant tumors can promote ischemia and necrosis of tissue because the tumor uses energy and nutrients needed by unaffected tissues. As stated previously, the term cancer is usually equated with malignant neoplasms.

Cancer Spread

Neoplasms invade locally by impinging on and moving into nearby tissues. **Local spread** is the proliferation of the neoplasm within the tissue of origin. Enlargement of tumors within the tissue or organ promotes loss of function and can result in obstruction, hemorrhage, and necrosis. Although the tumor is getting larger, it remains localized at this early stage. Obviously, confined neoplastic growths equate to a more favorable prognosis.

Direct extension is a process of tumor cells moving into adjacent tissues and organs. This aspect of invasion beyond the local tissues is a defining characteristic of malignancy. Penetration of the basement membrane is the first step for epithelial tumors. Those tumors located in areas without a basement membrane incur less resistance to invade distally. The neoplastic cells adhere to the extracellular matrix by expressing surface adhesion molecules. The tumor proceeds by releasing enzymes that dissolve the extracellular matrix. Once free of the confines of the local tissue or organ, the tumor travels to nearby structures, adheres to adjacent extracellular matrices, and again releases enzymes that degrade the neighboring matrix and allow the tumor to move into the nearby tissues and organs. **Seeding** is a form of direct extension in which neoplastic proliferation occurs within peritoneal and pleural cavities surrounding the affected tissue or organ. The malignant tumors move along these membranes and can gain easy access to other organs supported within these cavities.

Metastases occur when neoplasms are spread to distant sites often by way of the lymphatics or blood vessels (Fig. 7.7). The lethal aspect of cancer is metastatic growth. Once the neoplasm has moved to a distant site, detection and treatment become much more complex.

The mechanism for movement of neoplasms to distant sites is a process of adherence and degradation with the addition of access to the blood and lymphatics. The tumor cells accomplish this by:

1. Breaking through the basement membrane (if present) and extracellular matrix
2. Gaining access to and circulating within the blood vessels or lymph system
3. Leaving the blood vessels or lymph system and adhering to distant tissues
4. Establishing a new nutrient network at the distant tissues through a process of angiogenesis

Tumors can access distant sites most readily through the lymphatic system. Lymphatic capillaries and venules are thinner than other blood and lymphatic vessels and are therefore less resistant to invasion by neoplasms. The neoplasm binds to endothelial cells in the vessels, releases enzymes that degrade the vessel wall, and moves into the blood or lymph circulation. If the immune defense is unsuccessful, the tumor cells then travel through the circulation to distant sites, attach and move through vessel walls, exit the circulation, and move into the

■ **Figure 7.7** Metastatic spread of tumors through the vascular system. A primary benign tumor shows a slow-growing mass that has not invaded nearby tissues. A malignant tumor shows aggressive cell growth and invasion into nearby tissues and blood vessel.

distant site. Once inside the new location, the neoplasm must re-establish a nutrient network through a process of angiogenesis. The tumor secretes growth factors that allow the development of vascular flow to the proliferating neoplasm at the distant site. Vessels are generated, and the tumor continues to proliferate.

The preferred location of the newly settled neoplasm is somewhat predictable. Organ **tropism** is a term used to describe the affinity of a primary tumor to a specific distant site. Factors that promote preferential relocation include:

1. A favorable environment offered by the new tissue or organ
2. Adherence molecule compatibility between the neoplasm and the new tissue or organ
3. The location of the organ in relation to the path of blood flow

For example, tumors that originate in the colon are prone to metastasizing in the liver. This is related to easy access of colon tumor cells through the veins of the portal circulation, which travels directly to the liver, allowing adherence of tumor cells to this organ. Another common site for metastatic growth is the lung, where tumor cells adhere after being transported through the vena cava. Organ tropism is also demonstrated in tumors that move from the lung to the brain and from the breast or prostate to the bone.

Cancer Nomenclature

Identification of the tumor type based on the tissue of origin is a common method of naming neoplasms. Although not used consistently, the suffix "oma" is often employed to designate tumors based on cell or tissue of origin. The cell or tissue of origin is placed directly before this suffix in *benign* tumors. For example, a benign tumor of the squamous epithelium is referred to as an **epithelioma**. When the same cell origin presents as fingerlike projections, it is referred to as a **papilloma**. Benign tumors of glandular epithelial origin are termed **adenomas**; those that arise from germ cells are called **teratomas**; those that arise from bone cells are known as **osteomas**; and those stemming from chondrocytes are called **chondromas**.

When the tumor is *malignant*, the cell or tissue prefix and the suffix "oma" remain with one addition: "carcin" is placed in the middle to designate malignant epithelial cells, and "sarc" is placed in the middle to designate malignant connective tissue cells. For example, a malignant tumor of epithelial cells is called an **adenocarcinoma**. A malignant tumor of chondrocytes is a **chondrosarcoma**. As indicated, this nomenclature does not always follow a consistent pattern. Lymphoma, melanoma, leukemia, and hepatoma are all malignant neoplasms. Table 7.1 further distinguishes benign and malignant tumor nomenclature.

Carcinoma in situ is a unique term used to describe carcinomas confined to the epithelium that have not yet penetrated the basement membrane. These neoplasms remain "in situ" for an indefinite period. During this time, the tumor is often asymptomatic. Detection of tumors in situ represents a favorable prognosis. However, many carcinomas are not detected until the tumor cells penetrate the basement membrane and metastasize to distant organs.

CANCER CLASSIFICATIONS

Staging is a process of classifying the extent or spread of neoplasms and refers to the tumor size, location, lymph node involvement, and spread (Fig. 7.8). The higher the number, the more extensive the tumor size and spread. Treatment decisions are often based on staging criteria. The TNM classification system is frequently used to stage tumors (Table 7.2). TNM stands for:

- T = tumor size: indicates the presence and size of the primary tumor
- N = node (lymph) involvement: indicates involvement of regional lymph nodes
- M = metastases: indicates the extent of metastases

Tumor **grading** is a process of differentiating the level of anaplasia depicted by the tumor. Tumors are graded from I (well differentiated) to IV (highly undifferentiated). As the tumor grade increases, the cells become more deviant from the tissue of origin. Those that are graded lower (I or II) resemble the tissue of origin in terms of size, shape, structure, and mitotic activity. Those with a higher grade (III or IV) demonstrate little resemblance to the tissue of origin.

Table 7.1 Tumor Nomenclature

Tissue Type	Benign Tumors	Malignant Tumors
Epithelial		
Surface	Papilloma	Squamous cell carcinoma
Glandular	Adenoma	Adenocarcinoma
Endothelial		
Blood vessels	Hemangioma	Hemangiosarcoma
Lymph vessels	Lymphangioma	Lymphangiosarcoma
Connective		
Fibrous	Fibroma	Fibrosarcoma
Adipose	Lipoma	Liposarcoma
Cartilage	Chondroma	Chondrosarcoma
Bone	Osteoma	Osteosarcoma
Muscle		
Smooth muscle	Leiomyoma	Leiomyosarcoma
Striated muscle	Rhabdomyoma	Rhabdomyosarcoma
Neural		
Glial tissue	Glioma	Glioblastoma, astrocytoma, medulloblastoma, or oligodendroglioma
Meninges	Meningioma	Meningeal sarcoma
Blood		
Granulocyte		Myelocytic leukemia
Erythrocyte		Polycythemia vera
Plasma cells		Multiple myeloma
Lymphocyte		Lymphocytic leukemia or lymphoma

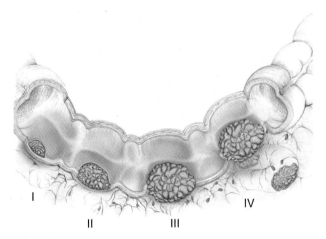

■ Figure 7.8 Tumor staging, I through IV. The size of the tumor and local to distant invasion increases with higher numeric staging. (Asset provided by Anatomical Chart Company.)

■ Cancer Prognosis

Many factors affect the likely course and outcome after a patient is diagnosed with cancer, including the type, location, and stage of the disease, as well as the person's age, overall health, and response to treatment. Cancer prognosis is typically communicated based on a 5-year survival rate. A 5-year relative survival rate is the percentage of persons who are living 5 years after diagnosis. The 5-year survival rate includes those who are cancer free, in

Table 7.2 TNM Classification System

Classification	Description
Primary Tumor (T)	
TX	Primary tumor cannot be evaluated
T0	No evidence of primary tumor
Tis	Carcinoma in situ (early cancer that has not spread to neighboring tissue)
T1, T2, T3, T4	Size or extent of the primary tumor
Regional Lymph Nodes (N)	
NX	Regional lymph nodes cannot be evaluated
N0	No regional lymph node involvement (no cancer found in the lymph nodes)
N1, N2, N3	Involvement of regional lymph nodes (number and/or extent of spread)
Distant Metastasis (M)	
MX	Distant metastasis cannot be evaluated
M0	No distant metastasis (cancer has not spread to other parts of the body)
M1	Distant metastasis (cancer has spread to distant parts of the body)

TNM, tumor size, node, metastases.

Reprinted with permission from Greene F, Page D, Morrow M, et al. *AJCC Cancer Staging Manual*. 6th ed. New York: Springer; 2002, with permission.

remission, or living with cancer. An example of variations in 5-year survival rates is illustrated by ovarian cancer. For patients diagnosed at stage III or IV in which the tumor could not be completely removed and treatment was suboptimal, the 5-year survival rate was less than 10%. In contrast, the 5-year survival approaches 50% for those with ovarian cancer who are diagnosed in earlier stages (prior to or at stage III) with surgical tumor removal.[5]

■ General Manifestations

Early general manifestations of neoplasms are often vague and ignored. Major general manifestations are related to the following:

1. Systemic inflammatory and immune responses
2. Increased metabolic rate induced by tumors
3. Paraneoplastic syndromes
4. Local effects of tumor encroachment or obstruction on neighboring tissues

General manifestations that are related to systemic inflammatory and immune responses include lymphadenopathy, fever, and anorexia. Lymphadenopathy, a condition of enlarged lymph nodes throughout the body, is a condition of lymph hyperplasia. Hyperplasia of the lymph nodes occurs in response to lymphocyte immunoreactivity, specifically against the developing neoplasm. Rapid, acute enlargement of lymph nodes often produces tenderness. The immunoreactivity that accompanies neoplasias is often a low-grade, chronic hyperplasia that is nontender. The supraclavicular nodes are often described as sentinel lymph nodes—these are often the first lymph nodes to receive lymphatic drainage from a malignant tumor.

Unexplained fever is also a common manifestation of cancer. Fever results from the release of pyrogens directly from cancer cells and other cells active in the inflammatory response (Chapter 3). Similarly, anorexia (loss of appetite) is a manifestation present within the inflammatory response caused by the presence of circulating chemical mediators. Anorexia can also result from changes in taste receptors (the mechanism is unclear) that can accompany tumor cell growth.

Inflammatory mediators, along with excess energy use by the proliferating neoplastic cells, can result in unexplained weight loss and tissue wasting, a syndrome called **cachexia**

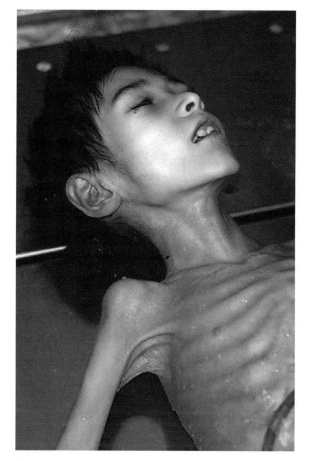

■ **Figure 7.9** Cachexia of malignancy. This photo is of a patient with pancreatic carcinoma. The wasting away of body tissue is not entirely a matter of lost appetite.

Box 7.1 ABCDE: The Warning Signs of Skin Cancer

The following characteristics warrant further examination by a health care practitioner:

Asymmetry: a mole that is irregularly shaped

Border: a mole with jagged edges without clear definition

Color: a growth that is multicolored or that changes color

Diameter: a sudden increase in a mole size, especially one that is greater than 6 mm across (the size of a pencil eraser)

Elevation: a flat mole that becomes elevated

provide clues to the presence of neoplasms. Constipation, diarrhea, and blood in the stool may be evident in colon cancer, and cough, hemoptysis (blood in sputum), and shortness of breath is often present in lung cancer. Visible changes in the skin are noticed in skin cancer (Box 7.1).

Tumors can also exert effects on the blood. High levels of circulating calcium (hypercalcemia) can result from breakdown of bone by tumor cells or as a paraneoplastic syndrome of excess parathyroid-like hormone secretion. Crowding of blood cells in the bone marrow can result in suppression of RBC and platelet production. Hemorrhage, also a common manifestation of tissue destruction caused by tumor-secreted enzymes, contributes to loss of blood cells. Anemia, bruising, and poor clotting are common effects of these alterations in the blood.

● **STOP** *and* **Consider**

How is delayed wound healing, as a clinical manifestation of cancer, explained by the deregulation of the destruction and regeneration/repair balance of the extracellular matrix during tumor invasion?

Diagnostic Tests

Coupled with a complete history and physical examination, the following diagnostic tests can be used to determine the presence and extent of neoplasms:

- Imaging studies
- Biopsy and cytology studies
- Tumor markers and other blood, urine, or tissue tests

Imaging studies allow direct visualization of tumor masses via radiographs (X-rays), endoscopic examination, ultrasound, computed tomography (CT), or magnetic resonance imaging (MRI) scans. These tests are useful in determining the presence, size, and location of tumors. Once the tumor has

(Fig. 7.9). Cachexia is believed to be a result of early feelings of fullness with eating coupled with the release of chemical mediators, such as tumor necrosis factor, that induce a lack of appetite. Tumor necrosis factor also suppresses the enzymes that are needed to release fatty acids from lipoproteins for use by tissues. The presence of high levels of tumor necrosis factor makes lipid energy unavailable to the tissues and promotes tissue wasting.

Local clinical manifestations are site dependent and are related to (1) the space occupied by the tumor that impinges on the local structures and (2) the loss of function in the tissue or organ that is being "taken over" by the tumor. Tumor cells are destructive to neighboring tissues and cause bleeding, bruising, and poor wound healing. A palpable mass is often the first clinical manifestation that may present in tumors such as those found in the breast, testicle, and lymph nodes. In later stages, compression on nearby structures can elicit a pain response, such as a chronic headache with brain tumors, bone pain with proliferating cells crowding in the bone marrow, and abdominal pain that can occur in pancreatic cancer. Loss of function may also been located, tissue samples can be removed (biopsy) and these cells examined (cytology) to determine the presence and stage of neoplasms. In most cases, a definitive diagnosis of cancer can be made only with a microscopic examination of tumor cells.

Tumor markers are substances that may be detected in cells or body fluids and can provide clues to the presence, extent, and treatment response of certain neoplasms. Tumor markers may be produced by the tumor itself or by unaffected cells in the body in response to the presence of a malignant or benign tumor. Hundreds of tumor markers are used to identify various types of tumors.

Tumor markers can be comprised of hormones, enzymes, and immunoglobulins. Many tumor markers are expressed as protein antigens. For example, prostate-specific antigen (PSA), produced by cells in the prostate, is present in low concentrations in adult males. Elevations of PSA may be found in the blood of men with inflammation (prostatitis), benign enlargement (benign prostatic hypertrophy), and malignant neoplasms of the prostate. Similarly, CA 125 is an antigen-expressed tumor marker for ovarian cancer, but it may also be increased in uterine, cervical, pancreatic, lung, colon, breast, and gastrointestinal cancers. This tumor marker can also be increased in noncancerous conditions, such as pregnancy, pelvic inflammatory disease, pancreatitis, liver disease, and inflammatory conditions of the lung. Measurement of carcinoembryonic antigen (CEA) is primarily used to monitor colorectal cancer disease and treatment; however, a wide variety of other cancers can also produce elevations in CEA, including cancer of the lung, breast, pancreas, stomach, cervix, bladder, kidney, thyroid, liver, and ovary. Inflammatory conditions, such as inflammatory bowel disease, pancreatitis, and hepatitis, can also cause elevations in CEA levels.

As indicated previously, tumor markers can also be expressed in some noncancerous conditions and are not elevated in every person with cancer, especially in the early stages. In addition, many tumor markers are not specific to one type of cancer; that is, a tumor marker level can be elevated by more than one type of cancer. Therefore, tumor marker results are interpreted with caution. The measurement of tumor marker levels alone is *not* sufficient to diagnose cancer. Rather, these tests are most informative after diagnosis when results are compared over time. Monitoring tumor marker trends allows the ability to determine treatment effectiveness and to determine recurrence of the tumor after treatment.

Other blood tests may also be needed to diagnose or monitor cancer treatment. Decreased hemoglobin levels may indicate anemia, a systemic manifestation of cancer. White blood cell (WBC), platelet, and RBC levels may also be decreased, particularly after chemotherapy.

Cancer Treatment

Treatment of cancer has three possible goals:

1. Completely eradicate the neoplasms
2. Control continued growth and spread
3. Reduce symptoms without curing the cancer

Major treatment strategies to achieve these goals include surgery, chemotherapy, radiation, hormones, and immunotherapy. Each of these therapeutic strategies can be used alone or in combination. Surgery, chemotherapy, and radiation are compared in Table 7.3. Bone marrow transplantation may also be used to replace or supplement blood cells in the bone marrow. Stem cell transplantation in the bone marrow has also shown promise as a therapeutic strategy for some types of cancer.

Although treatment of the tumor is important, care of the *patient* with cancer and his or her family involves the provision of psychosocial support needed to address the anxiety and depression that may accompany such a diagnosis. This support may include addressing sexuality, spirituality, and other personal issues related to the diagnosis, treatment, and coping with cancer. The health professional must also be aware of and open to discussing alternative, complementary, or experimental therapies.

Palliative care is another important aspect of cancer treatment. **Palliative care** is the term frequently used to describe

Research Notes

The use of alternative and complementary therapies for the treatment of cancer is relatively common. Alternative and complementary therapies include a diverse group of health care systems, practices, and products that are not presently considered to be part of conventional medicine. Examples of such therapies include acupuncture, herbal medicines, and homeopathy. In one study of 453 cancer patients with different types of cancer, 69% had used at least one form of complementary or alternative therapy.[6] Although conventional cancer treatment (chemotherapy, radiation, and surgery) approaches have undergone rigorous testing, much less is known about the safety and effectiveness of many alternative and complementary therapies. Clinical trials are underway to determine the safety and effectiveness of acupuncture to reduce symptoms of advanced colorectal cancer, the use of shark cartilage in the treatment of inoperable lung cancer, and the use of mistletoe extract and chemotherapy for the treatment of solid tumors.[7]

Table 7.3 Cancer Treatment Strategies

Treatment Strategy	Mechanism of Action	Adverse Effects/Complications
Surgery	Directly removing the tumor, organ, or affected lymph nodes through a variety of surgical techniques; pathologic specimens are examined for clear margins denoting complete tumor removal	Inability to remove all of the tumor cells, bleeding, infection
Chemotherapy	Administering medications systemically to interrupt tumor growth or kill tumor cells; combination therapy with two or more agents is common	Nausea, vomiting, hair loss, poor wound healing, immunosuppression, infections, and bleeding
Radiation	Using focal ionizing radiation to damage cell DNA and prevent further replication of the proliferating cells; external radiation (most common) is aimed at the tumor from outside of the body; internal radiation is implanted into or near the tumor in small capsules or other container; systemic radiation is a process of administering (oral or injected) unsealed radioactive materials that travel throughout the body	Skin penetration causes skin redness, irritation, itching, poor wound healing, skin ulceration, and, over time, hyperpigmentation and atrophy. Bleeding, infection, and anemia can result from loss of blood cells. Fibrosis of tissues and organs can occur, leading to diarrhea, esophageal or intestinal strictures, and fibrosis of the heart and lungs
Biologic response modifiers (BMRs)	Altering the biologic response of the host most often achieved through stimulating the host immune response	Few, if any, adverse effects; BMRs selectively aid in destroying tumor cells without affecting the host cells
Hormones	Manipulating tumors that depend on hormones by inhibiting RNA and protein synthesis and binding to receptor sites	Dependent on the expected response of the hormone used; The actions of the hormone are exaggerated

treating symptoms, such as pain, without curing the cancer. Common side effects of the treatment include fatigue, nausea, vomiting, pruritus, and diarrhea. Care of the patient includes addressing complications of treatment and providing nutritional support for optimal health.

Cancer Prevention

Prevention of cancer involves avoiding known carcinogens, participating in health promotion activities, such as exercising moderately and consuming a balanced healthy diet, accepting vaccinations when indicated, and taking measures to protect against chronic injury, including exposure to reactive oxygen species. Individuals with light skin are most at risk for basal cell carcinoma and melanoma. Those with darker skin are protected by melanin pigment. The melanin absorbs ultraviolet radiation. Although those with darker skin are more protected, the skin is still vulnerable to burn injuries, and cancer can develop. Using sunscreen and keeping exposed skin areas covered help protect against and prevent skin cancers.

Many other types of cancer are also considered preventable, including those caused by tobacco use, heavy alcohol consumption, infection with carcinogenic microorganisms, and obesity. Of the 564,000 deaths predicted to occur each year in the United States from cancer, the American Cancer Society estimated in 2009 that 180,000 cancer deaths were caused by tobacco use.[1] Approximately 170,000 preventable cancer deaths are predicted to be related to nutritional factors, physical inactivity, or obesity.[1] Vaccination against certain viral infections may also reduce the cancer incidence. For example, vaccination against hepatitis B virus should decrease the incidence of hepatocellular cancer.

Children and Cancer

Although rare, cancer is the leading cause of death by disease in children aged 1 through 14 years. Whereas most adult cancers involve tissues and solid organs with an epithelial origin (carcinomas), such as colon cancer, lung cancer, and breast cancer, most childhood cancers originate in the mesodermal germ layer, which develops into bone, blood, blood vessels, muscle, lymphatics, connective tissue, and kidneys. Therefore, the types of cancer most prevalent in childhood are leukemia (31%), brain/spinal cord tumors (21%), neuroblastoma (7%), Wilms tumor (6%), Hodgkin lymphoma (HL) (4%), non-Hodgkin lymphoma (NHL) (4%), rhabdomyosarcoma (3%), retinoblastoma (3%), osteosarcoma (3%), and Ewing sarcoma (2%). Neoplasms that resemble embryonic tissue can originate during embryonic and fetal development and persist to form tumors in the body. These embryonic tumors are most often manifested prior to age 5 years.

Research Notes

Gene therapy has been suggested as a viable therapy for childhood cancer. "Corrective" genes are implanted to overcome the genetic abnormalities present in neoplastic cells that are not yet considered malignant. Although limited success has occurred to this point, multiple mechanisms are suggested for the use of gene therapy in the treatment of childhood cancer. Some of these mechanisms include transferring genes into cells to inhibit neoplastic vascular growth or to render the malignant cell more sensitive to chemotherapeutic drugs. Another area of research is the use of genes to modify unaffected tissues to make them more resistant to the harmful effects of chemotherapeutic drugs or radiation, thereby allowing more intensive treatment of the malignant cells without such extensive damage to unaffected cells.[9]

The cause of childhood cancer more often has an inherited or developmental basis because children have had limited exposure to environmental exposures, such as chemicals, and limited time to participate in harmful health behaviors, such as smoking. Some childhood cancers are present at birth. Those with clear inheritance include retinoblastoma (retina), Wilms tumor (kidney), and osteosarcoma (bone). Children born with organ malformations and certain chromosomal aberrations, such as trisomy 21, are also more prone to the development of neoplasms.

Detection of cancer in children is often difficult. Unexplained clinical manifestations that should alert parents and health professionals to a potential problem include: unusual mass or swelling, pallor, persistent malaise, bruising, sudden and persistent pain, limping gait, fever, prolonged illness, headaches, vision changes, and excessive, rapid weight loss. Dramatic improvements in survival of children have occurred over the past 20 years because of advances in treatment. The average 5-year survival rates for all cancer types is greater than 75%.[8]

Module 3

Clinical Models

The following clinical models were selected to help apply knowledge related to altered cellular proliferation and differentiation. Note the commonalities of cellular autonomy and anaplasia. Recognize the differences in clinical manifestations and diagnosis based on the tumor types and locations.

Lung Cancer

Carcinoma of the lung is the leading cause of cancer deaths in the world. Smoking and other environmental toxin exposures are unequivocally implicated in the carcinogenesis.

PATHOPHYSIOLOGY

Lung carcinomas originate most frequently in the epithelial lining of the bronchi, bronchioles, and alveoli. Tumor growth is initiated by mutations that can trigger oncogenes, subdue tumor suppressor genes, or cause deletions in the short arm of chromosome 3. The development of lung cancer represents the end stage of multiple mutations and cellular transformations in the process of carcinogenesis.

As the tumor enlarges, the neoplasms can penetrate epithelial layers and move into the lung tissue, pleural cavity, chest wall, and beyond. The location of large lung tumors allows compression on lower cervical and upper thoracic nerves. Metastatic spread occurs via lymph channels and the vascular system. Lung carcinoma is organ tropic to the bone, liver, and brain and is divided into four subcategories:

- *Adenocarcinoma* (35%): Neoplasms develop in the peripheral bronchiolar and alveolar lung tissue leading to pleural fibrosis and adhesions

■ **Figure 7.10** Adenocarcinoma of the lung. Adenocarcinoma is the most common type of lung cancer and often begins in the peripheral bronchiolar and alveolar lung tissue. This tumor is found in the upper right lobe of the lung. (Image modified from Rubin E, Farber JL. *Pathology*. 4th ed. Philadelphia: Lippincott Williams & Wilkins; 2005.)

(Fig. 7.10). Adenocarcinoma is divided into subtypes based on the structure of origin, including acinar, papillary, and bronchioalveolar.

- *Squamous cell carcinoma* (30%): Begins with injury to the bronchial columnar epithelium (i.e., from smoking) and leads to squamous metaplasia, dysplasia, carcinoma in situ, and an invasive tumor. Tumor cells can be detected in expectorated sputum.
- *Small cell carcinoma* (20%): A highly malignant epithelial tumor that grows and metastasizes rapidly. Tumor cells invoke hemorrhage and necrosis. The etiology is strongly linked to smoking. This type was previously referred to as oat cell carcinoma.
- *Large cell carcinoma* (15%): Tumor cells are large, demonstrate high levels of anaplasia, and metastasize readily. Diagnosis is often based on exclusion of other types.

The subtypes of lung carcinoma vary in prevalence by gender. Adenocarcinoma is most common in women and nonsmokers. Small cell carcinoma historically has demonstrated a 10:1 male to female ratio, but currently is at 2:1 perhaps due to increased smoking behaviors in women. Squamous cell carcinoma is also found more prominently in men and is strongly linked to smoking.

CLINICAL MANIFESTATIONS

The most common clinical manifestations for all lung cancer subtypes are persistent cough, hemoptysis (bloody sputum), chest pain, and shortness of breath. These clinical manifestations are often ignored and explained away as "smoker's cough" or bronchitis. The common systemic and paraneoplastic manifestations discussed earlier also apply to lung carcinoma.

DIAGNOSTIC CRITERIA

Diagnosis is made through a variety of laboratory and diagnostic tests, including bronchoscopy, chest radiograph, tissue biopsy, cytologic tests of sputum, MRI, CT, and ultrasound. Lung tumor cells may present CEA. The presence, extent, and prognosis of lung carcinomas are often based on CEA levels, the ability to surgically remove the tumor, lymph node involvement, and the presence of distant metastasis. Factors that correlate with an adverse prognosis include the presence of pulmonary symptoms, large tumor size (more than 3 cm), nonsquamous histology, metastases to multiple lymph nodes, and vascular invasion.

TREATMENT

Treatment selection is based on identification of the tumor type as either small cell or nonsmall cell (adenocarcinoma, squamous cell, and large cell) lung carcinoma. Small cell carcinoma is more likely to respond to chemotherapy, yet is also more likely to be widely disseminated at diagnosis. Because patients with small cell carcinoma tend to develop distant metastases, surgical resection and radiation rarely contribute to long-term survival.

Treatment of nonsmall cell carcinomas is often based on the ability or inability to resect (surgically remove) all or part of the tumor. If nonsmall cell carcinomas (adenocarcinoma, squamous carcinoma, and large cell carcinoma) can be surgically removed, the cancer may be cured by surgery alone or by surgery and chemotherapy. If the tumor cannot be surgically removed, local control of the tumor may be achieved with radiation therapy, but cure is unlikely.

Small and large cell carcinomas carry the least favorable prognosis, although many lung carcinomas are not detected until the tumor is well advanced. Early symptoms, such as a chronic cough, are often ignored. The overall 5-year survival for lung carcinoma is 15%.[2]

Colorectal Cancer

Colorectal cancer is the third most common cancer diagnosed in men and women and the third leading cause of cancer-related death in the United States.[10]

Approximately, 75% of patients with colorectal cancer are unable to identify a clear cause and do not have evidence of inheriting the disease; the remaining 25% have familial colorectal cancer, suggesting a genetic inheritance (5 to 6%; autosomal dominant inheritance) or common environmental exposures among family members.[10]

PATHOPHYSIOLOGY

Although the exact cause is often not clearly established, the primary risk factor is age. More than 90% of cases are diagnosed in adults over the age of 50 years.[1] Other risk factors include family history of colorectal cancer, smoking, alcohol consumption, chronic inflammatory bowel disease, obesity and physical inactivity, and a diet high in fat and low in fruits and vegetables. Although this finding is controversial, higher amounts of fiber in the diet have been shown to bind to potential mutagens and move contents more quickly through the colon and therefore may prevent neoplasms. A reduced fat diet may decrease the secretion of bile into the intestine and limit the exposure of the bowel to the tumor-promoting effects of bile acids. Nutrients with a protective effect against colorectal cancer include selenium and vitamins E, C, and A, as well as vegetables such as broccoli, cauliflower, cabbage, and brussels sprout.

Tumors in the colon or rectum can range from benign polyps to invasive tumors and are most often of epithelial origin, termed adenomas or adenocarcinomas. These are classified according to three groups:

1. Nonneoplastic polyps (not generally considered a cancer precursor)

2. Neoplastic polyps (adenomatous polyps, adenomas; increased risk of developing carcinoma of colon/rectum)

3. Cancers (most often adenocarcinomas)

An average of nine major deleterious mutations are harbored within cancerous tumors of the colon/rectum and five to seven mutations are needed to promote the development of malignant tumors. At least two pathways have been identified that can lead from healthy epithelium to carcinoma:

1. A series of events triggering chromosomal instability (85%)

2. Replication errors (15%)

Chromosomal instability is based on alterations in chromosome number (aneuploidy) and chromosomal deletions, particularly of chromosomes 5q, 18q, 17p, and the mutation of the KRAS oncogene.[10] Chromosomal instability leads to a loss of tumor suppressor function, and impaired DNA repair is heavily implicated in the transformation to adenocarcinomas. Early activation of neoplasia is often related to a mutated loss of a tumor suppressor gene called *APC* (adenomatous polyposis coli) gene. Mutations in the *APC* gene lead to adenomatous polyps, which are considered a major precursor to malignant tumor development. Replication errors differ in that the chromosomes remain intact, but the patient has still acquired defects in DNA repair, allowing mutated neoplasia-promoting genes to promote cancerous transformations.

In both scenarios (chromosomal instability and replication errors), the cellular transformation that forms in the mucosal epithelium of the bowel begins at the base of the **crypts** or mucosal epithelial depressions (Fig. 7.11). This is the area where mitosis

■ **Figure 7.11**   From adenomatous polyps to adenocarcinoma. Cellular transformation begins at the base of the crypts where mitosis occurs. Tumor cells resist apoptosis and accumulate on the bowel surface. The cells continue to proliferate to form benign adenomatous polyps. Further mutations promote the transformation to adenocarcinoma. (Image modified from Rubin E, Farber JL. *Pathology.* 4th ed. Philadelphia: Lippincott Williams & Wilkins; 2005.)

Table 7.4 TNM Classification and Staging for Colorectal Cancer

Classification or Stage	Description
Primary Tumor (T)	
TX	Primary tumor cannot be assessed
T0	No evidence of primary tumor
Tis	Carcinoma in situ
T1	Tumor invades submucosa
T2	Tumor invades muscularis propria
T3	Tumor invades through and into subserosa, or into perirectal tissues
T4	Tumor directly invades other organs or structure, and/or perforates visceral peritoneum
Regional Lymph Nodes (N)	
NX	Regional lymph nodes cannot be assessed
N0	No regional lymph node metastasis
N1	Metastasis in one to three regional lymph nodes
N2	Metastasis in four or more regional lymph nodes
Distant Metastasis (M)	
MX	Distant metastasis cannot be assessed
M0	No distant metastasis
M1	Distant metastasis
Staging Based on TNM	
Stage 0	Tis, N0, M0
Stage I	T1 or T2, N0, M0
Stage IIA	T3, N0, M0
Stage IIB	T4, N0, M0
Stage IIIA	T1 or T2, N0, M0
Stage IIIB	T3 or T4, N1, M0
Stage IIIC	Any T, N2, M0
Stage IV	Any T, Any N, M1

TNM, tumor size, node, metastases.

Reprinted with permission from Greene F, Page D, Morrow M, et al. *AJCC Cancer Staging Manual.* 6th ed. New York: Springer; 2002, with permission.

occurs. As the cell matures, it moves up the crypt and eventually reaches the surface of the bowel where the cell then dies and is sloughed off and removed through the colon. With *APC* gene mutation, tumor cells in the bowel resist apoptosis and accumulate on the bowel surface. The cells continue to proliferate to form benign adenomatous polyps. Removal of benign adenomatous polyps can

reduce the risk of the development of adenocarcinomas. Other mutations further promote the transformation to a malignant tumor, such as the deletion of other tumor suppressor genes: the *DCC* ("deleted in colon cancer") gene and the *p53* gene. Disruption of the *p53* gene is implicated in three of four cases of colorectal cancer.[4]

The American Joint Committee on Cancer (AJCC) has designated staging of colorectal cancer using a modified TNM classification. Nodal and metastatic designations are identical to the classic TNM system. The tumor aspect of the classification depends on the extent of tumor progression through the bowel wall versus the size of the tumor. The modifications and staging for colorectal cancer are found in Table 7.4. Distant metastases, when present, are most often found in the liver.

CLINICAL MANIFESTATIONS

Clinical manifestations of colorectal cancer depend on the location and characteristics of the tumor. Early stages of tumor development are often asymptomatic. As the tumor enlarges, ulceration and hemorrhage can result in **occult**, or hidden, blood in the stool if the tumor is along the ascending colon. **Frank**, or visible, blood in the stool, abdominal pain, and bowel obstruction are more likely if the tumor is located along the descending colon or in the rectum. Anemia, caused by blood loss in the stool, or a change in bowel habits may be the first diagnostic clue. General systemic and paraneoplastic manifestations also apply for colorectal cancer.

DIAGNOSTIC CRITERIA

Early detection of rectal cancers is based on digital rectal examination, which should be performed annually for all individuals 40 years and older. Colon cancer detection involves the use of **colonoscopy**, direct visualization of the colon, which is recommended routinely for those over the age of 50 years. CEA levels are *not* a valuable screening test for colorectal cancer because of the large number of false-negative and false-positive results. For the same reason, the routine use of CEA for monitoring response to treatment is also not recommended.

From the Lab

Testing for occult blood in the stool involves taking a small sample of the stool and combining this with a chemically impregnated test strip. Guaiac or orthotolidine is an often-used chemical. These tests are often referred to as guaiac or Hemoccult tests. A positive test indicates the presence of occult blood in the stool and warrants further evaluation.

TREATMENT

Colorectal cancer is highly treatable and often curable when localized in the bowel. Surgical treatment is required and results in cure (with localized tumors) in about 50% of patients. Those with unresectable, locally advanced, or metastatic disease are treated with combination drug chemotherapy and radiation as indicated. The prognosis of colorectal cancer is directly related to the location and degree of penetration of the tumor through the bowel, the presence of bowel obstruction or perforation, lymph node involvement, and the presence of distant metastases. For patients with resectable hepatic metastasis at diagnosis (about 50% of patients), the 5-year survival rate is approximately 25 to 40%.[11]

Brain Cancer

In 2006, approximately 122,687 people were living with or in remission from brain and nervous system cancers in the United States.[12] Brain cancer is more likely to affect men than women (7.6 compared to 5.4 per 100,000 people) and white people are affected at a higher rate than other races/ethnicities. The exact cause of most brain tumors is largely unknown. Exposure to ionizing radiation, particularly for treatment of cancer, increases the risk of developing tumors in the nervous system.

PATHOPHYSIOLOGY

Brain metastases outnumber primary tumors at a ratio of at least 10 to 1.[12] These metastasis have primary tumors that originate most often in the lungs, breast, skin, or colon. These primary tumors then preferrentially relocate to the cerebral hemispheres (80%), cerebellum (15%), and brainstem (5%).

Primary CNS and peripheral nervous system (PNS) tumors originate from the following structures:

- *Glial cells:* Glial cells are the nonneurons in the CNS and PNS and include ependymal cells, astrocytes, oligodendrocytes, and microglia.
- *Meninges:* The membranous coverings of the brain; namely, the pia mater, arachnoid, and dura mater. Meningiomas emerge in middle to late adulthood, are slow growing, and tend to erode the cranium.
- *Schwann cells:* These cells produce myelin and collagen. Schwannomas arise within the brain, spinal nerves, and peripheral nerves and are rarely malignant.
- *Ectopic tissues:* Some tumors in the CNS originate in embryonic cells that have migrated to the brain and spinal cord and have proliferated. One example is the lipoma. Lipomas begin as embryonic adipose cells that have migrated to the CNS during embryogenesis. The tumor grows slowly and can go undetected for a lifetime.

Figure 7.12 depicts the distribution of these and other common intracranial tumors.

Gliomas, more specifically astrocytomas, are the most common tumor type originating in the brain. The specific genetic mutation or chromosomal aberration is variable depending on the subtype. For example, grade II diffuse astrocytomas most often occur in patients with inherited *p53* germline mutations or with a deletion of chromosome band 17p13.1.[12]

Astrocytomas most often present in the brainstem or cerebellum of the child, spinal cord of young adults, and cerebral hemispheres of the adult.

■ **FIGURE 7.12** The most common locations for select intracranial tumors. Tumors of *glial* (nonneurons) and *nonglial* origin are distinguished. Note that most tumors arise in the cerebral hemispheres. (Image modified from Rubin E, Farber JL. *Pathology.* 4th ed. Philadelphia: Lippincott Williams & Wilkins; 2005, with permission.)

Extracranial extension of meningioma

Lipoma (most commonly in corpus collosum)

Meningioma

Gliomas (cerebrum)

Pineal tumors

Astrocytoma (childhood)

Medulloblastoma

Pituitary adenoma

Acoustic schwannoma (VII cranial nerve)

Pontine glioma (childhood)

Ependymoma (fourth ventricle)

Astrocytomas vary in the level of differentiation at diagnosis. Approximately 20% are well differentiated, 40% are highly undifferentiated, and the remaining are somewhere in between. Gliomas can be benign or malignant. As gliomas enlarge, tumors impinge on vital brain structures and become fatal. Unlike other tumors, gliomas rarely metastasize outside of the CNS. Prognosis is based on the level of anaplasia; that is, the more undifferentiated the tumor, the poorer the prognosis.

The TNM classification is not used for brain tumors because of the following reasons:

- Tumor size is less relevant than the location and histology
- The brain and spinal cord have no lymphatics
- Most patients with CNS tumors do not live long enough to develop metastatic disease

Rather, the World Health Organization (WHO) classification of CNS tumors is often used as it incorporates morphology, genetics, and immunologic markers (Table 7.5).

CLINICAL MANIFESTATIONS

Clinical manifestations of intracranial tumors depend on the size and location of the tumor. Neurologic deficits are created when the tumor erodes functional neurons. This results in specific motor or sensory losses, such as vision changes, numbness, weakness, or paralysis. Cognitive, behavioral, and personality changes are also common and may manifest as irritability, forgetfulness, and depression. Pressure increase in the cranium from the growing tumor, along with inflammation and fluid accumulation, leads to headaches and

vomiting. Seizures can also result from irritation and the subsequent disorderly discharge of neurons. Tumor compression on the respiratory and cardiac centers can result in death.

DIAGNOSTIC CRITERIA

Diagnosis of brain tumors is based on history and physical examination, including a complete neurologic examination. This neurologic examination involves testing cranial nerves, reflexes, sensory function, and motor function. Direct visualization of tumor growth via brain scans, radiographs, CT, MRI, and cerebral angiography will also aid in the diagnosis and prepare for removal of the tumor. Positron emission tomography scanning and spectroscopic evaluations are current strategies for diagnosing metastasis in the cerebrum. These tests are also useful for differentiating the metastases from other lesions in the brain.

TREATMENT

The treatment of brain cancer varies depending on the location, extent, and nature of the neoplasms. Primary tumors are treated with surgical resection whenever feasible. The goal of surgery is to remove the tumor as completely as possible while still preserving neurologic function. Radiation therapy also has a major role in treatment and is almost universally indicated. Chemotherapy, often administered into the spinal canal, may also be used to treat certain chemosensitive tumor types, such as gliomas, medulloblastomas, and some germ cell tumors. Chemotherapy may also be placed directly in the brain during surgery as a local treatment. For patients with metastases to the brain, whole brain radiation therapy may be needed due to widespread tumors. Palliative care is essential and may include the use of anticonvulsants to treat seizures.

Leukemia

Leukemias are malignant neoplasms of the blood and blood-forming organs. Leukemia (literally, "white blood") is most often associated with overproliferation and lack of differentiation in WBCs, but it can also affect other cell types. Leukemia replaces cells in the bone marrow with immature, proliferating neoplasms. Immature cells are called **blast cells**. Nonfunctioning leukemic blast cells then circulate in the vascular system.

The etiology of leukemia is often unknown. Radiation and chemical exposure has been impli-

Table 7.5 World Health Organization Grading of Central Nervous System Tumors

Grade	Description
I	Lesions with low proliferative potential, discrete borders, and likely to be cured with surgical resection
II	Lesions that are generally infiltrating and low in mitotic activity but recur; may progress to higher grades of malignancy
III	Lesions with histologic evidence of malignancy associated with elevated mitotic activity are infiltrative and anaplastic
IV	Lesions that are mitotically active, necrosis-prone, and generally associated with rapid proliferation

Reprinted from Kleihues P, Burger P, Scheithauer B. The new WHO classification of brain tumours. *Brain Pathol*. 1993;3:255–268, with permission.

cated. Those who have been treated with chemotherapy for other types of cancer, such as lymphomas, are more prone to the development of leukemia. Those with Down syndrome are also more likely to develop leukemia, perhaps because of the damage caused by chromosomal translocations. Genetic predispositions have also been demonstrated in cases where multiple members of the same family are affected with leukemia.

The leukemias are classified as acute or chronic and are also classified according to cell type. Acute leukemias, as is the case with other acute conditions, are sudden and result in a rapid and noticeable loss of function. Chronic leukemias are more gradual in onset, and early symptoms, if any, are vague. The different cells affected by leukemia are either lymphoid or myeloid types. Lymphocytic leukemias involve immature lymphocytes that originate in the bone marrow. Myelogenous leukemias involve myeloid stem cells in the marrow. Myelogenous leukemias interfere with the maturation of all blood cells, including erythrocytes and platelets.

ACUTE LYMPHOCYTIC AND MYELOGENOUS LEUKEMIAS

Acute lymphocytic leukemia (ALL) is the most common cancer in children but can occur throughout adulthood as well. Immature B lymphocytes, and (infrequently) T lymphocytes, are the malignant cells in ALL (Fig. 7.13).

Pathophysiology

Over 80% of childhood ALL originates as a B-cell precursor and is expressed on CD79a, CD19, HLA-DR, CD10, and other B cell–associated antigens. ALL is

■ **Figure 7.13** Acute lymphoblastic leukemia. The lymphoblasts contain irregular, prominent, and indented nuclei. (Image from Rubin E, Farber JL. *Pathology.* 4th ed. Philadelphia: Lippincott Williams & Wilkins; 2005, with permission.)

associated with various alterations in the number of chromosomes and chromosomal translocations, and each specific alteration has prognostic significance. For example, a translocation involving the *MLL* (11q23) gene occurs in approximately 80% of ALL cases in infants and is associated with a poor treatment response.[13]

Acute myelogenous leukemia (AML) is the most prevalent acute leukemia and most commonly occurs in adults. In AML, immature myeloid cells proliferate in the bone marrow and lack the ability to differentiate into specific functional blood cells, resulting in anemia, leukopenia, and thrombocytopenia. Risk factors for the development of AML include male gender, smoking, previous chemotherapy or radiation treatment, history of ALL, exposure to atomic bomb radiation or benzene, and a history of myelodysplastic syndrome.[14] Similar to ALL, certain chromosomal aberrations in AML are associated with prognostic significance. For example, translocations of chromosomes 8 and 21 or 15 and 17, or an inversion of chromosome 16, are associated with a more favorable outcome.[14]

Clinical Manifestations

The clinical manifestations are similar in ALL and AML. They are sudden in onset and are related to:

1. Immaturity of WBCs and other cells originating in the bone marrow
2. Crowding of leukemic cells in the bone marrow
3. Infiltration of leukemic cells in the CNS, lymph nodes, liver, and spleen

Immaturity of WBCs leads to increased infections. Crowding of leukemic cells in the bone marrow can suppress erythrocyte and platelet production, leading to anemia, bruising, and bleeding problems, such as frequent **epistaxis**, or nose bleeds. Anemia leads to fatigue. Crowding also increases pressure and resorption within the bone and can result in bone pain. Infiltration into the CNS causes headaches, visual disturbances, nausea, vomiting, seizures, and coma. Infiltration in the lymph nodes, spleen, and liver causes enlargement and tenderness of these organs. Unexplained weight loss and fever are also common clinical manifestations.

Diagnostic Criteria

Diagnosis is based on patient history and physical examination. The blood cell count demonstrating blast (immature WBCs) cells greater than 20% and microscopic examination of blood cells is diagnostic. Further cytologic analysis differentiates the specific leukemia subtype.

Treatment

The most common treatment protocol for ALL includes a systemic combination of chemotherapy and specific prophylactic CNS intrathecal chemotherapy with or without cranial radiation. The treatment protocol is divided into stages that include induction, intensification, and maintenance. Close monitoring is required during treatment because of the myelosuppression and immunosuppression that is expected with intense chemotherapy. The goal is to achieve remission (blast cells less than 5%). Among children with ALL, more than 95% attain remission with an 85% 5-year survival rate.[1] Survival is increased in young children (aged 1 to 9 years), patients with lower WBC counts at diagnosis, the absence of CNS involvement, and female gender.

Treatment for AML also includes systemic combination chemotherapy in two phases: induction (to achieve remission) and postremission. Because only 5% of those with AML develop CNS disease, prophylactic CNS intrathecal chemotherapy is rarely indicated.[14] Approximately 70% of adults with AML can expect to attain complete remission after induction therapy.[1] Success with therapy is related to younger age, lack of CNS involvement, lack of systemic infection at diagnosis, and lower immature WBC counts.

CHRONIC LYMPHOCYTIC AND MYELOGENOUS LEUKEMIAS

Chronic leukemias have a more gradual onset and are found most commonly in middle and older adults. Chronic lymphocytic leukemia (CLL) results in overproliferation of B lymphocytes that are relatively mature but are not fully functional (Fig. 7.14). The cells do not readily form antibodies in the presence of antigens, and infection is common. Chronic myelogenous leukemia (CML) is similarly insidious in onset and impacts myelogenous cell types; again, these cells are relatively mature but not fully functional.

Pathophysiology

The chronic leukemias are differentiated by presenting certain B-cell antigens and other genetic and chromosomal aberrations. For example, the **Philadelphia chromosome** is found in approximately 95% of those with CML and represents a chromosome 9 and 22 translocation, which activates oncogenes. The *BCR-ABL* gene then becomes fused, allowing production of abnormal tyrosine kinase protein, leading to disordered myelopoiesis (formation of bone marrow).[15]

■ **Figure 7.14** Chronic lymphocytic leukemia. A peripheral blood smear shows numerous small-to-medium sized lymphocytes. (Image from Rubin E, Farber JL. *Pathology*. 4th ed. Philadelphia: Lippincott Williams & Wilkins; 2005, with permission.)

Clinical Manifestations

Clinical manifestations for the chronic leukemias are often subtle or not present until the disease is well advanced. When present, the clinical manifestations are similar to acute leukemias: fatigue, lymph node enlargement (particularly with CLL), hepatomegaly, splenomegaly, recurrent or persistent infections, low-grade fever, anemia, weight loss, bleeding, bruising, and bone pain.

Diagnostic Criteria

Diagnosis prior to the onset of recognizable symptoms is often made incidentally; the individual is seeking care for another purpose, a blood cell count is performed, an elevation in the WBC count is noted, and the patient undergoes further investigation. The patient may have detectable spleen enlargement on physical examination. A bone marrow biopsy is often performed and detects a greater proportion of immature myeloid cells. Cytologic analysis is used to determine specific chromosomal aberrations or genetic mutations. For example, CML is further distinguished by the presence of the Philadelphia chromosome.

Treatment

The optimal treatment for CML and CLL at diagnosis is still under investigation. More than half of patients may be cured with bone marrow or stem cell transplantation. However, eligibility is restricted by age, overall health status, and inability to locate a suitable donor. Patients with extremely high circulating WBCs (greater than 100,000/mm³) require immediate chemotherapeutic treatment to avoid death from obstructed blood perfusion to vital organs. Splenectomy may be required in those with physical discomfort and hematologic disorders related to massive splenic enlargement. The median survival is 4 to 6 years for those with CML and 8 to 12 years for those with CLL.[15]

Lymphomas

Lymphomas, malignant lymphocytes or lymphoblasts, are commonly classified as either HL or NHL. Lymphomas, like leukemia, are derived from WBCs (namely lymphocytes) and lymph tissues. Lymphomas form solid organ tumors in the lymph tissue and later in the bone marrow. Lymphomas can also be present in the spleen and liver.

Figure 7.15 Classic Reed–Sternberg cell. The Reed–Sternberg cell is derived from B lymphocytes and suggests the presence of Hodgkin lymphoma. The cell is large and binucleated or multinucleated with eosinophilic nucleoli. (Image from Rubin E, Farber JL. *Pathology*. 4th ed. Philadelphia: Lippincott Williams & Wilkins; 2005, with permission.)

HODGKIN LYMPHOMA

Hodgkin lymphoma is a malignant disorder of the lymphoid tissue often characterized by the painless, progressive enlargement of cervical (neck) lymph nodes. The exact cause of HL is unknown. Risk factors include exposure to viruses such as Ebstein–Barr virus, genetic factors, and immunosuppression. Incidence is highest in those between the ages of 10 and 30 years and in those older than 50 years. Interestingly, the childhood form of HL is similar in biology and pathogenesis to the adult-onset form. An estimated 82% of children with HL do not relapse within the first 5 years; the 5-year survival rate is 95%.[16] The mortality rate has declined dramatically for adults with HL at a greater pace than any other malignancy, also largely due to the effectiveness of contemporary radiation and chemotherapeutic treatments.

Pathophysiology

HL is characterized by the presence of multinucleated giant cells (macrophages), called Reed–Sternberg cells, or mononuclear giant cells, called Hodgkin cells, surrounded by multiple other inflammatory cells, such as neutrophils, eosinophils, plasma cells, small lymphocytes, and fibroblasts.

The pathogenesis of HL is still under investigation. The Reed–Sternberg or Hodgkin cell has been identified as the neoplastic origin, capable of clonal expansion. The **Reed–Sternberg cell** (Fig. 7.15) originates in the cell components of lymph nodes following a B-lymphocyte lineage; it is the neoplastic cell diagnostic for HL. Susceptibility to specific viral oncogenes or certain HLA subtypes suggest a multifactorial etiology with a genetic influence. HL typically arises in B cells that cannot synthesize immunoglobulin and are resistant to apoptosis. Speculation about a viral etiology is evidenced by Epstein–Barr virus (EBV) genetic material, which can often be detected in these affected cells. The risk of developing EBV-positive HL is increased significantly in those infected with this virus. Although rare, HL can be inherited. There is a seven-fold increase for the development of HL in siblings of parents with a history of this malignancy, and the risk is increased 100-fold when the sibling is an identical twin.[2] Once the primary tumor is established, the neoplasm may spread to connecting lymph channels and can also infiltrate the vascular system. HL is organ tropic to the lung, liver, bones, and bone marrow.

Classification of the histologic characteristics of the affected cells in HL is based on the WHO modification of the Revised European-American Lymphoma Classification (REAL). The two major categories differ based on B-cell immunophenotype:

1. Classic HL, with subcategories of nodular sclerosis HL, mixed cellularity HL, lymphocyte depletion HL, and lymphocyte-rich HL
2. Nodular lymphocyte-predominant HL

The staging of HL ranges from I (involvement of a single lymph node region) to IV (disseminated involvement of one or more organs outside the lymphatic system). These stages are further distinguished as A (absence of specific systemic manifestations) or B (presence with specific systemic manifestations). These specific manifestations are unexplained: weight loss (less than 10% in the previous 6 months), unexplained fever, and drenching night sweats.

Poor prognosis is based on the presence of systemic symptoms, the stage of the disease, the presence of large masses, treatment effectiveness, the extremes of age, expansive disease spread, and the presence of immunodeficiency. Even patients considered high risk (those who have several poor prognosis factors) demonstrate a 5-year survival of 42 to 51%.[16]

Clinical Manifestations

Approximately, 80% of individuals with HL present with a nontender enlarged lymph node or group of nodes often in the neck. The enlarged nodes are generally firm and rubbery in texture. Other manifestations, such as low-grade fever, fatigue, weight loss, pruritus, and night sweats, are associated with the release of lymphokines and cytokines (inflammatory mediators) by Reed–Sternberg or Hodgkin cells. Approximately, 20% of patients will have a mass at the mediastinum that is greater than one-third of the chest diameter. Splenomegaly and hepatomegaly may also be detected.

Diagnostic Criteria

The diagnosis and staging of HL is based on the patient history, physical examination, laboratory studies, and thoracic and abdominal CT scans. The most significant diagnostic feature of HL is the presence of Reed–Sternberg cells.

Treatment

Treatment is based on clinical staging of HL. Chemotherapy and radiation are the primary treatment modalities leading to a relapse-free survival of 77% in all patients newly diagnosed with HL.[16] Patients with stage IA or IIA disease are considered to have clinical early-stage disease and are treated with chemotherapy, combined chemotherapy–radiation therapy, or radiation therapy alone. Patients with stage III or IV disease or those with the presence of B symptoms at any stage require combination chemotherapy with or without adjunct radiation therapy. Reduced dosages, particularly lower-dose radiation, are used when treating children.

STOP *and Consider*

How are leukemias and lymphomas similar?

NON-HODGKIN LYMPHOMA

Non-Hodgkin lymphoma (NHL) is a generic classification made up of a broad range of B-cell and T-cell malignancies within the immune system. NHL occurs much more frequently than HL, does not exhibit the malignant Reed–Sternberg or

Hodgkin cell, and is more likely to affect noncontiguous (unconnected) lymph nodes. Similar to HL, the etiology of NHL is often unknown; however, viruses, immunodeficiency, and genetic factors are implicated.

Pathophysiology

The precise genetic susceptibility for NHL is highly variable, depending on the specific cell affected by neoplasia. For example, mutation of the *BCL-2* gene is present in more than 90% of patients with follicular lymphoma (a type of "indolent" NHL).[17] This mutation leads to an overexpression of the BCL-2 protein and is associated with the inability to limit apoptosis and subsequent overproliferation of lymph tissue. As with HL, spread can occur via the lymphatic and vascular systems. NHL is organ tropic to the liver, spleen, and bone marrow.

The staging system (I through IV) is similar to that of HL. Histologic classification is based on the WHO modification of the REAL classification, which recognizes three major categories of lymphoid malignancies based on morphology and cell lineage: B-cell neoplasms, T-cell/natural killer (NK)-cell neoplasms, and HL. Both the lymphomas (solid tumors in lymph) and leukemias (circulating neoplasms with immune cell lineage) are included in this classification. This inclusive classification does not put artificial boundaries around lymphomas and leukemias as both involve immune cell neoplasms. For example, B-cell CLL and B-cell small lymphocytic lymphoma are, in essence, the same neoplasm. Prognosis is based on the stage, cell characteristics, age, treatment response, tumor size, lactate dehydrogenase values, and the number of affected lymph node sites outside of those surrounding the primary tumor.

Clinical Manifestations

Clinical manifestations are variable depending on the tumor type and extent of disease. The most common occurrence, as with HL, is a painless enlarged chain of lymph nodes. Other lymph nodes throughout the body can also be affected. Those with NHL can experience systemic manifestations, an increased risk of infection, and paraneoplastic syndromes as are characteristic of malignant neoplasms.

Diagnostic Criteria

Diagnosis is based on patient history and physical examination, along with histopathologic analysis via biopsy of lymph node cells. Chest and abdominal

CT scans are also used to visualize the tumor size and location. Examination of the cells in the cerebrospinal fluid may be positive for metastases in patients with aggressive NHL.

Treatment

The future of NHL treatment is focused on identifying better methods to classify tumors based on genetic profiling as well as morphologic and biologic characteristics of the tumor. This will allow placing patients into targeted treatment groups to better predict survival after standard chemotherapy. Currently, treatment is based on categorizing the NHLs into two prognostic groups: the indolent (painless, passive) lymphomas and the aggressive lymphomas. Early-stage (stage I and stage II) indolent NHL can be treated effectively with radiation therapy alone with a relatively good prognosis. Later-stage indolent and aggressive NHLs require intensive combination chemotherapy regimens with or without radiation therapy. The remission rate for aggressive forms of NHL in adults is 60 to 80%. In general, with modern treatment of patients with NHL, overall long-term disease-free survival is approximately 30 to 50%.[17]

Summary

- Neoplasia is a disorder of cellular proliferation and differentiation.
- Mutations of genes that regulate cell growth, reproduction, and death are responsible for neoplastic transformations.
- Carcinogenesis is complex and involves multiple stages.
- Certain substances or exposures are known to cause or promote cellular mutations, such as radiation, exposure to reactive oxygen species (free radicals), hormones, tobacco, infectious microorganisms, and chemicals.
- Cancer often exhibits a prolonged latent period between the initiation and onset of clinical manifestations, making identification of a precise carcinogen difficult.
- Neoplastic cells are autonomous, anaplastic, and energy dependent. They undergo extensive angiogenesis, deprive unaffected tissues of oxygen and other nutrients, and secrete substances that can alter metabolic processes.
- General manifestations related to systemic inflammatory and immune systems include lymphadenopathy, fever, and anorexia.
- Local clinical manifestations are site dependent and are related to (1) the space occupied by the tumor that impinges on the local structures and (2) the loss of function in the tissue or organ that is being "taken over" by the tumor.
- Tumors spread locally and to distant sites through the vascular and lymphatic systems.
- Metastases are distant relocations of the tumor that contribute to the lethal aspect of cancer.
- Major treatment strategies for neoplasia include surgery, chemotherapy, radiation, hormones, and immunotherapy.

Case Study 7.1

M.T. is a 65-year-old Hispanic woman who recently underwent a mammogram offered by a community "health on wheels" clinic. The radiologist detected a breast mass on the right side. She has a younger sister who had breast cancer as well. Her sister died 2 years ago at the age of 62. M.T.'s menses began at age 11 and cessation of menstruation occurred around age 58. She is overweight and is on estrogen replacement therapy. She does not have any children.

1. *Outline the process that has occurred in her body.*
2. *What were the risk factors that she demonstrated?*
3. *What would you expect for clinical manifestations?*
4. *What additional diagnostic tests could be used?*
5. *What treatment measures would you anticipate?*

Log on to the Internet. Search for a relevant journal article or Web site (such as www.cancer.gov/cancertopics/pdq/genetics/breast-and-ovarian/healthprofessional) that details breast cancer to confirm your predictions.

Case Study 7.2

P.V. is a 51-year-old Caucasian man who is being evaluated for headaches, hypertension, severe skin itching, and liver and spleen enlargement. He has a ruddy complexion. Laboratory and diagnostic tests reveal that he has an elevated hematocrit and red blood cell count. He is diagnosed with polycythemia vera, an overproliferation of red blood cells. Although not described in your reading, use what you know about overproliferation/differentiation and apply this to what might happen if red blood cells were involved.

1. *Outline the processes that have mostly likely occurred in his body.*
2. *What would you expect for clinical manifestations?*

3. *What diagnostic tests were used and what do these tell you?*
4. *What treatment measures would you anticipate?*

Log on to the Internet. Search for a relevant journal article or Web site (such as http://www.cancer. gov/cancertopics/pdq/treatment/myeloproliferative/ HealthProfessional/page4) that details polycythemia vera to confirm your predictions.

Practice Exam Questions

1. A patient comes to the clinic concerned about a painless lymph node in the neck. A diagnosis of lymphoma is made. Which of the following would indicate that the lymphoma was Hodgkin lymphoma versus non-Hodgkin lymphoma?
   a. The location of the enlarged lymph nodes
   b. The presence of Reed–Sternberg cells
   c. Spread to the spleen, liver, and bone marrow
   d. The age of the patient

2. Which of the following genes, when mutated, is NOT implicated in the development of neoplasms?
   a. Cancinogenes
   b. Tumor suppressor genes
   c. Oncogenes
   d. Mutator genes

3. Which of the following cells is least likely to develop into a neoplasia?
   a. Epithelial cell
   b. Cardiac myocyte
   c. Lymphocyte
   d. Hepatocyte

4. Which gene has been implicated most frequently in the development of cancer?
   a. *p53* gene
   b. *Rb* gene
   c. *T21* gene
   d. None of these is implicated in the development of cancer

5. Which of the following is characteristic of benign neoplasms?
   a. Highly undifferentiated
   b. Invasive
   c. Destructive
   d. Cell overproliferation

6. Which is the most significant difference between acute lymphocytic and acute myelogenous leukemia?
   a. ALL affects adults and AML affects children most often
   b. Cell type affected
   c. Diagnostic tests used
   d. Clinical manifestations

7. Your grandfather has colon cancer but then it migrates to the liver. The affinity for movement to another specific organ is called:
   a. Tropism
   b. Migratism
   c. Magnitism
   d. Malignancy

8. You are a public health official and want to make the greatest difference in reducing cancer deaths across the globe. Which intervention would have the greatest impact?
   a. Smoking cessation programs
   b. Routine genetic testing
   c. Distribute sunscreen to all adults and children
   d. Eliminate unnecessary uses of radiation

9. What sign/symptom might indicate that you are experiencing a paraneoplastic syndrome?
   a. Bone pain
   b. Edema
   c. Cough
   d. Hematuria

10. Which type of cancer would most likely spread through the process called seeding?
    a. Lung
    b. Colon
    c. Ovarian
    d. Bone

Discussion and Application

1. What did I know about altered cellular proliferation and differentiation prior to today?

2. What body processes are affected by altered proliferation and differentiation? What are the expected functions of those processes? How does altered proliferation and differentiation affect those processes?

3. What are the potential etiologies for altered cellular proliferation and differentiation? How does altered proliferation and differentiation develop?

4. Who is most at risk for developing altered cellular proliferation and differentiation? How can altered proliferation and differentiation be prevented?

5. What are the human differences that affect the etiology, risk, or course of altered cellular proliferation and differentiation?

6. What clinical manifestations are expected in the course of altered cellular proliferation and differentiation?

7. What special diagnostic tests are useful in determining the diagnosis and course of altered proliferation and differentiation?

8. What are the goals of care for individuals with altered cellular proliferation and differentiation?

9. How does the concept of altered cellular proliferation and differentiation build on what I have learned in the previous chapters and in previous courses?

10. How can I use what I have learned?

RESOURCES

American Cancer Society:
http://www.cancer.org/docroot/home/index.asp

National Cancer Institute:
http://www.nci.nih.gov/

American Association for Cancer Research:
http://cancerres.aacrjournals.org/

Intercultural Cancer Council:
http://www.iccnetwork.org

REFERENCES

1. American Cancer Society. *Cancer Facts And Figures 2009*. Atlanta: American Cancer Society; 2009. Also available at: http://www.cancer.org/downloads/STT/500809web.pdf. Accessed June 25, 2010.
2. Rubin E, Gorstein F, Rubin R, et al. *Rubin's Pathology: Clinicopathologic Foundations of Medicine*. 4th ed. Baltimore: Lippincott Williams & Wilkins; 2005.
3. Ruddin R, ed. *Cancer Biology*. New York and Oxford: Oxford University Press; 1995:3–50, 141–276.
4. Carbone M, Klein G, Gruber J, et al. Modern criteria to establish human cancer etiology. *Cancer Res*. 2004;64:5518–5524.
5. National Cancer Institute. Ovarian epithelial cancer: Treatment. 2009. Available at: http://www.cancer.gov/cancertopics/pdq/treatment/ovarianepithelial/healthprofessional/. Accessed June 25, 2010
6. Richardson M, Sanders T, Palmer J, et al.. Complementary/alternative medicine use in a comprehensive cancer center and the implications for oncology. *J Clin Oncol*. 2000;18:2505–2514.
7. National Cancer Institute. Complementary and alternative medicine in cancer treatment: questions and answers. Available at: http://www.cancer.gov/cancertopics/factsheet/therapy/CAM. Accessed September 1, 2009.
8. Bleyer W. Cancer in older adolescents and young adults: epidemiology, diagnosis, treatment, survival and importance of clinical trials. *Med Pediatr Oncol*. 2002;38:1–10.
9. Biagi E, Bollard C, Rousseau R, et al. Gene therapy for pediatric cancer: state of the art and future perspectives. *J Biomed Biotechnol*. 2003;2003:13–24.
10. National Cancer Institute. Genetics of colorectal cancer. 2009. Available at: http://www.cancer.gov/cancertopics/pdq/genetics/colorectal/healthprofessional. Accessed August 1, 2009.
11. Steinberg S, Barkin J, Kaplan R, et al. Prognostic indicators of colon tumors: the Gastrointestinal Tumor Study Group experience. *Cancer*. 1986;57:1866–1870.
12. National Cancer Institute. SEER stat fact sheet: Brain and nervous system cancers. 2009. Available at: http://seer.cancer.gov/statfacts/html/brain.html. Accessed August 1, 2009.
13. Pui C, Relling M, Downing J. Acute lymphoblastic leukemia. *N Engl J Med*. 2004;350:1535–1548.
14. Grimwade D, Walker H, Harrison G, et al. The predictive value of hierarchical cytogenetic classification in older adults with acute myeloid leukemia (AML): analysis of 1065 patients entered into the United Kingdom Medical Research Council AML11 trial. *Blood*. 2001;98:1312–1320.
15. Goldman J, Melo J. Chronic myeloid leukemia: advances in biology and new approaches to treatment. *N Engl J Med*. 2003;349:1451–1464.
16. Mauch P, Weinstein H, Botnick L, et al. An evaluation of long-term survival and treatment complications in children with Hodgkin disease. *Cancer*. 1983;51:925–932.
17. Armitage J. Treatment of non-Hodgkin lymphoma. *N Engl J Med*. 1993;328:1023–1030.

Altered Fluid, Electrolyte, and Acid–Base Balance

LEARNING OBJECTIVES

1. Define and use the key terms listed in this chapter.
2. Compare and contrast the distribution of fluid in body compartments.
3. Differentiate between cations and anions, including expected concentrations within specific body compartments.
4. Identify the influences that promote fluid movement between and within compartments.
5. Outline the critical components that determine pH.
6. List four potential sources of body fluid loss.
7. Describe the clinical implications of alterations in electrolyte balance.
8. Compare and contrast mechanisms characterizing metabolic acidosis and metabolic alkalosis.
9. Apply concepts of altered fluid, electrolyte, and acid–base balance to selected clinical models.

INTRODUCTION

Have you ever been thirsty on a hot, sunny day? What about after a long workout or after eating a bag of pretzels? Thirst is the way the body communicates the need to increase fluid intake. Fluid intake must make up for fluid lost through sweating, breathing, and urinating. In addition to fluids, electrolytes and specialized compounds that control acid–base balance are necessary for cell and organ functioning. This chapter reviews the mechanisms involved in the dysregulation of fluid, electrolyte, and acid–base balance, presented in individual modules. It also covers interactions between these concepts and the clinical consequences that may result. Selected clinical models that highlight specific alterations are presented in Module 4 to allow the student to apply the learned concepts.

Module 1

Electrolyte Imbalance

Body fluid contains dissolved particles known as electrolytes. **Electrolytes** are electrically charged particles, or **ions**. Ions with a positive charge are called **cations** and include sodium (Na^+), calcium (Ca^{2+}), hydrogen (H^+), and potassium (K^+). Negatively charged ions are called **anions**, and include chloride (Cl^-), bicarbonate (HCO_3^-), sulfate (SO_4^{2-}), and phosphate (PO_4^{3-}). Ions with opposite charges are attracted to each other and form molecules. An example of this is the bonding of the cation Na^+ to the anion Cl^- to form the molecule NaCl, or sodium chloride.

The plasma within the vascular space and the interstitial fluid of the extracellular compartment are high in sodium, chloride, and calcium; low in potassium, magnesium, and phosphate; and contain moderate levels of bicarbonate. The intracellular fluid (ICF) contains extremely low levels of calcium, small amounts of sodium, bicarbonate, and chloride, and moderate amounts of phosphate and magnesium. Potassium is found in greatest concentrations in the ICF. Figure 8.1 illustrates the concentrations of electrolytes inside and outside of a cell.

Extracellular

Figure 8.1 Intracellular and extracellular distribution of ions. Distribution of electrical charge across the membrane. Electroneutrality of cations and anions promotes balanced charges across the membrane. (Image from Bear MF, Connors BW, Paradiso MA. *Neuroscience: Exploring the Brain.* 3rd ed. Baltimore: Lippincott Williams & Wilkins; 2006, with permission.)

between cellular compartments provides a homeostatic mechanism to maintain electrolyte and acid–base balance.

Electrolyte Transport

The cell membrane forms a barrier between the intracellular and extracellular compartments. Movement of electrolytes across the cell barrier occurs by transport mechanisms, some that require energy (active transport) and others that follow gradients determined by charge/electrical or concentration (passive transport), as detailed in Chapter 2. The transport of one positively charged ion for another in opposite directions across the cell membrane is called **cation exchange**. Similarly, when reciprocal transport of negatively charged ion occurs, it is called **anion exchange**. The exchange of like-charged ions

⬤ STOP *and Consider*

Calcium is one of the electrolytes important in muscle contraction. Large amounts of calcium must be available inside the cell to promote the development of tension in muscle cells. What must happen to intracellular calcium levels for this to occur?

Altered Electrolyte Balance

Regulation of electrolyte balance is critical to metabolic function of cells. Alterations in electrolytes can disrupt many processes, including generation of action potentials and maintenance of fluid and acid–base balance.

🔬 *From the Lab*

The amount of electrolytes in body fluids is described by the concentration of solute in a particular volume of fluid. Measurements are often described as milligrams per deciliter (mg/dL), the solute weight in one-tenth of a liter (dL), also equivalent to 100 microliters (μl) of solution. Electrolytes can also be expressed in measurements of milliequivalents per liter (mEq/L), which considers the charge equivalency for a specific weight of electrolyte. Based on electroneutrality, cations and anions must be balanced in the body. The combination of anions and cations results from the attraction based on ionic charge rather than molecular weight. Therefore, 1 mEq of sodium has the same number of charges as 1 mEq of chloride. Clinical measurements of electrolytes are determined by their concentration in the plasma.

ALTERED SODIUM BALANCE

Sodium is the most abundant cation in the extracellular compartment and serves as the primary determinant of blood osmolality.

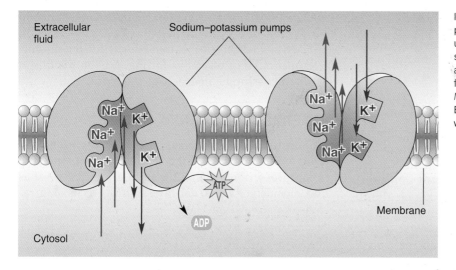

Transport of sodium out of the cell occurs against its concentration gradient, requiring active transport through the energy-dependent Na^+/K^+-2ATPase membrane pump (Fig. 8.2). Alterations in sodium balance can alter acid–base balance, fluid balance, and neural conduction. Dietary sources provide sodium, which is excreted mainly by the kidneys, along with water.

Hyponatremia

Hyponatremia is characterized by decreased levels of sodium in the blood. Sodium loss most often occurs through vomiting, diarrhea, and sweating. Blood sodium levels of less than 135 mEq/L are diagnostic of hyponatremia. Osmotic swelling of cells contributes to muscle twitching and weakness. Reduced extracellular circulating volume may lead to hypotension, tachycardia, and reduced or absent urine output (**oliguria** and **anuria**, respectively). Altered neuronal function may lead to nausea and vomiting, lethargy, confusion, seizures, or coma.

● STOP and Consider

Why is sodium balance especially critical to fluid balance?

Hypernatremia

Excessive dietary intake of sodium and loss of body water are the primary causes of hypernatremia. **Hypernatremia** is characterized by blood sodium levels of greater than 145 mEq/L. Cell metabolism is altered, as evidenced by agitation, restlessness, and decreased levels of consciousness. Fluid shifts caused by hypernatremia may result in thirst, hypertension, tachycardia, edema, and weight gain.

ALTERED POTASSIUM BALANCE

Potassium is the most abundant intracellular cation. Because most potassium is found in muscle, total body potassium is determined in large part by body size and muscle mass.

Hypokalemia

Loss of potassium may result from excessive loss due to diuretic use, severe vomiting, or diarrhea. Potassium levels of less than 3.5 mEq/L in the blood indicate **hypokalemia**. These levels of potassium alter membrane potential, which may result in dizziness, hypotension, cardiac arrhythmias, muscle weakness, and leg cramps. Decreased smooth muscle motility contributes to nausea, anorexia (loss of appetite), and abdominal distention.

Hyperkalemia

Potassium levels of more than 5 mEq/L in the blood are diagnostic of **hyperkalemia**. Causes of hyperkalemia are often iatrogenic; that is, caused by inappropriate use of drugs or their management, leading to increased potassium levels. Movement of potassium from the intracellular to the extracellular space may also lead to hyperkalemia. Inadequate excretion of potassium, as in renal failure (see Chapter 16), can also lead to hyperkalemia. These levels can alter membrane potential and are associated with the development of cardiac arrest, abdominal cramping, and flaccid paralysis because of their effects on sodium channels.

ALTERED CHLORIDE BALANCE

Chloride is a major extracellular anion. Chloride movement is often associated with sodium and plays a role in regulation of acid–base balance.

Hypochloremia

Hypochloremia is determined when blood chloride levels are less than 98 mEq/L. Common reasons for chloride loss include vomiting, diarrhea, and the use of diuretics. Hypochloremia is often associated with hyponatremia, hypokalemia, and metabolic alkalosis. Muscle effects include excessive tone and tetany (sustained contraction), weakness, and twitching. Shallow, depressed breathing, paralysis, or mental confusion may result.

Hyperchloremia

Hyperchloremia can result from severe dehydration, kidney failure, hemodialysis, and traumatic brain injury. Diagnosed by blood chloride levels of more than 108 mEq/L, hyperchloremia may result in hyperchloremic metabolic acidosis. Deep rapid breathing, weakness, headache, diminished cognitive ability, and cardiac arrest may result from hyperchloremia.

ALTERED CALCIUM BALANCE

Most calcium is contained within bones and teeth; only a small fraction is located in the extracellular fluid. Although the concentration of calcium in the extracellular fluid is relatively small, calcium plays an essential role in many metabolic processes, including activity of enzyme systems, generation of action potentials, and muscle contraction.

Hypocalcemia

Calcium blood levels of less than 8.5 mg/dL, indicative of **hypocalcemia**, lead to enhanced neuromuscular irritability. Medications, such as heparin and glucagon, can cause decreased blood calcium levels. In addition, thyroid disorders, severe burns (see Chapter 14), kidney failure, vitamin D deficiency (see Chapter 17), and sepsis may lead to hypocalcemia. Clinical manifestations include anxiety, irritability, muscle twitching, cramps, spasms, tetany, laryngospasm, and seizure. Hypotension and cardiac arrhythmia may occur because of decreased calcium entry into the cell.

Hypercalcemia

Blood calcium levels greater than 10.5 mg/dL indicate **hypercalcemia**. Increased blood calcium levels may result from excessive bone breakdown, thyroid disease, and excessive intake of calcium supplements, including calcium-containing antacids. Decreased neuromuscular irritability caused by increased threshold accounts for the main manifestations of hypercalcemia. These manifestations include confusion, fatigue, constipation, nausea and vomiting, muscle weakness, cardiac arrhythmia, headaches, and irritability.

ALTERED MAGNESIUM BALANCE

Magnesium has functions similar to the cations calcium and potassium. Much of the body's magnesium is contained in bone, similar to calcium. Soft tissues and muscle cells also contain significant concentrations of magnesium.

Hypomagnesemia

Hypomagnesemia, characterized by blood levels less than 1.5 mEq/L, usually occurs in association with hypokalemia and hypocalcemia. Inadequate intake of magnesium because of malnutrition, malabsorption syndromes, severe burns, or alcoholism is the most common cause of hypomagnesemia. Diuretic use is also associated with a risk of hypomagnesemia. Tetany, muscle cramping, and seizures are possible manifestations resulting from altered neuromuscular transmission. Cardiac arrhythmia and hypotension occur from the alteration of electrical currents because of the concurrent effects of sodium, potassium, and calcium imbalances.

Hypermagnesemia

Magnesium levels greater than 2.5 mEq/L measured in the blood define **hypermagnesemia**. This imbalance occurs with less frequency than other electrolyte imbalances, and it often results from excessive intake of magnesium-containing products or supplements or from end-stage renal disease. Neuromuscular transmission and cell excitability are reduced, resulting in hypotension, diminished reflexes, muscle weakness, flaccid paralysis, and respiratory depression. Cardiac arrhythmia and bradycardia may result, secondary to decreased movement of sodium into the cell.

ALTERED PHOSPHATE BALANCE

A component of ATP, phosphate is essential to cellular metabolism. Cellular functions of glycolysis and many enzyme reactions depend on phosphate. The major intracellular anion phosphate is stored in bones and teeth, in conjunction with calcium.

Hypophosphatemia

Blood phosphate levels less than 2.5 mg/dL are associated with **hypophosphatemia**. Often associated with hypomagnesemia and hypokalemia, hypophosphatemia may result from severe burns, malnutrition, malabsorption, alcoholism, kidney disease, vitamin D deficiency, or prolonged diuretic use. Manifestations of hypophosphatemia include muscle weakness, tremor, **paresthesia** (abnormal sensation such as tingling or burning), weight loss, and bone deformities.

Hyperphosphatemia

Hyperphosphatemia occurs when blood phosphate levels rise above 4.5 mg/dL, and it often occurs in tandem with hypocalcemia. Conditions resulting in hyperphosphatemia include fractures, bone disease, hypoparathyroidism, acromegaly (see Chapter 2), systemic infection (see Chapter 5), and intestinal obstruction (see Chapter 16). There are no associated symptoms of hyperphosphatemia, unless it is accompanied by other electrolyte imbalances.

Manifestations of electrolyte imbalances are summarized in Table 8.1.

Table 8.1 Manifestations of Electrolyte Imbalances

Electrolyte	Blood Level	Imbalance	Manifestations
Sodium	<135 mEq/L	Hyponatremia	**Muscle cramps, twitching, and weakness**
			Volume deficit, hypotension, and oliguria
			Headache, anxiety, and altered consciousness
	>145 mEq/L	Hypernatremia	**Thirst, dry skin, and mucous membranes**
			Decreased excretions
			Headache, restlessness, and altered consciousness
Potassium	<3.5 mEq/L	Hypokalemia	**Dizziness, muscle weakness, and leg cramps**
			Cardiac arrhythmia, hypotension
			Thirst, nausea, and anorexia
			Poorly concentrated urine, polyuria
	>5 mEq/L	Hyperkalemia	**Cardiac arrest**
			Abdominal cramping, flaccid paralysis
Chloride	<98 mEq/L	Hypochloremia	Increased muscle tone, twitching, weakness, and tetany
			Shallow, depressed breathing, and respiratory arrest
			Mental confusion
	>108 mEq/L	Hyperchloremia	Hyperchloremic metabolic acidosis rapid breathing
			Deep, rapid breathing
			Weakness, headache, and diminished cognitive ability
			Cardiac arrest
Calcium	<8.5 mg/dL	Hypocalcemia	Enhanced neuromuscular irritability
			Anxiety, irritability, and seizure
			Muscle twitching, cramps, spasm, tetany, and laryngospasm
			Hypotension, cardiac arrhythmia
	>10.5 mg/dL	Hypercalcemia	Decreased neuromuscular irritability
			Confusion, fatigue, headache, and irritability
			Constipation, nausea, and vomiting
			Cardiac arrhythmia
Magnesium	<1.5 mEq/L	Hypomagnesemia	Tetany, muscle cramping
			Seizures
			Cardiac arrhythmia, hypotension
	>2.5 mEq/L	Hypermagnesemia	Reduced neuromuscular transmission and cell excitability
			Flaccid paralysis, diminished reflexes, and muscle weakness
			Hypotension, respiratory depression
Phosphate	<2.5 mg/dL	Hypophosphatemia	Muscle weakness, tremor, and paresthesia
			Weight loss, bone deformity
	>4.5 mg/dL	Hyperphosphatemia	No associated manifestations

Fluid Imbalance

The body is mostly fluid, accounting for a significant percentage of body weight. Total body water can vary by gender, age, and amount of body fat. Sixty percent of the body is composed of fluids distributed between two compartments: 40% is located in the intracellular compartment and 20% is located in the extracellular compartment (Fig. 8.3). The **intracellular compartment** consists of the fluid inside the cells, containing approximately two thirds of the body water and accounting for 40% of body weight.

The smaller **extracellular compartment** contains the remaining one third, or 20%, of body fluid in the interstitial tissue and plasma outside the cells. Fluid in the plasma compartment accounts for 5% of body weight and the interstitial fluid accounts for 14% of body weight. A third, minor extracellular compartment is the transcellular compartment, separated by a layer of epithelium. The fluid in this compartment is contained in body spaces such as the spinal cord, peritoneal, pleural, pericardial, and joint spaces. This relatively small compartment of fluid is often referred to as a "third space" because it is unavailable for exchange between the other extracellular compartments.

Fluid Balance

Body fluid volume is regulated directly in the extracellular compartment and indirectly in the intracellular compartment by the kidneys. This process involves water and ion movement across the cell membranes of the renal tubules and close association with the vasculature of the kidneys (Fig. 8.4).

FLUID TRANSPORT

Water may move between compartments through special channels in the cell membrane, called **aquaporins**. Movement of water is stimulated by a concentration gradient, moving to an area of higher concentration of particles (less water content) from an area of lower concentration of particles (more water content). This process, **osmosis**, is regulated by the concentration of particles that do not diffuse across the semipermeable membrane. Some characteristics that make particles nondiffusible include large size or lipid solubility. **Osmotic pressure** is generated as water moves through the membrane. An **osmole** is the unit of measure reflecting the osmotic activity that nondiffusible particles exert in pulling water from one side of the semipermeable membrane to the other. **Osmolarity** is the osmolar concentration in 1 L of solution (mOsm/L) and is used when referring to fluids outside the body. **Osmolality** is the osmolar concentration in 1 kg of water (mOsm/kg of H_2O) and is used to describe fluids within the body.

Table 8.2 summarizes active and passive transport mechanisms.

Fluid also moves between extracellular compartments, with forces promoting fluid movement balance. **Hydrostatic forces** (pressure of fluid) can promote movement of fluid based on the pressure gradient, also known as **filtration pressure**. The pressure of the blood on the capillary walls (semipermeable membranes) can force fluid movement from within the vessel to the interstitial space; this movement is called filtration. Capillary filtration pressure is countered by interstitial fluid pressure, which opposes fluid movement out of the capillary. Conversely, capillary osmotic

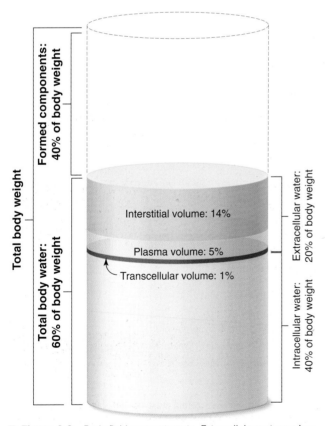

■ **Figure 8.3** Body fluid compartments. Extracellular water makes up 20% of body weight and intracellular water makes up 40% of body weight.

Figure 8.4 Renal regulation of fluid and electrolytes. Filtration, reabsorption, and secretion processes are illustrated between the renal structures and associated vasculature. Note the movement of ions and water along the tubules. ADH, antidiuretic hormone. (Image modified from Premkumar K. *The Massage Connection: Anatomy and Physiology*. Baltimore: Lippincott Williams & Wilkins; 2004, with permission.)

pressure caused by proteins or other molecules can pull fluid from the interstitial space into the intravascular space; this movement is called reabsorption. This force is countered by tissue osmotic pressure, which opposes such movement (Fig. 8.5). In vessels with intact endothelial cells, fluid moves out of the capillary at the arteriolar end of the capillary bed where the hydrostatic pressure is greater, and it moves back in at the venous end where osmotic pressure is greater. The small amount of fluid that remains in the interstitium is removed by the lymphatic system and returned to the circulation.

FLUID REGULATION

Mechanisms regulating total body water include those that promote thirst and water excretion. Neural and hormonal mechanisms work in concert to attain or maintain fluid balance.

Mechanisms to Promote Fluid Intake

Thirst is an important mechanism contributing to increased fluid intake. Thirst is characterized by a desire to drink fluids high in water content, which is prompted by uncomfortable sensations in the mouth and pharynx.[1] The sensory neurons known as

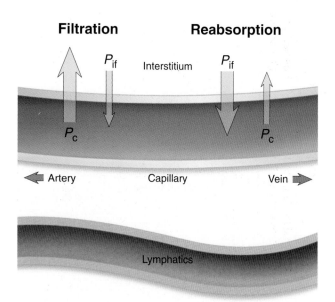

Figure 8.5 Forces for fluid movement across the capillary. P_c is the capillary lumen hydrostatic pressure and P_{if} is the interstitial hydrostatic pressure. When P_c is greater than P_{if}, filtration processes are dominant. When P_{if} is greater than P_c, reabsorption processes are "favored" or dominant.

Table 8.2 **Mechanisms of Membrane Transport**

Transport Mechanism	Type of Transport	Stimulus for Transport	Outcome of Transport
Diffusion	Passive	Chemical or electrical gradient	Particles are evenly distributed across the membrane
Osmosis	Passive	Concentration gradient	Flow of water is directed by osmotically active particles
Facilitated diffusion	Passive	Binding of substance to transporter	A carrier system moves particles across the membrane
Active transport	Active	Proteins using energy to pump ions across the membrane	Energy (ATP) moves particles against a gradient across the membrane

osmoreceptors in the hypothalamic thirst center that promote thirst are activated by:

- Cellular dehydration resulting from increased extracellular osmolality
- Decrease in blood volume

STOP *and Consider*

Are there any risks to drinking too much water?

Stretch receptors in the carotid and aorta (high-pressure baroreceptors) and the left atrium (low-pressure baroreceptors) sense change in arterial blood pressure and contribute to the development of thirst. The hormone, angiotensin II, also indirectly contributes to thirst in response to low blood volume and low blood pressure. The renal hormone, renin, is released from the kidneys and serves as an enzyme, converting angiotensinogen to angiotensin I. Angiotensin I is converted to angiotensin II by angiotensin-converting enzyme, primarily in the lungs. Angiotensin II also regulates aldosterone, a hormone produced in the adrenal cortex. The increase in sodium retention that results from the effects of aldosterone may have the indirect effect of increasing thirst.

Antidiuretic hormone (ADH) regulates fluid volume by controlling excretion of total body water. Produced in the hypothalamus, ADH is transported to the posterior pituitary where it is stored until needed. Production and release of ADH are stimulated by hypothalamic osmoreceptor detection of increased blood osmolality. Also known as vasopressin, ADH works at the level of the kidney to promote the reabsorption of water via aquaporins from the renal collecting ducts into the vasculature, reducing fluid loss through decrease in urine output. The mechanisms that promote fluid intake are illustrated in Figure 8.6.

Mechanisms to Promote Fluid Excretion

The most common method for increasing fluid excretion is the use of diuretics. **Diuretics** are drugs that increase urine production. The kidneys are the target of the effects of diuretics, which are designed to decrease reabsorption of sodium in the kidney. This mechanism is effective because water moves together with sodium.

Different types of diuretics work on different structures of the kidney. The **loop diuretics** reduce reabsorption of sodium in the thick ascending loop of Henle, causing a decreased osmolality in the interstitial fluid of the collecting ducts and impair the ability to concentrate urine at the loop. **Thiazide diuretics** prevent NaCl reabsorp-

tion in the distal convoluted tubule. This action is coupled with increased potassium loss in the urine and uric acid retention. Potassium-sparing diuretics, also known as aldosterone antagonists, reduce sodium reabsorption in the late distal tubule and collecting tubule, functions regulated by aldosterone. The effects of aldosterone at this site are inhibited, promoting excretion of sodium and water. The simultaneous effect of increased potassium reabsorption prevents the potential for excessive loss associated with other types of diuretics. The secretion of hydrogen ions may be altered, increasing the risk for metabolic acidosis, discussed later in this chapter.

Tonicity

The osmotic pressure or tension of a solution is known as tonicity.[1] Tonicity is determined by solutes that cannot cross the semipermeable cell membrane, producing an osmotic force that transports water. Cell size can be affected by tonicity, promoting fluid movement in or out of cells. **Hypertonic** solutions have a greater osmolality than the ICF. When cells are in a hypertonic solution in which the extracellular osmotic force is greater, water moves out of the cell causing cells to shrink. **Hypotonic** solutions have a lower osmolality than the ICF. The osmotic forces outside the cells are less than that of the intracellular environment, promoting water movement into the cell and causing cells to swell. An example of cellular changes in response to sodium concentration is shown in Figure 8.7, with hypernatremia serving as an example of a hypertonic solution, and hyponatremia representing a hypotonic solution. Cells in an **isotonic** solution, which has the same osmolality as the ICF, are unchanged with osmotic forces balanced within and outside of the cell.

Altered Fluid Balance

The imbalance of hydrostatic and osmotic forces can result in alterations in fluid balance. Total body fluid can also be altered by increases or decreases in

Research Notes

In addition to chemical diuretics, certain foods can have diuretic effects. The American Heart Association has long advocated the Dietary Approaches to Stop Hypertension (DASH) diet for blood pressure–lowering effects. The DASH diet is rich in fruits and vegetables. Although it was recognized that the DASH diet lowered blood pressure, the explanation for these effects was unknown until a group of researchers determined that the DASH diet promoted salt excretion and increased urine production, similar to the mechanism of action of diuretic drugs.[2]

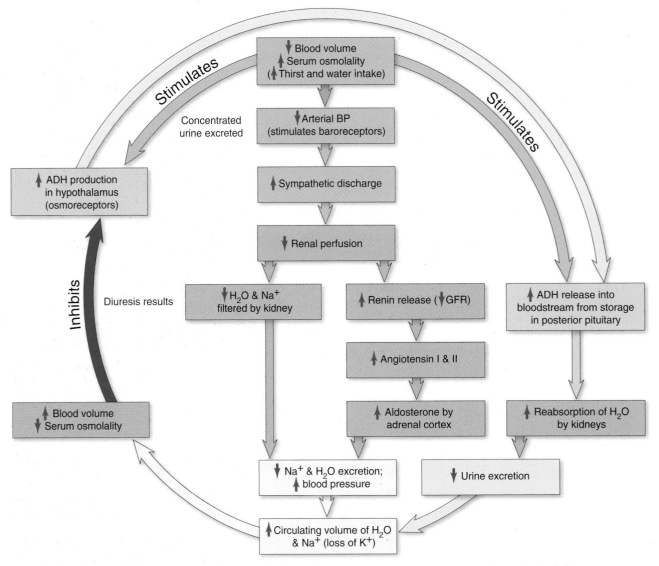

Figure 8.6 Fluid regulation cycle. Negative feedback mechanisms promote regulation of body fluid. Decreased blood volume and increased serum osmolality promote water intake via thirst. Decreased blood pressure (BP) increases sympathetic nervous stimulation, triggering reduced renal perfusion and the renin–angiotensin–aldosterone system (RAAS). Reabsorption of water through the actions of antidiuretic hormone (ADH) combined with reduced sodium and water secretion through the effects of aldosterone leads to increased circulating volume of water and sodium. Increased blood volume and low serum osmolality inhibit ADH production, promoting diuresis. (Image from Smeltzer SC, Bare BG. *Textbook of Medical-Surgical Nursing.* 10th ed. Philadelphia: Lippincott Williams & Wilkins; 2003, with permission.)

fluid ingestion and excretion. Excretion of bodily fluids, such as urine, emesis, sweat, or blood, as well as insensible fluid loss during respiration can significantly alter fluid balance. Fluid gain or loss can be measured by serial (repeated) measures of body weight, as 1 L of water weighs 1 kg or 2.2 lb.

WATER CONTENT

Alterations in water and sodium can affect total body fluid balance. Decreased vascular volume is known as **hypovolemia**, often the result of inadequate fluid intake or excessive excretion. **Hypervolemia**

is an excessive increase of fluid in the extracellular compartment.

Hypovolemia

Hypovolemia is a deficit of body fluid volume. Causes of hypovolemia can be attributed to excessive body fluid loss, reduction of fluid intake, or loss of fluid to a third space resulting in decreased extracellular fluid volume. Decreased intravascular volume results in decreased capillary hydrostatic pressure. Blood circulation and transport of oxygen and nutrients to tissues may be impaired.

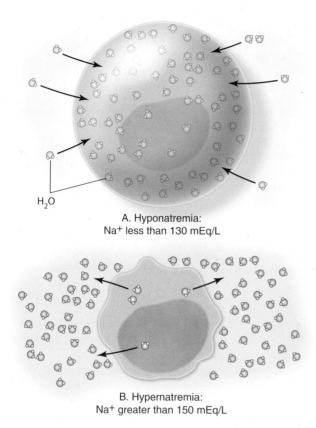

A. Hyponatremia:
Na+ less than 130 mEq/L

B. Hypernatremia:
Na+ greater than 150 mEq/L

H_2O

■ **Figure 8.7**   Effect of tonicity on cell size. **A:** The cell swells as water is pulled in from extracellular fluid. **B:** The cell shrinks as water is pulled out into extracellular fluid.

■ **Figure 8.8**   Skin turgor evaluation. After squeezing the skin together, release should result in the ridges immediately returning to a normal appearance. Dehydration should be suspected when evidence of ridges remains after release. (Image reprinted with permission from Lesha Studios.)

Clinical manifestations of hypovolemia, from least to most severe, include:

- Thirst
- Dry mucous membranes
- Weight loss
- Flattened neck veins
- Diminished skin **turgor** (fullness) (Fig. 8.8)
- Prolonged time for capillaries to refill after blanching (more than 3 seconds)
- Decreased urine output
- Increased heart rate
- Decreased blood pressure
- Altered level of consciousness

The body attempts to compensate with physiologic responses to counter the manifestations of hypovolemia. Decreased blood flow to the kidneys triggers the activation of the renin–angiotensin–aldosterone system (RAAS), increasing sodium and water reabsorption. Decreased blood pressure sensed by baroreceptors stimulates the sympathetic nervous system to increase heart rate, constrict arteries, and increase contractility of the heart. The expected response to compensate for decreased intravascular fluid volume is increased cardiac output and mean arterial pressure. ADH and aldosterone work together to decrease urine output and increase fluid intake by stimulating thirst. Failure to compensate adequately may impair cellular function significantly, resulting in multisystem failure.

The type of fluid loss that leads to hypovolemia may affect tonicity of the extracellular fluid. The diagnosis and management of alterations in fluid balance may depend on the circumstances contributing to hypovolemia. Laboratory testing of hemoglobin, hematocrit, blood urea nitrogen (BUN), serum creatinine, urine specific gravity, blood glucose, electrolytes, and plasma proteins can provide additional information to guide treatment strategies.

Hemorrhage

Hemorrhage, or excessive bleeding, may result in hypovolemia. Because water and sodium are lost at comparable rates, this condition is isotonic. Hemoglobin and hematocrit are decreased and BUN may be increased early in hemorrhage. Damage to other organ systems may be evident if hypovolemia is not corrected. Fluid replacement for volume expansion is often necessary and is determined by the amount of blood loss. Replacement of volume with blood products, either whole blood or packed (concentrated) red blood cells, provides the necessary extracellular fluid expansion as well as the cellular components lost with bleeding. The crystalloid solution **Ringer's lactate** intravenous fluid contains sodium, chloride, potassium, calcium, and lactate in concentrations that mirror those found in plasma and may also be an appropriate treatment in large-volume fluid resuscitation.[3] Fluid replacement with osmotically active fluids helps promote the movement of fluid from the interstitial space to the intravascular space.

Dehydration

Dehydration is the result of decreased extracellular fluid volume or increased sodium content in relation to water content, representing a hypertonic condition. Excessive watery diarrhea, sweating, and insensible respiratory water loss during hyperventilation or fever may lead to dehydration. Intravascular volume may become viscous, with evidence of an increase in hematocrit caused by hemoconcentration. Thirst may be stimulated, and urinary output decreased. Movement of fluid from the intracellular to the extracellular compartment promotes cell shrinkage. Dehydration of brain and nerve cells may result in headache, decreased reflexes, seizures, and coma. Expansion of extracellular volume with oral or intravenous rehydration, such as Ringer's lactate, is indicated to prevent organ damage. When chloride loss complicates dehydration, intravenous replacement with an isotonic solution of normal saline may be indicated to address the underlying ionic alteration.

Water Intoxication

Hypotonic hypovolemia, also known as water intoxication, results from decreased sodium concentration, often the result of water replacement after strenuous activity or excessive loss of sodium from diuretic therapy inhibiting ADH. Cellular swelling occurs because of movement of water from the extracellular space to the intracellular space. Increases in cellular water trigger clinical manifestations, including muscle weakness, cramps, and fatigue, and central nervous system involvement such as headache, confusion, and depression of deep tendon reflexes (DTRs). Treatments including limiting water or increasing sodium intake target the underlying cause of the condition. Hypertonic saline solutions and loop diuretics to increase water elimination are also optional treatments.

Hypervolemia

Hypervolemia is an expansion of extracellular volume involving the interstitial or vascular space.

When excess sodium and water are retained in similar proportions, the increased volume is isotonic. Causes of hypervolemia include:

- Heart failure
- Cirrhosis of the liver
- Kidney failure
- Excessive fluid replacement
- Administration of osmotically active fluids

Mean arterial blood pressure is increased in hypervolemia, inhibiting the secretion of ADH and aldosterone, resulting in increased urinary sodium and water elimination. In individuals who are unable to mount these compensatory mechanisms, heart failure and pulmonary edema may result.

Edema

Edema results from increases in the extracellular compartment of the interstitial fluid. Movement of fluid into the interstitial compartment can be driven by:

- Increased capillary filtration pressure: hydrostatic pressure forces water from capillaries into interstitial fluid
- Decreased capillary osmotic pressure: fluid moves to the interstitium across the concentration gradient
- Increased capillary permeability: altered integrity of the capillary wall allows proteins to leak from the capillaries into the interstitial space, increasing interstitial osmotic pressure
- Obstructed lymph flow (**lymphedema**): fluid in the interstitium cannot be returned to the systemic circulation

The mechanisms for the development of edema are depicted in Figure 8.9. Edematous tissues may be at risk for damage because of the resulting increased distance for diffusion and the compression of the vasculature supplying oxygen and removing waste. The clinical manifestations of edema are determined by the sites of occurrence. When located in the joints, pain and impaired movement may result. When located in the brain or lungs, function may be so impaired that death may result. When fluid accumulation in the peripheral interstitium exceeds the tissues' ability for absorption, the fluid becomes mobile when pressure is exerted upon it. When pressure over an edematous area forces fluid movement and leaves an indentation, the edema is referred to as **pitting** (Fig. 8.10). Edema may be recognized as a local area of swelling, increased body weight, and pain.

Body weight measurements provide an effective evaluation of edema, with increased body weight reflecting an increase in total body fluid. Visual inspection of extremities helps to identify peripheral edema. Evaluation of edema within organ systems not readily visible depends on the involved tissues. Auscultation of heart and lungs may reveal excessive fluid.

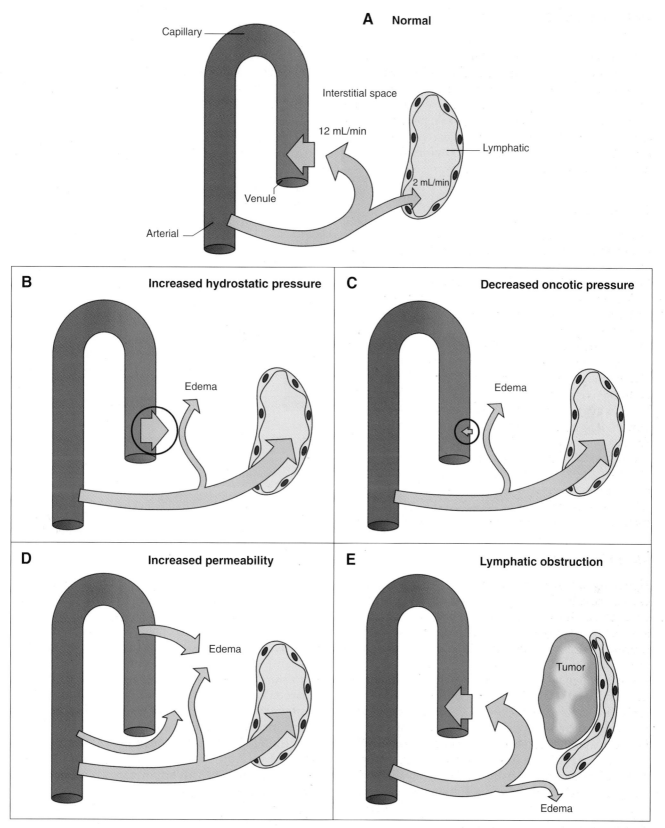

Figure 8.9 Mechanisms of edema in the capillary system. **A:** Normal. The differential between the hydrostatic and oncotic pressures at the arterial end of the capillary system is responsible for the filtration into the interstitial space of approximately 14 mL of fluid per minute. The fluid is reabsorbed at the venous end at the rate of 12 mL/min. Lymphatic capillaries drain fluid at a rate of 2 mL/min. **B:** Edema caused by increased hydrostatic pressure. Elevation at the venous end of the capillary decreases reabsorption. If the lymphatic capacity to drain fluid is exceeded, fluid accumulates. **C:** Edema caused by decreased oncotic pressure. Decreased oncotic pressure in the vascular space promotes reduced fluid reabsorption. **D:** Edema caused by increased permeability results from endothelial injury, allowing fluid to leak from the vascular space. **E:** Lymphedema results from accumulation of fluid caused by lymphatic obstruction. (Image from Rubin E, Farber JL. *Pathology*. 4th ed. Philadelphia: Lippincott Williams & Wilkins; 2005, with permission.)

■ **Figure 8.10**   Pitting edema. Palpation causes a depression when released because of movement of fluid in the interstitium. (Image from Rubin E, Farber JL. *Pathology*. 4th ed. Philadelphia: Lippincott Williams & Wilkins; 2005, with permission.)

Module 3

Acid–Base Imbalance

Regulation of acids and bases is critical to the metabolic activities of the body. A narrow physiologic pH range is required for the function of cells, tissues, and organs.

▍ Regulation of Acid and Base

Acids are substances that donate hydrogen ions and **bases** are substances that accept hydrogen ions. Weak acids in plasma include albumin and inorganic phosphorus. Strong ions almost completely dissociate, or separate, when in solution. In plasma, the strong cations include Na^+, K^+, Ca^{2+}, and Mg^{2+}. The strong anions are Cl^- and lactate.[3] The ratio between acids and bases in the extracellular fluid of the body is closely regulated to provide a favorable environment for metabolic cellular functions. The clinical measurement of this balance is known as **pH**. Hydrogen ion concentration represents the inverse of the pH, so that when the pH is low, there is a high amount of H^+; when the pH is high, there is a low amount of H^+.

The ions involved in acid–base balance are reflected in the determination of the anion gap.

The **anion gap** is a calculation of the major measured cations and anions in the plasma, providing an indication of acid–base balance. The clinical calculation of anion gap uses sodium (major measurable cation), chloride, and bicarbonate (major measurable anions), and it reflects the difference between the unmeasurable anions, including phosphates, sulfates, organic acids, and proteins. The difference in the concentrations of the cation sodium (140 mEq/L) and the anions chloride (102 mEq/L) and bicarbonate (26 mEq/L) in the blood is known as the anion gap. In other words, $Na^+(Cl^- + HCO_3^-)$ = 140 mEq/L − (102 mEq/L + 26 mEq/L) = anion gap (Fig. 8.11). Therefore, the anion gap is 12 mEq/L with a variation of 2 mEq/L, which results in a normal range of 10 to 14 mEq/L. The anion gap serves as a measurement of acid–base balance. Occasionally, other electrolytes may be considered, resulting in a different reference range distinguishing a normal from an abnormal value. An example of this variation includes the addition of the cation potassium to sodium, which changes the anion gap to 16 mEq/L (range 14 to 18 mEq/L).

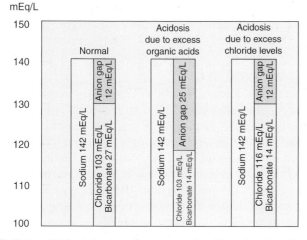

Figure 8.11 Anion gap. Excess organic acids replace bicarbonate in metabolic acidosis with increased anion gap. Rise in chloride is offset by decline in bicarbonate in hyperchloremic acidosis with normal anion gap.

BUFFER SYSTEMS

The balance of pH involves **buffer systems** (mixing of acid and base to resist pH change), which are responsible for trading stronger acids and bases for weaker varieties. Acid–base balance is regulated by the actions of buffer systems, working together to respond to conditions threatening acid–base balance. The onset of action in each system varies, leading to rapid responses to correct acute insults, followed by more prolonged correction via a slower onset of action. These buffer systems include the following:

1. *Plasma buffer system*: Reacts within seconds in response to hydrogen ion concentration
2. *Respiratory buffer system*: Reacts within minutes to excrete CO_2 through change in respiratory rate
3. *Renal buffer system*: Reacts within hours to days through the production, absorption, and excretion of acids, bases, and ions

Plasma Buffer Systems

Plasma buffer systems depend on rapid responses of chemical systems in the extracellular and intracellular compartments. The primary plasma buffer systems include the bicarbonate and protein buffer systems and the H^+/K^+ cation exchange system. The buffering of free hydrogen ions is central to the effectiveness of each of the plasma buffer systems. Hydrogen ion can be incorporated into substances, and this process reduces the amount of freely circulating H^+. Conversely, hydrogen ion can be released from substances to increase the amount of free H^+ circulating in the blood. In this way, changes in pH can be addressed in a rapid manner by simply regulating the amount of free H^+ in the blood. One of the primary chemical reactions that regulate these pro-

A. $HCL + NaHCO_3 \rightleftharpoons H_2CO_3 + NaCl$

B. $NaOH + H_2CO_3 \rightleftharpoons NaHCO_3 + H_2O$

Figure 8.12 Bicarbonate buffer systems. **A:** The strong acid HCl is substituted for the weaker acid H_2CO_3 through a reaction with the weak base $NaHCO_3$. **B:** The strong base sodium hydroxide (NaOH) is substituted for the weak base $NaHCO_3$ through a reaction with the weak acid H_2CO_3.

cesses involves water, carbon dioxide (CO_2), carbonic acid (H_2CO_3), and bicarbonate. The chemical alteration of water and carbon dioxide is catalyzed by the enzyme carbonic anhydrase, present in many body cells. The reaction is reversible and rapid, promoting immediate responses to large changes in pH.

$$H_2O + CO_2 \longleftrightarrow H_2CO_3 \longleftrightarrow H^+ + HCO_3^-$$

The immediate responses of these systems protect against major shifts in pH until the respiratory and renal buffer systems are activated.

Bicarbonate Buffer System

The bicarbonate buffer system is the primary extracellular buffer. The weak acid H_2CO_3 and the weak base sodium bicarbonate ($NaHCO_3$) are the primary substances involved in the bicarbonate buffer system (Fig. 8.12). The bicarbonate buffer system makes CO_2 available which can replace HCO_3^- lost as a result of added base or eliminated with the addition of acid.

Protein Buffer System

The protein buffer system responds to the moment-to-moment changes to retain pH in the narrow range necessary for optimal cell function. Proteins serve as the largest buffering system. The protein buffer system involves intracellular proteins and the proteins albumin and plasma globulins in the vascular compartment. Able to function as either acid or base, proteins are referred to as **amphoteric**. The protein buffers can both accept or donate H^+ ions. The H^+ and CO_2 ions that are released because of these reactions can then freely diffuse across cell membranes.

Potassium–Hydrogen Exchange

Ionic exchange of the potassium (K^+) and hydrogen (H^+) cations contributes to regulation of acid–base balance. Excess H^+ in the extracellular compartment can diffuse across the cell membrane inside the cell for buffering. The entry of H^+ prompts the exit of K^+ from within the cell to the extracellular space, potentially resulting in hyperkalemia. Conversely, if the extracellular level of K^+ falls, as in the case of hypokalemia, K^+ then moves out of the cell in parallel with H^+ entry into the cell, decreasing extracellular concentrations of H^+, thereby increasing pH. The regulation of acid–base and electrolyte balance is closely tied in an effort to maintain homeostasis.

Respiratory Buffer System

The respiratory buffer system is the second system that responds to changes in pH, contributing to regulation of CO_2. H_2CO_3 is an acid that is estimated by blood levels of dissolved CO_2. CO_2 in gas form is considered **volatile**, because it can be excreted by the lungs. Because CO_2 is excreted by the lungs, respiratory function contributes to H_2CO_3 levels. When pH levels fall (acidosis), increased respiratory rate increases excretion of CO_2 and lowers H_2CO_3 levels, promoting restoration of acid–base balance. In the case of an increase in pH (alkalosis), reduced respiratory rate promotes retention of CO_2, increasing H_2CO_3 levels. The respiratory buffer system is important in compensation for alterations in acid–base balance but is unable to completely restore homeostatic pH. Respiratory compensation is essential to provide the additional time needed for renal correction of acid–base imbalances.

Renal Buffer System

The kidneys are the primary regulators of the balance between acids and bases. Circulating fixed acids are considered **nonvolatile**, because they are unable to be excreted by the lungs and require buffering and excretion by the kidneys. Renal regulation of pH is accomplished through generating, buffering, and eliminating acids and bases. The main mechanisms of renal regulation of pH include hydrogen ion elimination/bicarbonate conservation, tubular buffer systems (phosphate, ammonia [NH_3]), potassium–hydrogen exchange, and chloride–bicarbonate exchange.

Hydrogen Ion Elimination/Bicarbonate Conservation

Excretion of excess H^+ promotes regulation of pH. When pH is low, excess H^+ ions are secreted from the blood into the renal tubular filtrate where they can ultimately be excreted in the urine. The kidney can regulate HCO_3^-, conserving it when excess acid is added and excreting it in the presence of excess base. The kidneys contribute to plasma regulation of HCO_3^- by the reabsorption of HCO_3^- from the urine into the bloodstream, or by the elimination of buffered hydrogen ions. Reabsorption of basic bicarbonate ions is among the ways the kidneys work to obtain a pH between 7.35 and 7.45, thereby promoting optimal cellular functioning. A pH of 7.4 requires a 20:1 ratio of bicarbonate (HCO_3^-) base to carbonic acid (H_2CO_3). Rather than the absolute concentration of a substance, the ratio of substances provides the balance, which serves as the determinant of pH.

Tubular Buffer Systems

The tubule structures of the kidney are protected by the regulation of urine pH. Intratubular buffers bind unbuffered H^+ to maintain local pH for kidney cell function. The phosphate buffer system uses HPO_4^{2-} to bind H^+, resulting in $H_2PO_4^-$, allowing the kidney to secrete H^+ ions. The ammonia buffer system promotes excretion of H^+ and generates HCO_3^- in a series of ion exchanges between ammonium (NH_4^+) and HCO_3^-. The secreted H^+ ions combine with ammonia (NH_3) and are then eliminated in the urine as NH_4Cl.

Potassium–Hydrogen Exchange

Cation exchange of K^+ and H^+ occurs in the renal tubular cells in a similar manner descibed in the discussion of plasma buffering systems. Hypokalemia promotes movement of K^+ out of the tubular cells in exchange for H^+ movement into the cells, promoting loss of circulating H^+ and increase in pH. A lowering of pH occurs in hyperkalemia, when K^+ moves into the tubular cells in exchange for H^+, leading to an increase in circulating H^+. The cation exchange between H^+ and K^+ is tightly aligned with changes in pH, with acidosis promoting an increase in H^+ excretion and decrease in K^+ excretion, while alkalosis promotes a decrease in elimination of H^+ and increase in elimination of K^+.

Chloride–Bicarbonate Exchange

Renal regulation of HCO_3^- can also be accomplished by anion exchange with Cl^-. Chloride typically is aborbed along with sodium in the renal tubule cells. Under certain conditions including volume depletion due to vomiting and other causes of chloride loss, anion exchange between HCO_3^- and Cl^- occurs. Anion exchange between HCO_3^- and Cl^- can lead to alterations in acid–base balance due to manipulation of HCO_3^-. In hypochloremia alkalosis, an excess HCO_3^- results from increased reabsorption of HCO_3^- from the filtrate to the blood due to low circulating Cl^- levels, increasing pH. A decrease in pH is the result of reduced HCO_3^- reabsorption due to an increase in circulating Cl^- levels, known as hyperchloremic acidosis. Because the change in HCO_3^- is offset by the change in Cl^-, the anion gap is normal in hyperchloremic acidosis (Fig. 8.11).

● **STOP** *and Consider*

What are the other organ systems important in the regulation of fluid, electrolyte, and acid–base balance?

◢ Altered Acid–Base Balance

Acid and base disorders can be respiratory or metabolic in origin. Respiratory acidosis is described in detail in Chapter 13. This chapter focuses on metabolic alterations in acid–base balance. Metabolic disorders result in an alteration in HCO_3^- caused by the addition or loss of nonvolatile acid or base in the extracellular fluid. **Metabolic acidosis** results in a reduction of HCO_3^-, prompting a decrease in pH. Increased levels of HCO_3^- result in an increase of pH, known as **metabolic alkalosis**. Initiating events that cause altered HCO_3^- levels trigger compensatory mechanisms to maintain acid–base balance. Kidneys compensate efficiently by conserving HCO_3^- or H^+ ions until the pH has returned to normal. These compensatory mechanisms adjust pH without altering underlying cause. Arterial blood gas (ABG) analysis is the lab test used to determine acid–base balance. Anion gap, **base excess** or deficit, CO_2 and HCO_3^- levels, and pH can be measured in an arterial blood sample. These variables not only determine balance but also point to causes that might result in altered balance. Base excess or deficit represents the amount of fixed acid or base needed to achieve a pH of 7.4 in the blood sample.

METABOLIC ACIDOSIS

A **base deficit** of HCO_3^- characterizes metabolic acidosis. Metabolic acidosis may occur secondary to an increase in strong anions (Cl^-) or to an increase in weak acids. The levels of circulating albumin must also be considered when determining the presence of metabolic acidosis. Hypoalbuminemia may mask the presence of metabolic acidosis caused by an alkalizing effect.[4] Mechanisms contributing to the development of metabolic acidosis include:

- Increased production of nonvolatile acids; caused by fasting, ketoacidosis, and lactic acidosis
- Decreased secretion of acids by the kidneys; associated with renal failure
- Increased loss of bicarbonate; caused by diarrhea, gastrointestinal suction

- Increase in Cl^-; caused by excessive chloride reabsorption in the kidney, sodium chloride infusion

The clinical manifestations of metabolic acidosis include anorexia, nausea, vomiting, weakness, lethargy, confusion, coma, vasodilation, decreased heart rate, and flushed skin. Laboratory findings include decreased pH (less than 7.35) and HCO_3^- less than 24 mEq/L. The anion gap may increase when the cause of the metabolic acidosis is due to excess metabolic acids. When acidosis is caused by increased chloride, the anion gap remains normal. Compensatory mechanisms in metabolic acidosis include increased breathing rate and depth, hyperkalemia, and increased ammonia in urine. Treatment is aimed to correct the primary cause of metabolic acidosis, replace fluid and electrolytes, and correct the pH.

METABOLIC ALKALOSIS

Increased pH caused by plasma excess of HCO_3^- characterizes metabolic alkalosis. Mechanisms contributing to the development of metabolic alkalosis include:

- Decreased H^+ ions
- Increased HCO_3^- ions
- Loss of Cl^- ions

Impaired excretion of excess HCO_3^- may be promoted by contraction of extracellular fluid volume, hypokalemia, and hypochloremia. Clinical manifestations of metabolic alkalosis may be asymptomatic or have signs related to extracellular volume depletion, or hypokalemia. Laboratory findings include increased pH (greater than 7.45) and HCO_3^- greater than 31 mEq/L. Treatment of the underlying cause is a primary target of therapy, in addition to correction of chloride deficit (if present) and circulating potassium in addition to volume replacement.

● **STOP** and *Consider*

Why can excessive, prolonged vomiting promote the development of metabolic alkalosis?

Module **4**

Clinical Models

The clinical models presented in this chapter incorporate the concepts of altered fluid, electrolyte, and acid–base balance. Each concept is individually highlighted, although clearly each is related to the other. When reviewing the clinical models, the student should apply the concepts he or she has learned about these alterations. An overview of the relationship between fluid, electrolyte, and acid–base balance is shown in Figure 8.13.

■ FIGURE 8.13 Concept map. Fluid, electrolyte, and acid–base balance.

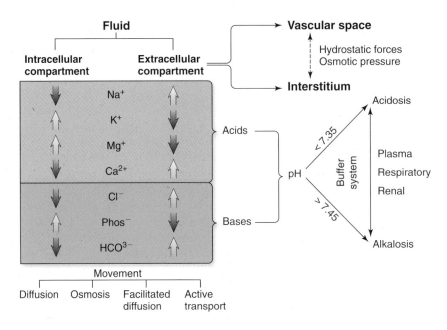

Altered Fluid Balance: Cirrhosis

Chapter 5 introduced the liver disease known as cirrhosis. In this chapter, the discussion of cirrhosis focuses on the implications of this disease related to alterations in fluid balance. Cirrhosis and chronic liver disease represent leading causes of mortality, although the rates are decreasing. From 1980 to 1989, hospitalization rates for women were less than that for men by one third. Hospitalization rates were 20% to 30% lower in whites as compared to blacks. Increasing age was associated with increased death rates in men (15.2 to 49 in 100,000) and in women (4.8 to 26.7 in 100,000) when rates for age-groups in the 35 to 44 and 65 to 74 (men) and 75 to 84 (women) range were compared.[5]

From the Lab

Urinary sodium concentration provides a measurement of renal sodium retention. In patients with large-volume ascites, urine sodium concentrations of 10 mmol/L are consistent with severe sodium retention. Analysis of ascitic fluid should be done to help determine etiology. Ascitic fluid analysis involves:

- Determination of serum-ascitic albumin gradient (SAAG): calculated from the difference between ascitic fluid albumin concentration and serum albumin concentration
  - Gradients greater than or equal to 1.1 g/dL indicate portal hypertension or transudative ascites
  - Gradients less than 1.1 g/dL indicate exudative ascites
- Amylase concentration: elevated in ascites of pancreatic origin
- White blood cell (WBC) count: increase indicates infection
  - Predominantly polymorphonuclear WBC indicates bacterial infection
  - Predominantly mononuclear WBC indicates fungal or tuberculin infection
- Red blood cell (RBC) count: increased concentration indicates hemorrhagic ascites, often caused by malignancy
- Gram stain and culture: determination of pathogen involved in infection
- Cytology: examination of cells for signs of malignancy

PATHOPHYSIOLOGY

As previously discussed, **cirrhosis** is a form of liver disease characterized by the interference of local blood flow and hepatocyte damage. Cirrhosis is often (but not always) the result of hepatitis and liver damage from alcohol exposure. The most common complication of cirrhosis is **ascites**, accumulation of fluid in the peritoneal cavity. This is an example of fluid loss to a "third space," making it unavailable for use in the remaining extracellular or intracellular compartments.

Ascites is the manifestation of the combination of hydrostatic pressure, oncotic pressure, and capillary permeability, similar to other forms of edema. Examples of conditions leading to ascites and the underlying causes include:

- Increased hydrostatic pressure
  - Budd–Chiari syndrome (hepatic vein obstruction)
  - Congestive heart failure
- Decreased colloid osmotic pressure
  - Malnutrition
  - Nephrotic syndrome
- Increased capillary permeability
  - Malignancy
  - Bacterial peritoneal infection

Increased vascular resistance to blood flow in the liver causes a condition known as **portal hypertension**, elevation in the portal (hepatic) pressure of the liver. Increased pressure promotes

Figure 8.14 Clinical evidence of ascites. Fluid accumulation in the abdominal cavity causes distention and bulging flanks and umbilicus. Tympany over the intestines and dullness over fluid in abdomen and flanks are also noted.

movement of fluid out of capillaries through hydrostatic mechanisms. The movement of fluid into the interstitium exceeds the ability of the lymphatic system to recirculate fluid to the systemic circulation, leading to accumulation. Increased vascular resistance triggers the production of vasodilators to decrease vascular resistance and increase blood flow. The dilation of the portal arteries eventually results in a decrease in blood volume and a drop in arterial pressure. To compensate for the drop in blood pressure, arterial pressure is maintained by activating mechanisms, which results in sodium and water retention and expands plasma volume. Intestinal capillary pressure and permeability are altered by the combination of portal hypertension and arterial dilation, promoting the transport of fluid to the abdominal cavity. In the advanced state, cirrhosis is associated with protein wasting. This leads to loss of albumin in the circulation, further altering fluid balance through loss of fluid to the extravascular space.

Progressive pathology may lead to renal impairment, including impaired free water excretion that leads to dilutional hyponatremia and renal vasoconstriction, which increases the risk of **hepatorenal syndrome** (renal failure caused by severe renal vasoconstriction). Increased levels of renin and aldosterone further contribute to altered fluid balance.

CLINICAL MANIFESTATIONS

The severity of ascites is related to the manifestation of clinical signs and symptoms (Fig. 8.14). Ascites can be described based on volume of fluid in the peritoneum (moderate to large volume) and is often associated with the following manifestations:

- Moderate to severe abdominal discomfort
- Increased abdominal girth
- Increased weight
- Severe sodium retention
- Dilutional hyponatremia
- Renal failure (oliguria and increase in serum creatinine)

DIAGNOSTIC CRITERIA

Physical examination and change in body weight are used to diagnose ascites. Measurement of abdominal girth or circumference may be useful. Evaluation of liver, renal, and cardiac function should be completed to determine systemic damage or dysfunction.

TREATMENT

The volume of ascites is a primary determinant of treatment. Diuretics are often used to promote ascitic fluid loss and normalize sodium balance. Caution must be used to avoid excessive diuresis, which results in hypovolemia and increases risk of renal failure. In severe cases, paracentesis may be necessary. **Paracentesis** is the insertion of a cannula into the peritoneal cavity to remove ascitic fluid (Fig. 8.15). Intravenous albumin may be administered to expand plasma volume in individuals who have had a large volume of fluid removed to reduce the risk of circulatory dysfunction and rapid recurrence of ascites.

● **STOP** and *Consider*

Why does ascites often return after fluid removal by paracentesis?

Research Notes

Ascites can lead to the development of shock, renal failure, respiratory failure, and hypoperfusion as a result of abdominal pressure. In a recent case report, a 67-year-old woman came into the emergency room who reported mild difficulty breathing. Her abdomen was obese and tense on examination. While being evaluated in the emergency room, the patient developed severe hypotension, oliguria (decreased urine output), and an increased serum creatinine level consistent with acute-onset renal failure. She required ventilatory support because of decreased oxygen saturation of her tissues. An ultrasound revealed severe ascites. Paracentesis was done with removal of 4500 mL of fluid, reducing abdominal pressure.[6]

■ **FIGURE 8.15** Paracentesis of the abdominal cavity. **A:** Midline approach. **B:** Lateral approach. (Image from Snell MD. *Clinical Anatomy.* 7th ed. Philadelphia: Lippincott Williams & Wilkins; 2003, with permission.)

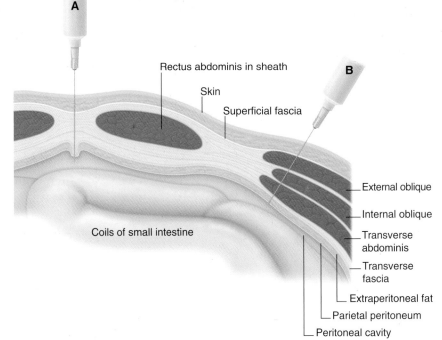

Altered Electrolyte Balance: Renal Tubulopathy

Hypokalemic salt-losing tubulopathies (SLTs) are a group of autosomal recessive disorders characterized by metabolic alkalosis. Many of the same physiologic abnormalities are common between the groups, although the age of onset varies between conditions. Four variants of this disorder are known:

1. Classic Bartter syndrome (cBS)
2. Gitelman syndrome (GS)
3. Hyperprostaglandin-E syndrome (HPS), also known as antenatal Bartter syndrome (aBS)
4. Hyperprostaglandin-E syndrome with sensorineural deafness (HPS + SND)

Bartter and Gitelman syndromes are characterized by hypokalemia and hypochloremic metabolic alkalosis.[7] The prevalence of Bartter syndrome worldwide is not currently known. Studies have been conducted in Australia, Europe, the Middle East, and the United States. A study of patients in Costa Rica revealed a high frequency of Bartter syndrome (1.2 cases per 100,000 live births). The incidence of Bartter syndrome is estimated to be 25.4 cases per 100,000 in preterm births.[8]

PATHOPHYSIOLOGY

In SLTs, electrolyte reabsorption in the renal tubules is impaired because of a gene defect altering five renal membrane proteins. The effects are related to specific protein alterations characteristic of each condition and have been likened to the effects of diuretics.[9] The cBS and HPS manifest alterations similar to those induced by the loop diuretics, inhibiting reabsorption of sodium and chloride in the loop of Henle. GS-associated electrolyte alterations mimic those induced by thiazide diuretics, blocking sodium reabsorption in the distal renal tubule. Inhibition of sodium reabsorption is desirable because excretion of sodium in the urine is accompanied by the excretion of water. Potassium may also be excreted, resulting in hypokalemia. Excessive loss of the strong cations sodium and potassium leads to the development of metabolic alkalosis.

From the Lab

As in evaluation of ascites, urinary sodium concentration can be used to provide a measurement of renal sodium retention. In patients with dehydration, urine sodium concentrations help determine etiology. Urinary sodium concentrations of less than 20 mEq/L indicate a nonrenal cause of fluid loss, such as ascites, vomiting, or diarrhea. Hypovolemia associated with urinary sodium concentration of more than 20 mEq/L indicates fluid loss of renal origin. Fluid loss of renal origin may be caused by drugs such as thiazide diuretics because they alter urine concentration. Renal causes of hypovolemia can also include excessive salt loss due to renal failure.

CLINICAL MANIFESTATIONS

Manifestation of HPS occurs in utero; neonates present with severe effects. The initial manifestation is maternal hydramnios (excessive amniotic fluid) due to increased fetal urine output. Bartter and Gitelman syndromes often present in early infancy through childhood and adolescence. The neonatal (first 28 days of life) course is complicated by polyuria (excessive urine output), hypercalciuria (excessive calcium excreted in urine), and effects from increased levels of prostaglandin, including fever, vomiting, and diarrhea, further contributing to altered fluid and electrolyte balance.[10]

Metabolic alkalosis is associated with contracted extracellular fluid volume because of sodium chloride loss. This decreased intravascular volume limits the space for distribution of bicarbonate, amplifying the hyperbicarbonatemia. Sodium chloride loss also contributes potassium loss and increased renal reabsorption of bicarbonate, further increasing blood pH and worsening metabolic alkalosis.[11]

DIAGNOSTIC CRITERIA

Renal structures can be evaluated with ultrasound. Determination of electrolyte and fluid imbalances can be evaluated by measurements of electrolytes in serum and urine. ABGs, anion gap, and base excess measures can be used to determine the presence of metabolic alkalosis and to guide treatment strategies. Fluid balance may be determined by urine specific gravity measurement. Laboratory evaluations to detect renal failure (discussed in more detail in Chapter 16) are done serially in these chronic conditions. In families with known risk for these disorders, DNA testing for the genetic defect located on chromosome number 1 can be accomplished on amniotic fluid in the antenatal period or from a cell sample taken directly from the neonate after birth.

TREATMENT

Treatment strategies are focused on the correction of renal salt and fluid losses. Sodium and potassium supplements are used to correct hyponatremia and hypokalemia. Diuretics that spare potassium excretion, including spironolactone and amiloride, may also be used. Indomethacin, a prostaglandin inhibitor, may be used to reduce prostaglandin production. Calcium and magnesium supplements may also be used to correct hypocalcemia and hypomagnesemia.

Research Notes

Salt transport depends on the recycling of potassium in the thick ascending limb of the loop of Henle. The genetic alterations associated with Bartter syndrome contribute to the loss of potassium channel secretory activity, accounting for the alteration in electrolytes characteristic of the syndrome.[12]

STOP and Consider

Why are potassium-sparing diuretics the preferred treatment of fluid and electrolyte imbalances associated with Bartter syndrome?

Altered Acid–Base Balance: Highly Active Antiretroviral Therapy (HAART)–Associated Acidosis

As discussed in Chapter 4, the treatment of HIV has been effective in prolonging life and decreasing the incidence and severity of many HIV-associated pathologies. Although HIV treatments have improved outcomes, there are known drug-related adverse effects. The use of nucleoside-analogue reverse transcriptase inhibitors (NRTIs) for the treatment of HIV has improved morbidity and mortality significantly. As more infected individuals take NRTIs and are on them for longer periods, some significant adverse drug effects are being uncovered. Among them is the development of **hyperlactatemia**, or an elevation of lactic acid in the blood. Many individuals who develop hyperlactatemia, also known as **lactic acidemia**, are not symptomatic, and they experience subclinical episodes that are self-limiting. Other individuals suffer from a life-threatening form of metabolic acidosis known as **lactic acidosis** that results from hyperlactatemia[13], a rare, but serious, complication of NRTI use. Asymptomatic lactic acidemia associated with elevated lactate levels and normal pH affects approximately 8 to 21% of individuals taking at least one NRTI, with lactic acidosis occurring in about 1.5 to 2.5%.[14]

PATHOPHYSIOLOGY

Inhibition of the enzyme DNA polymerase by NRTIs may lead to mitochondrial dysfunction and is believed to be responsible for the development of hyperlactatemia. Loss of mitochondrial DNA prevents production of the necessary components of the electron transport chain in the mitochondria. Oxidative phosphorylation is impaired, promoting the formation of lactic acid for use by the cells for energy. The buildup of lactic acid in the blood

Research Notes

The influence of mitochondrial DNA depletion and increases in serum lactate levels vary among different NRTIs. A study was done on patients taking NRTIs to determine the origin of hyperlactatemia. Blood samples were taken to determine serum lactate levels, and mitochondrial DNA concentrations were determined from liver biopsy samples. Depletion of mitochondrial DNA was increased by 47% in individuals taking the NRTIs zalcitabine, didanosine, and stavudine when compared to patients taking zidovudine, lamivudine, and abacavir. Increased lactate levels were also associated with the use of the drugs, which depleted mitochondrial DNA at a higher rate.[16]

reduces pH and predisposes affected individuals to developing lactic acidosis.

CLINICAL MANIFESTATIONS

Symptoms are related to the severity of the metabolic acidosis developing from hyperlactatemia. Most individuals with hyperlactatemia are asymptomatic and do not demonstrate any clinical manifestations.[14] Mild hyperlactatemia can induce symptoms such as nausea, vomiting, abdominal discomfort, and weight loss. **Hepatic steatosis** (fatty liver) is often associated with symptomatic hyperlactatemia, resulting from NRTI-stimulated fat deposition in the liver. Severe hyperlactatemia is the disease subtype associated with a form of metabolic acidosis known as lactic acidosis syndrome (LAS). Lactic acidosis is associated with pH levels of less than 7.3.[15] Liver involvement, including **hepatomegaly** (enlarged liver), elevated liver enzymes, and hepatic failure, is often associated with LAS. LAS may potentially result in coma and multiorgan failure.

DIAGNOSTIC CRITERIA

Early recognition and treatment of hyperlactatemia in HIV-infected individuals taking NRTIs are critical factors in decreasing morbidity and mortality due to this adverse drug effect. The clinical manifestations and laboratory determination of the amount of lactate in the blood assist in the diagnosis and form the basis of treatment strategies. Liver function tests may be completed to identify hepatic dysfunction. Electrolyte and blood pH levels may also be analyzed.

TREATMENT

Subclinical hyperlactatemia requires no treatment. This condition is usually transient and resolves without intervention. Drug selection may influence the development of hyperlactatemia; certain drugs deplete mito-

chondrial DNA more than others. NRTI treatment may be stopped or altered in individuals who develop symptoms of hyperlactatemia, but have not developed metabolic acidosis, in an attempt to prevent the development of LAS. NRTI treatment is stopped in individuals with LAS, although recovery cannot be assured. Intravenous administration of fluids can be used to expand intravascular volume, prevent cardiovascular collapse, and promote renal clearance of lactate. A period of weeks may be needed before lactate levels return to normal. Resolution of LAS is confirmed by:

- Normalization of sodium bicarbonate
- Normalization of pH
- Serum lactate of less than 3.0 mmol/L
- Normalization of liver function

⬤ **STOP** *and* **Consider**

How is lactic acidosis different from other types of metabolic acidosis?

▧ Altered Sodium Balance: Dehydration

Dehydration is characterized by negative fluid balance. Diarrhea is the most common cause of dehydration, although a variety of other conditions can lead to dehydration. According to the World Health Organization, dehydration secondary to diarrheal illness is the leading cause of infant and child mortality. It was estimated that between 2000 and 2003, diarrhea was the cause of death in 17% of children younger than 5 years and in 3% of babies younger than 28 days of age. A worldwide problem linked to 4% of all deaths, diarrhea kills approximately 2.2 million people in the world each year, mostly affecting children in developing countries.

PATHOPHYSIOLOGY

Fluid deficit associated with dehydration involves both intracellular and extracellular volume. Causes of dehydration resulting in fluid depletion include:

- Decreased fluid intake
- Increased fluid output
  - Renal
  - Gastrointestinal
  - Insensible
- Fluid shift between compartments
  - Ascites
  - Capillary leakage (burns and sepsis)

Table 8.3 Classifications of Dehydration: Sodium Considerations

Dehydration Category	Sodium Concentration	Frequency of Diagnosis	Type of Fluid Loss	Fluid Shifts
Hyponatremic	<(130 mEq/L	5–10%	Hypertonic	Intravascular to extravascular
Isonatremic	130–150 mEq/L	80%	Isotonic	None
Hypernatremic	>150 mEq/L	5–10%	Hypotonic	Extravascular to intravascular

Dehydration is categorized based on blood sodium concentration, providing information about the type of fluid loss and the potential complications associated with coexisting electrolyte imbalance. Categories of dehydration are described in Table 8.3. Volume deficit coupled with altered sodium balance stimulates further fluid shifts, determined by the amount of circulating sodium in the blood. In hyponatremic dehydration, the fluid lost contains more sodium than the amount contained in the blood, leading to a hypotonic state. Seeking equilibrium, fluid shifts from the intravascular compartment to the extravascular compartment because of the low level of sodium in the blood. This step results in further volume depletion of the intravascular space, exaggerating the effect of actual volume loss. Conversely, hypernatremic dehydration is associated with hypotonic fluid loss. Because less sodium is lost relative to the fluid amount, loss of hypotonic fluid leads to a hypertonic state, promoting fluid movement from the extravascular space to the intravascular space. This type of fluid shift actually minimizes the effects of the fluid loss, maintaining vascular volume and potential for perfusion.[17]

CLINICAL MANIFESTATIONS

Identification of clinical manifestations of dehydration helps to determine dehydration severity. Estimates of fluid deficit are based on age and body size. In newborns, dehydration is classified by loss of body weight, with 5% considered mild, 10% considered moderate, and 15% considered severe. In children who weigh more than 10 kg, mild dehydration is associated with a 3% weight loss, moderate is associated with a 6% loss, and severe equates to a 9% loss. Mild dehydration is associated with mild manifestations, with signs and symptoms worsening as the severity of dehydration increases. Manifestations of dehydration include:

- Decreased level of consciousness
- Prolonged capillary refill time
- Dry mucous membranes

- Decreased or absent tears
- Change in vital signs
  - Increased respiratory rate
  - Decreased blood pressure
  - Weak pulse
- Depressed fontanel (areas not enclosed by cranium, or "soft spots" on infants heads)
- Sunken eye
- Decreased or absent urine output

DIAGNOSTIC CRITERIA

A recent history helps determine the cause and severity of dehydration. Fluid intake, including volume and type (hypertonic or hypotonic), as well as fluid output, quantity, and characteristics (urine, stools, emesis, and sweat) are important in determining fluid balance. Appetite patterns and recent weight loss may provide an indication of malnutrition. Underlying medical condition, recent exposure to illness, or recent travel may point to an infectious cause of fluid imbalance.

History and evaluation of clinical manifestations provide the basis of diagnosis. Laboratory analyses are generally reserved for severe cases of dehydration. Blood concentrations of sodium, potassium, and chloride may indicate associated electrolyte and acid–base imbalances. Poor perfusion may promote buildup of lactic acid, consuming bicarbonate. Measures of circulating bicarbonate may provide another indication of acid–base balance. Hypoperfusion may also lead to renal damage, which can be determined by evaluation of BUN and creatinine. Urine can be evaluated for concentration by measurement of specific gravity and for electrolyte

From the Lab

Urine specific gravity measures the concentration of particles in the urine, comparing the weight of urine to the weight of water. A value between 1.010 and 1.025 suggests fluid balance. Concentrated urine contains more particles and has a higher specific gravity (more than 1.025). Dilute urine has a lower concentration of particles and has a lower specific gravity (less than 1.010). Urine osmolality measures indicate the kidney's ability to excrete or conserve water, or the ability to concentrate urine, providing additional information on the renal contributions to fluid and electrolyte balance.

Research Notes

Hyponatremia is becoming an increasing concern for marathon runners, contributing to race-related morbidity and mortality.[18] In a recent study of 488 athletes participating in the Boston Marathon, researchers found that 13% had hyponatremia and 0.6% had critical hyponatremia with extremely low serum sodium concentrations. Excessive fluid intake during the race was the strongest single predictor for the development of hyponatremia. The researchers found no association with the type of fluid intake among the runners (plain water or electrolyte solutions) and the risk for hypovolemia, emphasizing the greater role of volume in the development of fluid imbalance. The risk was significantly increased in women and in individuals with extremes of body mass index.

content (see From the Lab below). Results of the laboratory evaluation may assist in the treatment plan.

TREATMENT

Oral rehydration for mild to moderate dehydration helps restore fluid balance. Fluids intended for rehydration contain sodium, potassium, and glucose in the appropriate proportions, promoting ready absorption from the gastrointestinal system into the circulation. Rehydration fluids must be administered frequently and in small amounts. Severe dehydration with hypovolemia requires intravenous administration of Ringer's lactate or isotonic saline solution to promote intravascular volume. Ideally, volume replacement should be determined based on calculation of fluid deficit. Care must be taken to avoid rapid correction of hyponatremia, which is associated with neurologic complications. Rapid rehydration in hypernatremia may cause cellular swelling to the point of cellular rupture.

Summary

- Fluid, electrolyte, and acid–base balance are important to homeostasis and cellular function.
- Fluid represents 60% of body weight, with two thirds of body fluids contained in the intracellular compartment and the remaining one third contained in the extracellular compartment.
- Fluid transport is accomplished based on concentration and chemical gradients. Osmotic pressure is generated by charged particles and pressure gradients are generated by hydrostatic forces.
- Thirst, stimulated by hormonal mechanisms, is important in the regulation of fluid intake. Diuretics stimulate excretion of fluid through actions within the kidneys.
- Alterations in fluid balance may result from imbalance between hydrostatic and osmotic forces and from altered capillary permeability. Hypervolemia and hypovolemia are examples of altered fluid balance.

- Alterations in fluid, electrolyte, or acid–base balance can occur because of other diseases or can cause illness.
- Electrolytes contain positive charges (cations) or negative charges (anions) that determine attractive forces and movement caused by differing concentrations between compartments.
- Alterations in electrolyte balance may affect acid–base regulation, fluid balance, and neural conduction.
- Low blood levels of electrolytes are indicated by the prefix "hypo"; increased blood levels of electrolytes are indicated by the prefix "hyper," followed by the term for the specific electrolyte involved (i.e., -natremia [sodium], -kalemia [potassium], and -phosphatemia [phosphate]).
- Anion gap, based on calculation of measurable cations and anions, provides an indication of acid–base balance.
- Metabolic acidosis is characterized by a deficit in base. Metabolic alkalosis is characterized by an excess in base.
- Acid–base balance is regulated by buffer systems, working in concert to maintain pH balance.
- Correction of imbalances is critical to the maintenance of bodily functions.
- To correct imbalances in fluid, electrolyte, and acid–base, careful consideration must be given to the potential impact of one system on the other.

Case Study 8.1

Jenny, a 19-year-old college student, was injured in a fire resulting from a car accident. She experienced full-thickness burns over approximately 10% of her body. Consider the clinical model that is most related to this process. From your reading related to fluid, electrolyte, and acid–base balance, answer the following questions:

1. *What anatomic problem would most likely lead to fluid shifts because of burn injury?*
2. *What is the cause of fluid shifts in burn injury?*
3. *How would you manage fluid shifts in burn injury?*
4. *What would you expect for clinical manifestations?*
5. *What diagnostic tests might be used?*

Log onto the Internet. Search for a relevant journal article or Web site that details fluid resuscitation after burn injury to confirm your predictions.

Practice Exam Questions

1. Which of the following is an example of a strong acid?
   a. Albumin
   b. Inorganic phosphorus
   c. Sodium
   d. Lactate

2. An anion gap of 16 can be calculated by which of the following scenarios?
   a. Sodium 146, chloride 102, bicarbonate 26 mEq/L
   b. Sodium 140, chloride 102, bicarbonate 26 mEq/L
   c. Sodium 136, chloride 122, bicarbonate 30 mEq/L
   d. Sodium 148, chloride 100, bicarbonate 28 mEq/L

3. Fluid loss in response to hypervolemia is promoted by:
   a. Stimulating secretion of ADH, promoting urinary sodium and water elimination
   b. Inhibiting the secretion of aldosterone, promoting urinary sodium and water elimination
   c. Lowering mean arterial pressure
   d. Administering osmotically active fluids

4. Which of the following ions is most closely related to water movement?
   a. Potassium
   b. Sodium
   c. Chloride
   d. Calcium

5. A pH of 7.5 is defined as:
   a. Alkalosis
   b. Acidosis
   c. Acidemia
   d. Alkalemia

6. Which compartment contains the greatest amount of body water?
   a. Transcellular
   b. Plasma
   c. Interstitial
   d. Intracellular

7. Which of the following transport mechanisms is associated with movement of water across a semipermeable membrane?
   a. Diffusion
   b. Osmosis
   c. Facilitated diffusion
   d. Active transport

8. Which one of the following conditions will most likely result in edema?
   a. Intravascular filtration pressure greater than interstitial filtration pressure
   b. Intravascular reabsorption greater than interstitial reabsorption
   c. Intravascular oncotic pressure greater than interstitial oncotic pressure
   d. Increased lymphatic reabsorption

9. An example of anion exchange includes:
   a. Sodium and hydrogen exchange
   b. Sodium and chloride exchange
   c. Bicarbonate and chloride exchange
   d. Hydrogen and bicarbonate exchange

10. Hypokalemia is often associated with which one of the following conditions?
    a. Metabolic alkalosis
    b. Metabolic acidosis
    c. Hyperchloremia
    d. None of the above

11. Metabolic acidosis may be associated with
    a. Increased chloride levels
    b. Increased metabolic acids
    c. Decreased bicarbonate
    d. All of the above

12. Ascites is the primary mechanism of body fluid imbalance in which of the following conditions?
    a. Salt-losing tubulopathy
    b. Cirrhosis
    c. AIDS
    d. Isonatremic dehydration

13. Hyperlactatemia due to drug treatment is a complication in which of the following conditions?
    a. Salt-losing tubulopathy
    b. Cirrhosis
    c. AIDS
    d. Isonatremic dehydration

14. Hypokalemia is a hallmark of which one of the following conditions?
    a. Salt-losing tubulopathy
    b. Cirrhosis
    c. AIDS
    d. Isonatremic dehydration

15. Hypotonic fluid loss may result in:
    a. Hyponatremic dehydration
    b. Isonatremic dehydration
    c. Hypernatremic dehydration
    d. None of the above

Discussion and Application

1. What did I know about alterations in fluid, electrolyte, and acid–base balance before today?

2. What are the body processes affected by alterations in fluid, electrolyte, and acid–base balance? How do fluid, electrolyte, and acid–base imbalances affect those processes?

3. What are the potential etiologies for alterations in fluid, electrolyte, and acid–base balance? How do fluid, electrolyte, and acid–base imbalances develop?

4. Who is most at risk for developing fluid, electrolyte, and acid–base imbalances? How can these alterations be prevented?

5. What are the human differences that affect the etiology, risk, or course of alterations in fluid, electrolyte, and acid–base balance?

6. What clinical manifestations are expected during fluid, electrolyte, and acid–base imbalances?

7. What are the special diagnostic tests useful in determining the diagnosis and course of alterations in fluid, electrolyte, and acid–base balance?

8. What are the goals of care for individuals who have alterations in fluid, electrolyte, and acid–base balance?

9. How does the concept of alterations in fluid, electrolyte, and acid–base balance build on what I have learned in the previous chapter and in the previous courses?

10. How can I use what I have learned?

RESOURCES

AIDSinfo (a service of the U.S. Department of Health and Human Services):

http://aidsinfo.nih.gov

American Burn Association:

http://www.ameriburn.org/

REFERENCES

1. *Stedman's Electronic Dictionary*. Philadelphia: Lippincott Williams & Wilkins; 2004.
2. Akita S, Sacks FM, Svetkey LP, et al. Effects of the dietary approaches to stop hypertension (DASH) diet on the pressure-natriuresis relationship. *Hypertension*. 2003;42(1):8–13.
3. Leblanc M. Acid-base balance in acute renal failure and renal replacement therapy. *Best Pract Res Clin Anaesthesiol*. 2004;18(1):113–127.
4. Levraut J, Grimaud D. Treatment of metabolic acidosis. *Curr Opin Crit Care*. 2003;9(4):260–265.
5. Centers for Disease Control and Prevention (CDC). Deaths and hospitalizations from chronic liver disease and cirrhosis—United States, 1980–1989. *MMWR Morb Mortal Wkly Rep*. 1993;41(52–53):969–973.
6. Etzion Y, Barski L, Almog Y. Malignant ascites presenting as abdominal compartment syndrome. *Am J Emerg Med*. 2004;22(5):430–431.
7. Seyberth HW. An improved terminology and classification of Bartter-like syndromes. *Nat Clin Pract Nephrol*. 2008;4(10):560–567.
8. Madrigal G, Saborio P, Mora F, et al. Bartter syndrome in Costa Rica: a description of 20 cases. *Pediatr Nephrol*. 1997;11(3):296–301.
9. Reinalter SC, Jeck N, Peters M, et al. Pharmacotyping of hypokalaemic salt-losing tubular disorders. *Acta Physiol Scand*. 2004;181(4):513–521.
10. Jeck N, Reinalter SC, Henne T, et al. Hypokalemic salt-losing tubulopathy with chronic renal failure and sensorineural deafness. *Pediatrics*. 2001;108(1):E5.
11. Adrogue HJ, Madias NE. Management of life-threatening acid-base disorders. Second of two parts. *N Engl J Med*. 1998;338(2):107–111.
12. Lu M, Wang T, Yan Q, et al. ROMK is required for expression of the 70-pS K channel in the thick ascending limb. *Am J Physiol Renal Physiol*. 2004;286(3):F490–F495.
13. Izzedine H, Harris M, Perazella MA. The nephrotoxic effects of HAART. *Nat Rev Nephrol*. 2009;5(10):563–573.
14. McComsey GA, Yau L. Asymptomatic hyperlactataemia: predictive value, natural history and correlates. *Antivir Ther*. 2004;9(2):205–212.
15. Monier PL, Wilcox R. Metabolic complications associated with the use of highly active antiretroviral therapy in HIV-1-infected adults. *Am J Med Sci*. 2004;328(1):48–56.
16. Walker UA, Bauerle J, Laguno M, et al. Depletion of mitochondrial DNA in liver under antiretroviral therapy with didanosine, stavudine, or zalcitabine. *Hepatology*. 2004;39(2):311–317.
17. Huang LH, Anchala KR, Ellsbury DL. *Dehydration*. eMedicine. Available at: http://emedicine.medscape.com/article/906999-overview. Accessed on July 13, 2010.
18. Almond CS, Shin AY, Fortescue EB, et al. Hyponatremia among runners in the Boston Marathon. *N Engl J Med*. 2005;352(15):1550–1556.

Chapter 9

Altered Neuronal Transmission

LEARNING OBJECTIVES

1. Define and use the key terms listed in this chapter.
2. Describe outcomes related to altered voltage during the phases of action potential.
3. Differentiate between types of injury in the central and peripheral nervous systems.
4. Analyze potential targets of impaired function in altered reflex response.
5. Describe factors associated with altered synaptic transmission.
6. Compare and contrast neurologic transmission patterns and outcomes in the somatic, sympathetic, and parasympathetic nervous systems.
7. Identify common signs and symptoms of altered neuronal transmission.
8. Describe diagnostic tests and treatment strategies relevant to altered neuronal transmission.
9. Predict expected functional impairment from altered neurologic transmission based on type, severity, and site of neurologic injury.
10. Apply concepts of altered neuronal transmission to select clinical models.

INTRODUCTION

We often take for granted the simple things that are part of our daily life, such as putting one foot in front of the other, swallowing food, balancing a checkbook, or singing a favorite song. These activities are a reflection of the high-level functioning of nervous cells and tissues. This chapter highlights impaired neural function and the consequences of these alterations. A review of normal neural transmission is presented, followed by a discussion of the pathologic changes associated with impaired conduction of neural impulses in the various nervous system tissues and organs. Finally, these concepts are applied to selected models of clinical disease.

Module 1

Alterations in Neuronal Impulse Conduction

Neuronal transmission of impulses is critical to maintain vital functions. Disruption of any component required for conduction of nerve impulses may alter neural signaling. The basic structural components of the neuron must be intact to function properly. The organelles must support the function of neural cells through such things as the genetic regulation of essential functions and the production of proteins, neurotransmitters, and energy required for optimal cell functioning. The propagation of the neural impulses through development of synapses, availability of receptors, release and uptake of neurotransmitters, generation of action potentials, and target organ responsiveness is also required. The external environment, including ion concentrations and fluid balance, must be in harmony for optimal neural cell functioning. Neural impulse conduction requires a complex organization of neural structures for physiologic functioning.

Neurons

The **neuron** (nerve cell) is the fundamental functional unit of the nervous system. Composed of a central cell body, one axon, and a variable number of dendrites, neurons are excitable cells that contribute to the highly specialized cell function of the transmission of nerve impulses throughout the body. The **cell body**, or **soma**, is filled with cytoplasm and contains processes, including the nucleus, that support the metabolic demands of the cell. The cytoplasm of the cell body is also contained in the dendrites and axons. **Dendrites** are multiple, branched extensions of the cell body that transmit impulses to the cell body. The **axon** carries impulses away from the cell body. The transmission speed of nerve impulses from the dendrites to the synaptic terminals is enhanced by the myelin sheath, which is interrupted by the nodes of Ranvier. Figure 9.1 illustrates the structures of a neuron.

Neurons are categorized based on their highly specialized functions. **Sensory neurons**, also known as **afferent neurons**, carry impulses from receptors in the periphery to the brain and spinal cord in the central nervous system. **Motor neurons**, also known as **efferent neurons**, carry signals away from the spinal cord and brain to targets in the body that regulate activity. **Interneurons** are the most abundant neuron type. Interneurons provide connections between neurons, transmitting signals between afferent and efferent neurons.

Supporting Cells

The brain contains approximately 100 billion neurons and many trillions of **glia**, neural support cells. Glia, derived from the Greek meaning "glue," provide support and nutrition, maintain homeostasis, and form the myelin that covers the neurons of the brain. Support cells provide neurons with protection and metabolic support, and they help segregate neurons to promote optimal functioning. Support cell types vary depending on the component of the nervous system; that is, **central nervous system (CNS)** or **peripheral nervous system**, which is discussed further in the next section. The specific cell types are outlined in Table 9.1.

Myelin, a protein high in lipid content, is important to neural cell functioning. The insulating properties of myelin increase the speed of nerve impulse by containing the current in a small space surrounding the axon. The specific cell type supporting production and maintenance of myelin varies depending on the type of neuron involved. **Oligodendrocytes** are responsible for the formation of multilayered

�as **Figure 9.1**   Components of the neuron.

Dendrites

Nucleus

Axon

Synaptic terminals

Node of Ranvier

Myelin sheath

Cell body (soma)

Table 9.1 Supporting Cells of the Nervous System

Nervous System	Supporting Cell Type	Function
Central nervous system	Glial cells	
	Oligodendroglia (also known as oligodendrocytes)	Control myelin production and maintenance
	Astroglia (also known as astrocytes)	Provide transport mechanisms for the exchange of oxygen, carbon dioxide, and metabolites between blood vessels and neurons; stimulate phagocytosis; provide support to neural structures
	Microglia	Control phagocytosis of injured or damaged cells
	Ependymal cells	Line the ventricular system
Peripheral nervous system	Schwann cells	Stimulate myelin production and maintenance
	Satellite cells	Provide physical support of neurons

myelin segments around multiple axons in the brain, promoting the speed of nerve impulse conduction in the CNS. **Schwann cells** produce myelin on long, single axons of the peripheral nervous system. In myelinated axons, the myelin sheath is interrupted at intervals by the **nodes of Ranvier**. These nodes are rich in sodium channels and are necessary to promote the movement of the nerve impulse over long distances. Impulses traveling down the axon jump from node to node in a stepwise fashion in a process known as **saltatory conduction**.

Neuronal Transmission

Transmission of neuronal impulses requires complex coordination between neuronal structures and the surrounding environment. Alterations in any aspect of neuronal communication may result in manifestations of impaired function. Neurons communicate with other neurons and cells in the body through the generation of electrical signals called **action potentials**. Action potentials are electrical events that travel along the entire neuron by allowing charged ions to flood through channels in the semipermeable membrane around the nerve cell. Action potentials are regulated by changes in membrane potential. **Membrane potential** is the difference in electrical charge between the inside and outside of the cell. An excitable neuronal cell is **polarized** when at rest. The inside of the cell is more negative compared with the outside of the cell; the difference is measured at approximately −70 mV. Cell bodies and dendrites have few voltage-gated channels, which result in

changes in membrane potential that do not reach the threshold (**subthreshold**), or the point at which the cell is committed to an action potential. Voltage-gated channels are found in the **axon hillock**, the point at which the axon is joined to the cell body. Subthreshold potentials converge from the cell body and dendrites at the axon hillock, where a full action potential is generated and conducted down the length of the axon.

At rest, the neuron and the surrounding space act as a **capacitor**, storing current, which is released during the action potential. Myelin insulation reduces loss of current, limiting drift of sodium ions away from the neuron. Action potential is determined at the point when sodium channels open, allowing the flow of sodium into the cell. There are three components of the action potential in the neuron:

1. Resting membrane potential
2. Depolarization phase
3. Repolarization phase

The membrane potential of a cell at rest is known as the **resting membrane potential (RMP)**. RMP refers to the membrane potential (or state of tension) inside a cell membrane, measured relative to the fluid just outside in the absence of significant electrical activity. **Depolarization** is the result of rapid movement of sodium into the cell through sodium channels in the cell membrane. This inflow generates an electrical impulse. This impulse is transmitted along the axon to trigger the release of neurotransmitters. The **repolarization** phase is initiated by the flow of potassium ions out of the cell. The efflux of potassium ions promotes return of the cell to RMP (Fig. 9.2).

■ **Figure 9.2** Electrical charges at rest and with stimulation. Influx of sodium ions into the cell promotes depolarization and the development of an action potential. Efflux of potassium ions causes repolarization and return to resting membrane potential. (Image modified from Snell R. *Clinical Neuroanatomy*. Philadelphia: Lippincott Williams & Wilkins; 2003, with permission.)

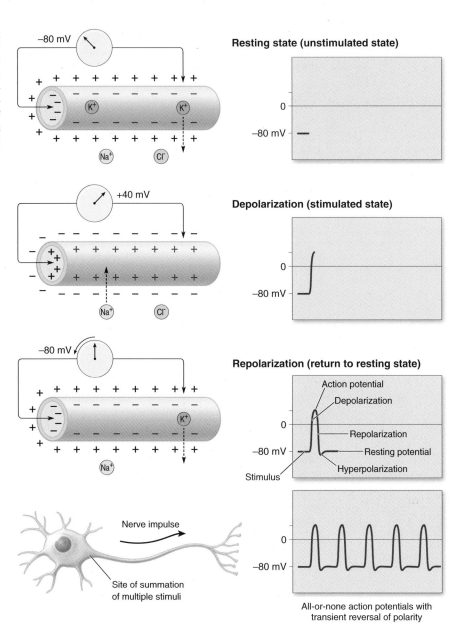

Communication between Neurons

Information from one neuron flows to another neuron across a **synapse**. The synapse is a small gap or junction separating neurons. Electrical and chemical synapses are typically found in the nervous system.

Electrical synapses transmit impulses by passage of current-carrying ions through small openings known as **gap junctions**. The transmission of electrical impulses through gap junctions is fast and direct. This mode of neural transmission is multidirectional. Gap junctions are commonly involved in the transmission of electrical impulses that lead to cardiac contractions.

Chemical synapses involve specific structures important for impulses stimulated by **neurotransmitters**, chemical agents affecting the function of

other nearby cell or cells. Neurotransmitters carry signals between nerve cells and other excitable cells, including other nerve cells and muscle cells, to trigger a response in another cell. The synaptic structures involved in this type of neural transmission include:

- Presynaptic terminals
- Synaptic cleft
- Postsynaptic membrane

Chemical synaptic transmission is unidirectional, limited to one-way communication between neurons. Synaptic arrangements can include contacts between axon and dendrite, axon and soma, and axon and axon. Presynaptic terminals contain neurotransmitters packaged in vesicles, mitochondria, and other cellular organelles. Release of neurotransmitters permits diffusion of these neurotransmitters into the synaptic cleft. Neurotransmitters released from vesicles at the synaptic cleft are then available to bind with specific receptors on the postsynaptic membrane, promoting excitation or inhibition of the postsynaptic neuron. These effects are caused by changes in membrane potential of the postsynaptic neuron induced by neurotransmitter-receptor binding, thereby resulting in hypopolarization or hyperpolarization. **Hypopolarization** changes membrane potential toward the point of **threshold potential** (less negative), promoting the excitatory effect of propagation of the impulse or neuron firing. **Hyperpolarization** has the opposite effect of moving the membrane potential away from threshold (more negative), promoting an inhibitory effect.

Neurotransmitter released into the synaptic cleft must bind to receptors on the postsynaptic neuron to achieve impulse generation. Interruption in neurotransmitter-receptor binding may result from reuptake of the neurotransmitter into the presynaptic neuron, diffusion of neurotransmitter out of the synaptic cleft, enzymatic breakdown of neurotransmitter in the synapse or postsynaptic receptor alteration that impairs neurotransmitter binding (Fig. 9.3). Alteration in the control of neurotransmitter-receptor binding impairs postsynaptic impulse generation and the physiologic outcome associated with neural conduction in the target cells.

Neural impulses require precise control, determined in part by the neurotransmitter type, the postsynaptic receptor with affinity for binding a specific neurotransmitter and modulators of neural transmission. Neurotransmitters are produced in the neuron, determined by the enzyme systems present in the neuron. Neurotransmitters can be grouped into three major types:

1. Amino acids (e.g., glutamic acid and gamma-aminobutyric acid [GABA])

2. Peptides (e.g., endorphins, enkephalins, substance P)

3. Monoamines (e.g., serotonin, dopamine, norepinephrine)

Neurons are classified by the primary neurotransmitter produced. For example, dopaminergic neurons produce dopamine as the primary neurotransmitter; norepinephrine is the primary neurotransmitter produced by adrenergic neurons; GABA is the primary neurotransmitter produced by GABAergic neurons.

Typically, there are multiple receptor types and subtypes that can bind a single neurotransmitter. The receptor determines the character of the neural impulse, either inhibitory or excitatory. The impulses generated by neurotransmitter-receptor binding are linked to a physiologic outcome in the target cells. For example, when norepinephrine binds to the α-adrenergic receptor, smooth muscle contraction results. Norepinephrine binding to the β-adrenergic receptor results in smooth muscle relaxation. In this way, a small number of neurotransmitters can induce multiple effects due to the much larger number of receptors available for binding. The effects of neurotransmitters can be altered by **neuromodulators**, released from axon terminals. The effects of neuromodulators may inhibit, potentiate, or prolong the effects of neurotransmitters.

Processes of Neuronal Injury

Mature neurons do not divide, a fact that is an important consideration when neurons are injured. Unlike most other cells, new neurons are not generated to replace those that have lost function through damage or death. Myelin that has been damaged is not

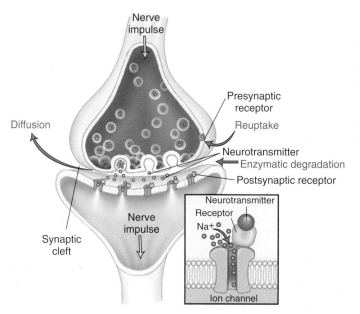

■ **Figure 9.3** The action potential generated at the axon hillock of the presynaptic neuron leads to release of neurotransmitter from the synaptic vesicle. Neurotransmitter enters the synaptic cleft and either binds to a receptor on the postsynaptic neuron, is taken back up into the presynaptic receptor, is degraded by enzymes in the synaptic cleft or diffuses away from the synapse. When neurotransmitter binding to a postsynaptic receptor occurs, a change in potential occurs. An inhibitory impulse results in a more negative potential, moving further away from threshold. An excitatory impulse raises voltage to a less negative membrane potential. When threshold is reached, an action potential results. The impulse is transmitted on the length of the postsynaptic neuron to the target cells, resulting in a physiologic outcome.

replaced, leading to permanent neurologic deficits. The loss of neurons through cell damage or as a process of aging contributes to disability and is the basis for a variety of neurologic disorders. Damage to neurons results from the following processes:

- **Chromatolysis**: the swelling of a neuron because of injury
- **Atrophy**: decrease in the size of the cell (neuron)
- **Neuronophagia**: phagocytosis and inflammatory responses caused by a dead neuron damaging neighboring cells
- **Intraneuronal inclusions**: distinctive structures formed in the nucleus or cytoplasm

Developmental Considerations

The neural tube develops early in embryonic life. Alterations in cellular differentiation, proliferation, or migration can result in significant neurologic impairment. At birth, almost all of the neurons necessary for functioning during adult life are present. By the age of 2 years, the brain achieves 80% of its adult size. The brain continues to develop and mature for the first few years of life. Glial cells divide and multiply, myelin deposition on neural fibers increases, and new connections are forged.

As individuals age, altered nervous system function may result from a decreased number of neurons, altered structure, or responsiveness of neural tissues. The characteristic brain changes that may occur with aging include:

- Enlargement in the size of the ventricle system
- Widening of sulci
- Decreased brain volume and weight
- Increase in the appearance of neurologic disorders, such as stroke, Alzheimer disease, and Parkinson disease
- Sensory changes, including cataract development, loss of focus, hearing, smell, and taste

Module 2

Alterations in Central Nervous System Function

The nervous system is divided into systems that connect and function as a unit. Functional distinctions are sometimes made, though it is important to recognize the broad scope of impact of neuronal impairment across systems. This chapter discusses the nervous system by organizing the nervous system into the CNS and the peripheral nervous system, which is further divided into the autonomic and somatic nervous systems. The **somatic nervous system** refers to voluntary nervous control in skeletal muscles. Involuntary nervous control is regulated by the visceral and autonomic nervous systems.

Central Nervous System Organization

The CNS is comprised of the brain and spinal cord. The brain weighs approximately 3 lb in an average adult and is composed of neurons and support cells. The brain receives and processes sensory information, initiating and coordinating motor responses. The spinal cord conducts sensory information from the peripheral nervous system and motor information from muscle to the brain for processing.

BRAIN

The brain is divided into lobes and hemispheres. Four separate lobes of the brain are divided by **sulci** (fissures), and **gyri** (irregular convolutions on the surface) have specialized functions (Fig. 9.4). The lobes and their functions include:

- Frontal lobe: reasoning, planning, speech, and movement
- Parietal lobe: perception of touch, pressure, temperature, and pain
- Temporal lobe: perception, memory, and recognition of auditory stimuli
- Occipital: vision

The brain is also divided into two halves, or hemispheres, each containing the four lobes of the brain. The right and left hemispheres communicate with each other through a bundle of nerve fibers known as the **corpus callosum**. Neural activity in the *right hemisphere* of the brain involves functional capacity of the left side of the body. The *left hemisphere* of the brain also demonstrates this contralateral pattern. Functions have been attributed to the control of specific brain hemispheres as follows:

- Left hemisphere
  - Speech and language
  - Calculations

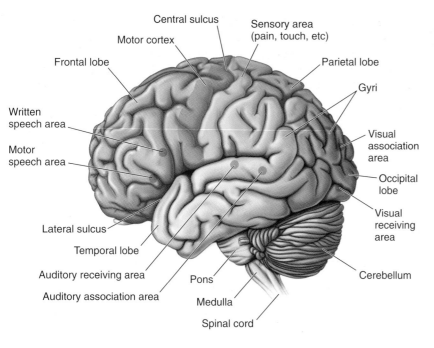

■ **Figure 9.4** Lobes of the brain. External view with motor and sensory areas. (Image modified from Bear MF, Connors BW, Parasido MA. *Neuroscience: Exploring the Brain*. 3rd ed. Philadelphia: Lippincott Williams & Wilkins; 2006, with permission.)

- Math
- Logical abilities
- Right hemisphere
  - Visual imagery
  - Face recognition
  - Music
  - Spacial abilities

Brain structures can be characterized further by their location. These categories include:

- Forebrain
  - Telencephalon
    - Cerebral cortex
    - Basal ganglia
    - Hippocampus
    - Amygdala
  - Diencephalon
    - Hypothalamus
    - Thalamus
- Midbrain
  - Mesencephalon
    - Tectum
    - Tegmentum
- Hindbrain
  - Metencephalon
    - Cerebellum
    - Pons
  - Myelencephalon
    - Medulla oblongata

The structures of the brain and related functions are outlined in Table 9.2. The cerebrum includes the telencephalon structures: cerebral cortex and basal ganglia. Figure 9.5 highlights the location of specific brain structures, which can be seen with a coronal view. The structure of the brain is also revealed by the composition of tissue in the lobes of each hemisphere. The tissue of the cerebral cortex, basal ganglia, hypothalamus, and thalamus is **gray matter**, primarily comprised of cell bodies; whereas other brain structures are comprised of **white matter**, tissue comprised primarily of myelinated axons and dendrites.

SPINAL CORD

The spinal cord serves as the primary pathway for communication of messages or impulses from the periphery and the brain. The spinal cord is also central to the control of reflex responses. The length of the spinal cord varies from an average of 43 cm in an adult female to 45 cm in an adult male. The vertebral column housing the spinal cord is approximately 70 cm long, far exceeding the length of the spinal cord. Because the spinal cord ends at the last of the thoracic vertebra, nerves branching from the spinal cord below the lumbar and sacral levels must extend for a distance before they exit the vertebral column. The extension of nerves in this portion of the vertebral canal is called the **cauda equina**.

The nervous tissue of the spinal cord is comprised of both white and gray matter, based on the presence or absence of myelin. The proportion of gray matter to white matter in the spinal cord is determined by the amount of tissue innervated. Differences in proportion of gray and white matter are seen in the various segments of the cord. The lower lumbar and upper sacral segment innervate the lower extremities and contain larger amounts of gray matter. The white matter proportion increases as the cord approaches the brain due to the greater number of ascending fibers.

Table 9.2 Brain Structures and Functions

Brain Structure	Anatomic Significance	Function
Cerebral cortex	Located in the telencephalon of the forebrain; convoluted layer of cerebrum that contains gray matter (unmyelinated cell bodies)	Controls higher-order functions including language and information processing
Basal ganglia	Located in the telencephalon of the forebrain; includes structures of the globus pallidus, caudate nucleus, subthalamic nucleus, putamen, and substantia nigra	Control voluntary movement; establish posture
Hippocampus	Component of the limbic system located in the telencephalon of the forebrain; convoluted structure located in the temporal lobe; forms the medial margin of the cerebral hemisphere	Controls impulses of emotion, hunger, sexual arousal, and aggression; involved in memory and learning
Amygdala	Component of the limbic system located in the telencephalon of the forebrain; almond-shaped structure of gray matter in the temporal lobe	Produces and responds to nonverbal signs of anger, avoidance, defensiveness, fear, and inspiring aversive cues
Hypothalamus	Located in the diencephalon of the forebrain; the hypothalamus is critical to the integration of homeostatic control of the internal environment; borders the posterior pituitary, the third ventricle, and the thalamus	Controls body temperature, appetite, water balance, secretion from the pituitary gland, emotions, and autonomic functions, including sleep and wakefulness
Thalamus	Located in the diencephalon of the forebrain; consists of two large egg-shaped masses of tissue, one on each side of the third ventricle	Relays sensory information (including pain) through an ascending pathway via the thalamus to the cerebral cortex, focusing of attention and organization of incoming stimuli
Tectum	Located in the dorsal region of the mesencephalon (midbrain); contains visual and auditory receptors	Controls auditory and visual responses
Tegmentum	Located in the ventral region of the mesencephalon (midbrain); consists of the cerebral aqueduct and reticular formation	Controls motor functions; regulates awareness, attention, and some autonomic functions
Cerebellum	Located in the metencephalon of the hindbrain; separated from the central hemispheres by a fold in the dura mater superior to the pons	Maintains muscle tone; coordinates muscle movement and balance
Pons	Located in the metencephalon of the hindbrain; serves as the connection between the cerebellum and the cerebrum and between the midbrain and the medulla oblongata	Assists in controlling autonomic functions, arousal, and sleep
Medulla oblongata	Located in the myencephalon of the hindbrain; a component of the brainstem, the medulla is the most caudal segment of the neural tube of the brain	Regulation of vasomotor, cardiac, and respiratory function
Reticular activating system (RAS)	A network of hyperexcitable neurons extending from the brainstem through the cerebral cortex	Routes incoming information to the appropriate location in the brain; RAS activity also involved in wakefulness

The gray matter contains synapses between sensory, motor, and interneurons. On cross section of the spinal cord, the gray matter has a butterfly-like appearance and contains nerve cell bodies. The posterior extensions are the **dorsal horns**, which contain sensory neurons that receive afferent impulses via the dorsal roots. The anterior extensions are known as the **ventral horns**, which contain efferent motor neurons that leave the cord through the ventral roots. **Upper motor neurons** (UMNs) include cell bodies in the motor cortex and the axons extending to the brainstem and spinal cord. **Lower motor neurons** (LMNs) are located in the ventral horns of the spinal cord. Interneurons connect UMNs with LMNs in the spinal cord.

Surrounding this gray matter is the white matter, comprised of the axons of the spinal cord. The white matter contains myelinated axons, giving the lighter-colored appearance reflected by its name (Fig. 9.6). Myelin produced by Schwann cells increases the velocity and survival of nerve impulses along longer neuronal processes.

The white matter contains ascending sensory and descending motor tracts with axons that communicate impulses within the CNS. The ascending tracts communicate sensory information from the periphery to the CNS and will be discussed in more detail in Chapter 10. The **pyramidal motor system**, comprised of the axons in the descending corticospinal and corticobulbar tracts, provides control of voluntary movement. Motor nerves of the pyramidal tract

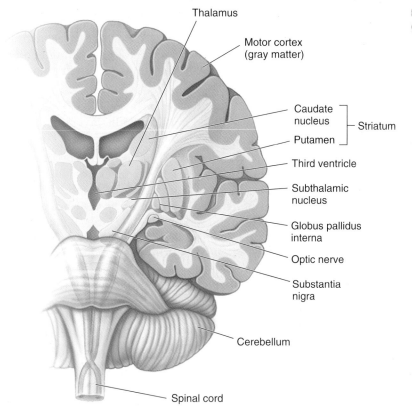

■ **Figure 9.5** Coronal view of the brain. (Asset provided by Anatomical Chart Company.)

originate in both hemispheres of the sensorimotor areas of the cerebral cortex and extend through the medullary brainstem, condensing to form pyramids. The majority of UMNs of the corticospinal tract cross over in the medulla, descending on the contralateral side. The UMNs synapse onto the LMNs, leaving the spinal cord via the ventral root. The UMNs that do not cross over in the medulla travel down the ipsilateral spinal cord, crossing over and synapsing on the LMN at the level of spinal cord exit. The LMNs synapse onto motor fibers in the peripheral nervous system, providing innervation and motor function to the legs. Injury to axons before they cross over results in spastic paralysis on the opposite side of the body, whereas injury to axons after they cross over exerts its effect on the same side of the body. Axons of the corticobulbar tract provide innervation to the muscles of the face, controlling motor neurons located in cranial nerve brain nuclei.

The **extrapyramidal system**, separate from the pyramidal motor system, modulates motor function, attenuating erratic motions and maintaining muscle tone and stability of the trunk. Functions associated with the extrapyramidal system are associated with the basal ganglia. The subcortical nuclei of the basal ganglia include the structures of the caudate nucleus, putamen, subthalamic nucleus, substantia nigra, and globus pallidus, which comprise the main structures of the extrapyramidal system.

Protective Structures of the Central Nervous System

The maintenance of a stable environment provides a source of protection for the neurologic system. The interconnected circulatory systems confer neurologic

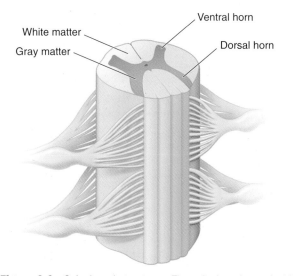

■ **Figure 9.6** Spinal cord structures. The spinal cord runs inside the vertebral column. Axons enter the spinal cord through the dorsal roots and exit by the ventral roots.

protection via the blood–brain barrier and cerebrospinal fluid.

NEUROCIRCULATORY SYSTEM

The nervous system is perfused by two parallel communicating systems. These systems include the cerebrovascular circulation and the cerebrospinal fluid circulation.

Cerebrovascular Circulation

The vascular supply of the CNS provides oxygenation and nutrients for optimal metabolism and function. Maintenance of perfusion to the brain is essential for prevention of cellular injury and death. Neurons in the brain are sensitive to hypoxia, requiring adequate perfusion. Arterial supply to the brain includes the vertebral, basilar, and carotid arteries. The circle of Willis is a cerebral arterial structure that connects the vertebral and carotid circulations. This structure is important as a route of collateral circulation in case perfusion is impaired in another arterial system. The primary vascular drainage of the brain occurs via the jugular veins. Perfusion to the spinal cord is supplied by the spinal arteries and drained by the spinal veins. Removal of excess fluid in the CNS occurs between the pia matter of the meninges and the blood vessels because typical lymphatics are absent in the brain.

● **STOP** *and Consider*

The preferred energy source for the brain is glucose. What manifestations can be expected when adequate levels of glucose are unavailable?

Blood–Brain Barrier

The brain is protected from exposure to potentially hazardous substances by reduced permeability in capillaries that supply the brain, known as the **blood–brain barrier (BBB)**. The BBB transports substances in a selective manner because of the tight junctions in the endothelial cells lining the capillaries of the brain. Transport across the BBB of large molecules, molecules with low lipid solubility, and molecules with high electrical charge are resisted. Substances that are small, highly lipid soluble, and have a low electrical charge are able to cross the BBB more readily. The BBB functions include:

- Protection of the brain from foreign substances
- Protection of the brain from hormones and neurotransmitters in the systemic circulation
- Protection against drastic environmental fluctuations

Cerebrospinal Fluid Circulation

The **meninges** of the CNS include three membranes that protect tissue surfaces, containing cerebrospinal fluid. These membranes and their relative locations include:

1. Dura mater (outer layer)
2. Arachnoid mater (middle layer)
3. Pia mater (inner layer)

The surface of the CNS is bathed by the **cerebrospinal fluid (CSF)**, which flows from four fluid-filled interconnecting cavities of the brain, known as the **ventricles**. CSF is produced by the **choroid plexus**, a structure located in the two lateral and single third and fourth ventricles of the brain. CSF flows from the lateral ventricle to the third ventricle through the **interventricular foramen** (also called the foramen of Monro). The third and fourth ventricles are connected by the **cerebral aqueduct** (also known as the aqueduct of Sylvius). CSF then flows into the subarachnoid space (Fig. 9.7). CSF protects the CNS by:

- Providing a cushion for brain structures
- Reducing the pressure on brain structures
- Removing harmful substances
- Transporting hormones to remote sites in the brain

The total volume of CSF in the CNS at any one time is approximately 125 to 150 mL. The choroid plexus produces 400 to 500 mL CSF per day to maintain a resting pressure of 150 to 180 mm H_2O. When CSF pressure exceeds venous pressure, CSF can be absorbed into the blood via the arachnoid. This movement of fluid from the CSF to the circulation is unidirectional, preventing the absorption of fluid from the blood into the CSF.

Pia mater
Arachnoid mater
Dura mater

Aqueduct of Sylvius
(cerebral aqueduct)

■ **Figure 9.7** Cerebrospinal fluid flow in the ventricular system. Arrows indicate the direction of cerebrospinal fluid flow.

STOP *and Consider*

How would CSF volume be altered if fluid could move directly from the blood into the CSF?

Central Nervous System Cellular Injury

Responses to injury vary based on the specific cell type involved. These responses mirror the major functional properties of the cells. In the CNS, astrocytes respond to local tissue injury through proliferation, forming a "glial scar." This process is known as **astrogliosis**. Common tissue injuries that are likely to cause this response include contusions, wounds, tumors, abscesses, and hemorrhages. Unchecked proliferation may result in neoplastic transformation responsible for the development of gliomas, as discussed in Chapter 7.

Microglia, like astrocytes, mount an immune response to areas of injury. Reactive changes seen in microglia include extension of the nucleus, leading to their description as "rod cells" when in this state. When joined together with astrocytes, microglia combine to form **microglial nodules**. Oligodendroglial damage leads to demyelination of axons. Ependymal cell damage is linked to alterations in CSF production and transfer, affecting intracranial pressure.

Neurologic transmission is impaired in the presence of significant neuronal damage or death. The manifestations of altered function reflect the site of injury and the functions that are controlled by those particular neurons. The nervous system responses to injury include degeneration of axons, demyelination, and **neuropathy**. Alteration in neuronal transmission underlies the manifestations that result from these types of injuries.

MECHANISMS OF INJURY TO THE CENTRAL NERVOUS SYSTEM

Functions of the brain and spinal cord can be impaired because of injury. Mechanisms of injury may result from trauma, ischemia, excitatory response to neurotransmitters, or pressure.

Traumatic Central Nervous System Injury

Traumatic injury can impair neurologic functioning locally or systemically. When injury is restricted to a structure innervating a specific area, a local effect may be seen. Injury to neural tissue responsible for the integrated transmission of impulses to multiple, distant sites is likely to have a more systemic effect.

Examples of these types of major injuries include trauma to the components of the CNS (the brain and spinal cord).

Traumatic Brain Injury

Automobile accidents, falls, sports-related accidents, and "shaken baby syndrome" are conditions that may result in traumatic brain injury. Groups of individuals at highest risk of brain injury from head trauma include children from birth to 4 years, males from 15 to 19 years, and the elderly.[1] Head trauma that results in brain injury may lead to changes in physical, intellectual, emotional, or social abilities. Head trauma from a **blunt force injury** (e.g., when the head strikes a hard surface or is struck by a rapidly moving object [coup/countercoup]) is an example of a **closed head injury**. The force of the acceleration impact causes injury to the tissue in the local area (coup), and the deceleration impact leads to injury on the opposite side of the skull (countercoup). Lacerations and contusions of the brain tissue may result from contact with the rough surface of the skull. The cerebral cortex may suffer effects of movement within the skull, increasing the likelihood of damage to the frontal, temporal, and occipital lobes of the brain as well as the upper midbrain. **Open traumatic injury** involves exposure of brain structures (e.g., dura, meninges, and brain tissue) to the environment. The risk of infection and injury to brain tissue is significant with this type of injury.

Traumatic brain injury may lead to seizure activity, concussion, contusion, hematoma (epidural, subdural, or intracerebral), edema, or skull fracture. Increased intracranial pressure (ICP), respiratory depression/failure, and herniation of the brainstem may also occur. Manifestations are caused by axonal injury from the original trauma and by spread of damage that causes secondary injury. Diagnosis is often made using brain imaging techniques, including computed tomography (CT) or magnetic resonance imaging (MRI). Brain activity can be determined with an electroencephalogram (EEG). Lumbar puncture (spinal tap) with removal and analysis of CSF may determine the presence of blood, indicating intracranial hemorrhage.

Treatment is directed toward the specific injury and diagnosis. Surgery may be necessary to evacuate a hematoma or to remove foreign fragments from brain tissue. Supportive care includes determination of the extent and progression of neurologic damage, reduction of increased ICP, pain control, provision of anticonvulsant medications to prevent seizures, respiratory support, and antibiotics to prevent or treat infection.

Traumatic Spinal Cord Injury

According to the National Spinal Cord Injury Statistical Center, spinal cord injury (SCI) primarily affects young adults. The average age at injury has increased from 28.7 years in the 1970s to an average age of 40.2 years in 2005. Most spinal cord injuries (approximately 81%) are among males. Although frequency among Caucasians has steadily decreased over the past two decades, the incidence of SCI has increased among African-Americans, Asians and Hispanics.[2] Spinal cord injuries may be the result of fractures, contusions, or compression of the vertebral column. These injuries may also stem from trauma to the head or neck. Neurologic damage resulting from pulling, twisting, severing, or compressing the neural tissue of the spinal cord is a serious, potentially life-threatening condition. The level of injury within the spinal cord is the determining factor for the clinical consequences. The most common spinal cord injuries occur at C5–7, T12, and L1.

Traumatic injury to the spinal cord is often secondary to motor vehicle accidents, falls, acts of violence and recreational injuries, similar to the events leading to brain injury. Injury often extends two segments above and below the site of damage. Diving into shallow water may also cause serious spinal cord damage. Damage results from hyperextension and hyperflexion due to rapid acceleration/deceleration, excessive pressure to the top of the head causing compression injury, and rotational forces causing trauma from twisting of the spinal cord. Hemorrhage in the gray matter and the pia mater/arachnoid may lead to necrosis. Extension of hemorrhage into the white matter and the development of local edema decrease perfusion to the cord, leading to ischemia. Phagocytic activity in the gray matter results in macrophage engulfment of axons, replacing neural tissue with nonfunctional connective tissue. Scarring and thickening of the meninges alters neural conduction and function.

A clinical manifestation of vertebrae fracture may be pain. When SCI results, responses can range from mild **paresthesia** (abnormal sensation, such as burning, pricking, tickling, or tingling) to **quadriplegia** (paralysis of all four extremities). The level of the SCI and the severity of injury (complete or incomplete transection) also contribute to the neurologic deficit. Table 9.3 presents the possible consequences of serious SCI.

Diagnosis of spinal cord injury can be made by radiograph (fracture),

neurologic examination, lumbar puncture, CT scan, or MRI scan. Immediate treatment includes immobilization of the spine to prevent further injury. Once the spine is stabilized, corticosteroids are given to lessen inflammation. Traction, casting, and surgery may also be necessary.

Ischemic Central Nervous System Injury

Ischemic injury occurs when there is inadequate perfusion to neurologic tissue, resulting in impaired oxygenation. Reduction in the supply of oxygen leads to tissue necrosis. The cause of decreased perfusion and oxygenation may be local or may be a systemic condition. For example, occlusion of blood supply may result from a thrombosis in a local vessel, embolism from a thrombus originating in a distant site, or from local hemorrhage. **Global ischemia** occurs when there is inadequate blood supply to meet the needs of the brain tissue. A global ischemic event results in hypoxia, as is seen in the case of cardiac arrest or profound hemorrhage (Fig. 9.8). Spinal cord ischemia is often due to occlusion of spinal blood vessels resulting from dissecting aortic aneurism or emboli. Malformations in the spinal vasculature may also impair perfusion leading to ischemia and neural injury.

The pathology underlying ischemic injury is related to oxygen and nutrient deprivation to neurologic tissue. Impaired blood flow for longer than a few minutes results in tissue infarction in brain tissue with high metabolic demands. Cellular function ceases because of the inability to use anaerobic metabolic processes or uptake glucose and glycogen. Infarction stimulates a response to tissue injury that results in an inflammatory

Table 9.3 Potential Results of Serious Spinal Cord Injury

Condition	Pathophysiology	Clinical Manifestations
Spinal shock	Loss of autonomic, reflex, motor, and sensory activity below the injury	Flaccid (without tone) paralysis
		Loss of deep tendon reflexes (DTRs)
		Loss of perianal reflexes
		Loss of motor and sensory function
Autonomic dysreflexia	Occurs after resolution of spinal shock	Alteration in heart rate
		Hypertension
	Associated with injuries at or above T6	Cold/gooseflesh skin below the lesion
	Stimulated by noxious stimuli (distended bowel or bladder, skin lesion)	
Neurogenic shock	Altered vasomotor response secondary to impaired sympathetic impulse transmission from the brainstem to the thoracolumbar region	Orthostatic hypotension
		Bradycardia
		Loss of ability to sweat below the level of injury
	Most common with cervical spinal cord injury	

Figure 9.8 Global ischemia. Consequences of global ischemia include lesions related to cerebral vasculature and the sensitivity of individual neurons. (Image from Rubin E, Farber JL. *Pathology.* 4th ed. Philadelphia: Lippincott Williams & Wilkins; 2005, with permission.)

Labels in figure: Anterior cerebral artery; Watershed zone of infarction; Middle cerebral artery; Laminar necrosis; Short penetrating arteries; Necrosis in Sommers sector of hippocampus; Necrosis of Purkinje cells of cerebellum

response and the development of edema, leading to increased ICP. Cell injury leads to changes in the transport of ions leading to local water and electrolyte imbalances and acidosis, as was discussed in Chapter 8. Calcium, sodium, and water build up in the area of cellular damage. Free radical formation and increased release of excitatory neurotransmitters may potentiate the effects of the ischemic injury.

Clinical manifestations of ischemic injury are related to the functional areas involved. Sensory and motor functions are often affected. When the injury occurs in the brain, the manifestations reflect the specific associated functions with motor deficits evident on the **contralateral**, or opposite, side of the body. Loss of consciousness, weakness, difficulty speaking or swallowing, impaired vision, and paresthesias may result.

CT scan, MRI, and angiography can be used to diagnose ischemic blockages. Altered metabolism in surrounding regions may be identified by positron emission tomography (PET) scanning. Treatment includes management of increased ICP, insertion of a stent to restore perfusion, thrombolytic therapy to dissolve the obstructive clot, and anticoagulation therapy to prevent future clot development.

Excitation Injury

Neurons that are easily depolarized or hyperexcitable may cause altered transmission of signals. Increased neuron impulse frequency, intensity, or cascade of transmission can lead to pathologic

consequences because of excitation injury. Injury to brain neurons may result from the effects of excitatory neurotransmitters, such as the amino acid glutamate. **Glutamate** is the main excitatory neurotransmitter in the body, active in the promotion of many higher-order functions. The effects of glutamate are exerted when it binds to its receptors, stimulating a cascade of signal transduction events. One receptor with affinity for glutamate is the ***N*-methyl-D-aspartate (NMDA) receptor**. When glutamate binds to the NMDA receptor, alterations in ion channel openings lead to prolonged action potentials. Damage to neurons from protein breakdown, free radical formation, DNA damage, and breakdown of the nucleus is stimulated by these prolonged action potentials.

Excitation injury may result from the inability to meet the metabolic demands of the cells. Oxygen needs dramatically increase with enhanced neurologic activity, increasing the risk of hypoxia development in affected tissues. Prolonged ischemia permits intracellular glutamate to move from the highly concentrated intracellular space to the extracellular environment, making more glutamate available for receptor binding, thereby intensifying the excitatory effects. In tissues sensitive to hypoxia, such as the brain, permanent brain injury may result.

The neurons of the hippocampus and cerebral cortex are particularly sensitive to the excitatory effects of glutamate and increases in calcium that result from changes in ion transport. The neurotoxic effects may be manifested by reductions in higher-order functions and cognitive and memory abilities. Neuronal cell death may result from prolonged exposure to the effects of glutamate.

Cell death may be prevented if the effects of glutamate can be blocked or the excessive level of glutamate removed from the neuronal synapses. Because glutamate is required by a wide variety of cells for normal functioning, the development of drugs to block or promote reuptake of glutamate has been hampered.

Excitatory responses may predominate during periods of deteriorating brain function. Loss of consciousness may promote the development of **decerebrate posturing**, the result of increased extensor muscle excitability, or **decorticate posturing**, the result of increased flexor muscle excitability (Fig. 9.9).

Central Nervous System Pressure Injury

The skull and vertebral column provide the rigid structure surrounding the brain and spinal cord, restricting the potential area of expansion. Increases in pressure may result in neuronal injury and cell death. Increased pressure in the brain and spinal cord may result from excessive CSF volume, cerebral edema, or space-occupying lesions.

Increased CSF volume is the result of increased production or decreased absorption of CSF. Obstruction of the ventricular system prevents CSF from reaching the arachnoid villi. Flow of the CSF may be obstructed by inflammation, tumor, hemorrhage, or congenital anomaly, promoting buildup in the ventricular system. Cerebral hemisphere enlargement and dilation of the ventricles result from pressure increases. Brain structures affected by the increased pressure respond with altered functional capacity. Responses may be altered by age and associated brain development.

Cerebral edema caused by abnormal water accumulation may also contribute to pressure injury. Edema may be a result of the transfer of water and protein from the vascular to the interstitial space, as discussed in Chapter 8. Edema may also be caused by an increase in intracellular fluid caused by a hypoosmotic state, such as occurs with water intoxication. Severe ischemia can also contribute to cerebral edema. Swelling of brain cells increases tissue volume, causing injury to cells. Manifestations of cerebral edema include disturbances in consciousness, intracranial hypertension, and neurologic deficit.

CNS tumors (discussed in Chapter 7) can also promote pressure injury. Brain and spinal cord compression, tumor infiltration, altered blood flow, and edema are often the sequelae of pressure injuries resulting from tumors. Tumors may obstruct CSF flow and promote brain displacement to an area of lower pressure, known as brain herniation. Stimulation of the vomiting center of the medulla may contribute to severe nausea. Personality and mental changes, including loss of memory and the development of depression, may result. The tumor location and site of pressure injury determine the specific signs and symptoms evidenced. Clinical manifestations of pressure injury are determined by the sites of injury and severity of damage, ranging from leg weakness to respiratory arrest.

A common response to pathologic events in the brain is ICP. Increased ICP can lead to blood flow reduction,

■ **Figure 9.9** Posturing in brain injury. **A:** Flexor, or decorticate posturing response, is characterized by flexion of elbows, wrists, and fingers. **B:** Extensor, or decerebrate posturing response, is characterized by neck extension and clenching of the jaw. Arms are extended with flexion of wrists and fingers.

death of brain cells, and damage to brain structures. Common symptoms of increased ICP include:

- Headache
- Vomiting
- **Papilledema** (edema of the optic disc)
- Mental deterioration

When increased ICP is caused by excessive CSF ventricular fluid volume, surgical shunting of CSF from the intraventricular spaces to the peritoneum may be required. A catheter is inserted into the left lateral ventricle and passed through the internal jugular vein into the right atrium (ventriculoatrial shunt) or the peritoneal cavity (ventriculoperitoneal shunt). For increased ICP caused by cerebral edema, osmotic diuretics such as mannitol are often used to promote fluid removal and excretion. Corticosteroids may also be used to stabilize cell membranes.

Module 3

Alterations in Peripheral Nervous System Function

The peripheral nervous system connects the CNS to limbs and organs, transmitting neural impulses via sensory pathways into the dorsal horn and extending motor pathways beyond the ventral horn. Located outside of the boundaries of the CNS, the peripheral nervous system is not protected by the BBB or bony support of the CNS, increasing the potential for damage due to toxic and mechanical injury.

Peripheral Nervous System Organization

Functionally, the peripheral nervous system includes the somatic and the autonomic nervous systems.

Motor and sensory nerves carrying nerve impulses to and from the periphery of the body are part of the peripheral nervous system, including the cranial and spinal nerves. Cranial nerves that mediate peripheral responses originate in the brain. There are 12 paired cranial nerves, each named, numbered, and specific in the sensory and motor functions they mediate (Table 9.4). There are 31 pairs of spinal nerves, each consisting of sensory/afferent and motor/efferent neurons. They are named for the vertebra immediately below their exit point from the spinal cord and include 8 cervical, 12 thoracic, 5 lumbar, 5 sacral, and 1 coccygeal nerve pairs. Table 9.5 provides further detail on the location and function of these nerves. Spinal nerves carry information to and from particular body regions, or **dermatomes** (Fig. 9.10). Manifestations of pain, numbness, or tingling can be linked to pressure or inflammation of the spinal nerves associated with specific dermatomes. Spinal nerves form together in an interconnection of fibers known as a **plexus**. Peripheral nerves arise in new combinations from each plexus. Common plexuses include the cervical, brachial, lumbar, and sacral.

● STOP *and Consider*

When having a heart attack, a common manifestation is pain in the left arm or shoulder. How are dermatomes related to this phenomenon?

SOMATIC NERVOUS SYSTEM

Coordination of body movement, reception of external stimuli and regulation of activities under conscious control are the primary functions of the somatic nervous system. The somatic nervous system includes the peripheral fibers that transmit sensory impulses including body position, pain, temperature, and touch to the CNS and motor impulses to skeletal muscle from cell bodies located in the brain or spinal cord. Targets for innervation include skeletal muscle, skin and sensory organs. A review of somatosensory function and dysfunction is included in Chapter 10.

AUTONOMIC NERVOUS SYSTEM

The **autonomic nervous system (ANS)** controls involuntary functions of organs. All internal organs are innervated by the ANS, which transmits messages from the brain and neuroendocrine system. The two major divisions of the ANS are the **sympathetic nervous system (SNS)** and **parasympathetic nervous system (PNS)**. These systems generally work in opposition to one another, working toward homeostatic balance.

Axon fibers extending from cell bodies in either the brain or spinal cord project to an autonomic **ganglion** (group of nerve cell bodies) known as **preganglionic neurons**. Fibers projecting from the autonomic ganglion to a target organ are known as **postganglionic neurons**. The SNS has short preganglionic fibers that synapse outside the spinal cord with secondary neurons. Long SNS postganglionic fibers

Table 9.4 Cranial Nerves

Number	Name	Location	Type	Function
I	Olfactory	Cerebral cortex Amygdala Hippocampus Basal ganglia (caudate nucleus, putamen, globus pallidus)	Sensory	Smell reflexes
II	Optic	Hypothalamus Thalamus	Sensory	Vision
III	Oculomotor	Basal ganglia substantia nigra, central gray matter	Motor	Extraocular eye movement (superior, medial, and inferior lateral), pupil constriction, upper eyelid elevation
IV	Trochlear	Pons	Motor	Extraocular eye movement (inferior medial)
V	Trigeminal	Pons	Sensory	Corneal reflex, transmission of stimuli from face to head
			Motor	Lateral jaw movement, chewing, biting
VI	Abducens	Pons	Motor	Extraocular eye movement (lateral)
VII	Facial	Pons	Sensory	Taste (anterior two thirds of tongue)
			Motor	Movement of facial muscles and muscles of expression in forehead, around eyes and mouth
VIII	Acoustic (vestibulocochlear)	Pons	Sensory	Hearing, balance
IX	Glossopharyngeal	Medulla	Sensory	Taste (posterior one third of the tongue), sensations of the throat
			Motor	Swallow
X	Vagus	Medulla	Sensory	Sensations of larynx, throat, abdominal (gastrointestinal tract), and thoracic viscera (heart, lungs, bronchi)
			Motor	Palate movement, swallow, gag, activity of thoracic and abdominal viscera (including heart rate and peristalsis)
XI	Spinal accessory	Medulla	Motor	Movement of shoulders, head rotation
XII	Hypoglossal	Medulla	Motor	Tongue movement

Table 9.5 Spinal Nerves

Spinal Nerves	Location	Function
Lower cervical	C5–8	Proprioception, deep tendon reflexes, movement, posture
Thoracic	T1–12	Proprioception, movement, posture, respiration, sensation, sympathetic reflexes (vasomotor control, sweating, piloerection)
Lumbar	L1–5	Proprioception, deep tendon reflexes, movement, posture, reflexes
Sacral	S1–5	Proprioception, reflexes, defecation, urination, erection
Coccygeal	Co1–2	Proprioception, posture

synapse on target organs. The exception to this pattern is in the case of the adrenal medulla. Here, the unusually long preganglionic fibers of the SNS synapse directly onto the adrenal medulla, with the adrenal medulla itself serving as the secondary fiber.

The PNS organization differs from the SNS, with long preganglionic fibers extending to the walls of target organs. There, they synapse with secondary neurons, extending short postganglionic fibers into the organ walls. PNS is often linked with *vagal stimulation* because approximately 75% of all PNS impulses travel along the vagus nerve (cranial nerve X). One of the differences between the ANS and the somatic nervous system is that the latter involves only one neuron, whereas the ANS requires two.

Sympathetic Nervous System

The **sympathetic nervous system** is also known as the **thoracolumbar nervous system** because of the location of the nerve exit sites. Spinal cord exit sites of the SNS neurons are located between the first thoracic and second lumbar vertebrae. The nerves leave the spinal cord to merge with ganglia. The preganglionic neurons enter ganglia near the cord, where the impulse is then carried to the postganglionic neurons (Fig. 9.11). Sympathetic activity is responsible for:

- Increased heart rate and contractility
- Smooth muscle relaxation of the bronchioles
- Decreased peristalsis of the gastrointestinal (GI) tract and constriction of anal sphincter

- Decreased bladder tone and constriction of urinary sphincter
- Vasoconstriction and elevated blood pressure
- Increased respiratory rate
- Pupil dilation and ciliary muscle relaxation
- Reduced secretion of the pancreas
- Increased sweat gland secretion

Parasympathetic Nervous System

The neurons of the PNS leave the CNS via the cranial nerves from the midbrain and the medulla, and with the spinal nerves between S2–S4 (craniosacral). The preganglionic neurons of the PNS are long, traveling close to organs or glands. The shorter postganglionic fibers innervate organs and glands, stimulating specific responses in the targets (Fig. 9.12). The typical effects of PNS innervation include:

- Decreased heart rate, contractility, and velocity of conduction
- Constriction of bronchial smooth muscle
- Increased peristalsis and GI tone with relaxation of anal sphincter
- Increased bladder tone and relaxation of urinary sphincter
- Vasodilation of arteries supplying external genitalia
- Constriction of pupils
- Increase in pancreatic, salivary, and eye secretions

■ **Figure 9.11** Distribution of sympathetic nerve fibers. (Image modified from Moore KL, Agur A. *Essential Clinical Anatomy.* 2nd ed. Philadelphia: Lippincott Williams & Wilkins; 2002, with permission.)

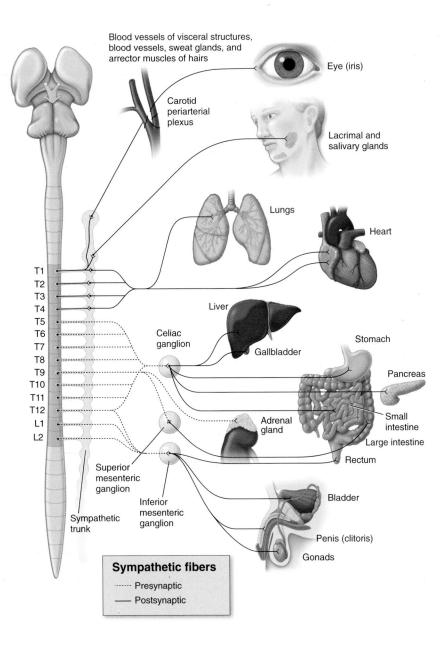

Blood vessels of visceral structures, blood vessels, sweat glands, and arrector muscles of hairs

Eye (iris)

Carotid periarterial plexus

Lacrimal and salivary glands

Lungs

Heart

Liver

Celiac ganglion

Gallbladder

Stomach

Pancreas

Small intestine

Adrenal gland

Large intestine

Rectum

Superior mesenteric ganglion

Inferior mesenteric ganglion

Sympathetic trunk

Bladder

Penis (clitoris)

Gonads

Sympathetic fibers

------- Presynaptic

——— Postsynaptic

▨ Reflex Arcs

Communication between various segments of the nervous system can be illustrated by the reflex arc. A basic functional pathway of the nervous system, the **reflex arc** represents the process by which stimuli are received and interpreted, and in turn stimulate a response. For example, the knee-jerk response, also known as the patellar or deep tendon reflex (DTR), is a basic reflex requiring one sensory neuron and one motor neuron with a synapse in the CNS. A tap on the patellar tendon causes a sudden contraction of the anterior thigh muscles through conduction of the nerve impulse through the sensory afferent to the dorsal horn of the spinal cord. There, the impulse is conducted to an interneuron, then to the motor neuron and away to the peripheral target,

which is the skeletal muscle spindle of the anterior thigh (Fig. 9.13). Using this simple test, the function of the following components of the nervous system can be determined:

- Peripheral afferent neuron
- Peripheral muscle sensory response
- Dorsal root ganglia
- Dorsal and ventral horn
- Motor neuron
- Neuromuscular synapse
- Muscle fiber contractile response
- Selected spinal and cranial nerves
- Brainstem

Although this example represents the reflex arc in its simplest form, stimulation of DTRs and other more complex reflex arcs are significant clinical tools used to quickly evaluate neurologic status.

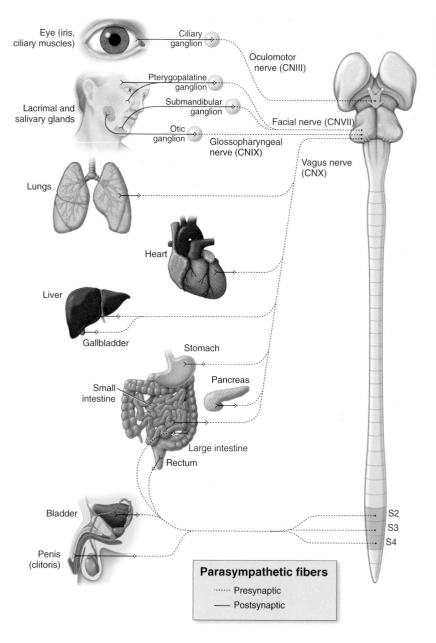

■ **Figure 9.12** Distribution of parasympathetic nerve fibers. (Image modified from Moore KL, Agur A. *Essential Clinical Anatomy*. 2nd ed. Philadelphia: Lippincott Williams & Wilkins; 2002, with permission.)

Peripheral Nervous System Cellular Injury

The peripheral nerves and their connective tissue support are vulnerable to injury due to the lack of protection afforded by the BBB and bony limits of the CNS. Peripheral nerve injury is often the result of damage due to trauma or pressure. Injury to the cells of the peripheral nervous system shows a more limited scope of responses, including degeneration of the axons and segmental demyelination. Responses of peripheral nervous system cells to injury differ from CNS cell responses in that peripheral nervous system cells have some capacity for regeneration, repair and reinnervation.

MECHANISMS OF INJURY TO THE PERIPHERAL NERVOUS SYSTEM

Axonal degeneration is caused by necrosis in response to significant injury to the cell body or axon of the neuron. In this process, an inflammatory response is stimulated, leading to phagocytosis of cellular debris by macrophages. **Distal axonopathy** occurs when the injury affects cells in distal areas of the body, such as the hands and feet. Regeneration of axons may be possible if the cell body and proximal axons are not damaged. When axonal degeneration occurs because of damage to the cell body (**neuronopathy**), the chance for regeneration is greatly reduced. When degeneration of the axon is caused by a crushing injury, it is known as a

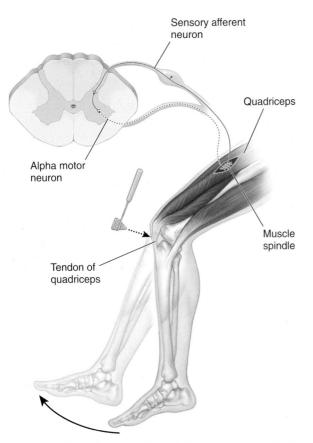

Figure 9.13 Reflex arc pathway. Reflex arc demonstrating the pathway of impulses between the receptor, spinal cord, and target organ. (Image from Bear MF, Connors BW, Parasido MA. *Neuroscience: Exploring the Brain*. 3rd ed. Philadelphia: Lippincott Williams & Wilkins; 2006, with permission.)

Wallerian degeneration. The clinical manifestations of damage to peripheral nerves are called **peripheral neuropathy**. Basic responses of peripheral nerves to injury are described in Figure 9.14.

Traumatic Peripheral Nerve Injury

Traumatic injury to peripheral nerves can occur because of the crushing or cutting of neurons. The area of nerve fiber that is severed from the cell body degenerates (Wallerian degeneration), stimulating the inflammatory processes induced by necrosis. Chromatolysis is induced in the injured neurons. Damage to peripheral nerves from traumatic injury manifests with sensory symptoms. These may include:

- Numbness
- Paresthesia
- Pain

The symptoms that result from peripheral nerve trauma are related to the number of axons involved and the ability of axons to regenerate. Regeneration

Figure 9.14 Basic responses of peripheral nerve fibers to injury. (Image from Rubin E, Farber JL. *Pathology*. 4th ed. Philadelphia: Lippincott Williams & Wilkins; 2005, with permission.)

of peripheral nerve fibers depends on the distance the regrowing fiber must go to restore communication. Because crushing injuries do not involve the complete separation of the axon and cell body from the target organ, regeneration success is much greater in these injuries than in fibers damaged by cutting injuries. When nerve trauma is limited to a single area (**mononeuropathy**), conditions such as nerve entrapment and compression may contribute to impaired functional responses. Sensory responses to traumatic nerve injury can result from scar tissue formation entrapping a regenerating nerve.

Peripheral nerve damage involving multiple axons is known as **polyneuropathy**. Polyneuropathy can occur secondary to disease processes such as multiple sclerosis, diabetes mellitus, nutrient deficiency, and toxic agents (arsenic). It contributes to multisystemic responses characterized by neural degeneration, neuroma formation, demyelination, and generation of abnormal, spontaneous nerve impulses from injured neurons. Responses may involve alterations in sensation, motor, or mixed responses. If the ANS is involved, systemic alterations affecting blood pressure, evacuation of bowel or bladder, and erectile function may result.

Peripheral Nervous System Pressure Injury

Pressure on peripheral nerves may also contribute to nerve injury and associated symptoms. Edema in constricted spaces may cause this type of injury. Symptoms may be mild, as in the case of carpal tunnel syndrome when edema causes pain and paresthesia in the hands. This damage is usually reversible by correcting the edema. Trauma may lead to edema formation impinging on a nerve plexus, as in the case of birth trauma leading to **brachial plexus palsy**. The brachial plexus provides innervation to the shoulder, arm, forearm, wrist, and hand. **Flaccid** paralysis of the affected arm, which is usually temporary, occurs from altered neural transmission caused by edema-induced compression. Neuroma may develop during the process of injury repair, resulting in more significant impairment.

● **STOP** and *Consider*

Why is it important to characterize specific types of altered movement?

◢ Peripheral Nervous System Motor Dysfunction

Disorders of motor function may be the result of peripheral nerve injury that alters reflex circuits. These disorders also can result from neuromuscu-

lar junction abnormalities, damage in skeletal muscle fibers, or SCI with damage to the corticospinal system or spinal nerve roots. Changes in skeletal muscle mass, such as occurs with atrophy or dystrophy, may contribute to impaired responses to adequate neural transmission. Movement disorders may be caused by excessive inhibitory or excitatory responses in nervous tissue that control functions such as coordination and proprioception. Movement disorders are characteristic of **extrapyramidal disorders**, which involve brain structures with the exclusion of the motor neurons, motor cortex, and pyramidal tract (corticobulbar and corticospinal). The extrapyramidal system (EPS) is often specifically referring to the structures of the basal ganglia, substantia nigra, and subthalamic nucleus. Neurotransmitter excesses or deficiency may also contribute to movement disorders. Box 9.1 lists terms used to describe specific disorders of movement. Motor deficits are discussed in more detail in Chapter 17. Sensory deficits may also result from altered neuronal transmission. These alterations are explored in Chapter 10.

● **STOP** and *Consider*

What are the challenges of maintaining a treatment plan for a person with clinical signs and symptoms related to altered neuronal transmission?

Box 9.1 Movement Disorders

Ataxia: inability to coordinate muscle activity

Athetosis: involuntary movements of flexion and extension, pronation and supination of hands, toes and feet; slow, writhing-type movements

Ballismus: jerking, swinging, sweeping motions of the proximal limbs

Bradykinesia/hypokinesia: decrease in spontaneity and movement

Chorea: irregular, spasmodic, involuntary movements of the limbs or facial muscles, often accompanied by hypotonia

Cogwheel: resistance to movement; rigidity decreasing to stiffness after movement begins

Dystonia: abnormal tonicity; difficulty maintaining posture

Hyperkinesis: excessive motor activity

Tic: repeated, habitual muscle contractions; movements that can be voluntarily suppressed for short period only

Tremor: oscillating, repetitive movements of whole muscles; irregular, involuntary contractions of the opposing muscle

Module 4

Clinical Models

Manifestations of neurologic alterations are often specific to the location of injury or damage. Alterations in mental status may include symptoms of altered consciousness, confusion, depression, anxiety, psychosis, inattentiveness, loss of rational thought, impaired memory, and poor judgment. Alterations in coordination lead to poor balance, injury from falls, difficulty in performing the **activities of daily living (ADLs)**, and movement disorders. Sensory deficits include blindness, deafness, pain, loss of the ability to smell or taste, and lack of sensation. Manifestations of motor deficits may involve paralysis, impaired voluntary movements, or enhanced involuntary movement.

A complete neurologic examination may be necessary to identify and diagnose neurologic disorders. When specific symptoms point to a particular injury or type of disorder, a more focused examination may be performed. Table 9.6 outlines the components of a general neurologic examination. Treatment of neurologic disorders is focused on curing, treating, or alleviating symptoms. Psychiatric disorders of altered mental status are often managed with behavioral, cognitive, and pharmacologic methods. Drugs most commonly used in the treatment of psychiatric disorders are described in Table 9.7. Synthetic drugs that alter neurotransmitter function may help manage psychiatric, motor, coordination, and sensory alterations.

Symptom management can include treatments to reduce spasticity, increase muscle strength and tone, and improve memory. A review of underlying mechanisms leading to manifestations of neuronal disease is summarized in Figure 9.15.

The clinical models presented in this chapter incorporate the concepts of altered neuronal transmission. Individual concepts are highlighted, although, clearly, each is related to the other. When reviewing the clinical models, apply previously learned concepts to each alteration.

Cerebral Palsy

Cerebral palsy (CP) is a group of disorders resulting from damage to UMNs. Symptoms appear during the first few years of life. The neuromuscular disorders that comprise CP stem from an event that occurs during the prenatal, perinatal (20 weeks' gestation through 28 newborn days), or postnatal (after birth) periods. According to the March of Dimes, CP affects approximately two to three per 1,000, diagnosed at the age of 3 years. Approximately 800,000 people of all ages in the United States have CP.[3]

PATHOPHYSIOLOGY

Central control of movement by the brain is altered in CP. Although the exact cause is not fully known, cerebral anoxia, hemorrhage, and other neurologic insults are likely involved. Classifications of CP can be based on the type of motor dysfunction or by the anatomy affected, as listed below:

- Motor dysfunction classifications
  - **Spastic**: inability of muscles to relax
  - **Athetoid or dyskinetic**: inability to control muscle movement
  - **Ataxic**: inability to control balance and coordination
- Anatomic classifications
  - **Hemiplegia**: involving one arm and one leg on the same side of the body
  - **Diplegia**: involving both legs
  - **Quadriplegia**: involving all four extremities, the trunk, and neck muscles

CLINICAL MANIFESTATIONS

Symptoms of CP vary among individuals, permanently altering body movement and muscle coordination.

Table 9.6 Components of a General Neurologic Examination

Examination Component	Findings
Mental status	Orientation: time, place, and person; memory, attention, judgment, reasoning
Language	Expressive aphasia; problems with expression: receptive aphasia; problems with understanding: dysarthria; problems with word formation
Sensory function	Vision: pupil responsiveness, acuity, visual fields, extraocular eye movements
	Hearing, touch, pain, temperature, pressure, taste, position sense, gag reflex
Coordination	Tremor, rapid alternating foot and hand movements, finger to nose, toe to finger
	Gait
Motor function	Movement: voluntary, reflexive
Muscle tone	Cogwheeling, spasticity, rigidity
Muscle strength	Hand grasp, strength of flexors and extensors

Table 9.7 Classification of Drugs for Treatment of Mental Health Disorders

Drug Classification	Drug Examples	Mode of Action	Anticipated Effect
Sedatives/hypnotics	Secobarbital Valium	Decrease CNS arousal	Relief of anxiety, general sedation and sleep
Stimulants	Ritalin (methylphenidate), Adderall	Suppress appetite, increase activity and alertness, general CNS arousal	Increased attention and focus
Opiate narcotics	Morphine, codeine	CNS depression	Pain relief, cough suppression
Antidepressants		Alter production, secretion, or reuptake of neurotransmitters	Improved mood
Monoamine oxidase inhibitors	Nardil, Parnate		
Tricyclics	Amitriptyline, Desipramine, Doxepin		
Selective serotonin reuptake inhibitors	Prozac, Zoloft, Paxil		
Mood stabilizers	Lithium, carbamazepine, gabapentin	Work at sites beyond the receptor, by modulating enzymes or regulating gene expression	Improved mood
Antipsychotics	Haloperidol, risperidone	Alteration in neurotransmitter effects	Resolution of severe psychosis

CNS, central nervous system.

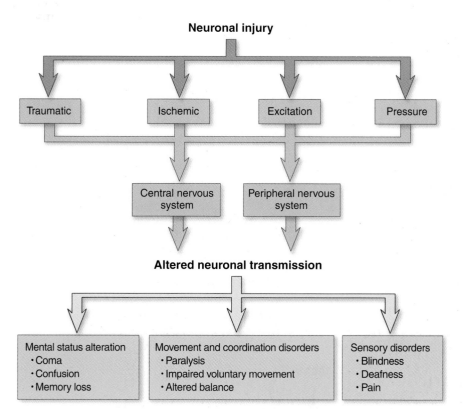

Figure 9.15 Concept map. Mechanisms of neuronal disorders.

Impairment may be manifested by mild motor dysfunction during physical activities, such as running, or by severe disability. Individuals with CP may have trouble with their fine motor skills or coordination for balance and walking. Cognitive function, speech and seizure disorders are also common manifestations associated with CP. Seizures and mental disorders represent the more severe consequences of CP. Signs of milder forms of CP may be seen during infancy, when developmental milestones are not achieved as expected. CP is not a progressive disease; therefore, worsening disabilities and deterioration of neural function are not expected with this diagnosis.

The development of seizures is often associated with CP, especially when the underlying event results in hypoxic insult. Excitotoxic injury of the brain caused by excessive glutamate-mediated transmission may represent sequelae of neonatal brain injury. Glial uptake of glutamate may be impaired, resulting in overstimulation of glutamate receptors, NMDA, and α-amino-3-hydroxy-5-methyl-4-isoxazole propionic acid (AMPA).[4]

The neonatal brain, still undergoing maturation, is extremely vulnerable to cell death because of this excitotoxic injury. Neonatal seizures may reflect the consequences of brain injury. Seizure disorder, or *epilepsy*, is the result of impaired chemical and electrical neurotransmission. Impulses are spread in a disorderly way resulting from abnormal firing of neurons in the cerebral cortex. During the neonatal period, seizures may be subtle, limited to eye movements, sustained eye opening, tongue movement, or lip smacking. Over time, seizure activity may become more obvious.

Partial seizures begin locally in a small group of neurons in one hemisphere, spreading impulses throughout that hemisphere or to the other side of the brain. *Simple partial seizures* are limited to the originating hemisphere and can involve either motor or sensory brain components. Symptoms are sensory and autonomic without promoting an altered state of consciousness. *Complex partial seizures* involve both hemispheres and result in loss of consciousness and lack of memory about events during and after seizure. Partial seizures are short lived, lasting a few seconds in simple seizures and a few minutes in complex seizures.

Generalized seizures are caused by a more generalized electrical transmission. Absence seizures, characterized by a brief change in level of consciousness (LOC) and eye and mouth movements, can occur up to 100 times a day. *Myoclonic seizures* are characterized by involuntary muscle movements of the extremities or body, and are not associated with LOC. *Tonic–clonic seizures* are convulsive and are associated with **tonic** (a state of continuous muscle contraction) or **clonic** (rapid successions of alternating muscle contraction and relaxation) motions. Loss of consciousness and traumatic injury related to a fall may result. The seizures resolve in 2 to 5 minutes, depending on the duration of the altered electrical current. Recovery from the seizure is manifested by extreme fatigue, headache, muscle pain and weakness, also referred to as the **postictal** state. *Status epilepticus* is a potentially life-threatening condition characterized by a continuous tonic–clonic seizure, which leads to hypoxia (Fig. 9.16).

DIAGNOSTIC CRITERIA

Pinpointing a specific time or event that resulted in the manifestations of CP is often difficult. The American College of Obstetricians and Gynecologists and the International Cerebral Palsy Task Force have attempted to define criteria to help determine the effects of a damaging neurologic event during labor or delivery.[5] These criteria include:

■ **Figure 9.16** Seizure activity in the brain. **A:** Simple and complex partial seizures. **B:** Generalized seizures.

1. Metabolic acidosis from the fetal umbilical cord blood at delivery. Base deficit 12 mmol/L or more and pH less than 7.
2. Early-onset of moderate to severe neonatal **encephalopathy** (brain disorder) in infants born at 34 weeks' or more gestation within 24 hours of birth. Disorders in cortical function (lethargy, coma, seizure).
3. Spastic quadriplegic or dyskinetic CP. Represents the only types of CP associated with acute hypoxic events during labor and delivery.
4. No other identifiable reasons for signs and symptoms. Must exclude events related to prenatal, maternal, or fetal factors before suggesting an event in labor or delivery.

Often, CP is diagnosed after excluding other possible diseases and conditions. No blood or diagnostic test can definitively diagnose CP. A combination of a thorough neurologic examination, including testing of motor skills and reflexes, along with a complete medical history, is adequate for a diagnosis of CP if other likely candidates have been excluded. Typical developmental milestones in infancy are based on motor function, including:

- Reaching for toy, 3 to 4 months
- Sitting, 6 to 7 months
- Walking, 10 to 14 months

Consideration of developmental milestones, evaluation of muscle tone, and presence of abnormal movements and reflexes contribute to the diagnosis of CP. Children are often as old as 18 months before a diagnosis can be made.

TREATMENT

No cure exists for CP. Individuals are treated based on the signs and symptoms they manifest. Drugs to control seizures (e.g., Dilantin, Tegretol, Depakote, Neurontin, Lamictal, and Topamax) and muscle spasms (e.g., Valium, Lioresal, and Dantrium) may be necessary. Mobility may be improved with the use of special braces and mechanical aids. Physical, occupational, emotional, and speech therapy may support maximal functioning and independence.

STOP *and Consider*

Why is it important to determine the timing of neurologic injury related to CP?

Multiple Sclerosis

Multiple sclerosis (MS) is a disease of the CNS neurons and is characterized by the degeneration of myelin, a process known as **demyelination** (Fig. 9.17).

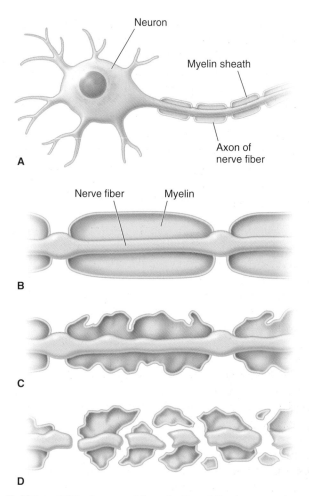

Figure 9.17 Process of demyelination. **A,B:** show normal nerve cells with intact myelin sheaths. **C,D:** show degenerating myelin, disrupting signal transduction in the axon.

MS is a progressive neurodegenerative disease affecting nerves in the CNS and peripheral nervous system. Although a great deal of research has been done to determine the exact cause of MS, currently none has been identified. Demographic characteristics of people most likely to develop MS include Caucasian women of northern European ancestry, aged 20 to 40 years. There are regional differences associated with the development of MS. Individuals who are born and continue to live in regions north of 40° latitude for the first 15 years of life have a higher risk (Fig. 9.18). Prevalence is highest in northern and central Europe; northern regions of North America; Italy; and southern Australia. Family history also contributes to an individual's risk of developing MS.

PATHOPHYSIOLOGY

MS is an autoimmune disease of multifactorial origin. Genetic and environmental factors play a role in an individual's risk for developing MS. Regional

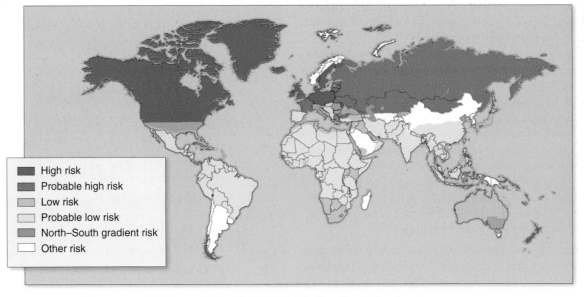

Figure 9.18 Worldwide distribution of multiple sclerosis.

variations may be caused by predominant pathogens of the regions, triggering MS through the process of molecular mimicry in genetically susceptible individuals, as discussed in Chapter 4. Factors including exposure to viral pathogens, vitamin D deficiency, exposure to sunlight and ultraviolet radiation, and genetic predisposition have been implicated in this complex disease of unknown origin.[6]

CLINICAL MANIFESTATIONS

The clinical manifestations of MS relate to the slowing of nerve conduction impulses down the nerve axon. Specific nerves are affected at different times, contributing to the variations seen in the time course and in the signs and symptoms of the disease. Four clinical courses are common in MS:

1. Relapsing-remitting (RR): characterized by periods of acute neurologic symptoms (flare-ups, exacerbations, relapses) alternating with periods of symptom relief or return of neurologic function (remissions)
2. Primary progressive: slow, chronic deterioration of neurologic function not associated with exacerbations or remissions
3. Secondary progressive: initially presenting with RR characteristics of exacerbations and remissions, followed by a pattern of slow, chronic deterioration as seen in primary progressive
4. Progressive relapsing: steady progression of a decline in neurologic function also associated with exacerbations and possible remissions

Symptoms in MS result from impairment in neurologic transduction. Common effects of MS are manifested by cognitive loss, bowel and bladder dysfunction, altered mobility, spasticity, paresthesias, slurred speech, fatigue, and pain. More rarely, a condition known as **pseudobulbar affect** (uncontrollable laughing or crying) can result from cerebral involvement, leading to altered control of emotional responsiveness. Impaired vision, one of the most common symptoms of MS, may be caused by optic neuritis or impaired extraocular eye movements, contributing to loss of visual fields, unilateral vision loss, altered color perception, **nystagmus** (irregular eye movements), and pain.

DIAGNOSTIC CRITERIA

Diagnosis of MS is based on the presence of signs and symptoms consistent with the disease. A complete medical history and a thorough neurologic examination are the first steps toward diagnosis. An MRI may be completed to detect scarring or plaques in the CNS (Fig. 9.19). It is also important to determine the response of the CNS to certain stimuli to induce *evoked potentials*. Additional testing using CT scans and lumbar puncture to evaluate CSF may be done. The revised McDonald Criteria combines subjective, objective, and diagnostic testing to diagnose MS using one of the following clinical scenarios:[7]

- Two separate acute exacerbations (flare-ups) and at least two objective lesions
- Two separate acute exacerbations (flare-ups), one objective lesion and confirmation by MRI, CSF evaluation or additional clinical attack
- One acute exacerbation (flare-ups), at least two objective lesions and confirmation by MRI or second clinical attack

Figure 9.19 Plaque formation in multiple sclerosis. Plaques in the white matter of the brain are indicated by arrows. (Image from Rubin E, Farber JL. *Pathology*. 4th ed. Philadelphia: Lippincott Williams & Wilkins; 2005, with permission.)

made in the use of drugs, known as disease-modifying drugs, to target symptoms and delay progression of the disease. In the most common form of MS (RR), early initiation of drugs is highly recommended. The immunomodulators Betaseron, Avonex, and Rebif, all forms of beta interferon (IFN-β), are the mainstays of treatment. In addition, Copaxone, a drug that mimics the effects of myelin, is commonly used. A treatment for the relapsing form of MS, Tysabri (natalizumab), is used under controlled conditions due to the risk of adverse effects. The immunosuppressant Novantrone (mitoxantrone) is the primary treatment for advanced or chronic MS. Table 9.8 provides a more thorough description of treatment options in MS.

STOP *and Consider*

How will regrowth of myelin help treat or cure other neurologic diseases?

- One acute exacerbation (flare-ups), one objective lesion and confirmation by MRI, CSF or second clinical attack
- Insidious progressive neurologic symptoms consistent with MS and MRI evidence multiple brain lesions or spinal cord lesions and abnormal visual evoked potential

TREATMENT

There is currently no cure for MS. A great deal of progress has been

From the Lab

Evoked potential testing provides information about the electrical activity in specific sensory nerve pathways. The altered transduction along these pathways may be too subtle to determine by routine neurologic examination. Stimulation of the pathways is measured by wires placed on the scalp over the areas of interest of the brain. There are three types of evoked potential tests:

1. Visual evoked potentials (VEP): stimulation induced by viewing an alternating checkerboard pattern
2. Brainstem auditory evoked potentials (BAEP): stimulation induced by clicking sounds in each ear
3. Sensory evoked potentials (SEP): stimulation induced by electrical impulses to the arm or leg

Table 9.8 Treatment Options in Multiple Sclerosis

Brand Name	Generic Name	FDA Approval Date	Indication	Administration Information	Common Side Effects
Avonex	Interferon beta-1a	1996	All relapsing forms	Weekly intramuscular injection	Flu-like symptoms
Betaseron	Interferon beta-1b	1993	All relapsing forms	Every other day subcutaneous injection	Flu-like symptoms
Copaxone	Glatiramer acetate	1996	Relapsing-remitting	Daily subcutaneous injection	Injection site reaction
Rebif	Interferon beta-1a	2002	All relapsing forms	Three times/week subcutaneous injection	Flu-like symptoms
Novantrone	Mitoxantrone	2000	Worsening relapsing-remitting, progressive relapsing or secondary progressive	Intravenous infusion four times/year, up to a maximum lifetime limit of 8–12 doses	Cardiac complications, nausea, hair loss
Tysabri	Natalizumab	2004/2006	All relapsing forms	Intravenous infusion	Headache, fatigue, urinary tract infection

FDA, Food and Drug Administration.

Hydrocephalus

Hydrocephalus, from the Greek "hydro" meaning water and "cephalus" meaning head, is a condition of increased ventricular accumulation of CSF. Hydrocephalus can be a congenital disorder identified soon after birth, or it can be acquired later in life. According to the National Hydrocephalus Foundation, approximately 1 in 500 births is affected by hydrocephalus in the United States. More than half of the cases of hydrocephalus are congenital. A long-term consequence of hydrocephalus is motor disability, estimated to affect up to three fourths of children with hydrocephalus. Intellectual disability is also a potential long-term risk. The incidence of acquired hydrocephalus is unknown because of the relationship to the underlying causes.

PATHOPHYSIOLOGY

Because of an imbalance between the amount of fluid produced and the rate of fluid reabsorption, the accumulation of CSF leads to ventricular enlargement and increased intracranial pressure. Classifications of hydrocephalus reflect the underlying cause and include **noncommunicating hydrocephalus** because of CSF flow obstruction and **communicating hydrocephalus** because of impaired CSF absorption.

Hydrocephalus can be congenital, often identified during fetal life or at birth. Congenital hydrocephalus may be caused by neural tube defects, including spina bifida, or by an alteration in the structure of the cerebral aqueduct or choroid plexus. Acquired hydrocephalus is secondary to another disease process. Common conditions resulting in acquired hydrocephalus include:

* Brain tumor
* Intraventricular hemorrhage
* Meningitis
* Traumatic injury to the head

Hydrocephalus often results from an episode of intraventricular hemorrhage in the newborn period, also a common consequence of prematurity.[8] Management strategies are directed toward controlling CSF volume to maintain ventricle size and normal ICP. Increased ICP is a common consequence of hydrocephalus. The pathology associated with increased ICP includes:

1. Impaired perfusion leading to ischemia and cell death
2. Atrophy caused by impaired circulation

CLINICAL MANIFESTATIONS

Age of onset, underlying pathology, and severity of brain tissue compression contribute to the clinical manifestations of hydrocephalus. The skull of the newborn is less restrictive because of the presence of fontanels (often referred to as soft spots) and the unfused sutures of the skull bones. These conditions allow for the increase in head circumference, a cardinal sign in a newborn with hydrocephalus. Scalp vein distention, bulging fontanels, separation of bony sutures, and vomiting may also be seen. Infants with hydrocephalus may have difficulty feeding and may have a shrill, high-pitched cry. Symptoms in older children and adults include impaired motor and cognitive function and incontinence (Fig. 9.20). Unresolved hydrocephalus may lead to impaired neurologic function and death because of increased ICP.

Signs and symptoms resulting from increased ICP include:

* Increased blood pressure in an attempt to promote perfusion in cerebral vessels
* Altered heart rate
* Initially increased (tachycardia) to increase cerebral blood flow; followed by a decreased heart rate (bradycardia) caused by stimulation of the baroreceptor reflex
* Headache resulting from stretching of the vessel walls or meninges
* Vomiting
* Decreased LOC
* Papilledema

DIAGNOSTIC CRITERIA

Diagnosis of hydrocephalus may be made by the noninvasive techniques of measurement of head circumference and transillumination. **Transillumination** is accomplished by shining a light against the head

Prominent scalp veins

Separated suture line

"Bossing" of forehead

Enlarged fontanelles

"Sunset" eyes

Increased head circumference

Shrill cry

Signs of increased intracranial pressure:
↓ Pulse
↑ Temperature
↓ Respirations
↑ Blood pressure

Lethargy or irritability

Hyperactive reflexes

■ **Figure 9.20** Clinical manifestations of hydrocephalus.

to see accumulations of fluid in the tissue. Other diagnostic techniques include CT or MRI scan of the head for examination of ventricle size and CSF flow; skull radiograph to determine separation of skull bones; and, less commonly, a spinal tap.

TREATMENT

The treatment of hydrocephalus includes establishing and maintaining normal CSF volumes and intracranial pressure. One of the most common treatments is the surgical placement of a ventriculoperitoneal shunt, a flexible tube placed into the ventricle to shunt excess CSF into the peritoneal cavity (Fig. 9.21). Another potential treatment option includes placement of a shunt that drains CSF fluid into the right atrium of the heart, called a ventriculoatrial shunt. The flow of CSF out of the ventricular system is controlled by a one-way valve, which helps control appropriate regulation. Observation of shunt-related complications, including infection,

blockage, and malfunction, must be carried out to promote maintenance of normal CSF volume and intracranial pressure.

A possible alternative treatment is a procedure known as endoscopic third ventriculostomy (ETV). This procedure involves surgically placing an opening in the floor of the third ventricle to allow free-flowing release of CSF into the basal cisterna for absorption. ETV is most appropriate for communicating hydrocephalus, most often in those older than 2 years of age. In one study that compared ETV to shunting in the resolution of hydrocephalus, ETV and shunting had similar results.[9]

From the Lab

The circulatory dynamics of both cerebral blood flow and cerebral spinal fluid contribute to intracranial pressure. Direct determinations of intracranial pressure measurements require invasive monitoring. This monitoring is achieved via an intraventricular drain connected externally to a transducer. Measurements are averaged over a minimum 30-minute period to take into account the dynamic fluctuations characteristic of CSF pressure.[10] Intracranial pressure should be monitored for a period of 24 to 48 hours to determine trends or effectiveness of treatments to reduce pressure.

Tube inserted into lateral ventricle through hole in skull

Drainage tube, usually introduced into peritoneal cavity, with extra length to allow for growth of child

Figure 9.21 Ventriculoperitoneal shunt placement in hydrocephalus. (Image from Bear MF, Connors BW, Parasido MA. *Neuroscience: Exploring the Brain*. 3rd ed. Philadelphia: Lippincott Williams & Wilkins; 2006, with permission.)

Incomplete Spinal Cord Transection

Many variables are associated with the degree of dysfunction experienced because of SCI. Spinal segmental level, type of injury, and degree of cord transection contribute to the manifestations and complications associated with SCI. An estimated 250,000 to 400,000 individuals live with SCI or spinal dysfunction. The condition of many individuals with SCI improves from the time of diagnosis, but few fully recover.

PATHOPHYSIOLOGY

SCI is due to nerve root or myelinated tract damage, impairing the transduction of afferent or efferent neural impulses. Damage to the gray matter of the central cord may result in loss of motoneurons and interneurons. The pathogenesis is related to the location, classification, type and severity of the injury. SCI may result from complete or partial transection (Fig. 9.22). In complete injury, sensation and motor functions below the level of injury are lost. Partial cord transections can be categorized into three types of syndromes (central cord, anterior cord, and Brown-Séquard syndrome), described in Table 9.9.

■ **Figure 9.22** Functional alterations in incomplete spinal cord injuries. **A:** Central cord syndrome. **B:** Anterior cord syndrome. **C:** Brown-Séquard syndrome. (Image from Hickey JV. *The Clinical Practice of Neurological and Neurosurgical Nursing.* 5th ed. Philadelphia: Lippincott Williams & Wilkins; 2003:420–421, with permission.)

Loss of motor power and sensation

Incomplete loss

C T S

L
T
C

Central area of cord damage

A

Loss of pain and temperature sensation on opposite side

Loss of voluntary motor control on the same side as the cord damage

Right　Left

Area of cord damage

C

Loss of motor power, pain, and temperature sensation, with preservation of position, vibration, and touch sense

Position and vibration, touch sense

Motor

Pain, temperature

Area of cord damage

B

Table 9.9 Categories of Partial Spinal Cord Transections

Syndrome	Area of Cord Affected	Cause	Manifestations
Central cord syndrome	Center cord affected	Usually caused by hyperextension injury	Motor deficits prominent in upper extremities
			Bladder dysfunction of variable severity
Anterior cord syndrome	Anterior cord affected	Occlusion of the anterior spinal artery	Loss of motor function, temperature, and pain below the level of injury
		Bone fragments	Sensations of touch, pressure, vibration, and position intact
Brown-Séquard syndrome	Hemisection of the anterior and posterior cord	Usually the result of stabbing or gunshot injury with damage localized to only one side of the cord	Ipsilateral (same side) complete or partial paralysis, loss of touch, pressure, vibration, and positions sense below the level of injury
			Loss of temperature sensations contralaterally

CLINICAL MANIFESTATIONS

SCI may be complicated by ischemia, hemorrhage, or necrosis. Injury to the neuronal fibers that carry impulses may be worsened by pressure from the edema related to the primary injury. The level of injury determines the nerves involved and helps anticipate the degree of functional loss. Loss of function in incomplete transection can be variable, based on the area and level of cord involved. In general, injuries to the cervical spine often result in quadriplegia. High injuries at the level of C1–2 may result in loss of involuntary function, including sweating, blood pressure regulation, and body temperature regulation. Respiratory support with artificial ventilation may be required for injuries above C4. Injury to lower cervical segments is associated with preservation of upper body function. C7 through T1 injuries allow individuals to straighten their arms, but they may result in impaired fine motor skills. Paraplegia usually results from injuries at the thoracic level. Trunk and lower body control are lost at T1, with return of sitting balance and abdominal muscle control from T9 through T12. Injuries in the lumbar and sacral segments result in loss of control of the lower extremities. Bowel, bladder, and sexual function may be affected with SCI.

DIAGNOSTIC CRITERIA

When SCI is suspected, it is important to diagnose, begin immediate treatment, and prevent further damage. SCI can be diagnosed in a conscious person based on findings from testing of cognitive, motor, and sensory function. If the injured individual has manifestations of neck pain or weakness or is unable to respond because of loss of consciousness, diagnostic testing may be done. Commonly used tests to diagnose SCI include radiograph, CT scan, MRI, and myelography (imaging after injection of dye into the spinal canal).

TREATMENT

Traction may be used to immobilize the spine in the acute phase of SCI in an attempt to prevent further damage. Corticosteroids may be given in large doses to decrease inflammation and pressure on the spinal nerves and are ideally begun within 8 hours of injury.

Promotion of functional abilities is a priority of treatment after the acute phase of injury. The work of many researchers is targeted toward a cure for SCI.

To achieve a return of motor, sensory, and autonomic function, the regeneration of axons and reestablishment of neuronal transmission must occur.[11] Current scientific efforts are directed toward:

- Stimulation of axon regeneration
- Neutralization of inhibitory factors
- Use of growth factors
- Establishment of an environment that promotes axon regrowth and conduction

Regeneration of the pyramidal, extrapyramidal, autonomic, sensory, and cerebellar pathways, integrated reflex responses, and the required neurotransmitters are necessary for return of function. The use of genetically engineered fibroblasts, grafts of peripheral nerves, transplant of Schwann cells, and the use of stem cells have shown great promise in efforts to achieve these results.[11]

From the Lab

Bowel and bladder storage require autonomic reflexes to coordinate involuntary smooth muscle activity of the urinary tract and voluntary contraction of the sphincter. Complex mechanisms involving the spinal and supraspinal nerve pathways may be impaired because of SCI. A process known as **functional electrical stimulation (FES)** may serve to generate artificial autonomic reflexes to promote mechanisms regulating bowel and bladder function. Electrical stimulation of efferent nerves to promote muscle contraction is accomplished through a process known as **neurostimulation. Microstimulation** provides electrical stimuli to preganglionic neurons and interneurons controlling bladder function via a microelectrode implanted within the spinal cord. Afferent fibers may be activated to adjust stimuli, a function known as neuromodulation.[12]

Normal intracranial pressure is considered to be 15 mm Hg or 150 to 200 mm H_2O.

Depression

Depression is a condition of altered mood, also referred to as an **affective disorder**. In addition to mood, depression involves altered thoughts and somatic complaints. Depression is a condition with a biologic basis, not resolved simply by a person's sheer desire or will, as many people believe. According to the Centers for Disease Control, more than 1 in 20 Americans over the age of 11 years indicate they are currently depressed. Rates were increased among individuals aged 40 to 59 years, women and non-Hispanic black individuals. Among the socioeconomically disadvantaged, the frequency of reports of current depression rises to one in seven Americans.[13]

PATHOPHYSIOLOGY

Triggers of depressive episodes may be influenced by genetic predisposition, associated responses of other medical illness, hormonal alterations, or major life events. Much is still unknown about the causes of depression and effective treatment, although researchers are continuing to provide better information for managing this debilitating disease.

Depression is believed to be a condition resulting from a deficiency in neurotransmitter in the synapses of critical areas of the brain. The specific neurotransmitter systems involved include those of the **monoamines** norepinephrine (NE), dopamine (DA), and serotonin (5-HT). Presynaptic neurons must release neurotransmitters at a normal rate and all the regulatory mechanisms in the neuron must be functional to obtain appropriate neurotransmitter release. This means that the proper amount and function of each of the following must be present:

- Enzymes that change the precursor substance into the active neurotransmitter
- Enzymes that break down the active neurotransmitter
- Functional membrane transporters involved in reuptake and recycling of the active neurotransmitters from the synaptic cleft
- **Autoreceptors** involved in the detection of neurotransmitters to control release and flow of impulse through the neuron

Postsynaptic neurons must have the appropriate receptors, which are able to bind the neurotransmitters available in the synaptic cleft. The postsynaptic neurons must also contain the regulatory mechanisms needed to promote signal transduction. The neurotransmitters released from the presynaptic neuron can bind with a variety of postsynaptic receptor types, each with specific signal transduction pathways that vary in the end responses of physiologic function and gene expression.

CLINICAL MANIFESTATIONS

Depression can be seen as a **syndrome**, or cluster of symptoms. One of these clusters is related to mood, and others reflect symptoms related to other aspects of life. These categories include:

- Mood features include degree of mood change and duration of abnormal mood
- Vegetative features include sleep patterns, appetite, weight and sex drive
- Cognitive features include attention span, memory, frustration, tolerance, and negative distortions
- Impulse control features include suicide and homicide ideations and actions
- Behavioral features include interests, motivation, pleasures, and fatigue
- Physical (somatic) features include muscle tension, headaches, and stomach aches

DIAGNOSTIC CRITERIA

Most people have felt sad at different times in their lives. It is important to distinguish emotional reactions to a particular life event from a response that is pathologic. Diagnostic criteria for depression are outlined in the *Diagnostic and Statistical Manual of Mental Disorders, Fourth Edition* (DSM-IV). This guide is the standard used in the United States for determining criteria for accepted diagnoses. The counterpart used in other countries is known as the *International Classification of Diseases*, 10th edition (ICD-10).

According to the DSM-IV, a major depressive episode must include five or more symptoms during the same 2-week period that reflect differences from prior functioning. One of these symptoms must reflect depressed mood or loss of interest or pleasure. A summary of possible symptoms include:

1. Depressed mood most of the day, on most days
2. Significant lack of interest in most activities most of the day, on most days
3. Significant weight loss without dieting, weight gain, or change in appetite (lack of or increased) most of the day, on most days
4. Sleeping too much (hypersomnia) or too little (insomnia) on most days
5. Increased agitation or activity "slowed down" on most days
6. Fatigue or loss of energy on most days
7. Feelings of excessive or inappropriate guilt or worthlessness on most days
8. Difficulty concentrating or decision making on most days
9. Recurrent suicidal thoughts or thoughts of death

In addition to the diagnostic criteria outlined, the diagnosis of depression should be based on a complete medical history to rule out any other organic causes.

TREATMENT

Treatment of depression can be evaluated based on the degree of response to medications, remission, recovery, relapse, or recurrence. Pharmacologic management is based on targeting what is known about the production of neurotransmitters (including their release and reuptake, enzymatic destruction, autoregulation, and postsynaptic receptor binding) and the events they induce (Fig. 9.23). The specific characteristics of the depressive episode may also be targeted for optimal response. Antidepressants are classified as follows:

- Selective serotonin reuptake inhibitors (SSRI)
- Selective norepinephrine reuptake inhibitors (SNRI)
- Norepinephrine and dopamine reuptake inhibitors (NDRI)
- Tricyclic antidepressants (TCAs)
- Monoamine oxidase inhibitors (MAOIs)

Antidepressants, especially those affecting multiple transmitters (TCAs and MAOIs), may have significant side effects. Typical side effects include dry

🔬 *From the Lab*

Clinical diagnosis of depression is aided by the use of depression inventory scales. These tools provide a statistically reliable method for detection of depression. Many of these scales are available for clinical use. They vary in length, depth, and scope. Some inventories target specific populations, including children, pregnant women, and older adults. Depression inventory scales can be used for initial screening of depression and for assistance in determining the individual alterations in mood, thought, and behavior consistent with criteria of the DSM-IV. A commonly used tool is the Beck Depression Inventory, a self-administered questionnaire that requires 10 minutes for a person to complete. Manifestations of depression, including attitudes and symptoms, can be determined based on item scoring.

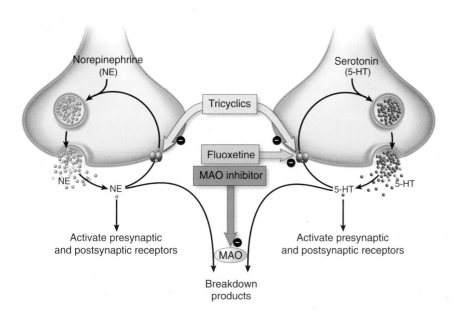

■ **Figure 9.23** Effect of antidepressants on neurotransmitter action. Monoamine oxidase inhibitors enhance the action of norepinephrine (NE) and serotonin (5-HT) by inhibiting their enzymatic destruction. Tricyclics block reuptake of NE and 5-HT, whereas selective serotonin reuptake inhibitors block reuptake of 5-HT, increasing effectiveness of these neurotransmitters. (Image from Bear MF, Connors BW, Parasido MA. *Neuroscience: Exploring the Brain*. 3rd ed. Philadelphia: Lippincott Williams & Wilkins; 2006, with permission.)

mouth, constipation, bladder problems, decreased sexual desire, erectile dysfunction, blurred vision, dizziness, drowsiness, headache, nausea, weight gain, anxiety, and insomnia. In addition, the beneficial effects of these drugs may take several weeks. Counseling and psychotherapy may contribute to improved response through directing efforts at resolving emotional triggers of depression.

● STOP *and Consider*

Why do TCAs have more side effects than other more selective antidepressants?

Summary

- The neuron is the fundamental unit of the nervous system; it has highly specialized functions in impulse transmission.
- Supporting cells provide neurons with metabolic support and protection.
- Impulse transmission is regulated by changes in membrane potential, induced by a variety of stimuli, including chemical, electrical, and mechanical.
- The nervous system is comprised of the CNS (brain and spinal cord) and the peripheral nervous system (spinal and cranial nerves; somatic and autonomic [sympathetic and parasympathetic] nervous systems).
- Nervous tissue of the CNS is comprised of both white and gray matter, based on the primary types of component neurons.
- Meninges (dura, arachnoid, pia) and the CSF provide protective and metabolic functions in the CNS.
- The brain is divided both by lobes (frontal, parietal, temporal, occipital) and hemispheres (right, left), each associated with highly specialized functions.
- The spinal nerves are categorized based on their relationship with spinal vertebrae (cervical, thoracic, lumbar, sacral).

- Autonomic functions are carried out by the sympathetic and PNS.
- Neuronal injury contributes to disability and is the basis for a variety of neurologic disorders. Peripheral nerves have limited capacity for regeneration and reinnervation.
- Trauma represents the most common cause of injury to the nervous system, leading to neurologic impairment because of brain, spinal cord, or peripheral nerve injury. Ischemic, excitation, and pressure injury may represent primary or secondary causes of neurologic impairment.
- Disorders of neurologic function may be characterized by specific manifestations, pointing to the origin of pathology.
- Altered neuronal transmission and conduction has implications for all body systems and whole body function.
- A thorough understanding of the concepts that govern neuronal transmission will promote your ability to apply your knowledge in a variety of conditions and pathologies.

Case Study 9.1

Jimmy, a 5-year-old, was having behavioral problems at school and at home. He also had some difficulty making and keeping friends. Upon the advice of his teacher, his parents decided to have Jimmy evaluated for attention deficit disorder (ADD).

1. *What are the clinical manifestations associated with ADD?*
2. *What is the underlying pathophysiology associated with ADD?*
3. *How is ADD diagnosed?*
4. *What are the possible treatments for ADD?*
5. *What are the issues related to appropriate management of ADD?*

Log onto the Internet. Search for a relevant journal article or Web site that details ADD to confirm your predictions.

Practice Exam Questions

1. Neurons that carry sensory information to distant parts of the brain and spinal cord are called:
   a. Efferent neurons
   b. Afferent neurons
   c. Interneurons
   d. Extraneurons

2. Depolarization involves:
   a. The rapid movement of sodium into the cell
   b. The movement of potassium ions out of the cell
   c. Movement of potassium ions into the cell
   d. The absence of electrical activity

3. The lobe of the brain primarily involved in functions related to vision is the:
   a. Frontal lobe
   b. Parietal lobe
   c. Temporal lobe
   d. Occipital lobe

4. Which of the following areas of the spinal cord contains 12 segments?
   a. Cervical
   b. Thoracic
   c. Sacral
   d. Lumbar

5. Which cell type has the most potential for regeneration after injury?
   a. Astrocyte
   b. Peripheral axon
   c. Glial cell
   d. Oligodendrocytes

6. Coup/contercoup occurs due to which type of injury mechanism?
   a. Traumatic injury
   b. Pressure injury
   c. Excitation injury
   d. Ischemic injury

7. Neurogenic shock is due to altered transmission in which conduction system?
   a. Sympathetic
   b. Parasympathetic
   c. Somatic
   d. Peripheral

8. Seizure disorders are associated with which type of injury mechanism?
   a. Traumatic injury
   b. Pressure injury
   c. Excitation injury
   d. Ischemic injury

9. Which type of spinal cord injury is associated with the clinical manifestation of ipsilateral loss of motor and sensory function?
   a. Anterior cord syndrome
   b. Central cord syndrome
   c. Brown-Séquard syndrome
   d. Complete cord transection

10. Which type of neuron synthesizes and secretes norepinephrine as the primary neurotransmitter?
    a. Serotonergic
    b. Cholinergic
    c. Nicotinic
    d. Adrenergic

Discussion and Application

1. What did I know about altered neuronal transmission before today?

2. What are the body processes affected by altered neuronal transmission? How do neuronal transmission patterns affect those processes?

3. What are the potential etiologies for altered neuronal transmissions? How do conduction defects develop?

4. Who is most at risk for developing altered neuronal transmission? How can these alterations be prevented?

5. What are the human differences that affect the etiology, risk, or course of altered neuronal transmission?

6. What are clinical manifestations expected in the course of altered neuronal transmission?

7. What are special diagnostic tests useful in determining the diagnosis and course of altered neuronal transmission?

8. What are the goals of care for individuals with altered neuronal transmission?

9. How does the concept of altered neuronal transmission build on what I have learned in the previous chapter and in previous courses?

10. How can I use what I have learned?

RESOURCES

Attention Deficit Disorder Association:
http://www.add.org

Massachusetts General Hospital Center for Women's Mental Health:
http://www.womensmentalhealth.org

March of Dimes:
http://www.modimes.org

National Hydrocephalus Foundation:
http://www.nhfonline.org/info.php

National Institute of Mental Health:
http://www.nimh.nih.gov

National Institute of Neurological Disorders and Stroke:
http://www.ninds.nih.gov/

REFERENCES

1. Centers for Disease Control and Prevention, National Center for Injury Prevention and Control. Traumatic brain injury. Bethesda: US Department of Health and Human Services. Available at: http://www.cdc.gov/ncipc/factsheets/tbi.htm. Accessed December 13, 2009.
2. National Spinal Cord Injury Association. Spinal cord injury: facts and figures at a glance. 2009; Birmingham: University of Alabama Department of Physical Medicine and Rehabilitation, Brain Rehabilitation Center. Available at: https://www.nscisc.uab.edu//public_content/facts_figures_2009.aspx. Accessed December 12, 2009.
3. March of Dimes. Cerebral palsy. Available at: http://www.marchofdimes.com/professionals/14332_1208.asp#howcommon. Accessed December 12, 2009.
4. Ferriero DM. Neonatal brain injury. *N Engl J Med.* 2004;351(19):1985–1995.
5. Hankins GD, Speer M. Defining the pathogenesis and pathophysiology of neonatal encephalopathy and cerebral palsy. *Obstet Gynecol.* 2003;102(3):628–636.
6. Milo R, Kahana E. Multiple sclerosis: geoepidemiology, genetics and the environment. *Autoimmun Rev.* 2010;9(5):A387–A394.
7. Polman CH, Reingold SC, Edan G, et al. Diagnostic criteria for multiple sclerosis: 2005 revisions to the "McDonald Criteria". *Ann Neurol.* 2005;58:840–846.
8. Garton HJ, Piatt JH Jr. Hydrocephalus. *Pediatr Clin North Am.* 2004;51(2):305–325.
9. Gangemi M, Maiuri F, Buonamassa S, et al. Endoscopic third ventriculostomy in idiopathic normal pressure hydrocephalus. *Neurosurgery.* 2004;55(1):129–134; discussion 134.
10. Czosnyka M, Pickard JD. Monitoring and interpretation of intracranial pressure. *J Neurol Neurosurg Psychiatry.* 2004;75(6):813–821.
11. Kakulas BA. Neuropathology: the foundation for new treatments in spinal cord injury. *Spinal Cord.* 2004;42(10):549–563.
12. Hickey KJ, Vogel LC, Willis KM, et al. Prevalence and etiology of autonomic dysreflexia in children with spinal cord injuries. *J Spinal Cord Med.* 2004;27(suppl 1):S54–S60.
13. Pratt LA, Brody DJ. Depression in the United States Household Population 2005–2006. National Center for Health Statistics Data Brief, 2008, no. 7. Available at: http://www.cdc.gov/nchs/data/databriefs/db07.pdf. Accessed December 12, 2009.

Chapter 10

Altered Somatic and Special Sensory Function

LEARNING OBJECTIVES

1. Define and use the key terms listed in this chapter.
2. Describe the mode of transmission of neural impulses involved with the sensations of pain, vision, and hearing.
3. Identify pathways for the integration of neural and sensory experiences.
4. Indicate common mechanisms of alterations in vision and hearing.
5. Determine processes that contribute to the perception of pain.
6. Describe alterations in sensory experiences and the associated pathophysiologic manifestations.
7. Identify common signs and symptoms of alterations in sensation.
8. Describe diagnostic tests and treatment strategies relevant to alterations in hearing, vision, and pain management.
9. Predict functional impairments resulting from alterations in sensation.
10. Apply concepts of sensory alterations to select clinical models.

INTRODUCTION

How do you feel when you see a beautiful sunset? Hear the voice of someone special? Smell your favorite meal cooking on the stove? Close your fingers in the car door? Many sensations cause responses such as wonder, happiness, contentment, and pain. Your perceptions of the world around you are shaped by the many sensory cues you take in, which stimulate predictable reactions. Alterations in these sensations can cause significant impairment in physical, psychologic, and social functioning. A basic understanding of the function of sensory systems promotes the ability to anticipate deficits that may occur when these systems are altered. The focus of this chapter is alteration in somatosensory and special sensory function. Table 10.1 provides a description of sensations resulting from stimulation of specific somatosensory and special sensory receptors. The modules target pain and alterations in the special senses of vision and hearing. The clinical models in this chapter are selected to help apply concepts of altered somatosensory and sensory function.

Table 10.1 Neurons of the Somatosensory System

Neuron Type	Receptor Location	Sensation
General somatic afferent neurons	Wide distribution with branches throughout the body	Pain, touch, and temperature
Special somatic afferent neurons	Muscle, tendons, and joints	Position and body movement
General visceral afferent neurons	Visceral structures	Fullness and discomfort

Module 1

Pain

Pain is a common, yet complex sensation. The typically unpleasant sensation is often associated with an emotional response and evidence of tissue damage. Protective reflex responses often limit the damage caused by an injury-provoking stimulus. Continued pain sensation reminds us of the damage and helps us to protect the injury during the healing process. Pain is transmitted by the somatosensory system, along with the sensations of touch, temperature, and body position.

Somatosensory System

Sensory systems relay information throughout the body from the periphery to the central nervous system (CNS) using sensory receptors, ascending pathways, and processing centers. Stimuli are received, which allow people to respond to the world around them. Afferent pathways, introduced in Chapter 9, promote communication from structures in the periphery to processing centers in the brain.

The diversity of the somatosensory system is the result of the receptors and pathways that are associated with the sensations of pain (nociception), touch, temperature, and proprioception (body position). A variety of receptor types result in specific somatosensory responses. These types include:

1. Mechanoreceptors: mechanical forces—receptor stretching alters membrane permeability
   a. Stretch receptors of muscles
   b. Skin receptors: touch, pain, cold, and heat

2. Thermoreceptors: radiant heat energy
3. Nociceptors: pain

Table 10.2 describes the neurons responsible for some of these specific functions.

● **STOP** *and* ***Consider***

Based on the sensations involved, what other nerves do you think are involved in the somatosensory system?

SOMATOSENSORY NEURONAL ORGANIZATION

Neurons are organized in an ordered series, and information is directed toward the processing cen-

Table 10.2 Sensory Receptor Forms and Functions

Receptor Type	Function	Example
Mechanoreceptor	Tactile skin sensation	Merkel's cells
	Deep-tissue sensation	Ruffini's endings
		Meissner's corpuscles
		Pacinian corpuscle
		Hair follicle end organ
		Free nerve endings
	Hearing	Cochlear sound receptors
	Proprioception	Merkel's cells
		Ruffini's endings
		Pacinian corpuscles
Photoreceptor	Vision	Rods and cones
Chemoreceptor	Taste	Taste bud receptors
	Smell	Olfactory epithelium receptors
Nociceptor	Pain	Free nerve endings

Third-order
neuron

Primary
somatosensory
cortex

Second-order
neuron

First-order
neuron

Thalamus

Receptors

Spinal cord

■ **Figure 10.1** Arrangement of first-, second-, and third-order neurons of the somatosensory system.

ters in the thalamus and cerebral cortex (Fig. 10.1). These neurons are categorized as follows:

- First-order neurons: communicate sensory information from the periphery to the CNS
- Second-order neurons: relay sensory input from reflex networks and sensory pathways directly to the thalamus
- Third-order neurons: communicate sensory information from the thalamus to the cerebral cortex

Interneurons are active throughout this network and modify the sensory information before it arrives at the processing centers. The numbers of neurons increase consistently with their order: third-order neurons are present in the greatest quantity.

SOMATOSENSORY NEURONAL TRANSMISSION

Somatosensory impulses are transmitted by a unique system of receptors and pathways. The sensory unit comprising the dorsal root ganglia (cell body, peripheral branch, and central axon) responds in distinct ways to different stimuli

because of the specific nature of their associated receptors and nerve fibers.

Dorsal Root Ganglia Fibers

Transmission of nerve impulses along the fibers of the dorsal root ganglia depends on the diameter of the nerve fiber and nerve fiber myelination. The three types of nerve fibers that are involved in the conduction of somatosensory impulses are types A, B, and C. Type A fibers have the largest diameter and are myelinated, accounting for their rapid rate of impulse conduction. The sensations transmitted by type A delta fibers include pressure, touch, cold sensation, and heat pain. Type A alpha and beta fibers may promote inhibitory effects, diminishing the sensation of pain. Type B fibers are also myelinated but have a smaller diameter than type A fibers, accounting for their slower rate of conduction. Mechanoreceptors in the cutaneous and subcutaneous areas of the skin stimulate nerve impulses along type B fibers. Type C fibers are unmyelinated and have the smallest diameter, leading to the slowest conduction rate of these three fiber types. Warm–hot sensation, as well as mechanical, chemical, heat-induced, and cold-induced pain sensations, is transmitted along type C fibers.

Dermatome Innervation

Dermatomes are innervated by a single pair of dorsal root ganglia and reflect the segmental organization of the spinal cord, as described in Chapter 9. Overlap of dermatome processes occurs in peripheral processes on the body surface and central processes in the spinal cord, providing some redundancy of the conduction system.

Two separate pathways are involved in the transmission of information involved in perception, arousal, and motor control. The **discriminative pathway** communicates sensory information, including discriminative touch and spatial orientation. This pathway integrates input from multiple receptors using the primary dorsal root ganglion neuron, the dorsal column neuron, and the thalamic neuron. Stimulation of this pathway results from vibration, touch, muscle, or joint movement. The discriminative pathway allows the identification of an object based on touch or the location of skin touch in two different areas, known as **two-point discrimination**. The **anterolateral pathway** involves both the anterior and the lateral spinothalamic pathways and is characterized by multiple synapses and slow conduction. The sensations of pain, temperature, crude touch, and pressure not requiring the specific location of the origin of the stimulus are transmitted along this pathway. Increased wakefulness stimulated by a "startle" reaction exists due to many fibers that travel to the reticular activating system by sensory conduction in this pathway. Autonomic responses, such as increased blood pressure and heart rate, activation of sweat glands, dilation of pupils, and constriction of blood vessels, are also stimulated when impulses are conducted along this pathway.

SOMATOSENSORY PROCESSING

The awareness, recognition, identification, and interpretation of stimuli involve processing. After stimuli reach the thalamus, further refinement occurs in the somatosensory cortex of the brain. The primary somatosensory cortex receives sensory information from the thalamus. This information is relayed to the somatosensory association areas, which interpret the stimuli into learned perceptions.

Somatosensory Modalities

Somatosensory modalities refer to the specific nature of the perception of various stimuli. The subjective interpretation of a stimulus, such as the difference between temperature and touch, is determined by the ability of a receptor to detect an impulse, the transmission of the impulse to the CNS, and the interpretation of the refined impulse.

Stimulus Discrimination

Acuity refers to the ability to locate the site of the initiation of a stimulus. High acuity allows for fine distinction and requires a greater density of neurons. Acuity reflects the threshold necessary for a neuron to achieve an action potential (see Chapter 9). Variations of acuity in sensory fields contribute to different levels of distinction between impulses.

Tactile Stimulation

Transmission of tactile stimuli usually occurs via large, myelinated nerve fibers. Touch, pressure, and vibration stimuli are recognized by receptors in and near the skin (Fig. 10.2) and include:

- Free nerve endings (detection of touch and pressure)
- Meissner's corpuscle (highly developed sense of touch)
- Merkel's disks (movement of light objects over skin, vibration)
- Pacinian corpuscle (detection of vibration)
- Hair follicle receptor (detection of movement on the surface of the body)
- Ruffini's ending (detection of heavy and continuous touch and pressure)

FIGURE 10.2 Cutaneous somatic sensory receptors. Distribution of sensory receptors in skin with and without hair. (Image modified from Bear MF, Connors BW, Parasido MA. *Neuroscience: Exploring the Brain*. 3rd ed. Philadelphia: Lippincott Williams & Wilkins; 2006, with permission.)

Thermal Sensation

Thermoreceptors (receptors that recognize thermal sensation) are located under the skin and include cold, warmth, and pain receptors. Thermal (warm and cold) receptors are sensitive to the differences in the temperature of objects that contact the skin. Thermal pain receptors respond to extremes in temperature. Transmission of thermal sensation is much slower than tactile impulse conduction.

Position Sensation

Limb/body movement and position sensation, independent of vision, are mediated by proprioceptive receptors, muscle spindle receptors, and Golgi tendon organs. Stretch receptors in the skin (Ruffini's endings, pacinian corpuscles, and Merkel's cells) also assist in proprioception. Somatosensory signals are transmitted via the posterior column and the vestibular system, and they are processed in the thalamus and cerebral cortex.

 ## Pain

The sensation of pain is disruptive to the quality of life. Determination of pain character provides clues to the underlying cause and provides a target for treatment.

CHARACTERIZATION OF PAIN

The sensation of pain is the result of a noxious stimulation of pain fibers. When the stimulus is initiated outside of the nervous system, the pain is characterized as **nociceptive**. Pain originating within the nervous system is termed **neurogenic** or **neuropathic**. Nociceptive pain involves specific receptors and pathways resulting in the sensation of pain. Neurogenic or neuropathic pain does not activate these receptors and does not follow a typical transmission pattern of impulse conduction.

CONDUCTION OF PAIN SENSATION

Nociception (pain sensation) involves free nerve endings stimulated by chemical, mechanical, or thermal

stimuli, inducing autonomic and motor reflexes, which result in the interpretation of the stimuli as pain (Fig. 10.3). Events involved in this process include transduction, transmission, modulation, and perception. Box 10.1 summarizes these processes.

THEORIES OF PAIN

The theoretic origins of pain are based on an understanding of the neurophysiologic events associated with the initiation, transmission, and perception of pain. Two well-accepted, traditional theories that attempt to explain the pain response include the pattern theory and the specificity theory, neither of which fully explains the origin, transmission, and perception of pain. The evolution of pain theory reflects the complexity of the pain sensation, incorporating the multiple dimensions and determinants of pain.

■ FIGURE 10.3 Mechanism of acute pain. Nociceptor stimulation is induced after tissue injury by release of inflammatory mediators. Impulses are transmitted to the dorsal horn of the spinal cord, synapsing with second-order neurons. Neurons cross and ascend via the spinothalamic pathway to the reticular activating system (RAS) and thalamus. The localization and perception of pain occurs in the somatosensory cortex.

Box 10.1 Processes of Nociception

Transduction of noxious stimuli into a nerve impulse and depolarization of the nerve stimulate the conduction of the sensory impulse

- The electrical impulses promote the release of algesic (causing pain) substances, including substance P, hydrogen and potassium ions, serotonin, histamine, prostaglandins, and bradykinin

Transmission of nerve impulses from tissues to the CNS

- Occurs along type A (delta) and type C fibers
  - Rapidly conducting type A fibers
    - Produce sensations of sharp, stinging, or pin-prick– type local sensations
    - Induced by mechanical or thermal stimuli
    - Impulses along type C fibers producing a dull ache or burning general response
    - Induced by chemical stimuli
- Responses of the brain resulting from the transmission of impulses must be delivered back to the original site of stimulation.

Modulation of the pain occurs during transmission of the impulse

- Substances released in response to pain stimuli result from activation of inhibitory processes
- Serotonin, norepinephrine, and endorphins
- Inhibit the transmission of the pain impulse by slowing the release of nociceptive neurotransmitters

Perception of the pain response

- Involves the sensory (somatosensory cortex), emotional (limbic system), and subjective reactions to the stimuli
- Perception is varied among individuals because of the influence of
  - Pain threshold: the intensity of the pain required to achieve a response
  - Perceptual dominance: the existence of pain at another location which is given more attention
  - Pain tolerance: the degree to which pain is endured (duration or intensity) before initiating a response

Pattern Theory

Pattern theory suggests that nerves transmitting pain impulses are shared with other senses. The shared pathways between pain and other somatosensory modalities influence the perceived sensation. The characteristics of receptor stimulation contribute to the specific somatosensory patterns, influenced by:

1. Duration of pain sensation
2. Quantity of tissue involved
3. The summation of impulses

An example of varying degrees of receptor stimulation and sensory perception includes the response of impulse generation through light touch and deep pressure. Slight, superficial skin pressure generates low-frequency receptor firing and the perceived sensation of light touch. Deep skin pressure generates high-frequency firing of the same receptor resulting in the perceived sensation of pain.

Specificity Theory

The **specificity theory** proposes that sensations of touch, warmth, cold, and pain involve distinct receptors and pathways. The specific nature of impulse generation is proposed to begin in a specific pain receptor, transmitted along pathways leading to pain centers in the brain where pain is perceived. Pain impulses travel from the periphery to the spinal cord, crossing to the opposite side at the synapses of the **substantia gelatinosa** (gray matter extending throughout the posterior horn of the spinal cord to the medulla oblongata). Impulses then ascend the specific pain pathways of the spinothalamic tract. The intensity of the pain is associated with the amount of tissue injured or damaged.

Gate Control Theory

The **gate control theory** is one of the most well-known theories on the physiologic basis of pain. According to the gate control theory, the substantia gelatinosa is a gate control system, regulating the transmission of pain impulses. This theory proposes that stimulation of the large type A beta and alpha inhibitory fibers "close the gate" at the substantia gelatinosa, preventing crossover and inhibiting pain impulse conduction along type A delta and type C fibers, diminishing pain perception. Stimuli thought to promote transmission along type A beta and alpha fibers needed to close the gate include electrical stimulation, massage, scratching, or rubbing of the skin.

Neuromatrix Theory

The **neuromatrix theory** suggests that pain is a multidimensional experience. Pain perception is the result of impulses generated along a widely distributed neural network in the brain (**body-self neuromatrix**), triggered either by sensory inputs or independent of identified stimulation.[1] The neuromatrix contains somatic, limbic, and thalamocortical

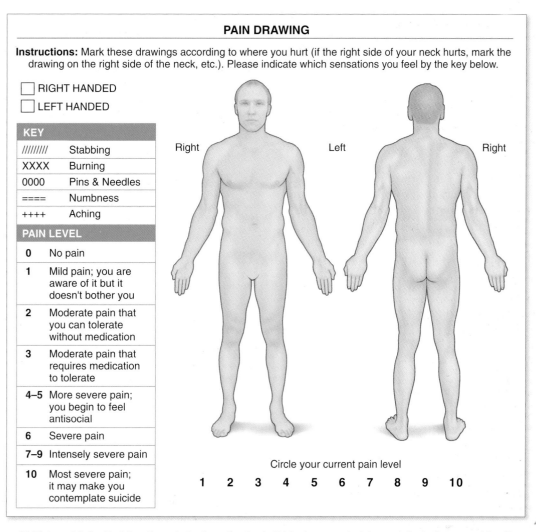

PAIN DRAWING

Instructions: Mark these drawings according to where you hurt (if the right side of your neck hurts, mark the drawing on the right side of the neck, etc.). Please indicate which sensations you feel by the key below.

☐ RIGHT HANDED
☐ LEFT HANDED

KEY	
////////	Stabbing
XXXX	Burning
0000	Pins & Needles
====	Numbness
++++	Aching

PAIN LEVEL	
0	No pain
1	Mild pain; you are aware of it but it doesn't bother you
2	Moderate pain that you can tolerate without medication
3	Moderate pain that requires medication to tolerate
4–5	More severe pain; you begin to feel antisocial
6	Severe pain
7–9	Intensely severe pain
10	Most severe pain; it may make you contemplate suicide

Right   Left   Right

Circle your current pain level

1   2   3   4   5   6   7   8   9   10

■ **Figure 10.4** Tool for characterization of pain. Individuals are asked to mark body figures to identify location, severity, and character of pain. (Image courtesy American Academy of Physical Medicine and Rehabilitation.)

components, integrating multiple sources of input resulting in the cognitive, affective, and sensory perceptions of pain. Variations in the synaptic architecture of the neuromatrix are thought to be influenced by genetic, emotional, cultural, past experience, and stress regulation influences, contributing to individualized pain responses. Sensation patterns may be induced in the absence of a sensory trigger. The neuromatrix theory can help explain phantom and chronic pain.

● **STOP** *and Consider*

Have you ever banged your head and began rubbing it in response to pain? How might this action decrease the pain sensation?

MANIFESTATIONS AND EVALUATION OF PAIN

Management of pain includes a careful evaluation of the subjective perception of pain. The nature, severity, location, initiating triggers, and patterns of radiation help to determine the cause and potential methods of treatment. Methods to objectively quantify an individual's pain, such as a pain drawing, can help determine severity of pain or evaluate pain control measures (Fig. 10.4). The classifications of pain are listed in Box 10.2.

TREATMENT OF PAIN

Pain relief, or analgesia, is the goal of pain treatment. Controlling pain to allow individuals to perform activities of daily living is another goal of treatment. Several mechanisms of pain control are available. Box 10.3 lists available methods of pain control in adults. Newborns have complex behavioral, physiologic, and biochemical responses to pain and require special considerations in pain management. Infants are commonly subjected to painful procedures, such as heel lancing and circumcision. Oral sucrose solution combined with nonnutritive sucking is a common nonpharmacologic strategy for relieving pain during invasive procedures. An interaction between gustatory and pain pathways is speculated to mediate the analgesic effect. The administration of oral sucrose to infants as pain management during invasive procedures is considered a safe, effective way to reduce procedural pain.[2]

Box 10.2 Classifications of Pain

Pain can be classified according to:
- Location
  - Cutaneous
  - Deep
  - Visceral
  - Referred
- Quality
  - Sharp
  - Burning
  - Diffuse
  - Throbbing
  - Stabbing
- Duration
  - Acute
    - Results from disease, inflammation, or injury to tissue
    - Sudden onset
    - Responsive to treatment
    - Self-limiting (lasting less than 3 months)
    - Associated with autonomic responses
    - Chronic
  - Persistent (lasting longer than 3 months)
    - Resistant to treatment
    - Associated with anorexia, insomnia, and depression

Box 10.3 Methods of Pain Control

- Nonpharmacologic
  - Cognitive behavior interventions
    - Relaxation
      - Focus on lessening muscle tension
    - Distraction
      - Focus attention on stimuli not associated with pain
    - Cognitive reappraisal
      - Self-distraction
      - Focus on the positive aspects of the experience
    - Imagery
      - Use of imagination to develop a soothing mental picture
    - Biofeedback
      - Awareness of bodily function on a cognitive level
  - Physical agents
    - Heat
      - Increase in local circulation, reducing local ischemia, and nociceptive stimulation
      - Modulation of pain
      - Release of endogenous opioids
    - Cold
      - Vasoconstriction to decrease swelling and stimulation of nociceptive pain fibers
      - Reduced afferent activity
- Transcutaneous electrical nerve stimulation
  - Transmission of electrical impulses across the skin to peripheral nerve fibers
  - Stimulation of large fibers to modulate pain transmission
- Acupuncture
  - Insertion of needles at specific points on the body surface
  - Stimulate secretion of endorphins
  - Stimulate large fibers to modulate pain transmission
- Pharmacologic
  - Nonnarcotic analgesia (e.g., aspirin [acetylsalicylic acid], nonsteroidal anti-inflammatories, or acetaminophen)
    - Central and peripheral blockade of nerve impulses
    - Inhibition of cyclooxygenase enzymes, decreasing production of prostaglandins
    - Decreased sensitivity to bradykinin and histamine
  - Opioid analgesics (e.g., morphine, codeine)
    - Bind to mu, delta, and kappa receptors, modulating pain at the level of the spinal cord
    - Stimulate release of endogenous opioids, including enkephalins, endorphins, and dynorphins
  - Adjuvant analgesics (tricyclic antidepressants)
    - Block reuptake of serotonin from the synaptic cleft
    - Particularly useful in chronic pain

Alterations in Vision

Vision is an important sensory function that informs us about the world around us. The processes resulting in sight are complex, involving the integration of eye structures, motor control, and neural control (Fig. 10.5).

Visual Structures and Function

Sight is achieved when light is reflected into the **cornea**, the clear, transparent structure that covers the exterior wall of the eye. Light then passes through the **pupil**, an opening in the **iris** (colored part of the eye). The pupil is able to control the amount of light that enters the eye, dilating to enhance light entry and constricting to decrease. Light entering the eye contacts the clear **lens**, responsible for fine-tuning of focus. The ability of the lens to change its shape, or **accommodate**, allows clear vision at a variety of distances. **Ciliary muscles** contract, promoting a rounder lens shape to focus on an object at close range. Relaxation of ciliary muscles allows flattening of the lens and the ability to see objects at a distance.

Chambers are compartments in the eye. The anterior chamber sits behind the cornea. The lens and the iris are the remaining boundaries. The posterior chamber is positioned directly behind the iris, in front of the lens. The anterior chamber contains the fluid, known as aqueous humor, that nourishes the lens and cornea. The vitreous body, a chamber containing clear, gelatinous fluid known as vitreous humor, is located behind the lens. The light that enters the eye passes through the lens and the vitreous humor where it is refracted, or bent, onto the retina.

● **STOP** *and Consider*

Why is it necessary to control the amount of light entering the eye?

The **retina**, located over the posterior two thirds of the eye, contains **photoreceptor** (receptor sensitive to light) cells called rods and cones. **Rods** produce a photopigment, **rhodopsin**, allowing vision in dim light. Opsin (a protein) and retinene (a vitamin A derivative) combine to form rhodopsin, which breaks down when in contact with light, stimulating a nerve impulse. Even low levels of light promote the breakdown of rhodopsin, allowing night vision.

● **STOP** *and Consider*

Why does a vitamin A deficiency cause the development of night blindness?

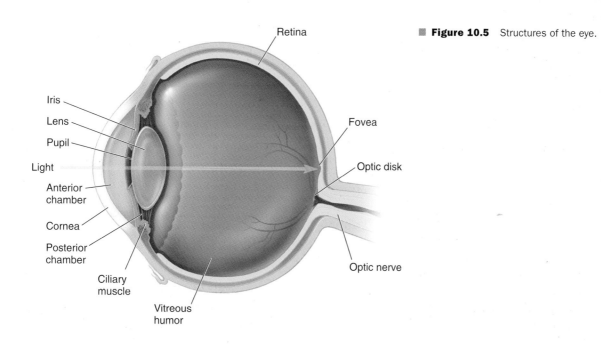

Retina

Iris
Lens
Pupil
Light
Anterior chamber
Cornea
Posterior chamber
Ciliary muscle
Vitreous humor

Fovea
Optic disk
Optic nerve

■ **Figure 10.5** Structures of the eye.

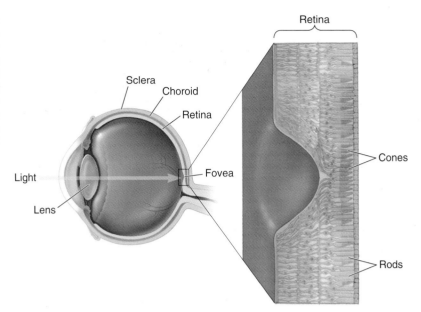

■ **Figure 10.6** Lateral view of the eye. Impulses initiated in the photoreceptors, rods, and cones are transmitted by the bipolar cells to the ganglion cells of the retina. The fovea in the center of the macula is made entirely of cones. Surrounding tissue and blood vessels are displaced from the central area, fovea centralis, allowing light to pass unimpeded to the cones. (Image modified from Bear MF, Connors BW, Parasido MA. *Neuroscience: Exploring the Brain.* 3rd ed. Philadelphia: Lippincott Williams & Wilkins; 2006, with permission.)

The photoreceptors called **cones** provide the ability to see bright light and color; these cones are involved in visual acuity (clarity). The photopigments in cones also contain retinene and opsins differing from the type found in rods. In contrast to rods, cone photopigments require bright light for breakdown and generation of nerve impulse. There are three types of retinal cones. Each contains a different combination of retinene and opsin, which results in absorption of light of different wavelengths and colors.

1. Erythrolabe: red cone absorbs light at 625-nm wavelength
2. Chlorolabe: green cone absorbs light at 530-nm wavelength
3. Cyanolabe: blue cone absorbs light at 455-nm wavelength

Color vision is determined by the combination of cones stimulated by light from a particular image. The absence of a single group of color-receptive cones results in the inability to distinguish particular colors from others, a condition commonly known as color blindness. This condition is caused by a sex-linked recessive genetic trait, and it predominantly affects males.

The center of the retina, the **macula**, is the area responsible for central vision, color vision, and fine detail. The **fovea**, an area in the center of the macula, is the site at which the cones are most dense. Cones are the only photoreceptors located in the fovea, increasingly interspersed with rods toward the retina periphery. Rods are most highly concentrated in the peripheral retina, promoting peripheral and night vision. Rods and cones convert light into electrical impulses, which are transmitted first to the bipolar neurons, then to ganglion neurons. The axons of the ganglion neurons meet at the optic disk and exit the eye as the optic nerve (Fig. 10.6). The impulse continues to the optic chiasm where the medial halves of the retinal nerves crossover. The impulse travels to the optic tract, the thalamus, and the occipital lobe for processing. Each eye transmits a slightly different image, focused upside down on the retina. Mirror reversal also occurs because of light reflected from the right side of an object to the left side of the retina and vice versa. Visual images are coordinated in the brain during **visual processing**.

CONTROL OF EYE MOVEMENT

Extraocular muscles are responsible for the rotational, horizontal, and vertical movements of the eyes (Fig. 10.7). A balance of contraction and relaxation of specific muscles allows controlled eye movement (Table 10.3). The six muscles that control eye movements are innervated by the oculomotor (III), trochlear (IV), and abducens (VI) cranial nerves. Eye movements can be described as follows:

- Saccades: looking from object A to object B
- Pursuit: smoothly following a moving object
- Convergence/divergence: both eyes turning inward/outward simultaneously
- Vestibular: eyes sensing and adjusting to head movement via connections with nerves in the inner ear
- Fixation maintenance: minute eye movements that position and accommodate both eyes

PROTECTIVE EYE STRUCTURES

The structures of the eye are protected by both physical and chemical barriers. Protective eye structures maintain, function, and promote optimal vision.

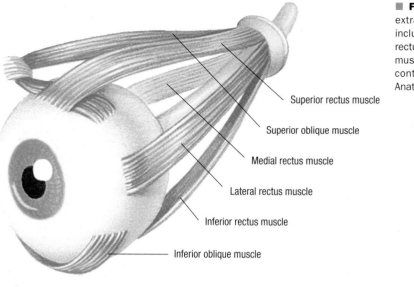

Figure 10.7 Extraocular eye muscles. Paired extraocular muscles control eye movement and include the superior/inferior rectus, medial/lateral rectus, and the superior/inferior oblique. The paired muscles have reciprocal responses, so that as one contracts, the other relaxes. (Asset provided by Anatomical Chart Company.)

External Structures

Eyelids provide a protective barrier for the eye. Opening and closing of eyelids (blinking) promotes the removal of debris and provides moisture for the eye surface. Eyelashes also protect the eye and remove small particles of debris. The conjunctiva is a mucous membrane lining the undersurface of the eyelid and front of the eye.

Tears

The **lacrimal glands** are the primary producers of tears. Tears protect the eyes by:

- Protecting against bacterial infection
- Providing nutrients and moisture
- Removing debris and waste from the eye

Closure of the eyelid forces tears downward, toward the nose and into the puncta (openings in the upper and lower lids). Tears are forced into the lacrimal sac through narrow channels. Upon muscle relaxation and eye opening, tears move from the lacrimal sac to the nasolacrimal duct and into the nose.

STOP *and Consider*

What is the most likely explanation for the runny nose that occurs during crying?

Aqueous Humor

The nutritive, watery fluid produced by the **ciliary body** is known as **aqueous humor** (Fig. 10.8). Released in the space between the iris and the lens (the posterior chamber), the aqueous humor maintains eye pressure and provides nutrients to the

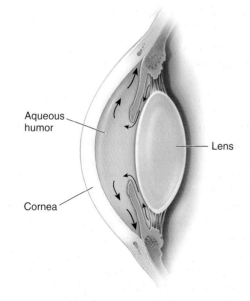

Figure 10.8 Aqueous humor. Aqueous humor flows from the posterior to the anterior chamber for reabsorption by the venous system to maintain eye pressure.

Table 10.3 Extraocular Muscle Function

Extraocular Eye Muscle	Eye Movement
Lateral rectus	Outward, away from nose
Medial rectus	Inward, toward the nose
Superior rectus	Upward, slightly outward
Inferior rectus	Downward, slightly inward
Superior oblique	Inward and downward
Inferior oblique	Outward and upward

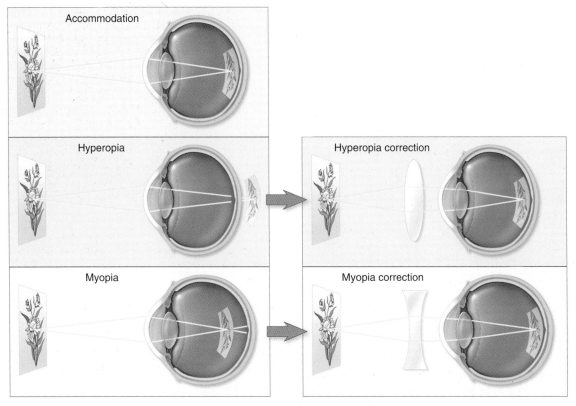

Figure 10.9 Error in refraction. Light entering the eye is focused onto the retina. Refraction errors misdirect light onto the retina, causing distortion of vision. (Image modified from Bear MF, Connors BW, Parasido MA. *Neuroscience: Exploring the Brain*. 3rd ed. Philadelphia: Lippincott Williams & Wilkins; 2006, with permission.)

cornea and the lens. Movement of aqueous humor from the posterior chamber to the anterior chamber occurs by diffusion via the pupil, allowing reabsorption into the venous system for removal. The primary mechanism for reabsorption occurs through the **trabecular network** (a meshlike structure) into the canal of Schlemm, promoting movement into the venous system. A smaller quantity of aqueous humor is reabsorbed directly into larger blood vessels through the anterior ciliary body, known as the **uveal-scleral outflow pathway**.

Alterations in Visual Function

Sight depends on the integration of multiple structures and processes within the eye and in surrounding tissues and organs. Alterations in vision can be induced by multiple causes, including damage to eye structures, motor dysfunction, and impaired neural conduction. Consequences can range from mild visual impairment amenable to correction or severe impairment resulting in blindness.

ERRORS IN REFRACTION

Bending of light, or refraction, can be altered at any step from light entry into the eye through the contact of light onto the retina (Fig. 10.9). One common error in refraction is **myopia**, commonly known as nearsightedness. In myopia, the eye focuses an image in front of the retina due to lens thickness. **Hyperopia**, commonly referred to as farsightedness, is caused by the focusing of an image behind the retina, which alters the transmission of light. These conditions are easily corrected with the provision of a lens that regulates light rays. A biconcave lens causes light to diverge, providing correction of myopia. A biconvex lens is the necessary correction for hyperopia, promoting the convergence of light rays. **Astigmatism**, caused by irregular curvature of the cornea or lens, prevents the focusing of images, blurring vision. Correction of astigmatism can be accomplished through glasses, contact lenses, or refractive laser surgery, discussed in more detail later in the chapter. **Presbyopia**, a condition of farsightedness associated with aging, results from the inability of the ciliary muscle and lens to accommodate for near vision. This condition is easily corrected with bifocals.

ALTERATIONS IN EYE MOVEMENT

Strabismus is a term that describes the lack of coordinated extrinsic eye muscle function that prevents the eyes from lining up in the same direction. Known commonly as "crossed eyes," the misalignment of visual axes results in the inability to focus on a single object. **Amblyopia**, commonly known as "lazy eye," may result from strabismus, leading to the loss of visual detail from uncoordinated eye movement and focus. When visual axes are misaligned in children, the brain is able to suppress one of the images, resulting in visual impairment in the ignored eye. The impairment may range from dimness of vision to the permanent loss of vision in one eye. Visual impairment resulting from amblyopia may not be fully correctable.

Diplopia, a condition often resulting from a lack of coordination of the extraocular muscles, may result in double vision. Images fall on noncorresponding areas of the retina, causing the visual defect. Involuntary oscillations of the eye, known as **nystagmus**, results from abnormal function in the brain, labyrinth of the inner ear, and vestibular pathways responsible for controlling eye movement. Congenital nystagmus often results from oculomotor abnormalities during neural development, manifesting at the age of 2 months. In the postnatal period, nystagmus can be acquired from a variety of visual input disruptions but is often the result of a head injury or space occupying lesion that interferes with vestibular pathways or cerebellar function. Other conditions known to contribute to the development of nystagmus include brainstem or cerebellar lesions, stroke, Ménière disease, multiple sclerosis, and drug or alcohol toxicity.

ALTERATIONS IN PROTECTIVE EYE STRUCTURES

Inflammation of the mucous membrane lining the eye, **conjunctivitis**, is commonly known as pink eye. Variations in categories of conjunctivitis are linked to the following causative factors:

- Viral conjunctivitis
  - Usually affects only one eye
  - Associated with excessive eye watering and a small amount of discharge
- Bacterial conjunctivitis
  - Usually affects both eyes
  - Associated with heavy discharge
- Allergic conjunctivitis
  - Usually affects both eyes
  - Associated with itching, redness, and excessive tearing

Cataracts result from the clouding of the lens, which alter vision focus by scattering the incoming light onto the retina (Fig. 10.10). Clouding often

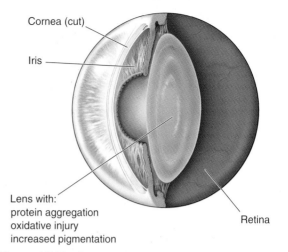

Cornea (cut)

Iris

Lens with:
protein aggregation
oxidative injury
increased pigmentation

Retina

■ **Figure 10.10** Cataract. Cross section of the cornea showing cloudy lens. (Asset provided by Anatomical Chart Company.)

results from the clumping or aggregation of the protein component of the lens. As the size of the opaque area increases, vision is increasingly impaired. Cataracts are classified into three types:

1. Nuclear
   a. Most common type
   b. Forms in the center, or nucleus, of the lens
   c. Is caused by the aging process
2. Cortical
   a. Forms in the lens cortex
   b. Extends from the outer lens toward the center
3. Subscapular
   a. Begins at the back of the lens
   b. May result from diabetes and severe hyperopia

◢ Manifestations and Evaluation of Alterations In Vision

Individuals often seek care when they notice that their vision has changed. Often, decreasing acuity or clarity of vision occurs over time. In the case of children, vision screening or change in academic performance may provide the impetus to seek further screening and diagnosis. A comprehensive vision screening is necessary to identify areas of deficit or dysfunction. The components of a vision screening are presented in Box 10.4.

Visual acuity, or sharpness, is commonly included in basic vision screening. It is important to evaluate both far and near vision. Evaluation of far distances is accomplished by using a standardized eye chart, such as the Snellen or E chart. The results are reported as a fraction, "20/X," with the numerator indicating what can be seen clearly at a 20-foot distance and the denominator indicating the distance at which the average eye can read the line. A report of 20/20 means that a person can see clearly at 20 feet what should be seen at 20 feet. A measurement of 20/40 means that what is seen clearly at 20 feet, the average person can read at 40 feet.

The results of a near vision test show a person's ability to see the details of near objects (within arm's distance from the body). Near vision is tested with a handheld card held at a comfortable distance. The patient reads the smallest line possible, which is recorded along with the distance. Some tests of near acuity use a standard handheld card at a prescribed distance. For example, when a Jaeger chart is used, it is placed 12 to 14 in. away. Individuals are asked to read the smallest of 10 available lines, ranging from 4- to 14-point type fonts, that they are able to read. The results are then converted to standards used in far vision evaluation.

Treatment Of Alterations In Vision

Treatment of alterations in vision is specific to the identified impairment. Muscle imbalances can be corrected by glasses, patching, or surgery, depending on the specific impairments identified. Errors in refraction may be corrected by glasses, contact lenses, or surgery. **Laser-assisted in situ keratomileusis (LASIK)** is a surgical procedure used to treat myopia, hyperopia, and astigmatism. Cataracts may also need to be surgically removed and replaced with a clear prosthetic lens. Glaucoma, covered in greater detail in the clinical model in this chapter, may require surgical or pharmacologic management.

Box 10.4 Components of Vision Screening

Vision evaluation often includes the following:

- Acuity-distance: visual acuity (sharpness, clearness) at 20 feet distance
- Acuity-near: clear vision for short distance (as in reading)
- Focusing skills: maintenance of clear vision at varying distances
- Eye tracking and fixation skills: the ability of the eyes to look at and accurately follow an object; a skill important in the process of reading
- Binocular fusion: the ability to use both eyes together at the same time
- Stereopsis: binocular depth perception
- Convergence and eye teaming skills: coordination of the eyes to aim, move, and work as a team
- Hyperopia: a refractive condition that causes difficulty in focus of near objects
- Color vision: the ability to distinguish colors
- Reversal frequency: confusing letters or words (b, d; p, q: saw, was)
- Visual memory: the ability to store and retrieve visual information
- Visual form discrimination: the ability to determine whether two shapes, colors, sizes, positions, or distances are the same or different
- Visual motor integration: the ability to combine visual input with other sensory input (e.g., hand and body movements, balance, and hearing); the ability to transform images from a vertical to a horizontal plane (such as from the blackboard to the desk surface)
- Intraocular pressure measurement: measurement of 10 to 21 mm Hg considered normal

---

Module 3

Alterations in Hearing and Balance

Hearing and balance involve a complex interaction between structural components of the ear and transmission of nerve impulses for sensory interpretation. The senses of hearing and balance are maximized by optimal function of both outer ear and inner ear structures.

Structural Components of the Ear

Structures of the outer, middle, and inner ear coordinate to funnel stimuli (sound) to the hearing receptors, initiating the signal that travels along the neural pathways to the brain. Figure 10.11 illustrates the structures of the ear.

OUTER EAR

The tissue that comprises what is viewed as the outer ear is known as the **pinna**. Composed of cartilage and soft tissue, the pinna maintains its shape, but it is also flexible and pliable. The pinna collects and funnels sound vibrations into the opening of the ear canal, or **external auditory meatus**. The ear canal is approximately 1 in. long in an adult and, similar to the pinna, is also composed of cartilage. The ear canal is covered with small hairs and glands

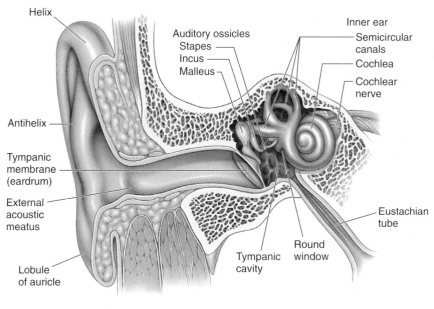

Helix
Auditory ossicles
Stapes
Incus
Malleus
Antihelix
Tympanic membrane (eardrum)
External acoustic meatus
Lobule of auricle
Tympanic cavity
Round window
Inner ear
Semicircular canals
Cochlea
Cochlear nerve
Eustachian tube

■ **Figure 10.11** Structures of the ear. (Asset provided by Anatomical Chart Company.)

that secrete wax (**cerumen**). These structures in the ear canal serve as protection against foreign bodies and environmental debris. At the distal end, the ear canal becomes bony with a tight skin covering.

MIDDLE EAR

The **tympanic membrane**, or eardrum, is located at the end of the ear canal opposite the external auditory meatus, marking the boundary of the middle ear. The middle ear contains three bones, or **ossicles**, that form a connection between the eardrum and inner ear. Sound waves that contact the tympanic membrane cause a back and forth movement. Tympanic membrane movement causes repositioning of the ossicles, which changes sound waves into mechanical vibration (Fig. 10.12).

The three bones comprising the ossicles are the **malleus**, **incus**, and **stapes**. These bones are also known as the hammer, anvil, and stirrup, respectively. Connections between the tympanic membranes and ossicles promote transduction of the mechanical vibration, producing sound. The progressive connections between the tympanic membrane, malleus, incus, and stapes cause an in-and-out movement at the base of the stirrup, or the stapes footplate. These in-and-out movements represent patterns matching the initiating sound waves.

The middle ear is located in the air-filled mastoid portion of the temporal bone of the skull. The eustachian tube connecting the middle ear to the nasopharynx runs along the front wall of the middle ear to the back of the nose and throat, providing pressure equalization on both sides of the tympanic

membrane. The eustachian tube is shorter and narrower in children, increasing the likelihood of eustachian tube blockage and pressure. The anatomic constraints in children may increase the risk of ear infection.

● **STOP** *and Consider*

What are the ways that we can voluntarily manipulate pressure changes in the ear?

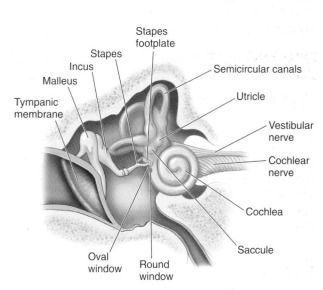

Stapes footplate
Stapes
Incus
Malleus
Tympanic membrane
Semicircular canals
Utricle
Vestibular nerve
Cochlear nerve
Cochlea
Saccule
Oval window
Round window

■ **Figure 10.12** Vestibular structures of the ear. Sound vibrations contact the tympanic membrane, causing vibration of the ossicles and footplate of the stapes at the oval window. Movement of the oval window promotes fluid movement against the cochlea stimulating nerve impulses, which are transmitted to the brain via the cochlear nerve.

INNER EAR

The stapes footplate of the middle ear fits into the **oval window**, marking the boundary between the middle ear and the beginning point of the inner ear. The inner ear is composed of the outer bony labyrinth and inner membranous labyrinth. Receptor stimuli results in signal transduction along the eighth cranial nerve (acoustic), composed of the cochlear nerve (hearing) and the vestibular nerve (balance).

Hearing Processes

The perilymph-filled bony labyrinth contains the **cochlea**, important for hearing. Within the cochlea, the **Organ of Corti** contains hair cells, the receptors responsible for the neural impulse that allows hearing. The membranous labyrinth is a closed system of endolymph-filled canals lying within the cochlea. The ionic concentration difference between perilymph fluid outside the membranous labyrinth and the internal endolymph fluid creates an endolymphatic potential, generating a current that sensitizes the cochlear hair cells in the Organ of Corti to sound. Cochlear hair cells are innervated by the cochlear portion of the acoustic nerve. Impulses are then transmitted to the visual cortex in the occipital lobe, regulating hearing.

Mechanical energy from the ossicles forces the oval window into the cochlea. The motion of the cochlea's fluid stimulates hair cells. Sterocilia on each hair cell contribute to the ability to respond to unique sound frequencies, or pitches. Movement of stereocilia leads to hyperpolarization or depolarization (Fig. 10.13). Depolarization of hair cells causes impulse generation and transmission to the brain via the acoustic (vestibulocochlear) VIII cranial nerve to the relay center in the midbrain, the cochlear nucleus. At that point, nerve fibers from each ear divide into two pathways. One pathway ascends directly to the auditory cortex on the same side hemisphere, while the second pathway crosses over and ascends to the auditory cortex on the contralateral hemisphere. This mechanism allows impulses from each ear to reach both hemispheres.

The central auditory system processes auditory information, supporting the following functions:

- Sound localization
- Auditory discrimination (recognizing differences between different sounds)
- Sound pattern recognition
- Time, or temporal, aspects of hearing
- Integration of multiple auditory stimuli by reduction in the auditory performance of competing or incomplete signals

Balance Processes

The three semicircular canals and vestibule (containing the utricle and saccule, connected membranous sacs) are also located in the bony labyrinth and are important for balance and equilibrium. The hair cell receptors in the semicircular canals and vestibule (vestibular apparatus) detect head position and acceleration, maintaining body position and stable visual fields. The perilymph in the semicircular canals senses motion caused by body movement, stimulating the hair cells lining the vestibular apparatus. Vestibular hair cells are innervated by the vestibular portion of the acoustic nerve. Impulses are then transmitted to the cerebellum via the vestibular branch of the acoustic nerve, regulating equilibrium and balance.

Alterations in Hearing and Balance

Most disorders of the ear are not fatal, but they significantly affect an individual's daily functioning. Ear disorders can result in impaired hearing, altered balance, discomfort, and pain.

DISORDERS OF THE EXTERNAL EAR

Disorders of the ear canal are frequently caused by inflammation, drainage, or obstruction. Obstruction can result from the accumulation of cerumen or the presence of a tumor, diminishing the movement of sound to the middle ear. Cerumen may be removed by a process of **irrigation**, or rinsing the external canal with warm water, after it is determined that

Figure 10.13 Hair cell. Hair cells hyperpolarize or depolarize depending on the direction in which the stereocilia bend.

Stereocilia

Hair cell

Sensory neuron

Normal   Hyperpolarization   Depolarization

the tympanic membrane is intact. In the case of an obstructive tumor, surgical excision is usually the preferred treatment.

● STOP *and Consider*

What are the risks to ear structures when the ears are irrigated?

Otitis externa, inflammation of the skin of the external ear, is a condition associated with pain and discomfort. Commonly known as "swimmer's ear," otitis externa often results from moisture in the ear canal or altered integrity of the skin in the ear canal. Manifestations include itching, redness, tenderness, and narrowing of tissues in the ear canal caused by swelling in response to inflammation. Mild hearing loss may result from drainage and from the reduced diameter of the ear canal.

ALTERATION IN THE MIDDLE EAR FUNCTION

Inflammation, trauma, and obstruction are often related to middle ear hearing loss. Eustachian tube dysfunction may lead to loss of hearing due to altered patency or obstruction, or as a contributing factor to other middle ear pathologies. Abnormally patent eustachian tubes promote movement of fluid from the nasopharynx into the middle ear. This particularly concerns infants and children because crying may precipitate the movement of secretions into the tube. Obstruction of the eustachian tube may promote the absorption of air from the middle ear, which is replaced by serous fluid escaping from surrounding capillaries. Hearing loss may result from the loss of mobility of the tympanic membrane caused by middle ear fluid, exudates compromising the conduction of vibration in the ossicles of the middle ear, or negative pressure in the middle ear resulting from eustachian tube obstruction.

Sudden changes in atmospheric pressure can result in **barotrauma**, or injury resulting from the inability of the ear to equalize barometric stress. Most commonly seen in air travel and sea diving, barotrauma results from middle ear pressure in parallel with atmospheric pressure. Persons at particular risk are those suffering from an upper respiratory infection with limited ability to normalize pressure in the eustachian tube.

● STOP *and Consider*

What strategies can a person use to avoid barotrauma caused by air travel during an upper respiratory infection?

Otitis media, infection of the middle ear, is one of the most common disorders of the middle ear. Hearing loss may result from immobility of the tympanic membrane, fluid accumulation of the middle ear, and scarring from rupture of the tympanic membrane, altering function. Otitis media may be acute or recurrent, and it is associated with effusion (fluid) in the middle ear. This condition may be seen across all age groups, but has the greatest prevalence in infants and children. The clinical model in this chapter provides a complete review of this condition. **Mastoiditis**, a bacterial infection causing inflammation of the air cells of the mastoid bone, may result as a complication of otitis media. Risks related to mastoiditis include meningitis, brain abscess, or facial palsy if it is not responsive to antibiotic therapy.

Otosclerosis, an autosomal-dominant condition, represents the most common cause of chronic, progressive, conductive hearing loss. Slow formation of spongy bone at the oval window immobilizes the footplate of the stapes, impairing the conduction of vibration. Most prevalent in females 15 to 30 years of age, affected individuals indicate a family history of this condition, consistent with the genetic basis of the disease. Surgical removal of the stapes with replacement of a prosthetic device restores partial or total hearing.

ALTERATION IN THE INNER EAR FUNCTION

Hearing loss caused by inner ear dysfunction is related to destruction of cochlear hair cells or damage to neural pathways. Tinnitus may be caused by noise-induced hearing loss, sensorineural hearing loss consistent with aging (**presbycusis**), hypertension, atherosclerosis, head injury, or cochlear infection/inflammation.

Balance and equilibrium are disturbed in altered function of the inner ear. **Ménière disease**, a condition associated with severe vertigo, sensorineural hearing loss, and tinnitus, is related to overproduction or decreased absorption of endolymph. Also known as endolymphatic hydrops or endolymphatic hypertension, hearing loss is caused by the progressive degeneration of vestibular and cochlear hair cells, described in greater detail in the clinical models. **Labyrinthitis**, or inflammation of the labyrinth of the inner ear, also precipitates severe vertigo and sensorineural hearing loss.

▨ Manifestations and Evaluation of Alterations in Hearing

Noticeable change in the ability to hear is why individuals commonly seek hearing evaluation. Difficulty hearing around groups of people, difficulty hearing competing sounds, or difficulty hearing specific types of pitches denote a potential for hearing loss. Hearing screening is routine in particular groups of individuals, such as newborns or those individuals working in areas that increase the risk for hearing loss. Hearing evaluation should include a thorough examination of all structural and functional auditory components. Deformities and lesions of the pinna and external auditory canal may indicate an acute, chronic, or congenital condition as the cause of hearing impairment. Audiometric testing can help determine the specific nature of hearing loss. Auditory acuity is the basic assessment of hearing, and provides a general sense of hearing sensation. Further testing can be pursued when evidence is present for hearing loss.

Screening procedures are performed to identify the type of loss (unilateral or bilateral, sensorineural, and/or conductive) and to quantify the degree of hearing loss. A thorough history should be completed to determine the duration, severity, and quality of the hearing loss. Associated symptoms should also be identified, such as pain or **tinnitus** (ringing or whistling in the ears).

Hearing Evaluation

The degree of hearing loss can be quantified using a unit of measure known as **decibels (dB)**. The frequency or pitch of the sound is referred to in **Hertz (Hz)**. Based on pure tone average, hearing levels can be categorized based on frequencies from 500 to 4,000 Hz. Individuals who have normal hearing are able to detect sounds at a minimal frequency of −10 to +15 dB. Individuals who have hearing impairment require sounds with increasing decibels for detection. Minimal decibels needed for sound recognition may help determine the degree of hearing loss, described as follows:

1. Minimal hearing loss: 16 to 25 dB
2. Mild hearing loss: 26 to 30 dB
3. Moderate hearing loss: 31 to 50 dB
4. Moderate to severe hearing loss: 51 to 70 dB
5. Severe hearing loss: 71 to 90 dB
6. Profound hearing loss: 91 dB or more

The type of hearing loss can be determined based on the identification of the event or structure involved. **Conductive hearing loss** is localized to the outer or middle ear, and it may be temporary or permanent. **Sensorineural hearing loss** is often permanent, resulting from disease, trauma, or genetic inheritance of a defect in the cochlea nerve cells. The inner ear or the auditory nerve is usually involved in sensorineural hearing loss. **Mixed hearing loss** refers to a combination of both sensorineural and conductive hearing loss. **Central auditory**

processing disorder is a disorder involving an alteration in auditory signal processing in the brain.

In addition to determining type and degree of hearing loss, auditory testing can determine whether the hearing loss is bilateral or unilateral, symmetric or asymmetric, or high or low frequency. Specific tests included in hearing evaluation include an audiogram, with the following three components:

1. Pure-tone audiometry
   a. Recognition of tones in the absence of background noise
   b. Results are graphed on an audiogram
2. Speech reception threshold
   a. Identification of the faintest level of speech heard
   b. Minimal decibel measurement of the "loudness" of speech required for detection recorded
3. Speech discrimination score
   a. Recognition of words at a normal level of speech
   b. Measured by the percentage of spoken words identified when spoken at a hearing level above threshold

Evaluation Of The Middle Ear

Tests that provide information about structures in the outer and middle ear are known as acoustic immittance measures. **Tympanometry** measures the degree of movement of the tympanic membrane to identify middle ear fluid, perforation, or cerumen blockage of the ear canal. **Acoustic reflex measurement** can be used to determine movement of the tympanic membrane in response to sound.

Evaluation Of The Inner Ear

The **pure tone bone conduction** hearing test can be used to evaluate the inner ear, independent of middle and outer ear function. A small vibrator is placed on either the forehead or the mastoid bone, directly stimulating the auditory nerve. This test is limited to the identification of sensorineural hearing loss. Air conduction tests can be used to identify both conductive and sensorineural hearing loss.

The vestibular evoked myogenic potential test uses evoked potential techniques (see Chapter 9) to stimulate a sound-induced reflex. This test allows evaluation of the saccule (a sensory organ of the inner ear), the vestibular nerve, the medial vestibulospinal tract, and the spinal accessory nerve. Generation of a response to sound is caused by acoustical stimulation of the saccule, resulting in transduction of the impulse beneath the stapes footplate.

Individuals who experience acute or chronic exposure to environmental noise are at risk for hearing loss. Exposure to noise and high-level sound can cause damage to outside hair cells, the main targets of high-level sound. Tests specific to outer hair cell function include **otoacoustic emission (OAE)**. OAEs are faint sounds produced by the outer hair cells in the cochlea of the inner ear. Sound recordings, obtained by a small microphone placed in the ear canal, may identify the specific reason for hearing loss. OAEs may occur spontaneously or may be induced by a stimulus, such as a click or a pure tone auditory stimulus.

Treatment of Alterations in Hearing

Alterations in hearing may be corrected by the use of hearing aids or assistive listening devices to amplify sound. When these devices provide little improvement in hearing, a cochlear implant may be considered. **Cochlear implants** are artificial devices surgically placed behind the ear. Using electrical stimulation of nerve endings, electrodes implanted in the cochlea transmit sounds to the auditory nerve, bypassing structures in the middle and outer ear. The device does not restore normal hearing, but it does provide a sense of sound that is processed into meaningful communication by the brain.

Hearing deficits in young children may be associated with impaired language and cognitive development. Early screening of hearing loss has provided an opportunity to treat loss at younger ages in an effort to promote language and cognitive development. Use of cochlear implants at younger ages has the potential to enhance cognitive development.[3,4]

Taste and Smell

The senses of taste and smell are linked such that if one is impaired, the other is also affected. While impairment of taste and smell is not life-threatening, alterations in these senses have the potential to negatively impact quality of life.

TASTE

The sensation of taste is also known as gustation. Taste is mediated by the chemoreceptors in the taste buds of the oral cavity. Taste or gustatory cells, one of the cell types that make up taste buds, are the sensory receptors responsible for triggering the impulse that is perceived as taste. Taste buds detect five types of basic tastes, including:

1. Sweet
2. Sour
3. Salty
4. Bitter
5. Savory

Substances must be dissolved in saliva to stimulate a taste response. Once dissolved, molecules released from food and drink by chewing, drinking, or digesting food penetrate the taste buds, bind to the taste receptor on the gustatory hairs of the taste cell, and transmit the taste signal via action potentials along associated dendrites. Impulses travel primarily along the facial nerve (cranial nerve VII) and glossopharyngeal nerve (cranial nerve IX) where they synapse in the medulla and the thalamus, then proceed to the gustatory cortex in the parietal lobe.

Taste is also indirectly affected by other stimuli. Visual, thermal, scent, and even pain receptors are stimulated to enhance the taste sensation. Of these, the olfactory stimulation of the sense of smell has the greatest influence. Receptor sensitivity of taste cells may be altered by environmental factors (such as cigarette smoking), drug reactions (chemotherapy), and clinical conditions (chronic liver disease).

Taste disorders often involve smell. Conditions of taste disorders include phantom taste perception (lingering, unpleasant taste), reduced ability to taste one or all of the five basic tastes, or distortion of flavor such as persistent metallic taste.

SMELL

The sense of smell is often pleasurable, enhancing enjoyment of the food we eat and the world around us. An intact sense of smell can also be protective, warning us of potential threats such as gas leaks or environmental toxins. **Olfaction**, or the sense of smell, is regulated by olfactory receptors located in each nasal cavity. A second olfactory pathway is through the roof of the throat region to the nose.

Olfactory hairs protrude from the receptor segments that extend through the nasal epithelium. Unmyelinated axons comprise the opposite end of the olfactory receptor, which merge with other olfactory axons to form the olfactory nerve (cranial nerve I). Afferent fibers ascend from the olfactory bulb to the olfactory cortex and are responsible for interpretation and processing of olfactory stimuli.

Alterations in olfactory sensation, while unpleasant, are not pathophysiologically significant. The most common smell disorders are associated with recent illness or injury. Conditions most frequently associated with smell disorders include upper respiratory infections, frontal head injuries, chemical exposure (including some medications), and smoking. Loss of smell acuity is also associated with aging.

Module 4

Clinical Models

The following clinical models have been selected to aid in the understanding and application of altered sensation. The student should pay attention to the commonalities and unique features of each condition when studying these models. Alterations in sensory functions often lead to physical and emotional distress and disruption of daily life (Fig. 10.14).

Fibromyalgia

Fibromyalgia, a condition of the soft tissues and muscles, is derived from the Latin words "fibro" for fibrous tissue and the Greek words "myo" for muscle and "algia" for pain. Estimated to affect 2% of the population, fibromyalgia is an increasingly recognized problem, which has lead to a renewed emphasis on improved management strategies. Fibromyalgia occurs in women seven times more frequently than in men. Women of childbearing age are most likely to suffer from fibromyalgia.

PATHOPHYSIOLOGY

Fibromyalgia causes significant pain and fatigue but is not linked to a well-defined pathogenesis.

The complexity of fibromyalgia pathogenesis involves genetics, developmental influences, triggering factors, and neurophysiologic and emotional variables.[5] Although there is no known cause or cure, research continues to determine the underlying mechanisms and effective treatments for the syndrome.

CLINICAL MANIFESTATIONS

A commonly diagnosed condition, fibromyalgia is characterized by disordered sleep, tenderness, stiffness and pain in the neck, shoulders, upper back, elbows, lower back, and hips.[6] Sleep disorders, consistent with manifestations of fatigue, often accompany fibromyalgia. Altered pain processing, psychologic stress, and poor physical condition caused by lack of exercise may be contributing factors.

Depression may coexist in individuals who have fibromyalgia. Serotonin levels are decreased in some individuals, consistent with symptoms of depression, pain, sleep alteration, anxiety, and altered muscle function. It is not known if this is a cause of or a response to fibromyalgia.

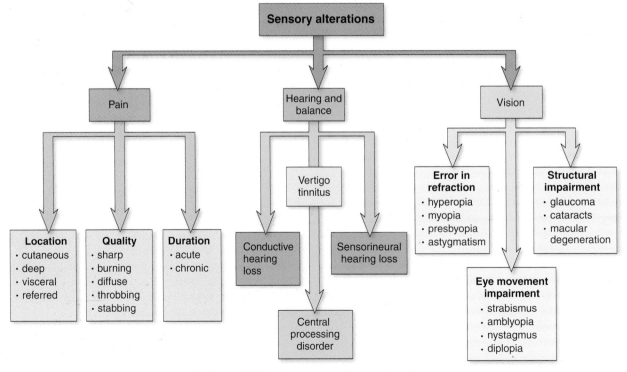

■ **Figure 10.14**   Concept map. Sensory alterations.

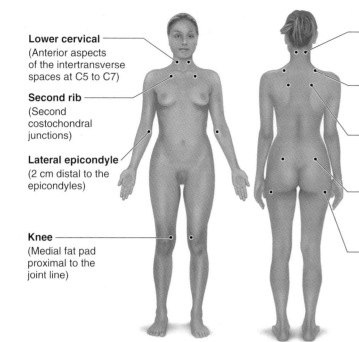

Lower cervical
(Anterior aspects
of the intertransverse
spaces at C5 to C7)

Second rib
(Second
costochondral
junctions)

Lateral epicondyle
(2 cm distal to the
epicondyles)

Knee
(Medial fat pad
proximal to the
joint line)

Occiput
(Suboccipital
muscle insertions)

Trapezius
(Midpoint of the
upper border)

Supraspinatus
(Above the medial
border of the
scapular spine)

Gluteal
(Upper outer
quadrants of
buttocks)

Greater trochanter
(Lower outer
quadrants of
buttocks)

■ **Figure 10.15** Tender points of fibromyalgia.

DIAGNOSTIC CRITERIA

Diagnostic criteria include subjective findings of fatigue and chronic musculoskeletal pain of at least 3 months' duration. Eighteen areas of pain, or tender point sites, located in the neck, shoulders, rib junctions, joints, gluteus, trochanters, and knees have been identified in patients suffering from fibromyalgia (Fig. 10.15). Pain must be present in 11 of the 18 tender point sites for diagnosis.[7] Some people with fibromyalgia develop trigger points or ropy bands occurring throughout the body.[8] The trigger points induce referred pain to other parts of the body, which is thought to be caused by pressure on blood vessels and nerves by fibrous bands causing tightening of **myofascia** (outer membrane of muscle tissue).

TREATMENT

Treatment of fibromyalgia is focused on symptom management, and it includes both nonpharmacologic and pharmacologic options.[8] Cognitive behavioral therapy, coupled with stress reduction methods and medication to promote sleep, is the most effective treatment regimen. Application of heat and cold, ultrasound, and deep massage may provide temporary relief of symptoms. Gentle exercise is critical to maintaining muscle fitness. Stretching and exercise promote muscle strength and facilitate

sleep. Alternative treatment options may include acupuncture, biofeedback, yoga, hypnosis, or other relaxation techniques.

Treatment with modulators of the neurotransmitters serotonin and norepinephrine, antiseizure medications, sedative hypnotics, and analgesics are the mainstays of pharmacologic management of fibromyalgia.[5] Medications that block serotonin (SSRI)[9] and norepinephrine (SNRI) reuptake have demonstrated effectiveness for relief of physical and emotional symptoms. Antiseizure medications have been shown to have pain-relieving effects, reducing severity of stiffness and joint discomfort. Sedative hypnotics that improve sleep often help alleviate fatigue symptoms. Nonsteroidal anti-inflammatory medications help reduce discomfort, particularly when combined with a tricyclic antidepressant.

● **STOP** and *Consider*

Why are anti-inflammatory medications preferred over narcotic analgesics in the treatment of fibromyalgia?

🔬 *From the Lab*

No diagnostic tests exist to confirm fibromyalgia. It is a diagnosis of exclusion, meaning that tests to confirm other likely diagnoses (including hypothyroidism or hyperparathyroidism) rule out other possibilities, leaving fibromyalgia as the most likely diagnosis.

Migraine Headache

Migraines are recurrent, moderate to severe headaches that last one to two days and are often associated with nausea, vomiting, and sensitivity to noise and light. The manifestations of migraine may be severe, resulting in significant loss of productivity and quality of life. Migraine is reported to be more common in women.[10]

PATHOPHYSIOLOGY

The precise cause of migraines is not clear. Alterations in certain cell groups in the brain triggered by inherited gene abnormalities is the explanation currently offered by scientists and researchers. Complex neurologic and biochemical events may initiate clinical symptoms. Neuromodulatory structures in the brainstem have been implicated in migraine pathogenesis.[11] Decreased serotonin levels may precipitate the release of chemical mediators from the trigeminal nerve, altering blood vessel function. The mineral magnesium may also be implicated because low levels prior to migraines may cause abnormal cellular communication. In susceptible people, migraines are often disabling and can be triggered by a variety of factors, including hormonal changes, anxiety, stress, and lack of food or sleep.

Individuals, particularly women of childbearing age, who experience migraines have an increased risk for early-onset ischemic stroke.[12] Although the association between migraine and stroke is accepted, it is unclear whether the migraines are the underlying cause of the stroke or were an expression of increased cardiovascular risk.

CLINICAL MANIFESTATIONS

The characteristics of migraine headaches are described as unilateral, pulsing, and throbbing. Some people experience symptoms, known as aura, that can predict the onset of a migraine. Auras may include visual disturbances such as flashing lights or temporary loss of vision. Loss of productivity and reduction in work and leisure time may result.

Migraines can be categorized based on the presence of aura. Most people suffer from common migraines without experiencing typical aura. Classic or uncommon migraines affecting approximately 15% of individuals include aura approximately 15 to 30 minutes before the onset of the migraine. Prodromal symptoms occurring 1 to 2 days before migraine onset are common and may include:

- Increased energy
- Sweet cravings
- Thirst
- Fatigue
- Irritability

Individuals who experience aura-associated migraines are at increased risk for cardiovascular disease.[13]

DIAGNOSTIC CRITERIA

Migraines are often diagnosed based on a thorough review of history and physical examination. If headaches develop acutely, other tests, such as computed tomography or magnetic resonance imaging scan, may be done to rule out other pathology such as meningitis, tumor, or increased intracranial pressure. The diagnosis of migraines associated with aura indicate increased risk for ischemic cardiovascular events.[14]

TREATMENT

Treatment of migraine headache includes nonpharmacologic and pharmacologic measures for prevention and treatment of existing pain. Prevention may be indicated when an individual:

- Experiences two or more migraines each month
- Uses pain-relieving medications more than two times a week
- Does not get relief from analgesic treatments
- Has uncommon migraines

Nonpharmacologic strategies effective in preventing migraines included avoidance of triggers, regular exercise, smoking cessation, and stabilization of hormone levels with oral contraceptives or hormone replacement therapy. Pharmacologic management for migraine prevention includes non-steroidal anti-inflammatory drugs (NSAIDs), antiseizure medications, beta-adrenergic receptor blockers, calcium channel blockers, and antidepressants that affect serotonin levels,[11] targeting the neuromodulatory etiology. The antihistamine cyproheptadine also affects serotonin activity and has been effective in preventing migraines in children. Injection of botulinum toxin (Botox) for facial wrinkles has been found to decrease the incidence of migraines. This incidental finding led to research on the effects of botulinum toxin on the prevention of migraines, effective in prevention of migraine headaches.[15] Surgical deactivation of migraine trigger sites is a treatment that has significantly reduced migraine symptoms.[16]

Pharmacologic treatment of migraines includes the use of NSAIDs, triptans, and ergots. Triptans mimic the action of serotonin, promoting constriction of blood vessels. The advantage of triptans is the rapid onset of action (within 15 minutes in the injectable form) and the high rate of effectiveness.

Treatment effectiveness is increased when initiated early prior to the onset of moderate to severe symptoms.[17] Ergots stimulate vasoconstriction, a potential contraindication in people with hypertension.

STOP *and* **Consider**

What is the most likely mechanism for the prevention of migraines with antiseizure medications?

Otitis Media

Otitis media is a commonly diagnosed condition in children. A complete history of illness combined with physical examination is important in determining an accurate diagnosis. Otitis media is a condition commonly diagnosed in infants and young children, although adults can also be affected. According to the National Institute of Deafness and Other Communication Disorders, 75% of children experience at least one episode of otitis media by their third birthday. The high prevalence of otitis media is estimated to cost approximately $5 billion per year in the United States.

PATHOPHYSIOLOGY

Acute otitis media (AOM), infection in the middle ear, is the most frequent diagnosis in febrile children in the United States and the world.[18] Most antibiotic agents for children are prescribed for AOM. The course of infection is associated with acute onset, fluid (effusion) in the middle ear, and inflammation. Otitis media with effusion (OME) is more common than AOM and is characterized by fluid/effusion in the middle ear without infection. OME results from the trapping of fluid in the middle ear by obstruction in the eustachian tube. AOM is considered recurrent when three or more episodes occur over 6 months or four or more episodes occur over 1 year.

Upper respiratory infections may lead to the development of AOM. Occlusion of the eustachian tubes caused by secretions and inflammation promote development of negative pressure and serous effusion in the middle ear. This environment presents an optimal medium for growth of upper airway viruses and bacterial pathogens, leading to AOM. Perforation of the tympanic membrane and spread of infection into the mastoid air cells are the most frequent complications.

CLINICAL MANIFESTATIONS

Clinical manifestations of otitis media include:
- Acute pain
- Enlarged periauricular lymph nodes
- Rhinorrhea (runny nose)
- Fever
- Impaired hearing

Examination of the ears using an otoscope may reveal gray or red tympanic membrane in OME and AOM, respectively (Fig. 10.16). Fluid may be visible behind the tympanic membrane, which may also appear to be bulging because of increased fluid volume. White areas on the tympanic membrane may be scarring from previous perforations. Discharge in the ear canal indicates possible acute perforation.

DIAGNOSTIC CRITERIA

Diagnosis of otitis media is usually made based on the history of symptoms and clinical findings, particularly those identified with otoscopic examination. It is important to distinguish OME from AOM for appropriate treatment. Criteria for diagnosis of AOM includes:[19]
- History of acute onset of signs and symptoms
- Presence of middle ear effusion
  - Bulging tympanic membrane
  - Limited or absent mobility of the tympanic membrane
  - Air-fluid level behind the tympanic membrane
  - Otorrhea (discharge in the ear canal)
- Signs and symptoms of middle ear inflammation
  - Redness/erythema of the tympanic membrane
  - Distinct otalgia (pain clearly referable to the ears) that interferes with normal activities or sleep

TREATMENT

Concerns about increasing rates of antibiotic resistance and lack of sound evidence for antibiotic effectiveness have encouraged a careful look at practice guidelines used in the treatment of AOM. According to clinical practice guidelines published jointly by the American Academy of Pediatrics and the American Academy of Family Physicians,[19] the following recommendations for treatment options were made:
- Observation without the use of antibiotics in uncomplicated AOM
- AOM unresponsive to observation may indicate the need for antibiotics
- Amoxicillin should be prescribed as the drug of choice if antibiotics are necessary
- Consider alternative antibiotic if unresponsive to initial antibiotic therapy (after 48 to 72 hours)

■ Figure 10.16   Classification of otitis media. **A:** Otoscopic examination in acute otitis media reveals infected fluid in the middle ear and a red tympanic membrane. **B:** Otitis media with effusion reveals middle ear fluid with a gray tympanic membrane. **C:** Tympanic membrane perforation reveals a hole in the tympanic membrane with possible fluid in the ear canal. (Assets provided by Anatomical Chart Company.)

Otoscopic view

Acute otitis media
- Infected fluid in middle ear
- Rapid onset and short duration

A

Otitis media with effusion
- Relatively asymptomatic fluid in the middle ear
B • May be acute, subacute, or chronic in nature

Perforation
- A hole in the tympanic membrane caused by chronic negative middle ear pressure, inflammation, or trauma   **C**

⬛ Ménière Disease

Ménière disease is a condition of altered vestibular function. The pathology is targeted to the labyrinth component of the inner ear, causing vertigo, tinnitus, hearing loss, pressure, and pain. Approximately 615,000 individuals are diagnosed with Ménière disease in the United States. Worldwide, the incidence of Ménière disease is estimated to range from 0.5 to 7.5 per 1,000, dependent on the diagnostic criteria applied. Age of onset is usually between 20 and 60 years, and the condition is equally common between genders.[20]

PATHOPHYSIOLOGY

The labyrinth is composed of two parts: the body and membranous components. The increased volume of endolymph (endolymph hydrops) causes dilation of the membranous labyrinth, altering hearing and balance. Rupture of the membranous labyrinth promotes the mixture of endolymph and perilymph, initiating symptoms. Onset and duration of symptoms are unpredictable with debilitating effects. Symptoms can occur as often as daily or as infrequently as yearly.

CLINICAL MANIFESTATIONS

Manifestations of Ménière disease are related to vestibular dysfunction, often unilateral. Severity of symptoms can vary from mild to disabling. Vertigo, a feeling of spinning, is a hallmark of Ménière disease and is often associated with nausea and vomiting. Nystagmus and tinnitus may also develop. A feeling of fullness and pain in the ear and sensorineural hearing loss may also complicate the condition.

DIAGNOSTIC CRITERIA

Auditory examination can provide the specific nature of hearing loss. Responses that measure electrical activity of the auditory nerve and the brainstem help to identify the type of hearing loss. Electrocochleography, a test that records sound-induced electrical activity in the inner ear, assists with diagnosis.

The **glycerol test** may also be used to identify inner ear volume excess typically seen in Ménière disease. A glycerol solution is orally ingested, promoting a condition of dehydration designed to reduce inner ear fluid volume. Serial audiometric testing after the glycerol ingestion shows evidence of improved audiometric score, consistent with the diagnosis of Ménière disease.

TREATMENT

Treatment of Ménière disease is symptomatic. Regulation of body fluid through reduction in salt intake or diuretic therapy, smoking cessation, and stress reduction may reduce symptom occurrence. Antiemetics to prevent nausea and drugs to reduce vertigo are the main pharmacologic treatments. Direct administration of the antibiotic gentamicin into the middle ear promotes ototoxicity, reducing vertigo while maintaining hearing.[21] Vestibular neurectomy, severing of the vestibular nerve, also helps reduce vertigo with no direct effect on hearing.[22] Labyrinthectomy, or surgical removal of the labyrinth, may help reduce vertigo; however, loss of hearing may result.

Macular Degeneration

Degeneration of the central portion of the retinal macula, the fovea, is the central pathology of macular degeneration (MD). Factors contributing to the development of MD include aging, inflammation, injury, and infection. Gene–gene and gene–environment interactions influence susceptibility of MD.[23] According to the American Macular Degeneration Foundation, MD is the leading cause of blindness among older Americans in the United States. Age-specific prevalence rates are comparable between races until age 75, when the prevalence increases significantly among White individuals, according to the National Eye Institute and Prevent Blindness America.

PATHOPHYSIOLOGY

MD can be categorized into two forms: **dry (atrophic) MD** and **wet (exudative) MD**. Most cases of MD are of the dry variety, with retinal deterioration resulting from deposition of **drusen**, small yellow deposits, under the macula next to the basement membrane of the retinal pigment epithelium (Fig. 10.17). Drusen thins and dries out the macula, promoting loss of function. Loss of vision is correlated with increases in drusen deposits.

Wet or exudative MD is caused by the formation of new blood vessels under the retina and macula, known as **choroidal neovascularization**. Choroidal neovascularization may be a compensatory response to poor perfusion of the arteries of the retina because of obstruction. Leakage of fluid and bleeding from these new vessels alter the shape of the macula, distorting central vision. Once choroidal neovascularization occurs in one eye, it will likely develop in the other, especially when the risk factors of more than five large drusen, pigmental clumping, and hypertension are present. The two categories of

From the Lab

Electronystagmography (ENG) is a group of tests that determine vestibular function based on eye movement. Nystagmus and other eye movements provide an evaluation of some brain functions. Eye movements are measured by small electrodes or are recorded by infrared video. Eye movements are evaluated as the eyes follow a target, when the head is positioned in different directions and during the caloric test. The caloric test uses warm and cool water or air irrigation to induce nystagmus, diagnostic of Ménière disease.

choroidal neovascularization include classic and occult:

1. Classic
   a. Well defined
   b. Associated with more leakage than occult
   c. Vision ranges between 20/250 and 20/800
2. Occult
   a. Poorly defined
   b. Associated with less leakage than classic
   c. Vision ranges between 20/80 and 20/200

CLINICAL MANIFESTATIONS

Dry, atrophic MD is characterized by fluctuating vision, difficulty in reading, and limited night vision. The progression of symptoms in the dry form of MD is usually slow. In wet, exudative MD, vision loss may be rapid and severe. Early symptoms are not always apparent, although some affected individuals may report a dark central spot. Consequences of MD include distortion of central vision; decreased ability to read, recognize faces or colors, or drive cars; and blindness.

Risk factors for development of MD include:

1. Age older than 50 years
2. White race
3. Smoking

Drusen
Macula
Optic disk
Hardening
and obstruction
of retinal arteries

■ **Figure 10.17**   Retinal changes in macular degeneration. (Asset provided by Anatomical Chart Company.)

DIAGNOSTIC CRITERIA

Regular eye examinations by an ophthalmologist or an optometrist are important to identify MD early. An examination with an ophthalmoscope can determine if the characteristic changes associated with MD are present. Because symptoms are not always apparent, a thorough eye examination, including dilation of the eyes for visualization of the retina and macula, is necessary in at-risk individuals, especially older adults. Dilation of the eyes and visualization of the retina allow detection of leakage, bulging macula, and drusen deposition. This examination component should complement the routine screening eye examination. If MD is suspected, further evaluation may include:

- Amsler's chart evaluation
  - Uses a grid (10 cm × 10 cm) containing twenty 5-mm squares to a side, with white lines on a black background containing a central black spot
  - Evaluates changes in vision consistent with progressive MD
- Fluorescein angiography
  - Colored dye is injected into a peripheral vein
  - As the dye passes through it, pictures of the retina are taken to detect the presence of abnormal fluid or progressive changes
- Color vision test
  - Determines an individual's ability to distinguish differences in color

TREATMENT

There are currently no treatment options for dry MD. Fortunately, dry MD is a slowly progressive

condition. Treatment of wet MD is targeted toward limiting progression of retinal damage and loss of vision. In wet MD, the goal of therapy is to reduce choroidal neovascularization, reducing lesion size and leakage. Intraocular use of drugs that block vascular endothelial growth factor (VEGF) is the primary pharmacologic treatment effective in blocking the formation of new blood vessels.[24] Laser or conventional photocoagulation can be used to target neovascularization, though reduction in vision is a potential risk. Photodynamic therapy involves irradiation of retinal neovascularization through activation of an injected drug by laser. Visudyne (verteporfin) was approved by the Food and Drug Administration for use in MD in 2000. Efficacy was based on the results of randomized, clinical trials of the efficacy of treatment of the wet form of age-related MD with photodynamic therapy in individuals with classic choroidal neovascularization.[25]

● **STOP** *and* **Consider**

Why do people with macular degeneration have difficulty with night vision and color differentiation?

▧ Glaucoma

Glaucoma is the second leading cause of blindness among the elderly and the leading cause of preventable blindness in the United States. According to the National Eye Institute and Prevent Blindness America, 2.2 million Americans over age 40 (approximately 1.9% of the population) are affected by glaucoma. Prevalence is increased among Blacks, Hispanics, and the elderly. Gender differences are evident—women are affected at increased prevalence rates up through the age of 65 years, after which time rates become comparable. Prevalence rate for White females aged 65 to 69 years is 1.6%, compared with a rate of 4.8% among Black females at the same age. It is often silent, with damage resulting in the absence of warning signs.

PATHOPHYSIOLOGY

Vision loss is the result of damage to the optic nerve. Increased intraocular pressure (IOP) is a risk factor, although glaucoma may be present despite normal IOP. Primary open-angle glaucoma is the most common form of glaucoma (Fig. 10.18). Angle refers to the point where the iris and cornea meet. A chronic disease, primary open-angle glaucoma is likely hereditary. The trabecular network draining the aqueous humor becomes obstructed or "clogged," causing an increase in IOP in most cases. IOP of 22 mmHg or more is considered abnormal, exceeding the expected normal pressure range of 14 to 16 mmHg.

Angle-closure glaucoma, also known as acute or narrow angle, is characterized by a rapid rise in IOP caused by blockage of aqueous humor drainage. This form is more common in people of Asian descent and in people with hyperopia. Angle-closure glaucoma is an inheritable trait. The trabecular network, situated in the angle where the cornea and iris meet, is narrowed, limiting drainage of the aqueous humor. Buildup of fluid and pressure promotes further narrowing of the angle. Complete closure is an acute crisis known as acute glaucoma.

Normal- (or low-) tension glaucoma is characterized by normal IOP and progressive optical nerve damage with loss of visual fields. Approximately, one third of individuals with open-angle glaucoma have normal IOP. The underlying pathology is related to poor blood flow to the optic nerve or increased sensitivity of the retina to ocular pressure (Fig. 10.19). Management is focused on lowering ocular pressure to below "normal" to reduce retinal damage.

CLINICAL MANIFESTATIONS

Risk factors in the development of glaucoma include:

1. Age
2. Black race
3. Diabetes
4. Eye trauma
5. Long-term steroid use

In primary open-angle glaucoma, the cornea adapts to the increasing pressure without swelling, thereby not causing subjective symptoms. If untreated, open-angle glaucoma can result in gradual, but irreversible, loss of vision. Manifestations of vision loss include "blind spots" in the field of vision.

From the Lab

Evaluation of the anterior chamber and angle can be accomplished by gonioscopy. Gonioscopy allows direct visualization of these structures via a special lens containing a mirror, eliminating the view-obstructing effects of the cornea and sclera. Indications for this evaluation include the need to visualize the anterior chamber, determine the angle, and classify glaucoma.

Initially limited to the periphery, central vision is soon affected. This form of glaucoma responds well to pharmacologic management.

An acute episode of angle-closure glaucoma may be induced by increased pupil dilation caused by drugs or by being in a darkened room, such as a movie theater. Symptoms may include eye pain, headache, nausea, blurred vision, and "rainbows" around lights at night. Scarring of the trabecular network may result in chronic glaucoma and cataracts. Damage to the optic nerve may result in permanent loss of vision. Surgical management is often indicated.

Normal optic disk

Optic disk

Central retinal artery and vein

Inferior macular artery and vein

Disk changes

Decreased blood supply to retina

Blood vessels displaced nasally

Enlarged physiologic cup

■ **Figure 10.19** Glaucoma-induced changes in the optic disk. Increased intraocular pressure reduces blood supply to the retina, leading to "blind spots" in the optic disk.

Obstruction distal to anterior chamber angle

■ **Figure 10.18** Open-angle glaucoma. Obstruction of the trabecular network leads to increased intraocular pressure.

DIAGNOSTIC CRITERIA

Early detection of glaucoma may promote effective treatment and management, decreasing associated loss of visual function. Efforts to determine the best screening type and frequency to detect early disease are ongoing. Pattern electroretinogram, electric potential derived from retinal ganglion cells, is used to evaluate IOP lowering after topical treatment in glaucoma patients with early visual field impairment.[26] Function of retinal ganglion cells may be at least partially restored after IOP reduction in early disease.

Screening for glaucoma is completed in at-risk individuals as a component of comprehensive vision screening, usually by optometrists or ophthalmologists. Common screening tests for glaucoma include:

- Tonometry
  - Measure IOP (e.g., the noncontact [air puff] device)
- Ophthalmoscopy
  - Detects changes in the optic nerve (cupping, pallor, hemorrhage) by using an ophthalmoscope in a funduscopic examination
- Perimetry
  - Determines response to visual stimuli at multiple locations in the visual field

TREATMENT

Treatment of glaucoma may be pharmacologic or surgical.

- Pharmacologic
  - Miotics: increase outflow of fluid
  - Epinephrine-based: increase the outflow of fluid
  - Beta blockers: decrease fluid levels
  - Carbonic anhydrase inhibitors: decrease fluid levels
  - Alpha-adrenergic agonists: decrease fluid levels
  - Prostaglandin analogs: increase fluid flow through secondary drainage
- Laser surgery
  - Trabeculoplasty: correction of the trabecular network to promote fluid outflow from the eye in open-angle glaucoma
  - Iridotomy: incision into the iris to promote fluid outflow
  - Cyclophotocoagulation: correction of ciliary tissue to decrease the production of fluid
- Conventional surgery
  - Trabeculectomy: surgical removal of a small portion of the trabecular meshwork under the lid to create new drainage

STOP *and* *Consider*

What are the implications for older Americans who develop glaucoma? What lifestyle changes can they expect to experience?

Retinopathy of Prematurity

Retinopathy of prematurity (ROP) is the leading childhood cause of blindness. As the name implies, infants born prematurely have the highest risk for developing ROP. Premature infants born at or less than 31 weeks gestation and those with low birth weight of less than 1250 gm (2.75 lbs) are at highest risk for the development of ROP. In the United States, it is estimated that of the 10,000 infants born with a birth weight of less than 1250g, 68% of them will develop ROP, with approximately one third progressing to severe ROP and nonreversible loss of vision.[27]

PATHOPHYSIOLOGY

The retina is one of the last organs to develop the vascular blood supply. In fetus, retinal development begins at 16 weeks gestations in a low-oxygen intra-uterine environment and continues until birth. During that period, the retinal blood vessels grow out from the optic nerve toward the periphery, providing the retina with essential oxygen and nutrients. Rapid development of retinal blood vessels occurs in the final 12 weeks of gestation (28 to 40 weeks) and continues for the first few weeks of postnatal life. When delivery occurs early in gestation, retinal blood vessel development is interrupted resulting in the lack of oxygen and nutrient supply to the nonvascularized peripheral retina.

When retinal blood vessel growth is prematurely stopped with early delivery, retinal blood vessel growth is impaired. Further retinal blood vessel development must now occur in the high oxygen extra-uterine environment. As most infants at risk for ROP also have respiratory risks due to inadequately developed lungs, supplemental oxygen is provided to assure adequate ventilation and oxygen delivery to cells and tissues. The result is arrested growth of retinal blood vessels, the first phase of ROP.

The second phase of ROP is characterized by unregulated growth of retinal blood vessels into the vitreous cavity. The release of VEGF and other angiogenic factors promotes excessive growth of abnormal, leaky blood vessels. Hemorrhage and contraction of scarred, fragile blood vessels pulls the retina away, leading to retinal detachment and vision loss.

According to the National Eye Institute, ROP is classified in five stages based on disease severity. The stages are:

- Stage I: mildly abnormal blood vessel growth
- Stage II: moderately abnormal blood vessel growth
- Stage III: severely abnormal blood vessel growth
- Stage IV: partially detached retina
- Stage V: completely detached retina

CLINICAL MANIFESTATIONS

The identification of clinical manifestations is challenging. Among infants at risk for ROP, a thorough ophthalmological examination is necessary to detect the subtle changes associated with ROP. Manifestations of severe ROP may include:

- Leukocoria (white pupils)
- Nystagmus (abnormal eye movements)
- Strabismus (crossed eyes)
- Myopia (severe nearsightedness)

DIAGNOSIS

Ophthalmologic examination targets retinal blood vessels. In mild ROP, there may be evidence of normal growth of retinal blood vessels. Abnormalities of retinal blood vessels are evident in severe cases of ROP and include dilation, tortuosity, and venous congestion of retinal blood vessels. Evidence of scarring and retinal detachment is observed in the most severe stages of ROP.

TREATMENT

The initial lessons about prevention of ROP came as a result of an epidemic that occurred in the 1940s and 1950s. At that time, hospital nurseries began using high concentrations of oxygen to manage the other critical problems of prematurity related to impaired ventilation. It is now recognized that delivery of high concentrations of oxygen to premature infants increases the risk of ROP. That risk for ROP must be balanced with the need to oxygenate other cells and tissues in the premature infant with impaired ventilation. Today, oxygenation of premature infants is monitored to provide concentrations of oxygen that do not exceed what is necessary to support the metabolic requirements of the infant, reducing risk for ROP.

In stages I and II, spontaneous resolution will result in children not requiring treatment. Children with stage I and II disease will likely develop normal vision. In stage III, some infants improve and develop normal vision without treatment. Others with abnormal growth patterns of enlarged or twisted retinal blood vessels require treatment, the stage referred to as stage III plus.

If initiated early, retinal detachment may be prevented. Retinal detachment in stages IV and V requires immediate treatment to increase potential for maximal vision. Treatment of infants with stage III plus through stage V ROP involves invasive surgical intervention on the eye with either laser treatments or cryotherapy (freezing treatment). Later stages of ROP may require other treatments that are targeted toward correction of retinal detachment. Application of a scleral buckle, a silicone band tightened around the eye, reduces traction of the vitreous humor on the retina. The retina can relax onto the wall of the eye. A vitrectomy, replacement of the vitreous humor with saline, may also be done in stage V disease. The removal of retinal scar tissue during the procedure is done to promote flattening of the retina onto the eye wall.

Summary

- Sensory systems relay information from the periphery to the CNS.
- The sensations of pain, touch, pressure, temperature, and proprioception are transmitted by the somatosensory system via specialized receptors and pathways.
- Vision results from light entry through the pupil, stimulating photoreceptors in the retina and generating a nerve impulse. Vision processing occurs in the occipital lobe of the brain, where visual images are coordinated.
- Hearing results from connections between the tympanic membrane and the ossicles, leading to the transduction of the mechanical vibration, producing sound.
- Balance and equilibrium are regulated by the semicircular canals of the ear, generating an impulse, which is then transmitted to the cerebellum via the vestibular branch of the acoustic nerve.
- Pain sensation is generated by stimulation of nociceptors, the impulse transmitted and modulated along pain fibers until it reaches the brain for processing.
- Alterations in vision may result from errors in injury or damage to visual structures, errors in refraction, impaired eye movement, and alterations in protective structures.
- Disorders of hearing are affected by outer, middle, and inner ear structural and functional integrity. Hearing loss may be conductive, sensorineural, mixed, or caused by a central auditory processing disorder.

- Pain can be characterized by location, quality, and duration. Management of pain is reflected by pain characteristics and is based on regulation of impulse inhibition. Options for pain treatment include non-pharmacologic and pharmacologic measures.
- Altered sensory transmission and conduction have implications for all body systems and whole body function. A thorough understanding of the concepts that govern neuronal transmission promotes the ability to apply knowledge in a variety of conditions and pathologies associated with sensory deficit.

Case Study 10.1

A 75-year-old man discusses vision concerns with his ophthalmologist at his yearly visit. After a careful history and physical examination, he is diagnosed with bilateral cataracts.

1. What are the clinical manifestations associated with cataracts?
2. What is the underlying pathophysiology associated with cataracts?
3. How are cataracts diagnosed?
4. What are the possible treatments for cataracts?
5. What are the issues related to appropriate management of cataracts?

Log onto the Internet. Search for a relevant journal article or Web site that details cataract to confirm your predictions.

Practice Exam Questions

1. Which sensory receptor is responsible for impulses resulting in the sensation of touch?
   a. Mechanoreceptor
   b. Chemoreceptor
   c. Nociceptor
   d. Osmoreceptor

2. Which somatosensory neurons are responsible for communication of sensory information from the thalamus to the cerebral cortex and are present in the greatest quantity?
   a. First order   c. Third order
   b. Second order   d. Interneuron

3. The most likely site of pathology leading to alterations in balance is:
   a. The outer ear
   b. The middle ear
   c. The inner ear
   d. The tympanic membrane

4. Which type of pain involves a typical pattern of impulse conduction and originates outside of the nervous system?
   a. Neurogenic   c. Neuropathic
   b. Nociceptive   d. Analgesic

5. Hyperopia is a condition characterized by:
   a. Alterations in eye movement
   b. Infection of the conjunctiva
   c. Increased sensitivity to light
   d. Error in refraction

6. Infection of the middle ear is also known as:
   a. Mastoiditis   c. Otitis media
   b. Vestibulitis   d. Labyrinthitis

7. Sensorineural hearing loss is:
   a. Often permanent, resulting from disease, trauma, or genetic defect
   b. Localized to the middle ear and is often temporary
   c. Caused by alteration in auditory signal processing in the brain
   d. A response to immobility of the tympanic membrane

8. The mechanism of action of opioid analgesics is:
   a. Blockade of serotonin reuptake at the synaptic cleft
   b. Inhibition of cyclooxygenase enzymes and prostaglandin production
   c. Stimulation of large fibers to modulate pain transmission
   d. Modulate pain at the level of the spinal cord by binding to mu, delta, and kappa receptors

9. Which one of the following eye conditions is the result of increased intraocular pressure?
   a. Retinopathy of prematurity
   b. Glaucoma
   c. Wet macular degeneration
   d. Dry macular degeneration

10. Balance and body position are the function of
    a. Utricle
    c. Semicircular canals
    b. Saccule
    d. All of the above

11. Damage to the cochlear hair cells may result in
    a. Hearing loss
    b. Loss of balance
    c. Lack of proprioception
    d. None of the above

12. Fibromyalgia is diagnosed by
    a. Loss of bone mass
    b. Muscle inflammation
    c. Weight loss
    d. Multiple tender points

13. Which of the following is a symptom?
    a. Pain
    b. Hearing loss
    c. Loss of proprioception
    d. None of the above

14. Which of the following reports of pain level (0 to 10) is considered moderate, requiring medications?
    a. 1
    b. 2
    c. 3
    d. 4

15. Neuromatrix pain theory states
    a. Specific stimuli cause predictable pain responses
    b. Specific stimuli results in prevention of impulse crossing in spinal cord
    c. Neural network integration of multiple inputs determines pain perception
    d. Pain perception is determined by duration of impulse and amount of tissue involved

Discussion and Application

1. What did I know about pain and alterations in sensation before today?

2. What body processes are affected by pain and alteration in sensation? How do pain and alteration in sensation affect those processes?

3. What are the potential etiologies for pain and alteration in sensation? How do pain and alteration in sensation develop?

4. Who is most at risk for developing pain and alteration in sensation? How can these alterations be prevented?

5. What are the human differences that affect the etiology, risk, or course of pain and alteration in sensation?

6. What clinical manifestations are expected in the course of pain and alteration in sensation?

7. What special diagnostic tests are useful in determining the diagnosis and course of pain and alteration in sensation?

8. What are the goals of care for individuals with pain and alteration in sensation?

9. How does the concept of pain and alteration in sensation build on what I have learned in the previous chapters and in the previous courses?

10. How can I use what I have learned?

RESOURCES

American Academy of Physical Medicine and Rehabilitation: http://www.aapmr.org/condtreat/pain/paindrawing.htm. (provides information about pain management)

American Macular Degeneration Foundation: http://www.macular.org/disease.html

American Speech, Language and Hearing Association: http://www.asha.org/public/hearing/disorders/types.htm. (provides information on types of hearing loss)

National Eye Institute (NEI): http://www.nei.nih.gov. (conducts and supports research on eye diseases and vision disorders)

National Institute for Deafness and other Communication Disorders (NIDCD): http://www.nidcd.nih.gov/health/hearing/index.asp. (provides information about hearing disorders)

National Institute of Neurologic Disorders and Stroke: http://www.ninds.nih.gov/disorders/chronic_pain/chronic_pain.htm (provides information on chronic pain)

Prevent Blindness America: http://www.preventblindness.org

U.S. Food and Drug Administration, Center for Drug Evaluation and Research: http://www.fda.gov/cder/drug/analgesics/QandAanalgesics.htm. (provides information about over-the-counter analgesics)

REFERENCES

1. Melzack R. Evolution of the neuromatrix theory of pain. The Prithvi Raj Lecture: presented at the Third World Congress of World Institute of Pain, Barcelona 2004. *Pain Pract.* 2005;5(2):85–94.
2. Thompson DG. Utilizing an oral sucrose solution to minimize neonatal pain. *J Spec Pediatr Nurs.* 2005;10(1):3–10.

3. Cohen NL. Cochlear implant candidacy and surgical considerations. *Audiol Neurootol.* 2004;9(4):197–202.

4. Khan S, Edwards L, Langdon D. The cognition and behaviour of children with cochlear implants, children with hearing aids and their hearing peers: a comparison. *Audiol Neurootol.* 2005;10(2):117–126.

5. Mease PJ, Choy EH. Pharmacotherapy of fibromyalgia. *Rheum Dis Clin North Am.* 2009;35:359–372.

6. Bennett RM. Clinical manifestations and diagnosis of fibromyalgia. *Rheum Dis Clin North Am.* 2009;35:215–232.

7. Wolfe F, Smythe HA, Yunus MB, et al. The American College of Rheumatology 1990 criteria for the classification of fibromyalgia. Report of the Multicenter Criteria Committee. *Arthritis Rheum.* 1990;33(2):160–172.

8. Peterson J. Understanding fibromyalgia and its treatment options. *Nurse Pract.* 2005;30(1):48–55.

9. Samborski W, Lezanska-Szpera M, Rybakowski JK. Effects of antidepressant mirtazapine on fibromyalgia symptoms. *Rocz Akad Med Bialymst.* 2004;49:265–269.

10. Patel N, Bigal ME, Kolodner KB, et al. Prevalence and impact of migraine and probable migraine in a health plan. *Neurology.* 2004;63(8):1432–1438.

11. Sprenger T, Goadsby PJ. Migraine pathogenesis and state of pharmacological treatment options. *BMC Med.* 2009;7:71.

12. Chang CL, Donaghy M, Poulter N. Migraine and stroke in young women: case-control study. The World Health Organisation Collaborative Study of Cardiovascular Disease and Steroid Hormone Contraception. *BMJ.* 1999;318(7175):13–18.

13. Scher AI, Terwindt GM, Picavet HS, et al. Cardiovascular risk factors and migraine: the GEM population-based study. *Neurology.* 2005;64(4):614–620.

14. Dodick DW. Review of comorbidities and risk factors for the development of migraine complications (infarct and chronic migraine). *Cephalalgia.* 2009;29(suppl 3):7–14.

15. Cady RK. OnabotulinumtoxinA (botulinum toxin type-A) in the prevention of migraine. *Expert Opin Biol Ther.* 2010;10(2):289–298.

16. Guyuron B, Kriegler JS, Davis J, et al. Comprehensive surgical treatment of migraine headaches. *Plast Reconstr Surg.* 2005;115(1):1–9.

17. Valade D. Early treatment of acute migraine: new evidence of benefits. *Cephalalgia.* 2009;29(suppl 3):15–21.

18. Bluestone CD. Studies in otitis media: Children's Hospital of Pittsburgh-University of Pittsburgh progress report—2004. *Laryngoscope.* 2004;114(11 pt 3 suppl 105):1–26.

19. American Academy of Pediatrics Subcommittee on Management of Acute Otitis Media. Diagnosis and management of acute otitis media. *Pediatrics.* 2004;113(5):1451–1465.

20. da Costa SS, de Sousa LC, Piza MR. Ménière's disease: overview, epidemiology, and natural history. *Otolaryngol Clin North Am.* 2002;35(3):455–495.

21. Perez N, Boleas M, Martin E. Distortion Product otoacoustic emissions after intratympanic gentamicin therapy for unilateral Ménière's disease. *Audiol Neurootol.* 2005;10(2):69–78.

22. Perez R, Ducati A, Garbossa D, et al. Retrosigmoid approach for vestibular neurectomy in Ménière's disease. *Acta Neurochir.* 2005;147(4):401–404.

23. Katta S, Kaur I, Chakrabarti S. The molecular genetic basis of age-related macular degeneration: an overview. *J Genet.* 2009;88(4):425–449.

24. Karagiannis DA, Ladas ID, Parikakis E, et al. Changing from bevacizumab to ranibizumab in age-related macular degeneration. Is it safe? *Clin Interv Aging.* 2009;4:457–461.

25. Photodynamic therapy of subfoveal choroidal neovascularization in age-related macular degeneration with verteporfin: one-year results of 2 randomized clinical trials—TAP report. Treatment of age-related macular degeneration with photodynamic therapy (TAP) study group. *Arch Ophthalmol.* 1999;117(10):1329–1345.

26. Ventura LM, Porciatti V. Restoration of retinal ganglion cell function in early glaucoma after intraocular pressure reduction: a pilot study. *Ophthalmology.* 2005;112(1):20–27.

27. Penn JS, Madan A, Caldwell RB, et al. Vascular endothelial growth factor in eye disease. *Prog Retin Eye Res.* 2008;27(4):331–371.

Chapter 11

Altered Hormonal and Metabolic Regulation

LEARNING OBJECTIVES

1. Define and use the key terms listed in this chapter.
2. Identify features that characterize hormones.
3. Discuss the role of the hypothalamic–pituitary axis in regulating hormone levels.
4. Identify pathways for mediating cell-to-cell communication.
5. Describe the role of the neuroendocrine system in the stress response.
6. Analyze the mechanisms of impairment that can lead to altered hormonal and metabolic regulation.
7. Discuss common measures to diagnose and treat hormone dysfunction.
8. Apply concepts of altered hormonal and metabolic regulation to select clinical models.

INTRODUCTION

Consider the phone calls, texts, e-mails, and instant messages that people send and receive in a day. In each of these communications, there is a sender, a message, a receiver, and (usually) a response. Communication between cells relies upon neuronal and endocrine signals for the regulation of body functions. This chapter reviews basic mechanisms for cell-to-cell communication, particularly as it relates to hormone-driven messages. You are already familiar with this idea through your reading on inflammation (Chapter 3) and altered neurologic function (Chapter 9). This chapter builds on that learning. A basic understanding of communication mechanisms within the body will help to predict the impact of high or low hormone levels on the function of endocrine glands. Clinical models are presented to help understand specific disease conditions affected by hormone alterations.

Function and Regulation of Hormones

Hormones are chemicals, formed originally in tissues or organs, which affect the growth and/or function of other target tissues or organs. The structure of hormones can vary in composition from a single amino acid, such as with thyroid hormone, to a complex of proteins, carbohydrates, or lipids, as occurs with cortisol. Hormones have many important regulatory functions, including energy metabolism, growth and development, muscle and fat distribution, fluid and electrolyte balance, sexual development, and reproduction (Chapter 12). Hormones are also instrumental in the stress response. Table 11.1 outlines the functions specific to select hormones and should be referred to frequently as hormone processes are discussed.

⬤ **STOP** *and Consider*

In Table 11.1, hormones are organized alphabetically. How else could you organize this table? What type of organization is most useful to you as a learner?

◪ Integrating Endocrine, Neuronal, and Defense Mechanisms in the Body

Hormones are commonly connected with the **endocrine system**, a collective group of tissues capable of secreting hormones (Fig. 11.1). The pancreas and thyroid are examples of endocrine glands. Note, however, that endocrine glands are not the only tissues capable of secreting hormones. Neurons can synthesize and release hormones. Neurotransmitters, such as epinephrine, dopamine, serotonin, and norepinephrine, are chemical messengers, synthesized by neurons, which rapidly stimulate a neuronal response. In this regard, neurotransmitters act as hormones (Chapter 9). Inflammatory and immune cells release chemical mediators, such as cytokines, leukotrienes, and prostaglandins, which also function as hormones. The inflammatory and immune responses require these substances to trigger the mechanisms of defense. Some tumor cells also synthesize and release ectopic hormones, which ignore the body's control and feedback mechanisms and ultimately contribute to a loss of homeostasis (Chapter 8).

Like an orchestra, the neurologic, inflammatory, immune and endocrine systems collaborate in a unified symphony. Neurotransmitters act quickly,

whereas endocrine hormones often take days to exert their maximum effect on target tissues. Yet these systems are highly dependent on one another. Regulatory processes integrate with an overall goal of protecting the body from injury and maintaining homeostasis.

◪ Regulating Hormones

Several features are common to all hormones. Each of these features is discussed below:

- *Control:* Hormone synthesis and release is controlled by tissues and organs; the hypothalamic–pituitary axis in the brain is an important control-center for many hormones.
- *Patterns:* Hormones exhibit predictable patterns of secretion, metabolism, and elimination.
- *Feedback:* Hormones listen and adjust based on negative or positive feedback loops.
- *Action:* Hormones exhibit two primary functions: (1) to act on target organs to achieve an effect or (2) to act on glands to produce another hormone.
- *Receptor binding:* To exert an effect, hormones must locate and attach onto target tissues.

THE HYPOTHALAMIC–PITUITARY AXIS

The **hypothalamic–pituitary axis** controls the synthesis and secretion of many hormones. The *hypothalamus* contains neurons that synthesize prolactin, inhibiting hormones, and releasing hormones to act on the anterior pituitary gland. The inhibiting and releasing hormones include:

- Releasing hormones
  - Growth hormone-releasing hormone (GHRH)
  - Thyrotropin-releasing hormone (TRH)
  - Corticotropin-releasing hormone (CRH)
  - Gonadotropin-releasing hormone (GnRH)
- Inhibiting hormones
  - Somatostatin (inhibits growth hormone [GH] and thyroid-stimulating hormone [TSH])
  - Dopamine (inhibits prolactin)

The *pituitary* gland responds to these hypothalamic triggers and acts accordingly. It is important to understand that the pathways and hormones released from the *anterior* pituitary gland are different than the hormones released from the *posterior* pituitary. More specifically, to get from the hypothalamus to the anterior pituitary, prolactin releasing or inhibiting

Table 11.1 Functions of Select Hormones

Hormone	Source	Target	Function
Androgens	Testes	Reproductive organs	Control the development of reproductive organs, (testosterone) sperm production, and secondary sex characteristics and growth in males
Antidiuretic hormone (ADH)	Hypothalamus–posterior pituitary	Kidney	Promotes water reabsorption (retention of fluids)
Adrenocorticotropic hormone (ACTH)	Anterior pituitary	Adrenal cortex	Stimulates release of hormones from the adrenal cortex (primarily aldosterone and cortisol)
Corticotropin-releasing hormone (CRH)	Hypothalamus	Pituitary gland	Controls release of pituitary hormones
Epinephrine and norepinephrine	Adrenal medulla	Sympathetic nervous system	Transmits neural impulses
Estrogen	Ovaries	Reproductive organs	Promotes development of reproductive organs and secondary sex characteristics in women
Follicle-stimulating hormone (FSH)	Anterior pituitary	Reproductive organs	Stimulates growth of ovarian follicle and ovulation in women; stimulates sperm production in men
Glucagon	Pancreatic islet cells	Blood glucose	Stimulates glycogen breakdown in the liver to increase glucose in the blood
Glucocorticoids (cortisol)	Adrenal cortex	Multiple targets	Affects metabolism of all nutrients and growth; regulates blood glucose levels; has anti-inflammatory properties
Gonadotropin-releasing hormone (GnRH)	Hypothalamus	Pituitary gland	Controls release of pituitary hormones
Growth hormone-releasing hormone (GRHR)	Hypothalamus	Pituitary gland	Controls release of pituitary hormones
Growth hormone (GH)	Anterior pituitary	Bone, muscle, organs, and other tissues	Stimulates growth, protein synthesis, and fat metabolism; inhibits carbohydrate metabolism
Insulin	Pancreatic islet cells	Blood glucose	Facilitates glucose transport into the muscle, adipose, or liver cell to use for energy and growth
Luteinizing hormone (LH)	Anterior pituitary	Reproductive organs	Stimulates release of oocyte and production of estrogen and progesterone in women; stimulates secretion of testosterone in men
Mineralocortico-steroids (aldosterone)	Adrenal cortex	Kidney	Increases sodium reabsorption and potassium loss
Oxytocin	Hypothalamus—posterior pituitary	Uterus and breasts	Stimulates contraction of the uterus during labor and milk release from the breasts after childbirth
Parathyroid hormone (PTH)	Parathyroid glands	Bone, blood	Regulates calcium levels in the blood
Progesterone	Ovaries	Reproductive organs	Affects menstrual cycle; increases thickness of uterine wall; supports/maintains pregnancy
Thyroid hormones: triiodothyronine (T_3) and thyroxine (T_4)	Thyroid gland	Multiple targets	Increases metabolic rate, needed for fetal and infant growth and development
Thyrotropin-releasing hormone (TRH)	Hypothalamus	Pituitary gland	Controls release of pituitary hormones
Thyroid-stimulating hormone (TSH)	Anterior pituitary	Thyroid gland	Stimulates synthesis and secretion of thyroid hormones (TH: T_3 and T_4)

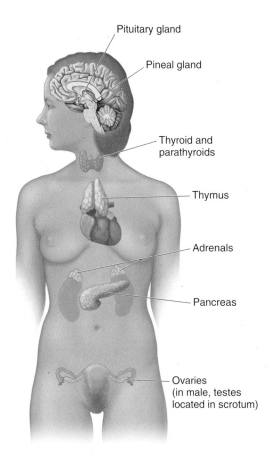

Pituitary gland

Pineal gland

Thyroid and parathyroids

Thymus

Adrenals

Pancreas

Ovaries
(in male, testes
located in scrotum)

■ **Figure 11.1** Organs of the endocrine system. (Asset provided by Anatomical Chart Company.)

Box 11.1 Release of Hormones from the Hypothalamus to the Anterior Pituitary

Action 1:

- The hypothalamus produces the hormone
- The hormone travels to the anterior pituitary
- The hormone is released unchanged into the circulation

Example: prolactin

Action 2:

- The hypothalamus produces a releasing hormone
- The releasing hormone travels to and acts upon the anterior pituitary
- The pituitary is stimulated to produce and release a different hormone into the circulation

Example: growth hormone

Action 3:

- The hypothalamus produces a releasing hormone
- The anterior pituitary is activated to release a stimulating hormone
- The stimulating hormone acts on the gland to produce and secrete a final hormone that is released into the circulation

Example: thyroid hormone

hormones (those listed above) travel through the hypophyseal portal system (blood vessels) to the anterior pituitary gland. Three possible scenarios that characterize release through the anterior pituitary are illustrated in Box 11.1. Each scenario demonstrates increasing complexity in the process and an example is provided. In contrast, the hypothalamus produces antidiuretic hormone (ADH) and oxytocin, which then travel along nerve axons to the posterior pituitary for unchanged release into the systemic circulation. This pathway through the posterior pituitary is not nearly as complicated as the anterior pituitary scenarios.

● STOP *and Consider*

What are the major differences and similarities between the actions of the hypothalamus on the anterior pituitary gland versus the posterior pituitary gland? Why would this difference matter? What is an effective way to remember this difference?

A few hormones are secreted without initiation through the hypothalamus and come directly from

the pituitary. One example is melanocyte-stimulating hormone, which is a hormone that regulates skin pigment. Pathways and actions for select hormones are depicted in Figure 11.2.

FEEDBACK MECHANISMS

What triggers the hypothalamus or pituitary to initiate a hormone release? Multiple mechanisms, such as neurotransmitters, injury and the resulting release of chemical mediators, and neuroendocrine signals, provide input to the hypothalamus to regulate body functions. This most commonly occurs through a **negative feedback loop** (Fig. 11.3). The mechanism of negative feedback has been equated to temperature regulation with the use of a thermostat.[1] When the temperature gets too hot, the thermostat shuts down the heat source; when the temperature is too cool, the furnace is stimulated to release heat. Amazingly, the hypothalamus and pituitary act as sensors that are constantly gauging the levels of hormones in the body. When levels rise above the expected range, the stimulation, production, or secretion of hormone is decreased. When levels fall, stimulation, production, or secretion of hormone is increased. The negative feedback mechanism is affected by environmental and body temperature, stress, nutrition, and the presence of specific body substances. For example, aldosterone levels adjust based on sodium and potassium

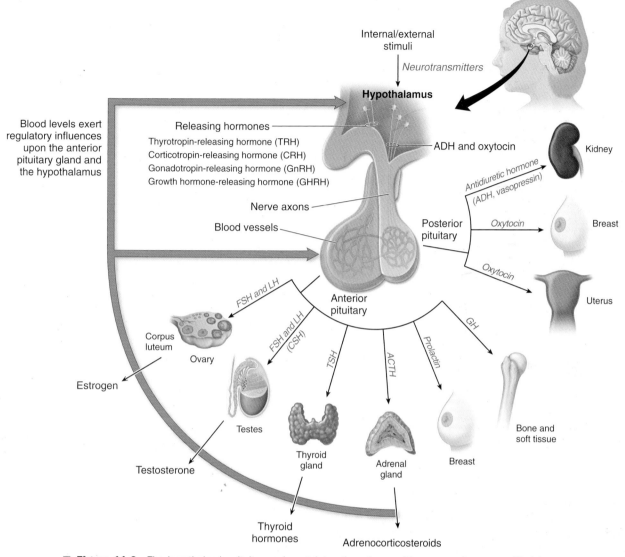

■ **Figure 11.2**   The hypothalamic–pituitary axis regulates the release of hormones. (Image modified from Smeltzer SC, Bare BG. *Textbook of Medical-Surgical Nursing*. 10th ed. Philadelphia: Lippincott Williams & Wilkins; 2003, with permission.)

levels in the body. ADH is responsive to fluid levels in the body.

Although much less common, a few hormones are regulated by a **positive feedback loop**. In positive feedback, presence of the hormone stimulates increased production of the hormone until there is an interruption of the cycle. Oxytocin is one example (Fig. 11.4). Specific feedback mechanisms for each hormone are discussed in depth within the clinical models.

HORMONE SECRETION, METABOLISM, AND ELIMINATION

Many hormones exhibit predictable patterns of secretion. For example, a 28-day cyclic secretion of

estrogens, progesterone, luteinizing, and follicle-stimulating hormones (FSHs) regulates the female menstrual cycle. Some hormones have 24-hour diurnal patterns of secretion. For example, GH levels increase during sleeping hours and decrease during waking hours. Secretion patterns highlight the complex, fluctuant, and responsive nature of hormones.

The accumulation of hormones is prevented through a process of inactivation and elimination. A common mechanism for inactivation is through enzymes that break down the hormone after attaching to the cell receptor and exerting an effect. Some hormones are also inactivated in the liver. Elimination commonly occurs through the urine or along with bile, via the feces.

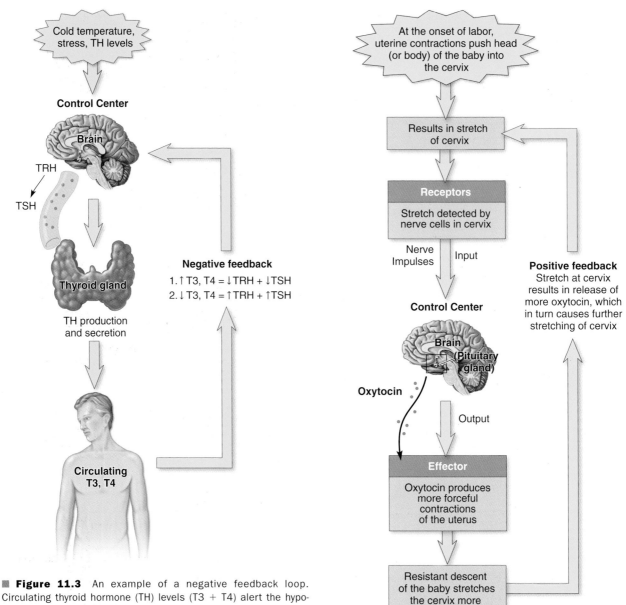

■ **Figure 11.3** An example of a negative feedback loop. Circulating thyroid hormone (TH) levels (T3 + T4) alert the hypothalamus and anterior pituitary to increase or decrease thyrotropin-releasing hormone (TRH) and thyroid-stimulating hormone (TSH) secretion.

■ **Figure 11.4** An example of a positive feedback loop. Oxytocin levels during labor and delivery increase release of additional oxytocin until the birth of the baby decreases stretching of the cervix and the cycle is interrupted. (Image from Premkumar K. *The Massage Connection: Anatomy and Physiology*. Baltimore: Lippincott Williams & Wilkins; 2004, with permission.)

RECEPTOR BINDING

Receptor binding allows hormones to act selectively on certain cells. The number of receptors on each cell can reach up to 100,000 or more. To access the cell, hormones seek out and attach to specific receptors, similar to a key that must fit a certain lock. Hormones can bind to a surface or inner receptor of a cell (Fig. 11.5). A surface receptor requires a second messenger to elicit a response from the cell. Without the appropriate receptor, the hormone moves along and has no impact on that cell. For example, skeletal muscle cells have receptors for GH but are unresponsive to ADH. Receptor binding

is altered when the number of receptors is reduced, as may occur with autoimmune conditions, or when the affinity, or attraction, for the hormone is reduced. The affinity can be reduced by many

■ **Figure 11.5** Two types of hormone-receptor interactions: the surface receptor **(A)** and the intracellular receptor **(B)**. (Image from Porth CM. *Essentials of Pathophysiology: Concepts of Altered Health States*. Philadelphia: Lippincott Williams & Wilkins; 2003, with permission.)

factors such as genetics, hormone levels, and body fluid pH.

Mediating Cell-to-Cell Communication

Five major pathways characterize cell-to-cell communication, where hormones move from production and section, to response (Fig. 11.6):

- *Paracrine pathway:* Hormones are produced in a cell, secreted, and act directly on nearby receptive cells.
- *Autocrine pathway:* The same as the paracrine pathway except that the receptor cells are also secretory cells so, in essence, the cell is able to produce the hormone and exert an effect on itself.
- *Endocrine pathway:* Hormones are produced in a cell, secreted, and travel through blood vessels to distant cells, attach to receptors, and act on that cell.
- *Synaptic pathway:* Hormones are produced in the neuron, secreted, and travel along the axon

■ **Figure 11.6** Hormonal mechanisms of mediating cell-to-cell communication. **A:** Paracrine pathway. **B:** Autocrine pathway. **C:** Endocrine pathway. **D:** Synaptic pathway. **E:** Neuroendocrine pathway.

to the synapse where they are released and taken up by a nearby neuron with the appropriate receptors to exert an effect.

- *Neuroendocrine pathway:* Hormones are produced in a neuron, secreted, travel along the axon to the synapse, are released, are taken up into the vascular system, and travel to distant cells with the appropriate receptors to exert an effect.

Module 2

The Stress Response

Cell-to-cell communication is an integral part of the stress response. **Stress** is the body's reaction to harmful forces (stressors) capable of disturbing homeostasis. An individual's response depends on many factors such as age, general health, type of stressor, the persistence of the stressor, perception of the stressor, social support, and genetic influences. Homeostasis is dependent on an adequate response to stress through mobilizing energy, activating defense mechanisms, and repairing any damage. An inadequate or even excessive response to stress can result in destruction of body tissues. The neuroendocrine response and hormones play a vital role in this process. Figure 11.7 details how the stress response involves neurologic and hormonal influences.

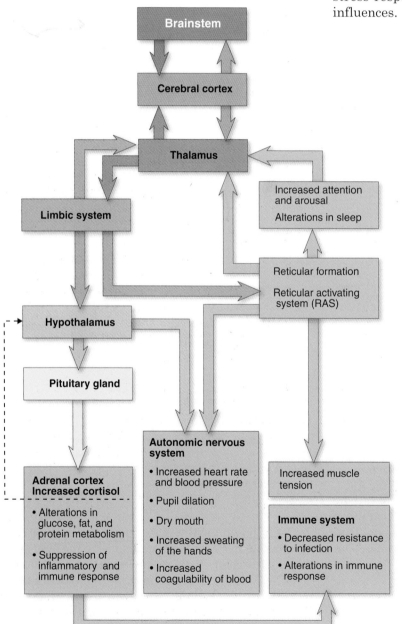

■ **Figure 11.7** Concept map. Stress pathways. The broken line represents negative feedback. (Image modified from Porth CM. *Essentials of Pathophysiology: Concepts of Altered Health States*. Philadelphia: Lippincott Williams & Wilkins; 2003, with permission.)

Neurologic Response to Stress

Neurologic influences, particularly the central nervous system (CNS), are instrumental in the stress response. The brainstem coordinates the performance of the autonomic nervous system, cerebral cortex, limbic system, and hypothalamus and produces norepinephrine so the body can quickly defend against the stressor. Specific structures in the CNS that play a major role include:

- *Autonomic nervous system:* Increases heart rate, blood pressure, respiratory rate, pupil dilation, and sweating. Blood flow is increased to the muscles, heart, and lungs in preparation of "fight or flight." Gastric function decreased to shunt blood to vital organs. Altered blood flow, decreased oxygenation to gastric tissues, and prolonged cortisol exposure may result in "stress ulcers" of the gastrointestinal tract.
- *Cerebral cortex:* Regulates cognitive activities such as intense focus, planning, attention, and persistence.
- *Limbic system:* Regulates emotional activities, such as fear, anxiety, anger, and excitement, and stimulates the reticular activating system.
- *Thalamus:* Intensifies sensory input related to the stressor such as vision, hearing, and smell.

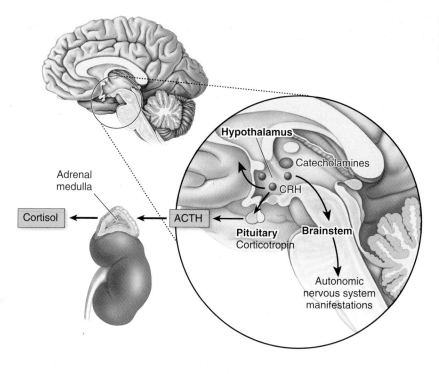

■ **Figure 11.8** Stimulation of cortisol and catecholamines in the stress response. ACTH, adrenocorticotropic hormone; CRH, corticotropin-releasing hormone.

- *Hypothalamus:* Releases hormones to initiate the neuroendocrine response; acts on the autonomic nervous system.
- *Reticular activating system:* Increases alertness and muscle tension and contributes to stimulation of the autonomic nervous system.

Hormonal Response to Stress

Four major hormones or groups of hormones are instrumental in the endocrine response to stress. First, stress stimulates the release of CRH from the hypothalamus. CRH stimulates the pituitary to secrete adrenocorticotropic hormone (ACTH), which in turn stimulates the adrenal glands to secrete cortisol. As depicted in Table 11.1, cortisol is needed to increase metabolism and regulate blood glucose levels for energy and also acts as a potent anti-inflammatory. Second, release of the catecholamines (epinephrine, norepinephrine, and dopamine) is triggered by the sympathetic nervous system, which also acts on the adrenal glands (Fig. 11.8). Catecholamines induce a neurologic response to receptive organs. For example, blood flow is shunted to vital organs such as the heart, brain, and lungs. As a result, heart rate increases, blood pressure increases, respiratory rate increases, and the person becomes much more alert. The skeletal muscles also become activated to allow a rapid escape. Blood is shunted away from the skin and stomach. So, the person will look pale or ashen and digestion is decreased.

● **STOP** *and Consider*

How do you usually respond to stress? Think about the last time you were in a haunted house or were really scared. How did your body respond? How does this correlate to the neuroendocrine response described in this section?

General Adaptation Syndrome

The neuroendocrine response is often initiated by a stressor. **General adaptation syndrome** is a term used to describe this neuroendocrine response and the corresponding physiologic changes. General adaptation syndrome is divided into three major stages: (1) the alarm stage, (2) the resistance stage, and (3) the exhaustion stage.[2] In the alarm stage, catecholamines and cortisol are released in response to stimulation of the sympathetic nervous system, the hypothalamic–pituitary axis, and the adrenal glands. This stage is often referred to as the "fight or flight" stage. These hormones prepare the body for defense against the stressor. In short-term and mild-stress situations, the response may resolve within the alarm stage and may be limited in intensity and duration.

Other hormones are also at play early in the stress response. Suppression of certain hormones, such as GH, thyroid hormone, and the reproductive hormones, is necessary to conserve energy that will be needed to fend off the stressor. ADH is increased to retain fluid, thereby maintaining the blood pressure needed to perfuse vital tissues. Once the stress is resolved, prestress hormone levels are resumed.

Persistent stress is followed by the resistance stage, whereby cortisol levels decrease through negative feedback mechanisms. Excess cortisol is helpful in the early stages of stress to increase metabolism by breaking down proteins, releasing lipids, and increasing circulating glucose. This gives the body energy for fight or flight. However, over time, hypercortisolism is detrimental, leading to exhaustion of inflammatory and immune responses, excessive loss of body proteins and breakdown of tissues, and glucose intolerance. Therefore, cortisol secretion is not an effective method of adapting to prolonged stress. As indicated, some hormone levels are suppressed with stress and remain so during the resistance stage. This also has detrimental effects. Loss of circulating thyroid, growth, and reproductive hormones can have long-term affects on linear growth, metabolism, and reproduction. The persistent increase in ADH through prolonged stress is manifested by excessive fluid retention and subsequent hypertension (high blood pressure).

Chronic overwhelming stress leads to exhaustion. The exhaustion stage is characterized by energy depletion and degeneration of cells, tissues, organs, and organ systems. Severe, prolonged stress contributes to poor health and marks a significant loss to homeostasis.

Module 3

Altered Hormone Function

A number of mechanisms can impact hormones (Box 11.2). Most commonly, hormone excesses or deficits arise from impairment of the endocrine (secreting) gland, lack of hormone synthesis, excessive hormone synthesis, impaired receptor binding, impaired feedback mechanisms, or an altered cellular response to the hormone. Problems with hormone function can manifest through inadequate or excessive production, composition, secretion, receptor binding, uptake, metabolism, or elimination.

Damage to the Hypothalamic–Pituitary Axis

Damage to the hypothalamic–pituitary axis due to infection, inflammation, tumors, degeneration, hypoxia, hemorrhage, or genetic defects can lead to problems with the production and secretion of multiple hormones. Refer to Table 11.1 to review which hormones are synthesized and secreted through the hypothalamic–pituitary axis. **Hypopituitarism** is a generic term indicating decreased secretion of one or more pituitary hormones. Hyperpituitarism is an excess of pituitary hormone secretion. **Panhypopituitarism** indicates a decrease in pituitary hormones. Because the pituitary secretes ACTH, TSH,

Box 11.2 Process of Altering Hormone Function

The following questions address the potential problems that can alter hormone function:

1. Is there impairment of the hypothalamic–pituitary axis?
2. Is there impairment of the endocrine gland?
3. Is there too little or too much hormone that is being produced and secreted?
4. Is the gland producing active hormone?
5. Is receptor binding adequate?
6. Is the target cell responding to the hormone?
7. Is the negative feedback loop impaired?
8. Is hormone being produced ectopically?
9. Is hormone metabolism (inactivation) and elimination impaired?

GH, FSH, luteinizing hormone (LH), and prolactin, damage to the pituitary has a broad range of clinical manifestations related to the loss of thyroid, adrenal, and reproductive glands and problems with growth.

Damage to Endocrine Glands

Destruction of endocrine glands or the lack of active hormone secretion can also lead to problems with target-tissue function. Endocrine glands can be impaired through genetic defects, autoimmune conditions, degeneration, atrophy, infection, inflammation, neoplastic growths, hypoxia, radiation, certain medications, and other types of injuries. The gland becomes incapable of adequately responding to neuroendocrine messages, and hormone secretion is depressed or absent. Excessive stimulation of the endocrine gland can result in hyperplasia and an excessive amount of hormone production and secretion. In some cases, the endocrine gland is functioning appropriately, but the hormone may lack the necessary biologic activity to elicit the cellular response. This often occurs when antibodies destroy biologically active hormone even after the hormone is secreted from the gland.

Damage to Cell Receptors

Receptor binding and cell-to-cell communication is required to elicit a cellular response. Disorders of receptor binding may involve one or more of the following:

1. A decreased number of receptors
2. The lack of receptor sensitivity to the hormone
3. The presence of antibodies that block receptor sites or occupy the receptor site and mimic the hormone
4. The presence of tumor cells with receptor activity that deprives the unaffected cells of the hormone

Impaired receptor binding is manifested through circulating levels of hormones that are incapable of eliciting an appropriate cellular response. Likewise, problems within the cell can lead to impaired cell-to-cell communication and hormone responsiveness. Intracellular disorders involve malfunction of the inner mechanisms of the cell. For example, if hormone mechanisms were a relay race, the baton would have been passed from several runners (the hypothalamus, the pituitary, the secreting gland, the vascular system, and the receptor on the target cell) and then dropped once inside the cell. Intracellular inadequacies most often involve impaired enzyme or protein production or usage within the cell.

Damage to Feedback Mechanisms

Feedback mechanisms may fail to respond to hormone levels and continue to suppress or stimulate hormone production and secretion. This impairment can occur at any point along the hypothalamic–pituitary axis, at the level of the secreting gland, the receptors, or target tissues. Impairment of feedback mechanisms may be a problem of ectopically produced hormone. Some neoplasms are capable of producing and secreting ectopic hormones. The tumor is not part of the negative feedback mechanism and continues to produce and secrete excessive hormones despite high serum levels. Removal of the tumor will often result in resolution of hormone hypersecretion. The most common ectopically produced hormones are ADH and ACTH.

Damage to Metabolism and Elimination Mechanisms

The metabolism (inactivation) and elimination of hormones is essential to maintaining homeostasis. The impaired ability to metabolize or eliminate hormones, such as that which may occur with liver or kidney disease, will result in excess circulating hormone.

General Manifestations of Altered Hormone Function

Hypopituitarism, a deficit of one or more pituitary hormones, usually has a gradual onset, and clinical

From the Lab

Hormone function is measured directly or indirectly. In the past, radioimmunoassay was a common technique used to detect minute quantities of hormones present in the blood. They are not widely used today because of the radioactive waste resulting from such assays. Current detection of hormone activity is now assayed with nonradioactive immunoassays with fluorescence labels, enzymes, and other techniques. Chemiluminescence is one such technique that uses light-producing chemical reactions to detect amounts of hormone in ligand-binder assays.

manifestations are not evident until most of the pituitary gland has been destroyed. The general manifestations are often vague and may include fatigue, weakness, anorexia, sexual dysfunction, growth impairment, dry skin, constipation, and cold intolerance. Hyperpituitarism, an excess of one or more pituitary hormones, also has a wide range of manifestations depending on which hormones are elevated. Table 11.2 details general manifestations of specific hormone excesses and deficits.

Table 11.2 General Manifestations of Select Hormone Excesses and Deficits

Hormone	Excess	Deficit
Antidiuretic hormone	Fluid retention, low urine output, and hyponatremia	Excessive water losses through the urine, leading to nausea, vomiting, fatigue, muscle thirst, dehydration, can progress to shock twitching; can progress to convulsions and death
Glucocorticoids (cortisol)	Truncal obesity, moon face, buffalo hump, glucose intolerance, atrophic skin, striae, osteoporosis, psychological changes, poor wound healing, and increased infections	Hypoglycemia, anorexia, nausea, vomiting, fatigue, weakness, weight loss, and poor stress response
Growth hormone	Before puberty (called gigantism): excessive skeletal growth. After puberty (called acromegaly): bony proliferation of spine, ribs, face, hands, and feet; enlarged tongue, edema, overactive sebaceous glands, coarse skin, and body hair; pain, weakness, and inflammation related to excessive growth; hypertension and left heart failure may also occur	Short stature, obesity, immature facial features, delayed puberty, hypoglycemia, and seizures in children; obesity, insulin resistance, and high circulating lipids in adults
Mineralocorticoids (aldosterone)	Hypertension, hypokalemia, hypernatremia, muscle weakness, fatigue, polyuria, polydipsia, and metabolic alkalosis	Weakness, nausea, anorexia, hyponatremia, hyperkalemia, dehydration, hypotension, shock, and death
Thyroid hormone	Hypermetabolism, weight loss, diarrhea, exophthalmos, anxiety, and goiter	Hypometabolism, weight gain, constipation, goiter, dry skin, and coarse hair
Parathyroid hormone	Hypercalcemia, excessive osteoclastic activity and bone resorption, pathologic fractures, and formation of renal calculi	Hypocalcemia, muscle spasms, hyperreflexia, seizures, and bone deformities

Diagnosing and Treating Altered Hormone Function

Diagnosing alterations in hormonal or metabolic function begins with a complete patient history and physical examination and often relies on measuring hormone levels or other indicators in the blood or urine. Hormone suppression or stimulation tests can be used to detect hormone responses. Because secretion rates can fluctuate over time, urine hormone levels are often collected over a 24-hour period. Serum electrolyte, glucose, calcium, and other lab tests may provide indirect information on hormone functioning. Imaging studies, such as computed tomography or magnetic resonance

imaging scans, may be needed to locate a tumor that could be suppressing or stimulating hormone secretion. Genetic testing may also be needed to identify a genetic alteration that is affecting hormone function.

Treating hormone alterations varies depending on the cause. Hormone elevations require eliminating the excess hormone. This often occurs by removing tumors that may be secreting ectopic hormone, removing all or part of the corresponding endocrine gland, or administering medications that block the effects of the hormone. Low hormone levels often require lifelong replacement through exogenous medication administration.

Module 4

Clinical Models

The following clinical models have been selected to aid in the understanding and application of altered hormonal processes and effects. The structure, function,

and altered function of the reproductive organs and the endocrine pancreas have been reserved for Chapters 12 and 18, respectively.

Hypothalamus

Serum osmolality

Blood volume

Posterior pituitary

Thirst

Secretion of ADH

Water Ingestion

Reabsorption of water by the kidney

Extracellular water volume

■ **Figure 11.9** Pathways for regulation of extracellular fluid volume by thirst and antidiuretic hormone. ADH, antidiuretic hormone. (Image modified from Porth CM. *Essentials of Pathophysiology: Concepts of Altered Health States*. Philadelphia: Lippincott Williams & Wilkins; 2003, with permission.)

Antidiuretic Hormone Function

ADH is produced in the hypothalamus, travels to the posterior pituitary, and is released into the circulation. ADH controls fluid balance by regulating reabsorption of water by the kidneys (Fig. 11.9). Secretion rates of ADH are based on serum osmolality and extracellular fluid volume. The hypothalamus senses changes in serum osmolality and alters secretion of ADH. Similarly, sensors in the blood vessels recognize changes in blood volume and can affect ADH secretion. High levels of ADH stimulate water retention; low levels of ADH trigger water loss through urination.

Syndrome of Inappropriate Antidiuretic Hormone

The **syndrome of inappropriate antidiuretic hormone (SIADH)** is a condition of excessive production and release of ADH despite changes in serum osmolality and blood volume. Although ADH levels can transiently increase with certain medications and stressful stimuli, such as trauma, exposure to temperature extremes, pain conditions, surgery, or infection, the diagnosis of SIADH is typically reserved for those without such stimuli to explain excessive ADH release. The most common cause of

SIADH is a tumor, somewhere in the body, which is secreting ectopic ADH.

PATHOPHYSIOLOGY

ADH promotes water retention by increasing the permeability of the nephrons in the kidneys. Most of the body water accumulates intracellularly and alters cell function. The CNS is most sensitive to these changes. Because water initially accumulates intracellularly, edema or fluid overload in the vascular system is uncommon. The excess circulating fluid within cells increases total body water concentration and eventually dilutes the sodium concentration in the extracellular space.

CLINICAL MANIFESTATIONS

Clinical manifestations are related to hypotonic hyponatremia and include a decreased and concentrated urine output. The severity of symptoms depends on the serum sodium level and the rate of onset. Significant symptoms usually do not manifest until serum sodium is less than 115 to 120 mEq/L. A more rapid onset of hyponatremia leads to greater severity of symptoms. Initially, these symptoms include anorexia, nausea, vomiting, headache, irritability, disorientation, muscle cramps, and weakness. As the serum sodium level drops below 110 mEq/L, additional symptoms emerge, including psychosis, gait disturbances, seizures, or coma.

DIAGNOSTIC CRITERIA

Diagnosis is based on the following clinical and laboratory findings:

- Hyponatremia (serum sodium less than 135 mEq/L)
- Hypotonicity (plasma osmolality less than 280 mOsm/kg)
- Decreased urine volume
- Highly concentrated urine with a high sodium content
- Absence of renal, adrenal, or thyroid abnormalities

TREATMENT

Treatment focuses on removing the cause of SIADH if possible. For patients with mild symptoms of hyponatremia, water restriction is often the only necessary therapy. Severe hyponatremia generally requires isotonic or hypertonic saline administered intravenously. Hypertonic intravenous (IV) solutions are reserved for those individuals with severe hyponatremia who display alterations in mental status. Medications may be administered to block the effects of ADH or to increase urine output if removing the cause is not feasible.

Diabetes Insipidus

Diabetes insipidus (DI) is a condition of insufficient ADH that results in the inability of the body to concentrate or retain water (Fig. 11.10). Three major causes of DI include:

- Insufficient production of ADH by the hypothalamus or ineffective secretion by the posterior pituitary

- Inadequate kidney response to the presence of ADH, also called nephrogenic DI
- Ingestion of extremely large volumes of fluids and decreasing ADH levels; water intoxication can sometimes be attributed to a psychiatric disturbance

PATHOPHYSIOLOGY

Impairment of hypothalamic osmoreceptors after trauma or surgery to a region at or near the hypothalamus is the most common cause. Nephrogenic DI can be observed in those with chronic renal insufficiency, lithium (a drug used to treat manic-depressive disorder) toxicity, hypercalcemia, hypokalemia, or with disease of the renal tubules. Rarely, nephrogenic DI is inherited as an X-linked disorder.

● **STOP** *and* **Consider**

What effect do you think that drinking alcohol has on ADH levels?

CLINICAL MANIFESTATIONS

Manifestations depend on the severity of DI. Loss of ADH or inadequate kidney response to ADH results in **polyuria** (large volume urine output) and excessive thirst. The urine is highly dilute with a low specific gravity. Loss of fluids leads to serum hyperosmolality and severe dehydration. Shock and death can occur if untreated.

DIAGNOSTIC CRITERIA

Diagnosis is made through a careful patient history and physical examination. The patient history often includes recent surgery to remove a tumor of the brain, or other cranial surgery, or head trauma. The physical examination may detect signs of dehydration and possibly an enlargement of the bladder due to constant overfilling. Laboratory measurement of serum solute concentration, ADH levels, and urine-specific gravity is used to confirm the diagnosis. A urine specific gravity of 1.005 or less and a urine osmolality less than 200 mOsm/kg are often found in DI.

TREATMENT

Except for those without access to water, most patients can drink enough fluid to replace urine losses. Hydration is an important aspect of treatment. In some cases, particularly in those with inadequate thirst, IV hydration with a hypotonic solution

Figure 11.10 The mechanism of diabetes insipidus. ADH, antidiuretic hormone. (Image modified from Rubin E, Farber JL. *Pathology*. 4th ed. Philadelphia: Lippincott Williams & Wilkins; 2005, with permission.)

is required. Pharmacologic treatment may include the use of desmopressin (DDAVP), a synthetic vasopressin analogue, which acts as a potent antidiuretic. If the cause cannot be corrected, this drug may be required for the individual's lifetime.

Thyroid Hormone Function

The production of thyroid hormone is a multistep process. TRH from the hypothalamus triggers the release of TSH from the anterior pituitary, which in turn stimulates the production and release of the thyroid hormones from the thyroid gland (see Fig. 11.3). The thyroid hormones are produced in the follicular (epithelial) cells of the thyroid. The follicles use iodide from dietary intake of iodized salt, combine this with tyrosine (an amino acid) and secrete this combination into the central colloid portion of the follicle to form the thyroid hormones: tetraiodothyronine (T_4), also referred to as thyroxine, and triiodothyronine (T_3). When needed, T_3 and T_4 are reabsorbed into the follicular cells and then released into the circulation. T_4 is reduced by deiodination in the peripheral tissues to T_3, the active form of the hormone. Circulating thyroid hormone provides feedback to the hypothalamus and pituitary gland. TSH is suppressed or activated depending on circulating thyroid hormone levels. Stress and cold environmental temperatures also act to stimulate thyroid hormone production.

⬤ **STOP** *and* **Consider**

What would happen if you had a diet that did not include iodized salt?

Thyroid hormone has an impact throughtout the body and plays a critical role in stimulating metabolism. Other functions include facilitating the breakdown of carbohydrates, proteins, and fats for energy, stimulating heat and glucose production, producing structural proteins, enzymes, and other hormones, and promoting growth and development in children. As a result of thyroid hormone release, there is:

- Increased glucose absorption
- Release of lipids from adipose tissue
- Metabolism of proteins from muscle tissue
- Increased cholesterol breakdown in the liver
- Increased production of metabolic by-products
- Increased oxygen consumption
- Increased body heat production
- Increased cardiac output
- Increased gastric motility
- Increased muscle tone and reactivity
- Increased activation of cognitive processes

Hyperthyroidism

Hyperthyroidism is a state of excessive thyroid hormone. Hyperthyroidism can result from excessive stimulation to the thyroid gland, diseases of the thyroid gland, or excess production of TSH by a pituitary adenoma. Certain medications contain large amounts of iodine, such as cough expectorants, health food supplements that contain seaweed, and iodinated contrast dyes, which can induce hyperthyroidism in thyroid-sensitive individuals.

PATHOPHYSIOLOGY

Graves disease, an excessive stimulation of the thyroid gland, is the most common cause of hyperthyroidism and is the most common autoimmune condition in the United States. Women are 7 to 10 times more likely to develop Graves disease than are men.[3] As with many autoimmune conditions, the triggering event is often unknown; genetic (e.g., family history or gender) and environmental (e.g., stress or smoking) factors are implicated. In Graves disease, IgG antibodies bind to the TSH receptor on thyrocytes (thyroid cells) and stimulate excessive thyroid hormone secretion, causing a state of **thyrotoxicosis**. Chronic thyrotoxicosis can be complicated by progressive thyroid failure and result in hypothyroidism. The thyroid gland undergoes hyperplasia due to excessive stimulation. **Thyrotoxic crisis**, or thyroid storm, is a sudden, severe worsening of hyperthyroidism that may result in death.

CLINICAL MANIFESTATIONS

Major clinical manifestations are related to enlargement of the thyroid gland and the excessive metabolic rate of the body (Fig. 11.11). Weight loss, agitation, restlessness, sweating, heat intolerance, diarrhea, tachycardia, palpitations, tremors, fine hair, oily skin, irregular menstrual cycle in women, and weakness are common findings. The development of a **goiter** (enlargement of the thyroid gland) may occur because of follicular epithelial cell hyperplasia. **Exophthalmos** (a protrusion of the eyeballs) is also characteristic of Graves disease. This protrusion is usually bilateral and results from the interaction of TSH-sensitized antibodies interacting with fibroblast antigens found in extraocular muscles and tissues. The interaction results in lymphocyte infiltration, edema, and fibroblast accumulation, which displaces the eyeballs forward. Exophthalmos often persists despite treatment of hyperthyroidism.

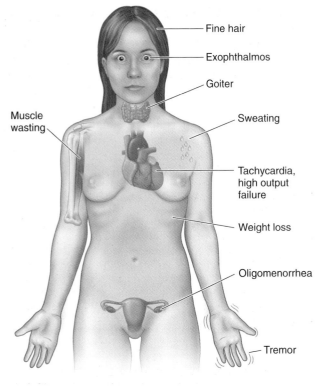

Fine hair

Exophthalmos

Goiter

Muscle wasting

Sweating

Tachycardia, high output failure

Weight loss

Oligomenorrhea

Tremor

■ **Figure 11.11**   Major clinical manifestations of Graves disease.

DIAGNOSTIC CRITERIA

Diagnosis of Graves disease is based on the patient history and physical examination; common clinical manifestations are noted. The patient history may be significant for a family history of autoimmune disease, thyroid disease, or emigration from an iodine-deficient location. The physical examination often

TSH levels are greatly suppressed. This is caused by the negative feedback loop, which communicates high thyroid hormone levels to the hypothalamic–pituitary axis and causes suppression of TSH. Laboratory studies may also reveal elevated serum levels of T_3 and T_4. Increased uptake of radioactive iodine by the thyroid gland confirms the diagnosis.

TREATMENT

Treatment measures are based on reducing thyroid hormone levels often through gland destruction via radioactive iodine, medications that block thyroid hormone production, or, less commonly, surgical removal of all or part of the gland. Full ablation (removal) of the thyroid gland requires lifelong supplementation with oral thyroid hormone replacement therapy.

▨ Hypothyroidism

Hypothyroidism is a state of deficient thyroid hormone. Hypothyroidism can be congenital or acquired. Congenital hypothyroidism occurs during fetal development and results in a lack of thyroid gland development, a lack of appropriate synthesis of thyroid hormone, or problems with TSH secretion. In utero, maternal T_4 crosses the placenta; therefore, the newborn appears unaffected at birth. If the child is untreated after birth, the lack of thyroid hormone production and secretion results in mental retardation and impaired growth, a condition referred to as **cretinism**. Neonatal screening, when instituted, detects congenital hypothyroidism, allowing treatment with thyroid hormone replacement to be initiated.

reveals an enlarged and slightly firm thyroid gland as well as protrusion of the eyes. Measurement of serum TSH level is a useful screening test for the presence of hyperthyroidism; however, the diagnosis of hyperthyroidism must be confirmed by the measurement of serum-free thyroxine.[4] In thyrotoxicosis,

PATHOPHYSIOLOGY

Acquired hypothyroidism can result from (1) deficient thyroid hormone synthesis, (2) destruction of the thyroid gland, or (3) impaired TSH or TRH secretion. Common causes of acquired hypothyroidism include autoimmunity, iodine deficiency, surgical removal of or radiation therapy to the thyroid gland, medications that destroy the thyroid gland, and genetic defects that affect the thyroid hormones. Autoimmune processes attack the thyroid gland or may block the TSH or the TSH receptor without activating the thyroid gland, as in hyperthyroidism. Hashimoto thyroiditis is an autoimmune

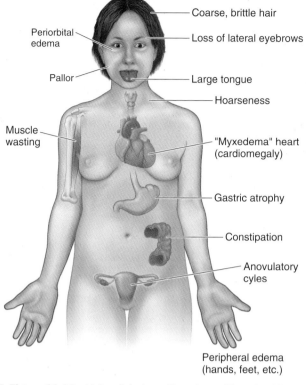

Coarse, brittle hair

Loss of lateral eyebrows

Periorbital edema

Pallor

Large tongue

Hoarseness

Muscle wasting

"Myxedema" heart (cardiomegaly)

Gastric atrophy

Constipation

Anovulatory cyles

Peripheral edema (hands, feet, etc.)

■ **Figure 11.12** Major clinical manifestations of hypothyroidism.

hypothyroidism that can result in total destruction of the thyroid gland. This condition affects women up to 10 times more frequently than men.[3]

CLINICAL MANIFESTATIONS

Clinical manifestations are often gradual and include fatigue, cold intolerance, weakness, weight gain, dry skin, coarse hair, constipation, lethargy, impaired reproduction, and impaired memory (Fig. 11.12). Goiter may also be present in hypothyroidism as the gland enlarges in an effort to increase function. Dietary iodine deficiency, excess, or the use of medications that suppress thyroid hormones can stimulate the development of hypothyroid goiter. **Myxedema** is a unique characteristic finding of hypothyroidism. Protein–carbohydrate complexes accumulate in the extracellular matrix drawing water into the tissues, resulting in boggy, nonpitting, edematous tissues, especially of the face and mucous membranes, hands, and feet.

DIAGNOSTIC CRITERIA

Diagnosis of hypothyroidism is based on patient history and physical examination, during which

characteristic clinical manifestations are noted. Laboratory studies include the sensitive TSH assay, free T_4, total T_4, and T_3 uptake, thyroid autoantibodies, and antithyroglobulin tests to confirm the diagnosis and provide evidence as to causality. Serum thyroid hormones may be decreased, and TSH is often elevated.

TREATMENT

Treatment focuses on replacing the deficient hormone with the goals of normalization of TSH, T_4, and T_3 levels, along with alleviation of the clinical signs and symptoms. Lifelong thyroid hormone replacement therapy is initiated and increased gradually until optimal hormone levels and clinical improvement are achieved. The most common drug used to treat hypothyroidism is levothyroxine (Synthroid, Levoxyl). Levothyroxine is a synthetic form of T_4.

Adrenal Hormone Function

The adrenal glands are located at the apex of the kidneys and contain two distinct parts: (1) an outer adrenal cortex and (2) an inner adrenal medulla (Fig. 11.13). The adrenal hormones play a critical role in the stress response. The adrenal medulla secretes epinephrine and norepinephrine. Table 11.3 illustrates the three categories and functions of steroid hormones secreted by the adrenal cortex.

STOP *and* *Consider*

Would loss of the adrenal cortex or the adrenal medulla be more problematic?

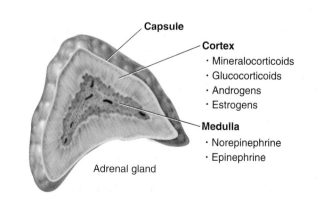

Capsule

Cortex
· Mineralocorticoids
· Glucocorticoids
· Androgens
· Estrogens

Medulla
· Norepinephrine
· Epinephrine

Adrenal gland

■ **Figure 11.13** Hormone secretion from the adrenal cortex and adrenal medulla.

Table 11.3 Categories of Steroid Hormones Secreted by the Adrenal Cortex

Category	Major Example	Functions
Mineralocorticoids	*Aldosterone* (secretion stimulated by the renin-angiotensin system and serum potassium levels)	Regulates sodium and potassium levels; regulates water balance and blood pressure
Glucocorticoids	*Cortisol* (secretion stimulated by corticotropin-releasing hormone from the hypothalamus and adrenocorticotropic hormone from the anterior pituitary)	Regulates metabolism, inflammatory/immune responses, and the stress response
Adrenal sex	*Androgens* (secretion; see *Cortisol*)	Contribute to pubic and axillary hair growth hormones in women; minimally impact sexual function

Adrenal Cortical Excess: Cushing Syndrome

Cushing syndrome refers to a condition of excess glucocorticoids secreted from the adrenal cortex. **Cushing disease** is hypercortisolism specifically related to pituitary cortisol-producing tumors. Women are five times more likely than men to develop Cushing disease. Glucocorticoids contribute to metabolic function, the inflammatory and immune responses, and the stress response. More specifically, glucocorticoids function to:

- Stimulate glucose production
- Decrease tissue glucose utilization
- Increase breakdown and circulation of plasma proteins
- Increase mobilization of fats
- Prevent the release of chemical mediators that trigger the inflammatory response
- Decrease capillary permeability and inhibit edema formation
- Inhibit the immune response
- Inhibit bone formation
- Stimulate gastric acid secretions
- Contribute to emotional behavior
- Contribute to an effective stress response

PATHOPHYSIOLOGY

Four major processes can lead to Cushing syndrome:

1. Long-term administration of corticosteroid medications (such as prednisone)
2. Tumors of the pituitary gland that stimulate excess ACTH production
3. Tumors of the adrenal gland that stimulate excess cortisol production
4. Ectopic production of ACTH or CRH from a tumor at a distant site, such as small cell carcinoma of the lung

Long-term administration of corticosteroid medications is indicated for a wide variety of chronic inflammatory and autoimmune conditions. Exogenous corticosteroids suppress the inflammatory and immune responses and can decrease the deleterious effects of chronic inflammation. Long-term use of these medications will result in suppression of cortisol production by the adrenal cortex and should not be discontinued abruptly.

● **STOP** *and Consider*

You are on a 1-week hiking trip and one of your friends forgets her glucocorticoid medication that she takes for severe asthma. Should she go back and get the medication or is she OK without it for that week?

Excessive ACTH production, through pituitary or ectopic tumors, overstimulates the adrenal cortex. This results in adrenal hyperplasia and excess cortisol production. This form of hypercortisolism depends on ACTH, and reduction of cortisol levels may require removal of the ACTH-secreting tumor or CRH-secreting tumor if this is stimulating the excess ACTH production. Adrenal tumors, however, hypersecrete cortisol directly and are not directed by ACTH.

● **STOP** *and Consider*

Map out how the negative feedback loop is impacted by an ACTH-dependent hypercortisolism versus a non–ACTH-dependent hypercortisolism.

CLINICAL MANIFESTATIONS

Excess secretion of glucocorticoids can result in metabolic alterations, excessive circulating glucose and subsequent glucose intolerance, suppression of the inflammatory and immune responses, behavioral changes, and an impaired stress response. Mobilization of fats and changes in fat metabolism leads to obesity of the trunk, face, and upper back. Obesity of the face and posterior neck and back have been characterized by the terms "moon face" and "buffalo hump" (Fig. 11.14). Striae, or stretch marks, can develop from truncal obesity. Protein degradation results in extremity weakness and muscle wasting. The skin becomes atrophic and thin. Bones exhibit osteoporosis. Suppression of the inflammatory and immune responses leads to increased infections, skin ulcerations, and poor wound healing. Glucose intolerance, from excess circulating glucose and loss of tissue utilization, can lead to diabetes mellitus. Changes in behavior can range from euphoria to minor emotional disturbances to psychosis.

Stimulation of the adrenal cortex to overproduce cortisol can also stimulate the production of the other adrenal cortex hormones, primarily androgens and aldosterone. Clinical manifestations can reflect elevations of these hormones. Excess aldosterone results in hypertension and hypokalemia. Excess androgens can result in **hirsutism**, the development of excessive body and facial hair, or changes in patterns of pubic and axillary hair growth (primarily in women).

DIAGNOSTIC CRITERIA

Diagnosis of Cushing syndrome is often based on a 24-hour urine collection during which elevations in cortisol excretion are noted. False-positive tests may result in those with obesity, alcoholism, chronic renal failure, anorexia, or bulimia, because these also raise cortisol secretion. Imaging studies are needed to locate tumors that may be secreting excess ACTH or cortisol.

TREATMENT

Treatment is focused on removing the cause of excess hormone production. Surgery or radiation may be needed to remove tumors. Corticosteroid medications may be needed to avert an adrenal crisis during acute illness and then they must be gradually withdrawn.

STOP *and Consider*

How would a deficiency of cortisol present in terms of clinical manifestations?

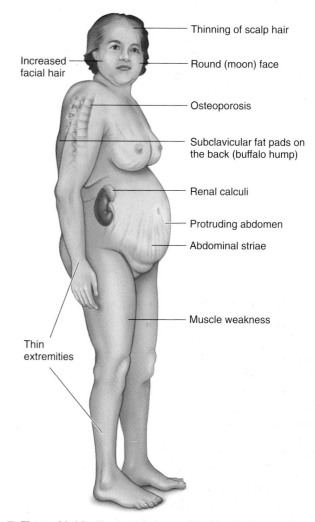

■ **Figure 11.14**   Dominant features of Cushing syndrome.

Labels on figure:
- Thinning of scalp hair
- Increased facial hair
- Round (moon) face
- Osteoporosis
- Subclavicular fat pads on the back (buffalo hump)
- Renal calculi
- Protruding abdomen
- Abdominal striae
- Muscle weakness
- Thin extremities

Research Notes

Scientists have noted that somewhere between 5 and 13% of cases of hypertension are caused by abnormally high aldosterone levels. Research continues to explore the long-term effects of excess aldosterone, particularly on cardiovascular function. Improved treatment of hypertension may rely on blocking aldosterone when indicated, preventing hypertension, and limiting harmful cardiovascular effects of hyperaldosteronism. The high prevalence of hypertension in Black individuals may be explained, in part, by the role of aldosterone in maintaining the antioxidant–oxidant balance. Aldosterone decreases the activity of the enzyme glucose-6-phosphate dehydrogenase (G-6-PD). This enzyme has a role in antioxidant defenses. A deficiency of G-6-PD is seen in 10 to 15% of Black people, perhaps related to high aldosterone levels. This may also explain the levels of high blood pressure in this population.[6]

▨ Adrenal Cortical Insufficiency: Addison Disease

Acute ACTH deficiency is considered one of the most serious endocrine disorders because it can lead to severe hypotension, shock, and death. Adrenal cortical insufficiency can result from lack of CRH or ACTH, or lack of secretion of hormones from the adrenal cortex.

PATHOPHYSIOLOGY

Lack of ACTH production from the pituitary is most often caused by destruction of the pituitary gland from tumors, hemorrhage, trauma, radiation, or surgical removal. Adrenal cortical insufficiency can also result from lack of hormones secreted from the adrenal cortex. Autoimmune destruction of the layers of the adrenal cortex is the most common cause of **Addison disease**. This destruction leads to the inability of the adrenal gland to produce any glucocorticoids, mineralocorticoids, or androgens. As a result, ACTH levels are elevated to increase the secretion of these three major steroid hormones from the adrenal glands.

CLINICAL MANIFESTATIONS

Clinical manifestations are based on insufficient levels of the steroid hormones as depicted in Table 11.4. Elevations in ACTH levels stimulate skin melanocytes, resulting in a characteristic hyperpigmentation, or darkening, of the skin and mucous membranes.

DIAGNOSTIC CRITERIA

Diagnosis of Addison disease is based on the clinical presentation and laboratory analysis of electrolyte levels demonstrating hyponatremia and hyperkalemia. Serum corticosteroid levels can also be measured, and results will show corticosteroid levels that remain depressed after administration of ACTH.

TREATMENT

In acute illness, isotonic IV fluid replacement is infused along with hydrocortisone sodium succinate or phosphate. Improvement in blood pressure should occur within 4 to 6 hours. Gradually, the IV infusion

Table 11.4 Clinical Manifestations of Addison Disease

Deficient Hormones	Clinical Manifestations
Glucocorticoids	Hypoglycemia, weakness, poor stress response, fatigue, anorexia, nausea, vomiting, weight loss, and personality changes
Mineralocorticoids	Dehydration, hyponatremia, hyperkalemia, hypotension, weakness, fatigue, and shock
Androgens	Sparse axillary and pubic hair in women

of hydrocortisone is tapered and oral replacement of glucocorticoid and mineralocorticoid hormones ensues for the remainder of the individual's life. Because of elevations in sodium excretion, salt intake may need to be increased in hot weather. The exception to this is for those patients with Addison disease caused by tuberculosis. The tuberculosis bacteria can also destroy the adrenal gland. Treatment of the bacteria with antibiotics is required, and adrenal function resumes without lifelong glucocorticoid and mineralocorticoid replacement.

▨ Summary

- Hormone messengers have many important regulatory functions, including energy metabolism, growth and development, muscle and fat distribution, fluid and electrolyte balance, sexual development, and reproduction.
- Hormones are instrumental in the stress response and are essential for maintaining homeostasis.
- The initiation of hormone secretion and regulation for many hormones relies on neuronal control through the hypothalamic–pituitary axis, receptor binding, intracellular communication, and feedback mechanisms.
- Functional deficits usually arise from impairment of the endocrine (secreting) gland, lack of or excessive hormone synthesis, impaired receptor binding, impaired feedback mechanisms, or an altered cellular response to the hormone.
- Problems with hormone function can manifest through inadequate or excessive production, composition, secretion, receptor binding, uptake, metabolism, or elimination of hormones.
- The general manifestations of hypopituitarism are often vague and may include fatigue, weakness, anorexia, sexual dysfunction, growth impairment, dry skin, constipation, and cold intolerance; likewise, hyperpituitarism also has a wide range of manifestations depending on which hormones are elevated.
- Diagnosing alterations in hormonal or metabolic function begins with a complete patient history and physical examination and often relies on measuring hormone levels or other indicators in the blood or urine; imaging studies, such as CT or MRI scans, may be needed to locate a tumor that could be suppressing or stimulating hormone secretion. Genetic testing may also be needed to identify a genetic alteration that is affecting hormone function.
- Treating hormone alterations varies depending on the cause; hormone deficits often require exogenous replacement and hormone elevations require eliminating the excess hormone. This often occurs by removing tumors that may be secreting ectopic hormone, removing all or part of the corresponding

endocrine gland, or administering medications that block the effects of the hormone.

Case Study 11.1

J.W. is a 43-year-old male who was diagnosed with a somatotrope adenoma. Somatotropes are pituitary cells that secrete growth hormone. As a result, he is diagnosed with **acromegaly**, or an excess of growth hormone that occurs after puberty.

1. *Outline the process that is most likely occurring in this man's body.*
2. *What hormone is altered?*
3. *What would you expect for clinical manifestations?*
4. *What diagnostic tests could be used?*
5. *What treatment measures would you anticipate?*

Log on to the Internet. Search for a relevant journal article or Web site (such as http://www.emedicine.com/med/topic27.htm) that details acromegaly to confirm your predictions.

Case Study 11.2

J.W. in the first case study has noticed that his child is quite a bit shorter than the other kids of his age. P.W., now 2 years old, was of normal birth length. Over time, though, he has not kept up with the linear growth of other children of his age. He appears to learn new things without difficulty but is overweight and has immature facial features. He does have a history of hypoglycemia and seizures. He is diagnosed with congenital growth hormone deficiency.

1. *Outline the process that is most likely occurring in this child's body.*
2. *What hormone is altered?*
3. *What would you expect for clinical manifestations?*
4. *What diagnostic tests could be used?*
5. *What treatment measures would you anticipate?*

Log on to the Internet. Search for a relevant journal article or Web site that details congenital growth hormone deficiency to confirm your predictions.

Practice Exam Questions

1. Which of the following is *not* a major role of hormones?
   a. Growth stimulation
   b. Erythrocyte synthesis
   c. Fluid balance and regulation
   d. Metabolic rate regulation

2. The release of hormones from glands is most often controlled by:
   a. Negative feedback mechanisms
   b. Nephrogenic mechanisms
   c. Ectopic hormone production
   d. Active transport

3. The most common cause of endocrine disorders is:
   a. Surgical removal of endocrine glands
   b. Infection
   c. Adenomas
   d. Immunodeficiency

4. Excess cortisol is represented by which condition?
   a. Addison disease
   b. Cushing syndrome
   c. Diabetes insipidus
   d. Hyperthyroidism

5. Diabetes insipidus, if left untreated, will rapidly develop into:
   a. Malignant hypertension
   b. Diabetic coma

   c. Dehydration
   d. Metabolic alkalosis

6. A patient is asked to collect a 24-hour urine test to check a hormone level. Why is the 24-hour urine needed?
   a. To measure female reproductive hormone levels
   b. To obtain a measurement of hormone secretion over time
   c. It is easier than obtaining a blood sample
   d. Urine is not an effective method of measuring hormone levels

7. You are experiencing constipation, dry skin, weight gain, and cold intolerance. Which condition are you most likely experiencing?
   a. Hyperthyroidism
   b. Addison disease
   c. Cushing syndrome
   d. Hypothyroidism

8. Which of the following occurs with elevated levels of cortisol?
   a. Fatty acids are mobilized
   b. Glucose levels are suppressed
   c. Plasma protein levels increase
   d. Inflammation increases

9. Which type of hormone is not produced in the adrenal cortex?
   a. Mineralcorticoids
   b. Glucocorticoids
   c. Adrenal sex hormones
   d. Neurotransmitters

10. Diagnosis of SIADH is based on which of the following?
    a. Hyponatremia
    b. Hypertonicity
    c. Increased urine volume
    d. Dilute urine with a low sodium content

Discussion and Application

1. What did I know about altered hormonal and metabolic regulation prior to today?

2. What body processes are affected by altered hormonal and metabolic regulation? What are the expected functions of those processes? How does altered hormonal and metabolic regulation affect those processes?

3. What are the potential etiologies for altered hormonal and metabolic regulation? How does altered hormonal and metabolic regulation develop?

4. Who is most at risk for developing altered hormonal and metabolic regulation? How can altered hormonal and metabolic regulation be prevented?

5. What are the human differences that affect the etiology, risk, or course of altered hormonal and metabolic regulation?

6. What clinical manifestations are expected in the course of altered hormonal and metabolic regulation?

7. What special diagnostic tests help determine the diagnosis and course of altered hormonal and metabolic regulation?

8. What are the goals of care for individuals who have altered hormonal and metabolic regulation?

9. How does the concept of altered hormonal and metabolic regulation build on what I have learned in the previous chapters and in previous courses?

10. How can I use what I have learned?

RESOURCES

The Hormone Foundation is a public affiliate of the endocrine society. The Hormone Foundation is dedicated to serving as a resource for the public by promoting the prevention, treatment, and cures for hormone-related conditions. The Web site can be accessed at:
http://www.hormone.org/

REFERENCES

1. Porth C. *Essentials of Pathophysiology: Concepts of Altered Health States*. Baltimore: Lippincott Williams & Wilkins; 2004.
2. Selye H. *The Stress of Life*. New York: McGraw-Hill; 1976.
3. Rubin E, Gorstein F, Rubin R, et al. *Rubin's Pathology: Clinicopathologic Foundations of Medicine*. 4th ed. Baltimore: Lippincott Williams & Wilkins; 2005.
4. Weetman A. Graves' disease. *N Engl J Med*. 2000;343:1236–1248.
5. Gussekloo J, vanExel E, deCraen A, et al. Thyroid status, disability and cognitive function, and survival in old age. *JAMA*. 2004;292:2591–2599.
6. Mikta M. Scientists probe aldosterone's role in hypertension and heart disease. *JAMA*. 2004;292:2704–2705.

Chapter 12

Altered Reproductive Function

LEARNING OBJECTIVES

1. Define and use the key terms listed in this chapter.
2. Identify structures and processes required for effective reproductive function.
3. Analyze the mechanisms of impairment that can lead to altered reproductive function.
4. Discuss common measures to diagnose and treat altered reproductive function.
5. Apply concepts of altered reproductive function to select clinical models.

INTRODUCTION

Consider the complexity of creating a new human being. Reproductive function is reliant upon structural integrity, neurologic, and hormonal processes of males and females. Both are needed and they must work together in order to be successful. This chapter focuses on structural and functional expectations in order to reproduce and processes that can alter reproductive function.

Module 1

Function and Regulation of Reproduction

▨ Female Reproductive Hormone Function

Structural integrity is required to achieve reproduction. For females, this includes the external genitalia and internal reproductive structures. External genitalia features the mons pubis, labia majora, vestibule, Bartholin glands, labia minora, clitoris, Skene glands at the urethral opening, and the vaginal orifice (Fig. 12.1). The primary purpose of external structures is protection and lubrication. The clitoris, analogous to the male penis, is highly sensitive and distends during sexual stimulation.

Internal reproductive structures include the vagina, uterus, fallopian tubes, and ovaries, located in the pelvic cavity (Fig. 12.2). The vagina is needed as an outlet for menses and other secretions and also serves the function of sexual fulfillment and entry for sperm from the male penis. The cervix forms the inlet to the uterus. Secretions from the cervix offer some protection from infection and allow increased or decreased receptivity

to sperm depending on hormone influences. The uterus, a muscular organ, has three layers, an inner endometrium, a middle myometrium, and an outer perimetrium. The functional layer of the endometrium proliferates as the uterine lining builds and sloughs as menses each month. The muscular myometrium contracts to expel menses and in uterine contractions during childbirth. Fallopian tubes extend from the uterus to a funnel-shaped opening with finger-like projections toward the ovaries to attract the ovum (Fig. 12.3). The fallopian tubes form an important connective passageway for the ova and sperm. The almond-shaped ovaries have four parts:

- Stroma, the supporting tissue
- Interstitial cells, which secrete estrogen
- Follicles, which contain the ova (germ cells)
- Corpus luteum, forms after the ovum has been released from the ovarian follicle

Led by the hypothalamus, pituitary, and ovaries, hormonal processes are also needed to facilitate reproduction (Fig. 12.4). The ovaries produce the female sex hormones: estrogens, progesterone, and androgens. These hormones are secreted in a monthly cyclical pattern under the direction of the hypothalamus (gonadotropin-releasing hormone [GnRH]) and the anterior pituitary (follicle-stimulating hormone [FSH], luteinizing hormone [LH]).

If pregnancy occurs, three additional hormones come into play. Human chorionic gonadotropin (hCG) appears within 2 to 3 days after the zygote implants into the endometrium. hCG is produced by the zygote and acts on the corpus luteum to maintain its estrogen and progesterone-secreting function. Home pregnancy tests measure the presence of hCG in the urine. The anterior pituitary also secretes prolactin during and after pregnancy to allow lactation to occur. Oxytocin is a hormone secreted from the posterior pituitary that stimulates contractions during labor and milk ejection during lactation.

As indicated, the interstitial cells of the ovary secrete estrogens. The estrogens (estradiol, estrone, and estriol) are the primary female sex hormones. These are secreted throughout the monthly menstrual cycle and dominate from the end of menses to ovulation. The major actions of the estrogens include:

- Female reproductive organ development
- Female body fat contour distribution

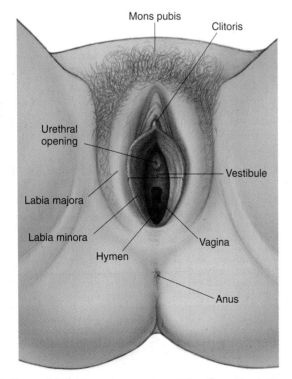

■ **Figure 12.1** Female external genitalia. (From Westheimer R, Lopater S. *Human Sexuality.* Baltimore: Lippincott Williams & Wilkins; 2003, with permission.)

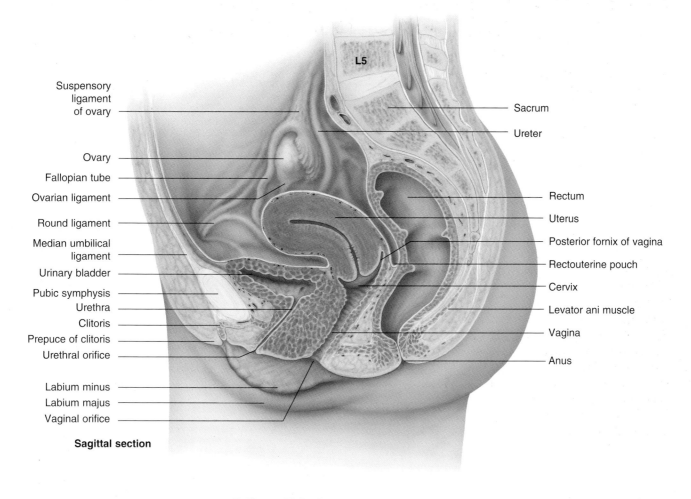

Suspensory ligament of ovary

Ovary

Fallopian tube

Ovarian ligament

Round ligament

Median umbilical ligament

Urinary bladder

Pubic symphysis

Urethra

Clitoris

Prepuce of clitoris

Urethral orifice

Labium minus

Labium majus

Vaginal orifice

Sagittal section

L5

Sacrum

Ureter

Rectum

Uterus

Posterior fornix of vagina

Rectouterine pouch

Cervix

Levator ani muscle

Vagina

Anus

■ **Figure 12.2** Female reproductive structures.

- Breast development and skeletal growth during puberty
- Ovulation and support of pregnancy and lactation
- Cervical mucus alterations (copious, thin, watery, and more receptive to sperm)
- Axillary and pubic hair growth
- Female skin maintenance
- Decreased bone resorption; maintenance of bone integrity
- Retention of sodium and water

Progesterone is another important female sex hormone, secreted in large amounts from ovulation to the onset of menstruation. The corpus luteum of the ovary secretes progesterone and estrogen. Progesterone thickens the lining of the uterus to support implantation and nourishes the embryo in early pregnancy. Progesterone also helps to maintain the pregnancy by relaxing smooth muscles in the uterus to avoid expulsion of

the embryo. Progesterone elevates the core body temperature slightly and can induce nausea, headaches, constipation, indigestion, and swelling in pregnancy.

Ovulation is the process of releasing an oocyte from an ovarian follicle. Ovulation occurs once every 21 to 40 days for most women (the average is approximately 28 days). Ovulation relies on hormone regulation and is typically divided into two parts: (1) the follicular phase in the first half of the ovulatory cycle and (2) the luteal phase in the second half of the ovulatory cycle (Fig. 12.5). Follicles are epithelial capsules that hold oocytes. Follicles are further distinguished as primary and secondary follicles. Primary follicles are inactive. During each ovulatory cycle, approximately 10 primary follicles are stimulated by FSH and LH and become secondary, or active, follicles.

During the follicular phase, secondary follicles enlarge, further develop, and become capable of

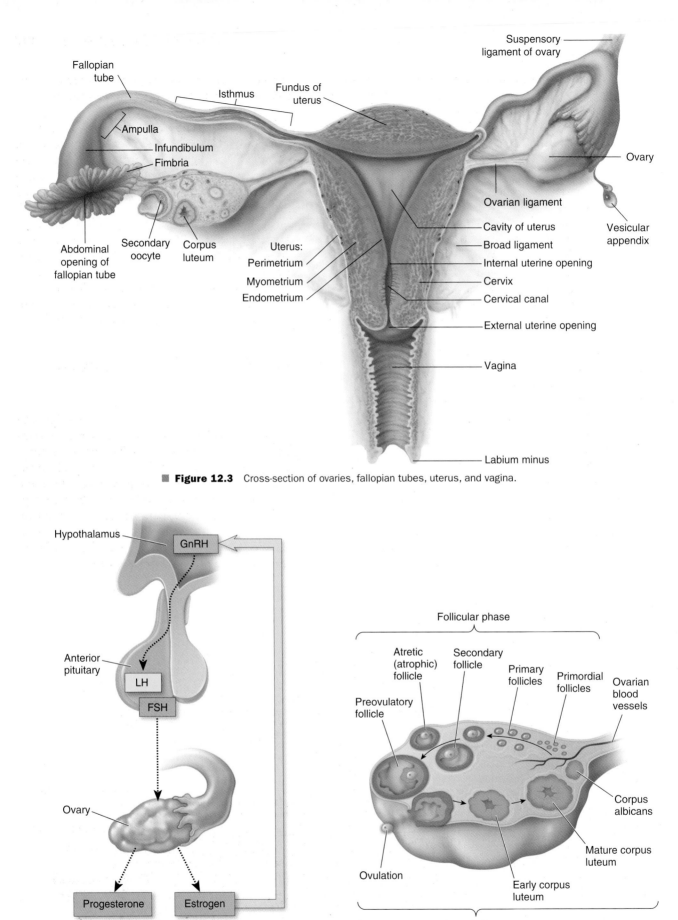

Figure 12.3 Cross-section of ovaries, fallopian tubes, uterus, and vagina.

Figure 12.4 Feedback regulation of ovarian function. FSH, follicle-stimulating hormone; GnRH, gonadotropin-releasing hormone; LH, luteinizing hormone. (Image modified from Premkumar K. *The Massage Connection: Anatomy and Physiology*. Baltimore: Lippincott Williams & Wilkins; 2004, with permission.)

Figure 12.5 Sequence of ovulatory events showing ovarian follicle origin, growth, and rupture and the formation and degradation of the corpus luteum. The atretic (atrophic) follicle was one that did not fully mature.

secreting estrogen and progesterone. In a process that is not completely understood, one of these follicles becomes dominant by secreting large amounts of estrogen, and the remaining follicles subsequently become **atretic** (atrophic). The dominant follicle continues to secrete estrogen, which alerts the pituitary to decrease FSH. LH levels remain elevated and then surge at the peak of estrogen secretion from the dominant follicle, causing the oocyte to break through the fluid-filled follicle. This is the point of ovulation.

The ruptured follicle forms a corpus luteum in the luteal phase of ovulation. The corpus luteum secretes large amounts of progesterone and estrogen. If pregnancy occurs, the progesterone from the corpus luteum hormonally supports the pregnancy until the placenta has developed (approximately 12 weeks). If pregnancy does not occur, progesterone and estrogen levels drop within about 14 days after ovulation and menstruation begins.

Corresponding to the ovulatory cycle is the growth of the endometrium, or lining of the uterus (Fig. 12.6). The growth of the endometrium, also under the direction of hormones, allows zygote implantation and nourishment. Endometrial growth is divided into three phases:

- *Proliferative* (end of menstruation to ovulation) phase: At the end of menstruation the endometrium is thin. Estrogen acts to support growth (proliferation) of the superficial layer of the endometrium. The endometrium

thickness increases to six to eight times greater than that found at the end of menstruation.

- *Secretory* (ovulation to the beginning of menstruation) phase: Progesterone, in addition to estrogen, further supports proliferation of the endometrium. The lining becomes thick, vascular, and swollen. The fertilized ovum can embed into this thick lining.

- *Menstrual* phase: In the absence of fertilization of the ovum, the corpus luteum becomes useless. Disintegration of the corpus luteum results in cessation of estrogen and progesterone production from these cells. This leads to shedding of the superficial endometrial layer, which is also called the menstrual period.

Male Reproductive Hormone Function

The male reproductive organs and tissues include the testes, epididymis, vas deferens, seminal vesicles, prostate, and penis (Fig. 12.7). The male genitourinary system is responsible for urine elimination, sexual function, and reproduction. Androgens, the male sex hormones, promote metabolism and growth. The pattern of male sex hormone secretion does not follow a cyclical pattern as seen with females; the hormone secretion rates remain fairly constant throughout the male's adult life.

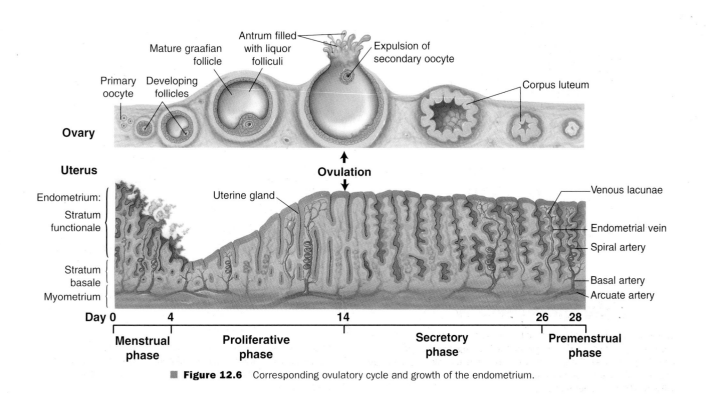

Figure 12.6 Corresponding ovulatory cycle and growth of the endometrium.

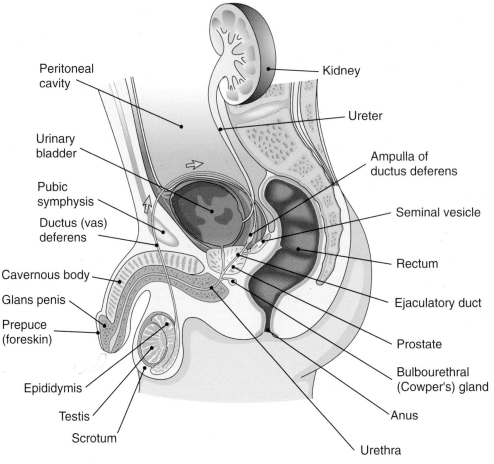

Peritoneal cavity

Kidney

Urinary bladder

Ureter

Pubic symphysis

Ampulla of ductus deferens

Ductus (vas) deferens

Seminal vesicle

Cavernous body

Rectum

Glans penis

Ejaculatory duct

Prepuce (foreskin)

Prostate

Epididymis

Bulbourethral (Cowper's) gland

Testis

Anus

Scrotum

Urethra

■ **Figure 12.7**   Male reproductive structures.

Stimulation of androgen production and release begins in the hypothalamus (Fig. 12.8). The hypothalamus releases GnRH, which stimulates the anterior pituitary to release LH and FSH. LH acts on the Leydig cells in the testes to produce testosterone, the primary male sex hormone. Testosterone has multiple effects, including:

- Development and function of male reproductive organs
- Sperm production and maturation
- Protein metabolism
- Muscle mass promotion
- Skin thickness promotion
- Sebaceous gland activity
- Growth of pubic, chest, and facial hair
- Maturation of the larynx resulting in a deeper voice tone

Excess testosterone levels alert the hypothalamus to decrease secretion of GnRH and the pituitary to decrease production of LH.

The second major sex hormone secreted from the pituitary is FSH. When gonadotropin (FSH, LH) levels increase, FSH acts on the Sertoli cells within the seminiferous tubules to secrete inhibin, a hormone that alerts the pituitary to suppress secretion of the gonadotropins. Sertoli cells also play a role in spermatogenesis.

Spermatogenesis occurs in the seminiferous tubules of the testes. Spermatozoa are released from the epithelial lining of the tubules into the lumen. Sertoli cells play an active role in releasing sperm into the lumen. Spermatogenesis requires a 2 to 3° cooler scrotal temperature than that found with the core body temperature. Failure of the testes to descend into the scrotum or excessive heat to the scrotum, such as occurs when sitting in a hot tub, can impair spermatogenesis. Testosterone production is not affected by temperature. Maturation of the sperm takes place within approximately 60 days. Spermatozoa then transit to the epididymis (the reservoir), then eventually to the vas deferens, and then exit the body through the urethra (Fig. 12.9). The accessory glands, seminal vesicles, prostate, and Cowper's glands facilitate the transport of spermatozoa during the ejaculatory process and aid in spermatozoa survival.

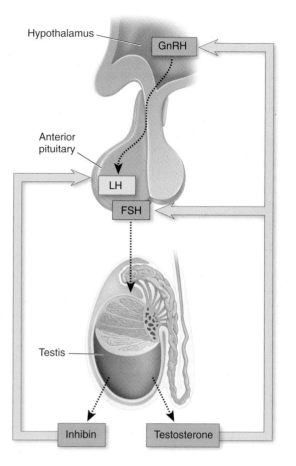

Figure 12.8 Feedback regulation of testicular function. FSH, follicle-stimulating hormone; GnRH, gonadotropin-releasing hormone; LH, luteinizing hormone. (Image modified from Premkumar K. *The Massage Connection: Anatomy and Physiology*. Baltimore: Lippincott Williams & Wilkins; 2004, with permission.)

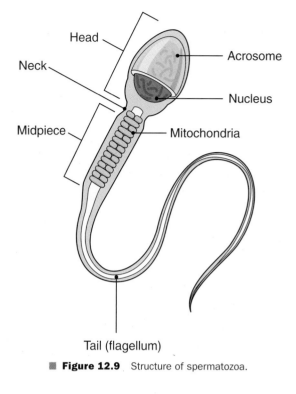

Figure 12.9 Structure of spermatozoa.

Module 2

Altered Reproductive Function

Achieving pregnancy is a complex interaction of ovulation, spermatogenesis, intercourse, ejaculation, conception, implantation, and embryo growth. Infertility, defined as the inability to achieve pregnancy after 1 year of unprotected intercourse, can result from problems in any of these steps. About 10% to 15% of couples are considered infertile. In many cases, the exact cause of infertility is not identified.

Altered reproduction can result from a functional impairment in the male or female partner, or both. Figure 12.10 illustrates causes of acquired infertility impacting females. Factors involved with altered reproduction may include:

- *Hormonal* imbalance causing the absence of, or infrequent, ovulation, which impairs oocyte development and release; testosterone losses result in impaired sperm production.
- *Motility* impairment caused by adhesions or obstruction in the pathway from the cervix to the ovary, which results in problems with oocyte or sperm transit and block the joining of these cells. Examples include inhospitable cervical mucus that blocks sperm from entering the uterus or previous or current infection that results in adhesions and obstruction of reproductive structures. **Leiomyomas**, fibrous tumors that may form in the uterus, distorts the endometrial cavity.
- *Immune* problems caused by antibodies to the male sperm, which quickly destroy sperm, rendering it unable to reach the oocyte.

Figure 12.10   Causes of acquired infertility in females. (Image from Rubin E, Farber JL. *Pathology*. 3rd ed. Philadelphia: Lippincott Williams & Wilkins; 1999, with permission.)

General Manifestations of Altered Reproductive Function

The inability to conceive and maintain pregnancy is a universal clinical manifestation. In many cases, particularly in men, there are no individual clinical manifestations. With hormone alterations, irregular menstrual periods or **amenorrhea** (absent menstrual periods) may be reported. This often signifies **anovulation**, the absence of ovulation manifested by the excess or deficit of one or more reproductive hormones. Amenorrhea can also result from pregnancy, emotional stress, or prolonged strenuous exercise. With the exception of pregnancy-induced amenorrhea, absent menstrual periods is often the result of CNS alterations that affect the release of GnRH from the hypothalamus and therefore suppress or overstimulate the production of reproductive hormones. For example, a pituitary adenoma may induce hyperprolactinemia, a condition that results in anovulation and subsequently produces amenorrhea.

Pain is another possible clinical manifestation. Testicular/scrotal pain in men or pelvic pain in women may occur with infection or inflammation

of reproductive structures. **Dysmenorrhea**, or severe pain with menstrual periods, **dyspareunia**, or pain with intercourse, and other forms of pelvic pain, may be present with infections or structural problems in women. **Endometriosis**, a condition involving endometrial tissue that is located outside of the uterus, can result in pelvic adhesions, distortion of pelvic structures, and dysmenorrhea (Fig. 12.11).

Diagnosing and Treating Altered Reproductive Function

The diagnosis of altered reproduction is based on the couple's inability to conceive or the presence of clinical manifestations described above. Determining the cause requires a systematic history, physical examination, and specialized diagnostic tests. Initially, a semen analysis must be completed in the male along with an analysis of ovulation in the female. Determination of ovulation can involve observing for cervical mucus changes at the time of ovulation, measuring the basal body temperature over 2 to 3 months, noting the 0.5°F increase at the

■ **Figure 12.11** Endometriosis implants on the ovary appear as red-blue nodules. (Image from Rubin E, Farber JL. *Pathology*. 3rd ed. Philadelphia: Lippincott Williams & Wilkins; 1999, with permission.)

time of ovulation as progesterone levels rise, or using a home ovulation predictor kit, which measures the LH surge just prior to ovulation. Patency of the reproductive structures can be visualized using hysterosalpingography (Fig. 12.12). This procedure involves injecting a radiopaque material into the uterus and fallopian tubes, then using a fluoroscope and radiograph to determine the presence of obstructions through the reproductive pathway. Laparoscopy, a scope placed through an incision in the abdomen, can view peritoneal and abdominal structures outside of the uterus and fallopian tubes.

General treatment involves supportive counseling, education about intercourse frequency, avoidance of lubricants that can act as a spermicide, and basic health maintenance. Focused treatment is aimed at the cause, if identified. Sexually transmitted or other pelvic infections place the female at high risk for infertility and must be treated quickly and completely. Obstructive processes, such as leiomyomas, endometriosis, or pelvic adhesions, may require surgical intervention. Ovulatory failure requires a determination of the endocrine problem and a corresponding treatment. Some individuals may require clomiphene citrate, a medication that induces ovulation. In those with hyperprolactinemia, medications may be needed to reduce prolactin and therefore induce ovulation. Artificial

■ **Figure 12.12** Anteroposterior radiograph of the female pelvis after injection of radiopaque compound into the uterine cavity (hysterosalpingogram). (From Snell RS. *Clinical Anatomy*. 7th ed. Lippincott Williams & Wilkins; 2003, with permission.)

insemination may be used to inject sperm into the uterus if cervical mucus is thick or if the sperm quantity or quality is compromised. Some couples seek advanced reproductive technologies such as in vitro fertilization. The evaluation and treatment of infertility is highly complex and emotionally charged. Sensitivity to the range and intensity of emotions is an important aspect of care.

Module 3

Clinical Models

Pelvic Inflammatory Disease

Pelvic inflammatory disease (PID) is the result of a sexually transmitted infection of the reproductive tract (Fig. 12.13). The most frequent cause is a combination of sexually transmitted microorganisms including *Chlamydia trachomatis* and *Neisseria gonorrhoeae*. In women, sexual intercourse propels microorganisms into the vagina where the infection then ascends to the cervix, uterus, fallopian tubes, ovaries, and even into the peritoneal cavity.

PATHOPHYSIOLOGY

After attaching to the epithelial cells lining the reproductive tract, the offending microorganisms elicit acute inflammatory and immune responses. The reproductive tract becomes hyperemic and edematous. The fallopian tubes become obstructed with purulent exudate. Repeated or chronic infection results in scar formation. This scarring is particularly problematic in the fallopian tubes and ovaries, where ovulation and free movement of the ovum to the uterus is prohibited. Ectopic pregnancy, tubo-ovarian abscess, pelvic adhesions, and infertility are potential complications of PID. In the male reproductive tract, sexually transmitted infections can result in a similar problem in the urethra, epididymis, and testes.

CLINICAL MANIFESTATIONS

Early infection is often asymptomatic, increasing the likelihood of transmission to others. As the infection ascends and the inflammatory and immune responses become more intensified, common clinical

Figure 12.13 Clinical manifestations and complications of pelvic inflammatory disease.

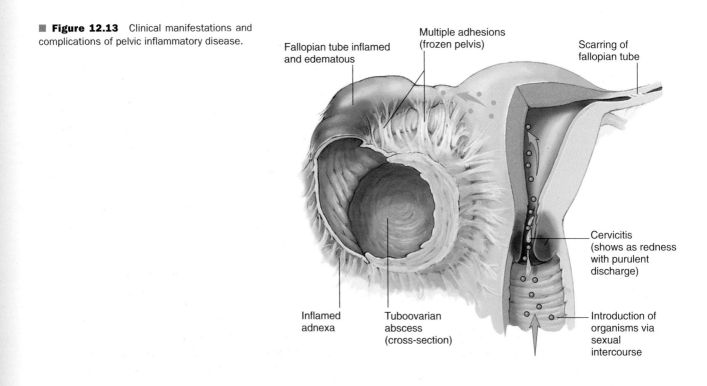

manifestations include pelvic and lower abdominal pain, purulent cervical discharge, cervical tenderness, fever, and malaise.

DIAGNOSTIC CRITERIA

Diagnosis of PID is based on history, physical examination, and laboratory studies. The minimum criteria for the diagnosis of PID include lower abdominal tenderness on palpation, adnexal (tissues supporting the uterus) tenderness, and cervical motion tenderness. Cervicitis and a purulent discharge from the cervix may be visualized during pelvic examination. The presence of fever, elevation in the erythrocyte sedimentation rate or C-reactive protein (nonspecific tests of inflammation), and positive bacterial cultures of infected genitourinary secretions provide additional clues for diagnosis. Laparoscopy may be used to confirm the diagnosis as needed.

TREATMENT

Treatment of PID requires an immediate and often prolonged course of oral or intravenous antibiotics. Hospitalization with intravenous antibiotics and fluids is required if the patient is:

- Pregnant
- Immunodeficient
- Presenting with severe illness, nausea, vomiting, or a high fever
- Unable to follow or tolerate the outpatient treatment with oral antibiotics
- Potentially in need of emergency surgery, such as if appendicitis cannot be excluded
- Diagnosed with a tubo-ovarian abscess

Treatment of sexual contacts is also important to avoid reinfection. The patient must abstain from intercourse during the treatment regimen and until partners are treated and cure is achieved. The goal of treatment is to prevent complications such as pelvic adhesions, ectopic pregnancy, abscesses, and infertility.

Polycystic Ovarian Syndrome

A common cause of anovulation is a condition known as **polycystic ovary syndrome (PCOS)**. About one in ten women of childbearing age has PCOS. PCOS is a condition of excess androgen production from the ovaries and occurs in about three-quarters of women with anovulatory infertility (Fig. 12.14). Excess androgen exposure results in:

- Multiple immature ovarian follicles
- Decreased progesterone production

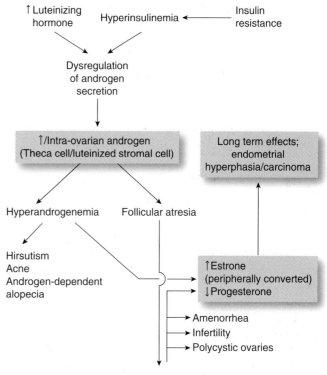

■ **Figure 12.14** Concept Map. Pathogenesis of polycystic ovary syndrome. (Image from Rubin E, Farber JL. *Pathology*. 3rd ed. Philadelphia: Lippincott Williams & Wilkins; 1999, with permission.)

- Increased acyclic (constant) estrogen production
- Anovulation
- Obesity from conversion of androgens to estrogen in adipose tissues
- Hirsutism and acne

PATHOPHYSIOLOGY

The exact cause of PCOS is unknown. A genetic cause has been suggested and those with PCOS are more likely to have a mother or sister also with PCOS. The reproductive cycle is regulated by changing hormone levels produced by the pituitary and by the ovaries. In PCOS, the pituitary gland secretes high levels of LH and the ovaries make excess androgens. The continued presence of FSH allows for follicle development, but maturation of the follicles does not occur. In the absence of ovulation, estrogen alters GnRH resulting in high LH levels with elevation of androgen release and suppression of FSH. The menstrual cycle is disrupted. Chronic anovulation produces bilaterally distended and cystic ovaries. A relationship has been noted between high androgen levels and insulin resistance, where insulin excess promotes excessive androgen production by the ovaries. Insulin sensitizing drugs have been shown to promote ovulation and, ultimately, pregnancy in some cases.

■ **Figure 12.15** Polycystic disease of the ovary. Cut sections of an ovary show numerous cysts embedded in a sclerotic stroma. (Image from Rubin E, Farber JL. *Pathology.* 3rd ed. Philadelphia: Lippincott Williams & Wilkins; 1999, with permission.)

CLINICAL MANIFESTATIONS

Clinical manifestations with PCOS are associated with menstrual irregularities, excess androgen production, and, in many cases, polycystic ovaries (Fig. 12.15). Prolonged menstrual periods and menstrual intervals longer than 35 days or fewer than eight menstrual cycles per year are not uncommon. Excess androgen production may result in physical signs, such as hirsutism (excess facial and body hair), acne, and male-pattern baldness, with some variability based on ethnicity. Obesity is present in about half of women with PCOS. Acanthosis nigricans (darkened, velvety skin) on the nape of the neck, armpits, inner thighs, vulva, or under the breasts can occur as a result of insulin resistance. In some cases, PCOS is identified only when fertility is desired but not achieved.

DIAGNOSTIC CRITERIA

There are no definitive diagnostic tests for PCOS. Clinical manifestations often lead to a suspected diagnosis and hormone levels are altered. Laboratory tests can be used to rule out hyperprolactinemia and ovarian or adrenal tumors. Enlarged ovaries containing numerous small cysts can be detected by ultrasound, but are not diagnostic in isolation of other manifestations. Some women with PCOS do not exhibit visibly cystic ovarian changes. Additionally, fasting cholesterol and triglyceride levels are needed to determine hypercholesterolemia and a glucose tolerance test is needed to determine the level of insulin resistance.

TREATMENT

Treatment is aimed at suppressing androgen production and managing the clinical manifestations. To induce pregnancy, treatment with antiestrogen medications to induce ovulation, such as clomiphene citrate, is needed. Caution must be used because of the risk for ovarian hyperstimulation. Metformin is an oral medication that lowers insulin levels and improves ovulation, thereby regulating menstrual cycles. This drug is often used in combination with clomiphene citrate. If unsuccessful, injectable FSH and LH (gonadotropins) may be used. Laparoscopic laser surgery to puncture the multiple ineffective follicles may improve follicular function.

If pregnancy is not desired, low-dose birth control pills decrease androgen production and correct irregular bleeding. Progesterone can also be taken for 10 to 14 days each month to regulate menstrual periods, but does not improve androgen levels. Managing obesity, high cholesterol, diabetes, and hypertension are important to prevent long-term cardiovascular risks. Spironolactone may be used to block the skin effects of androgens, including the reduction of excessive hair growth and acne. Shaving, waxing, depilatory creams, and even electrolysis are also used to reduce excessive hair.

◢ Ovarian Cancer

Neoplasia can occur anywhere throughout the reproductive tract. Uncommonly, women can develop cancer of the vulva or vagina. More commonly, neoplasias can be found in the cervix (Chapter 2), uterus, and ovaries. Endometrial cancer of the uterus is the most common invasive cancer in reproductive tract for women. Epithelial carcinoma of the ovary is the second most common genitourinary cancer and the fifth most frequent cause of death in women and is discussed here. More than 48% of all cases occur in women over the age of 65.[1]

PATHOPHYSIOLOGY

There are several types and variations of ovarian cancer, the most common being serous adenocarcinoma (Fig. 12.16). Approximately 5% to 10% of ovarian cancers are inherited as one of the three patterns: ovarian cancer alone, ovarian-breast cancer, or ovarian-colon cancer. In these types, the most important risk factor is a family history of a first-degree relative (mother, daughter, or sister) with the disease. This risk increases in women with two or more first-degree relatives with ovarian cancer. The *BRCA-1* gene, located on chromosome 17q21, has been linked to families affected with ovarian cancer and in the

Figure 12.16 Ovarian cancer. A cross-section of the enlarged ovary shows a solid tumor with focal hemorrhages. (Image modified from Rubin E, Farber JL. *Pathology*. 4th ed. Philadelphia: Lippincott Williams & Wilkins; 2005, with permission.)

ovarian-breast cancer combination. *BRCA-2*, located on chromosome 13q12, is also responsible for some instances of inherited ovarian-breast cancer.[2]

For those without a clear familial inheritance pattern, ovarian cancer development appears correlated with increased trauma to the ovaries. Monthly ovulation results in the ovum breaking through the epithelial surface of the ovary, causing an inflammatory response and culminating in tissue repair. Over time with repeated ovulation, the risk for ovarian cancer increases. Pregnancy, the use of contraceptives, and other events that suppress ovulation may have a protective effect.

Classification of ovarian cancer is based on the tissue of origin and includes:

- *Epithelial tumors:* arise from the surface of the ovary. Serous adenocarcinoma, an epithelial tumor that resembles the epithelial tissue of the fallopian tube, is the most common type.
- *Germ cell tumors:* comprise 25% of ovarian tumors but are mostly benign in adult women. Germ cell tumors can also occur in children but are more often malignant in children and young adults. Germ cell tumors resemble embryonic tissues. Development is similar to that of testicular cancer.
- *Sex cord tumors:* comprise 10% of ovarian tumors. These tumors arise from primitive sex cord or connective tissue of the developing ovary.

The spread of ovarian cancer occurs via local shedding into the peritoneal cavity with seeding and implantation on the peritoneum. This is followed by local invasion of the bowel and bladder. Infiltration of the pelvic lymph nodes is common, and its incidence increases with greater severity of disease. At the time of diagnosis, ovarian cancer is staged on a I to IV scale:

I. Limited to one or both ovaries
II. Extends into pelvis
III. Metastases in peritoneum outside the pelvis
IV. Distant metastases

As with other types of cancer, metastases can relocate in the ovaries from a primary tumor that originates elsewhere. A more favorable prognosis is based on younger age at diagnosis, cell type other than mucinous or clear cell, lower stage, greater cell differentiation, small size of tumor, absence of ascites (fluid accumulation in the peritoneum), and an adequate response to surgical, radiation, or chemotherapeutic treatment. Ovarian cancer is curable in a high percentage of patients if detected in the early stages. Unfortunately, at the time of diagnosis, three of every four women have local spread to the pelvis or distant metastases, making ovarian cancer one of the most lethal female reproductive cancers. More than half of these individuals are at stage III or greater at diagnosis. For stage III or IV tumors that cannot be removed adequately via surgery, the 5-year survival rate is less than 10%. The composite 5-year survival rate for all patients diagnosed with ovarian cancer is 35%.[3]

CLINICAL MANIFESTATIONS

Ovarian cancer is often asymptomatic in the early stages. Vague abdominal bloating may be noticed in some. As with pregnancy, the peritoneum allows for growth of tumors without immediate obstruction on other nearby structures. Therefore, most patients have widespread disease at the time of diagnosis. Large tumors may manifest as abdominal distention, pressure, or pain.

DIAGNOSTIC CRITERIA

Diagnosis is based on patient history, physical examination (bimanual palpation of the ovaries), laparoscopic or other surgical exploration of the

From the Lab

The serum CA-125 level, a tumor marker (antigen), indicates a high probability of epithelial ovarian cancer. However, CA-125 has no prognostic significance when measured at diagnosis. This tumor marker has greater utility in monitoring treatment efficacy and determining recurrence of disease in those with an elevated CA-125 at diagnosis. This test can also be elevated in other malignant and non-malignant conditions, such as endometriosis.

peritoneal cavity, and cytologic examination of ovarian epithelial cells. If the tumor appears to be isolated to the ovary or pelvis, laparotomy is used to examine the peritoneum and obtain ovarian, lymph, and surrounding tissues for analysis. Serum tumor marker levels are also obtained at diagnosis.

TREATMENT

Treatment is based on the stage of ovarian cancer at diagnosis. For those diagnosed at stages I or II, a tumor that is well differentiated or moderately well differentiated is treated through surgical removal of the uterus, both ovaries, and surrounding omentum. The diaphragm is biopsied along with multiple lymph nodes to detect spread. In those patients considering childbearing with stage I well-differentiated tumors, the removal of reproductive organs may be limited to the affected ovary and fallopian tube. In all stages with a less differentiated tumor and greater spread, surgery is accompanied by extensive internal and external radiation therapy and local and systemic combination chemotherapy. The goal of therapy is removal of neoplastic cells and complete remission.

Menopause

Menopause, the complete cessation of ovarian activity, is an expected biological stage marking the end of a woman's reproductive life. This occurs generally around 48 to 55 years of age. **Perimenopause**, also known as climacteric, is the 4- to 5-year gradual transition between predictable reproductive cycles and menopause. Subtle changes in bleeding patterns are the earliest manifestation of the perimenopausal period.

PATHOPHYSIOLOGY

From **menarche** (the time leading to the first menstrual period) onward, the cells of the reproductive system respond to trophic signals produced by the ovarian steroid hormones, estrogen and progesterone. The feedback mechanisms of the hypothalamus–pituitary axis acting upon the ovaries regulate both the stimulation and suppression of estrogen to allow for adequate physiologic functioning. The loss of the trophic stimulation of the hormones associated with ovarian cycles precipitates atrophic changes in the cells of the reproductive organs and the symptoms commonly associated with menopause.

As the ovaries age, the follicles become exhausted and unable to respond to functional demands despite adequate stimulation. Reduced release of ovarian hormones triggers the hypothalamus to increase secretion of GnRH. As a result, the anterior pituitary secretes additional FSH and LH yet this activity is ineffective in producing the desired effect because the aging ovaries are no longer unable to produce estrogen and progesterone.

CLINICAL MANIFESTATIONS

The clinical manifestations of menopause become clearer when the complete activity of estrogens on target tissues is discussed. Estrogens circulating in the body enter cells by diffusing through the plasma membrane. Estrogen enters the nucleus of the cell, binding to one of the two forms of estrogen receptor, the alpha (ER-α) and beta (ER-β) receptors. Distribution of these receptors in organs and tissues vary. The dominant locations of each receptor type include:

- Alpha (ER-α) receptor
  - Breasts
  - Kidney
  - Endometrium
  - Ovaries
  - Vagina
- Beta (ER-β) receptor
  - Brain
  - Ovaries
  - Bladder
  - Lungs

The clinical manifestations are best explained by the loss of the estrogen effect on cells of these target organs. Estrogen deprivation can cause obvious effects leading to acute symptoms, and can also cause changes that are not detected until much later. The full effects of estrogen deprivation may not be detected for many years but includes effects on the menstrual cycle, internal and external genitalia and sexual functioning, breasts, vasomotor response, mood, sleep, and bone mineralization.

Uterine effects of decreased steroid hormone levels include alterations in menstrual pattern. Decreased menstrual frequency (**oligomenorrhea**) with ultimate cessation of menses occurs. During this time, some women also experience other menstrual alterations, including:

- **Menorrhagia** (excessive flow or prolonged duration; regular interval)
- **Metrorrhagia** (irregular intervals)
- **Polymenorrhea** (increased frequency; shortened interval)
- **Metromenorrhagia** (shortened interval, heavy bleeding)

Atrophic changes also occur in other estrogen-stimulated tissues. Breast size is decreased because of atrophy of internal breast structures, including the ducts and lobes. Skin elasticity reduces. Body hair and subcutaneous fat levels decrease. The ovaries and uterus atrophy. The walls of the vagina become thin. Dyspareunia (painful intercourse) is often a consequence of vaginal atrophy because these cells can no longer produce adequate amounts of lubrication for comfort. Urinary difficulties, such as urgency and stress incontinence, can be attributed to atrophy of bladder cells as a result of the loss of hormonal stimulation necessary for optimal cell functioning.

Hot flashes or flushes are the common description of the vasomotor symptoms associated with menopause. Localized in the upper half of the body, hot flashes are described as a sudden feeling of warmth and are associated with reddened skin and sweating. Vasomotor symptoms are brief, lasting between 30 seconds to 5 minutes. Frequency and severity can vary from mild to severe and can be quite disruptive. Although the physiologic explanation is not completely understood, vasomotor symptoms are likely the result of altered thermoregulation.

Alterations in sleep and mood, including symptoms of depression and fatigue, have been associated with menopause. Although this is not a universal manifestation, women with a prior history of depression are more likely to develop symptoms, especially in early perimenopause. Irritability, mood lability, and anxiety are also common. Trouble falling asleep or disrupted sleep may be a response to hot flashes, depression and other mood changes, or chronic pain and lead to severe fatigue.

Sexual functioning may be affected by the hormonal changes of menopause. In addition to the physical changes of the reproductive organs described previously, motivation to engage in sexual activities (libido) may be affected. Women report less frequent sexual activity and less satisfaction during this developmental period.

Bone demineralization occurs with advancing age but is more rapid after menopause. Menopausal bone loss, the manifestation of bone atrophy, results from the effects of cytokines in the absence of the protective effects of the ovarian hormones. This imbalance promotes delayed apoptosis of cells that breaks down bone (osteoclasts) and enhances apoptosis of cells favoring bone growth (osteoblasts).

Cardiovascular disease is the leading killer of women older than 50 years. Markers of cardiovascular disease are altered after menopause, increasing risk of stroke and heart attack. Cholesterol levels, including the components high-density lipoprotein (HDL) and low-density lipoprotein (LDL), are altered in favor of an increased ratio of LDL:HDL, increasing cardiovascular risk.

DIAGNOSTIC CRITERIA

There is no single, reliable biological marker to diagnose menopause. In the average time it takes to reach menopause, the pituitary-stimulating hormone FSH becomes elevated, with a gradual decline in the ovarian hormones estrone and estradiol. Menopause is often confirmed through absence of menses for a 12-month period with a corresponding increase in FSH. Pregnancy must be ruled out as the cause for amenorrhea.

From the Lab

There is no one reliable laboratory test to diagnose menopause. Hormonal markers are of limited usefulness due to the significant fluctuation of levels among individual women. The diagnosis of menopause is based on the history of manifestations and physical findings on examination. General limits for specific hormones involved in the physiology of menopause are provided for review:

- Estradiol
  - Premenopausal levels: 20 to 400 pg/mL
  - Postmenopausal: 2 to 25 pg/mL
- FSH
  - Premenopausal: 5 to 30 IU/L
  - Postmenopausal: >30 IU/L
- LH
  - Premenopausal female: 5 to 20 IU/L
  - Postmenopausal female: >20 IU/L

TREATMENT

Treatment is often initiated when clinical manifestations become disruptive to functioning. Although many women do not require treatment, others rely on treatment for the management of undesirable symptoms. Treatment is best targeted toward the specific concern. Most often, pharmacologic hormonal therapies are used to manage manifestations. Combined estrogen and progesterone are used in women who have a uterus, because treatment with estrogen alone increases the risk of endometrial cancer. Hormone treatment can be provided in the form of oral contraceptive pills or hormone replacement therapy (HRT). Until 2002, HRT was the standard treatment for women in menopause for amelioration of symptoms and prevention of long-term health risks, including cardiovascular disease. Based on the results of studies on the use of HRT on health outcomes, including the Heart and Estrogen/Progestin Replacement Study (HERS) and the

Women's Health Initiative (WHI), routine treatment of menopausal women with combined hormone therapy was curtailed. The studies revealed a lack of evidence to support the use of hormones for the expected protective effects, and the determination of poor health outcomes combined to alter standard treatment practices.

Treatment of menopausal symptoms with combined hormone therapy remains an option. Treatment is instituted based on specific criteria rather than on routine usage. Current practice includes hormonal treatments based on the following criteria:

- Severe symptoms requiring treatment
- Short-term duration
- Lowest effective dose

Hormone delivery systems may affect the risk profile in women treated with HRT. Transdermal patch delivery of HRT is effective for vasomotor symptoms and maintenance of bone mineral density.[4] Vaginal estrogen cream in low-dose applications can effectively manage vaginal atrophy and urinary symptoms, without stimulating systemic effects. Vaginal ring delivery is also effective for local symptoms without the undesired systemic effects. Local progestin delivery, using an intrauterine device, results in both local and systemic effects. Testosterone treatment may be useful in the treatment of altered sexual desire, although it is not currently approved by the Food and Drug Administration (FDA). Topical estrogen cream may be an effective treatment for menopause-related decrease in skin thickness and aging.[5] Initiation of HRT in women older than 65 years is not recommended because of the increased associated risk of dementia in this age group.

Research Notes

HRT using a combination of estrogen and progesterone can be administered to synthetically increase ovarian hormone levels, reverse the atrophic changes, and decrease symptoms associated with menopause. The WHI studied major causes of death and disability in women on HRT. A major recruitment goal of WHI was to enroll 20% of study participants from minority groups.[6] Recent findings from the WHI indicated evidence for increased risk of breast cancer, venous thrombosis, coronary heart disease and stroke, prompting the U.S. Preventative Services Task Force to recommend discontinuation of HRT as the risks outweighed the benefits.

Tissue-targeted therapies are also useful when managing specific manifestations. Because of the specificity of hormone binding to selective receptors, drug effects can be modulated based on the targeting of specific receptors located predominantly in a certain tissue type. Selective estrogen receptor modulators (SERM) are drugs designed to capitalize on these pharmacologic principles. The drug raloxifene is often used for prevention of osteoporosis in post-menopausal women. Raloxifene binds to the ER-β receptor and results in antagonist effects in the endometrium and breast tissue, decreasing bone breakdown, total cholesterol, and LDL levels.

Nonpharmacologic strategies should be considered in the management of menopausal symptoms. The following measures may help minimize the discomfort and unpleasantness associated with many common menopause-related concerns:

- Dress in layers
- Avoid spicy foods
- Avoid caffeine and alcohol
- Initiate deep breathing measures at the start of a hot flash
- Use relaxation techniques
- Incorporate soy products containing phytoestrogens in the diet
- Perform pelvic floor exercises to strengthen muscles of the pelvis and vagina
- Use water-based lubricants for more comfortable intercourse

STOP *and Consider*

What other tissue types can be affected by decreased trophic signals of ovarian hormones? What other tissue types can be similarly affected?

Erectile Dysfunction

Sexual dysfunction is one of the most common health problems affecting men and includes such problems as low sexual interest, **erectile dysfunction (ED)**, premature ejaculation, and physical abnormalities of the penis.[7] ED is the inability to achieve or maintain an erection sufficient for satisfactory sexual performance. ED is one of the main types of sexual dysfunction in men, and the prevalence increases with age. In one US study, around 52% of men between the ages of 40 and 70 years reported experiencing ED. Other countries throughout the world have demonstrated a similar prevalence.[8]

PATHOPHYSIOLOGY

Achieving an erection is a complex interaction of arousal and parasympathetic nervous stimulation at the S2–4 level, signaling increased blood flow that becomes trapped in the corpora cavernosa of

A

B

■ **Figure 12.17** Anatomic depiction of penile erection. **A:** Innervation and arterial and venous blood supply to the penis. **B:** Cross-section of corpora cavernosa.

the penis (Fig. 12.17). This trapping of blood in the corpora cavernosa depends on smooth muscle relaxation that occludes the veins and does not allow blood flow out. The erection is reversed under the influences of the sympathetic nervous system. All of these activities are facilitated by androgen activity on the hypothalamus and anterior pituitary.

CLINICAL MANIFESTATIONS

The inability to achieve and maintain an erection is the primary clinical manifestation. The complexity of ED is illustrated by several causes that may lead to other manifestation. These causes include:

- *Hormonal factors:* hypogonadism, hypothyroidism, or adrenal cortical hormone dysfunction resulting in inadequate hormonal "priming" of the sexual centers of the brain
- *Neurological factors:* spinal cord or perineal nerve injury resulting in inadequate nerve signaling to the penile vessels
- *Psychological factors:* anxiety, low self-esteem, or depression resulting in inadequate arousal

- *Vascular obstruction:* hypertension, atherosclerosis, vascular obstruction, and smoking disallow blood flow to the corpora cavernosa and spongiosa, thereby preventing erection from occurring
- *Impaired veno-occlusive ability:* the inability to trap blood within the corpora cavernosa
- *Certain medications*, such as antihypertensives, can inhibit hormone and erectile function

DIAGNOSTIC CRITERIA

Diagnosis of ED is based on a comprehensive history and physical examination to identify the potential cause. Laboratory measurement of testosterone, LH, thyroid, and prolactin levels may suggest a hypothalamic, pituitary, or hormonal problem. Hypogonadism—specifically, a reduction in the levels of testosterone—can contribute to ED.

TREATMENT

Treatment is individualized and directed by the etiology (physical, psychological, or both). Testosterone replacement therapy, or other hormone intervention, may be indicated. Psychological influences may be addressed and treated by a mental health professional. Medications, such as sildenafil (Viagra), vardenafil, and tadalafil, are often prescribed for men with ED. These drugs act to promote smooth muscle relaxation and vascular congestion in the corpora cavernosa, thereby maintaining an erection. Penile implants or other devices may be used to help maintain an erection.

Research Notes

Lifestyle, most notably obesity, smoking, and alcohol use, affects the development of ED. One study aimed to determine the impact of lifestyle changes (weight loss and physical activity) on male erectile function. After a 2-year diet and exercise intervention, those men who had significant decreases in body weight, body mass index, waist-hip ratio, blood pressure, glucose levels, and total cholesterol demonstrated a statistically significant improvement in sexual function. The researchers suggested that obesity resulted in a state of chronic oxidative stress and inflammation throughout the body. The inflammation was responsible for blood vessel lining obstruction. Weight reduction saw a corresponding decrease in inflammatory markers and a subsequent improvement in sexual function.[9]

Benign Prostatic Hyperplasia

The prostate gland is a small organ about the size of a walnut, which lies below the bladder and surrounds the urethra. The prostate tissue produces prostate-specific antigen (PSA) and prostatic acid phosphatase, an enzyme found in seminal fluid. The major role of the prostate is to secrete a fluid, which combines with semen, to increase sperm motility and decrease vaginal acidity. Benign prostatic hyperplasia (BPH) affects more than 50% of men over age 60 and as many as 90% of men over age 70.[10] BPH is a condition of aging; nearly all men over the age of 50 have some level of enlargement of the prostate.

PATHOPHYSIOLOGY

The cause of BPH is unknown. Hormone changes associated with aging have an impact on prostatic cell growth. Over time, lowered testosterone levels result in higher proportions of estrogen, which promotes prostatic cell proliferation. In all men, testosterone is converted to dihydrotestosterone (DTH) and estradiol in certain tissues. DTH is involved in prostate growth and may accumulate over time, also resulting in overproliferation of prostatic epithelial cells of the acini and ductules, smooth muscle cells, and stromal fibroblasts. The cell proliferation occurs primarily in the periurethral part of the gland. BPH is not considered a precursor to prostate cancer.

CLINICAL MANIFESTATIONS

Clinical manifestations of BPH are related to urethral obstruction from the enlarged prostate, which impedes the flow of urine from the bladder to the urinary meatus. This results in urinary frequency, dribbling, hesitancy, incontinence, urgency, and retention. Complete obstruction leads to acute urinary retention and an absolute inability to urinate. This leads to severe pain and can progress to renal failure and death if not treated.

DIAGNOSTIC CRITERIA

Diagnosis is based on patient history, physical examination, laboratory tests, and evaluation of symptoms. The physical examination includes a digital rectal examination. This procedure allows the health practitioner to determine the size, shape, and consistency of the prostate gland, as palpated through the rectal wall (Fig. 12.18). Benign enlargement of the prostate tissue is soft; malignant tissue is hard, asymmetrical, and often has a cobblestone texture. PSA is often measured to determine elevations that may indicate prostate hyperplasia or dysplasia. Elevations in PSA are followed by a biopsy to confirm or rule out malignancy. The American Urological Association (AUA) Symptoms Index may

■ **Figure 12.18** Digital rectal examination noting enlargement of prostate characteristic of BPH. (From Weber J, Kelley J. *Health Assessment in Nursing*. 2nd ed. Philadelphia: Lippincott Williams & Wilkins; 2003, with permission.)

be used. This index is a seven-question survey on a 1 to 5 scale related to the presence and frequency of symptoms related to BPH. A higher point total (i.e., 20 to 35) equates to greater severity of symptoms. Urodynamic tests can be used to measure the volume and pressure of urine in the bladder and to evaluate the flow of urine.

TREATMENT

Treatment is reserved for those men with significant symptoms. Pharmacologic treatments may be prescribed that relax the smooth muscles of the arteries, prostate, and bladder neck to relieve urinary obstruction. Because the prostate also depends on hormonal stimulation, drugs may be prescribed that inhibit the action of testosterone by restricting conversion to DTH. The lack of hormonal stimulation results in prostate atrophy. Laser or other heat-based treatments may also be applied to destroy all or part of the prostate gland. Surgical intervention may also be included in the treatment regimen, depending on the severity of symptoms and potential risks to the patient. The most common procedure is the transurethral resection of the prostate (TURP). In this procedure, part of the prostate is removed using a surgical instrument placed into the urethra via the penis. For patients who are not appropriate candidates for pharmacologic, laser, or surgical treatments, a stent may be placed in the urethra. A stent is a small, rigid tube that holds the urethra open and allows urine to drain. The disadvantages to stents are that they can elicit irritation, frequent urination, pain, and incontinence, and they are difficult to remove if removal is necessary.

Prostate Cancer

During a man's lifetime, the risk of developing prostate cancer is 1 in 6, making it the second leading cause of cancer death in men, exceeded only by lung cancer. About 85% of men with prostate cancer are diagnosed after the age of 65.

PATHOPHYSIOLOGY

Similar to BPH, carcinoma of the prostate is predominately a disease of older men. Prostate cancer is extremely common; it is estimated that a 50-year-old American man has a 40% chance of developing prostate cancer during his lifetime.[11] The exact cause is often unknown. Risk factors for the development of prostate cancer include advancing age, family history of prostate cancer, Black race, smoking, and nutritional factors, such as high intake of fats and meat, low intake of lycopene (found primarily in tomato-based products) and fruit, and high dietary calcium.

The malignant transformation of prostate epithelial cells, as with other forms of cancer, is a result of a complex series of initiator and promoter events with genetic and environmental influences. Approximately 5% to 10% of prostate cancer cases are estimated to be related to inherited genetic factors or prostate cancer susceptibility genes.[12] One major locus of susceptibility is found at chromosome 1q24, designated as *HPC1* (hereditary prostate cancer). This mutation is associated with a younger age at diagnosis, a higher tumor grade, and more advanced stage at diagnosis. Several other chromosome regions, which have been linked to susceptibility in inherited and sporadic forms of prostate cancer, have also been identified.

More than 95% of primary prostate cancers are classified as adenocarcinomas. Androgens and estrogens are two hormones that appear to support carcinogenesis by influencing prostate epithelial proliferation, although elevations in androgens are not found universally in those with prostate cancer. Premalignant changes in patients with prostate cancer are designated as prostatic intraepithelial neoplasia (PIN) and are characterized by atypical lumen cells lining the prostatic ducts. These PIN lesions are believed to progress to prostate adenocarcinoma, with the neoplasm arising in the peripheral portion of the gland (Fig. 12.19). This peripheral location is clinically significant in

Figure 12.19   Digital rectal examination noting mass characteristic of prostate cancer. (From Weber J, Kelley J. *Health Assessment in Nursing.* 2nd ed. Philadelphia: Lippincott Williams & Wilkins; 2003, with permission.)

that the tumor does not compress the urethra until later in its progression.

CLINICAL MANIFESTATIONS

Prostate cancer is often asymptomatic and is found incidentally after a digital rectal examination and PSA screening. When clinical manifestations are present, the tumor has often expanded and is obstructing the urethra. In this case, the manifestations are identical to that of BPH and include urinary frequency, dribbling, hesitancy, incontinence, urgency, and retention. Common systemic manifestations, paraneoplastic syndromes, and manifestations significant for metastatic spread, such as pain as the tumor spreads to the bone, also apply to prostate cancer.

From the Lab

PSA in the blood may be bound to proteins or may exist in an unbound state. Total PSA is the sum of levels of both forms. Free PSA measures only the levels of unbound PSA. Some studies suggest that malignant prostate cells produce more *bound* PSA; therefore, a low level of free PSA compared to total PSA may indicate malignant prostatic neoplasia. A high level of free PSA compared to total PSA might indicate BPH or an inflammatory condition of the prostate.

DIAGNOSTIC CRITERIA

Digital rectal examination, transrectal ultrasound, and PSA levels are used to screen for prostate cancer. Diagnosis is confirmed through a cytologic analysis of prostate tissue (biopsy) via fine needle aspiration usually performed transrectally. Pelvic lymph node dissection during surgical treatment for those undergoing radical prostatectomy is often required to determine lymph node involvement. Radionucleotide bone scans are used to detect metastases to the bone, the most common site of distant spread. Once diagnosed, prostate cancer is staged using the TNM classification system, with slight modifications in the tumor designation:

- T1: a clinically inapparent tumor not palpable or visible by imaging
- T2: the tumor is confined to the prostate
- T3: the tumor extends through the prostate capsule
- T4: the tumor is fixed or invades adjacent structures other than the seminal vesicles

Survival rate and prognosis is based on the histologic features (differentiation and distribution) of the tumor and staging. The 5-year survival is more than 99% for patients with local or regional disease spread. The 5-year survival drops significantly to 33.5% in those patients with distant metastases.[2]

TREATMENT

Treatment is based on tumor grading, TNM classification, age, and health status. Radical prostatectomy (removal of the entire prostate) is often used to treat prostate cancer, particularly in younger men (less than 70 years of age) without other health complications or surgical risk factors. Radiation therapy and chemotherapy may be used as a surgical adjunct or for those who are not surgical candidates. Androgen-deprivation hormone therapy may also be used to decrease prostate cell proliferation. Because prostate cancer is considered a slow-growing tumor and is typically diagnosed later in life, "watchful waiting" may be the treatment of choice in those without clinical symptoms. This approach avoids the complications inherent with surgical, radiation, and chemotherapeutic interventions, and it appreciates the reality that many men with clinically undetectable prostate cancer die from other causes.

Testicular Cancer

Testicular cancer is a highly treatable and often curable cancer, which is most commonly found in men between 20 and 40 years of age. Testicular cancer is five times more common in Americans of European descent than in African Americans.[3] Approximately 90% of tumors arise from germ cells. The remaining tumors are of sex cord cell origin or metastases from other sites.

PATHOPHYSIOLOGY

Germ cell tumors are classified according to cell origin and include the following:

- *Seminomas:* malignant germ cells that resemble primitive sperm cells
- *Nonseminomas:* malignant germ cells that do not resemble primitive sperm cells and actually appear as embryonic or undifferentiated somatic (e.g., skin, muscle, glands, etc.) components

The germ cell divides through mitosis and differentiates into a primitive sperm cell, called a **spermatogonia**, and finally into a mature spermatocyte. Seminomas are the most common type of testicular cancer. Seminoma formation begins with a germ cell mutation, more than likely during fetal development, which has stagnated sperm cell development and has resulted in proliferation of immature spermatogonia. The spermatogonia proliferate and the testicular tissue becomes enlarged and fibrotic.

Nonseminomas are a complex derivative of embryonic development. Notable subcategories of nonseminomas include embryonal carcinomas, yolk sac tumors, choriocarcinomas (arising from the chorion), and teratocarcinomas (Fig. 12.20). **Embryonic carcinomas** resemble primitive undifferentiated embryonic tissue. **Teratocarcinomas** are a combination of embryonic carcinomas and undifferentiated somatic (e.g., skin, muscle, bone, and glands) tissues. The undifferentiated somatic tissue arises from stem cell embryonic tissue origin that then differentiates into the embryonic germ layers (ectoderm, mesoderm, and endoderm). These tissues then further differentiate into various somatic tissues. In other words, teratocarcinomas appear as undifferentiated embryonic tissue and skin or bone cells where mature spermatocytes should be found. The origin of some nonseminomas may result from misplaced fetal germ cells that did not migrate to seminiferous tubules during fetal testicular organogenesis. The nonseminomas grow faster, are more invasive, and are more likely to metastasize than the seminomas.

Although the exact cause is often unknown, an alteration in chromosome 12 may be implicated in those with testicular cancer. A major risk factor is **cryptorchidism**, or undescended testis, and other problems with testicular development. Those with cryptorchidism are 20 to 40 times more likely to develop testicular cancer. One theory of carcinogenesis indicates that an initiating event and mutation occurs during fetal development. Autonomy and anaplasia are then promoted through hormonal stimulation during puberty. Tumor development often progresses through two major stages: (1) carcinoma in situ and (2) invasive carcinoma. The carcinoma in situ, common with testicular cancer, is confined to the seminiferous tubules. Testicular cancer is often malignant at diagnosis.

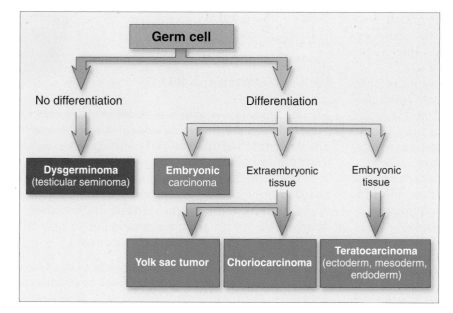

■ **Figure 12.20** Classification of germ cell tumors of the testes. (Image modified from Rubin E, Farber JL. *Pathology.* 4th ed. Philadelphia: Lippincott Williams & Wilkins; 2005, with permission.)

Although testicular cancer is highly treatable and curable, the prognosis for testicular cancer is less favorable when the following factors exist:[13]

- The presence of bone, liver, or brain metastases
- High serum tumor markers
- The presence of a primary mediastinal nonseminoma
- A large number of lung metastases

The largest proportion of patients with seminomas (90%) is diagnosed with primary tumors without metastases or elevations in tumor markers. Patients with seminomas at a primary site without metastases or elevations in tumor serum markers demonstrate a 5-year survival of 86%.[13] In contrast, those patients with mediastinal nonseminomas with metastasis or elevated tumor markers have a 48% 5-year survival. Even with widespread metastases, those with primary testicular cancer may also be cured and should be treated as such.

CLINICAL MANIFESTATIONS

Common clinical manifestations include a small painless testicular mass, slight enlargement of the testicle, heaviness or enlargement of the scrotum, and mild testicular discomfort.

DIAGNOSTIC CRITERIA

Self-testicular examination is an important aspect of early detection and should be practiced by all men on a monthly basis. Diagnosis of the primary tumor is through physical examination and radical orchiectomy (removal of the testicle). Transscrotal biopsy is not recommended because it may result in seeding of the tumor into the scrotum or spread to inguinal lymph nodes. Tumor markers provide additional clues to the diagnosis and treatment efficacy. Imaging studies, such as ultrasound, CT scan, and MRI, can identify the tumor location and spread.

TREATMENT

Treatment of testicular cancer involves surgical removal of the tumor and affected testicle or testicles. Radiation and chemotherapy may also be used in treatment. The risks involved with radiation and chemotherapeutic treatment in testicular cancer include infertility, secondary leukemias (or other types of cancer), and possible renal function impairment. This type of cancer is often curable.

▨ Summary

- Reproductive function is reliant upon structural integrity, neurologic, and hormonal processes of males and females.
- Female reproductive organs include the vagina, uterus, fallopian tubes, and ovaries. The ovaries produce the female sex hormones: estrogens, progesterone, and androgens. These hormones are secreted in a monthly cyclical pattern under the direction of the hypothalamus (GnRH) and the anterior pituitary (FSH, LH).
- The male reproductive organs and tissues include the testes, epididymis, vas deferens, seminal vesicles, prostate, and penis. Androgens, the male sex hormones, promote metabolism and growth.

The pattern of male sex hormone secretion does not follow a cyclical pattern as seen with females; the hormone secretion rates remain fairly constant throughout the male's adult life.

- Stimulation of androgen production and release in males begins in the hypothalamus. The hypothalamus releases GnRH, which stimulates the anterior pituitary to release LH and FSH. LH acts on the Leydig cells in the testes to produce testosterone, the primary male sex hormone.
- Achieving pregnancy is a complex interaction of ovulation, spermatogenesis, intercourse, ejaculation, conception, implantation, and embryo growth.
- Infertility, defined as the inability to achieve pregnancy after 1 year of unprotected intercourse. About 10% to 15% of couples are considered infertile. In many cases, the exact cause of infertility is not identified. Potential causes, when identified, include hormone imbalance, motility impairment, and immune problems.
- Clinical manifestations are sometimes absent. With hormone alterations, irregular menstrual periods or amenorrhea may be reported often as a result of anovulation. Testicular/scrotal pain in men or pelvic pain in women may occur with infection or inflammation of reproductive structures.
- The diagnosis of altered reproduction is based on the couple's inability to conceive or the presence of clinical manifestations. Initially, a semen analysis must be completed in the male along with an analysis of ovulation in the female. Patency of the female reproductive structures can be visualized using hysterosalpingography or laparoscopy.
- Treatment involves supportive counseling, education about intercourse frequency, avoidance of lubricants that can act as a spermicide, and basic health maintenance. Sexually transmitted or other pelvic infections place the female at high risk for infertility and must be treated quickly and completely. Obstructive processes, such as leiomyomas, endometriosis, or pelvic adhesions, may require surgical intervention.
- Some individuals may require clomiphene citrate, a medication that induces ovulation. In those with hyperprolactinemia, medications may be needed to reduce prolactin and therefore induce ovulation. Artificial insemination may be used to inject sperm into the uterus if cervical mucus is thick or if the sperm quantity or quality is compromised. Some couples seek advanced reproductive technologies such as in vitro fertilization.
- The evaluation and treatment of infertility is highly complex and emotionally charged. Sensitivity to the range and intensity of emotions is an important aspect of care.

Case Study 12.1

A couple seeks reproductive counseling for inability to achieve a pregnancy after 14 months of unprotected intercourse. After multiple diagnostic tests with both individuals, the male partner is determined to have a moderately decreased sperm count and motility. Upon physical examination of the scrotum, enlargement of scrotal veins is determined, described by the clinician as feeling like "a bag of worms." The condition is termed varicocele.

1. *Outline the process that has occurred in his body.*
2. *What were the risk factors that he demonstrated?*
3. *What would you expect for clinical manifestations?*
4. *What additional diagnostic tests could be used?*
5. *What treatment measures would you anticipate?*

Log on to the Internet. Search for a relevant journal article or Web site (such as http://www.bing.com/health/article.aspx?id=articles%2fmayo%2f49350764eff4162f5819541a0b2313f0.html&br=lv&q=varicocele) that details varicocele to confirm your predictions.

Case Study 12.2

J.T. is a 62-year-old woman who has been on estrogen therapy without progesterone for menopausal symptoms for the past 6 years. She is seeking medical care for unexplained vaginal bleeding. She is obese and has been menopausal for 8 years and has not had any menstrual bleeding until a week ago. She does not have any pelvic discomfort. After examination, she is scheduled for a dilatation and curettage (D&C) with biopsy. The biopsy reveals endometrial cancer.

1. *Outline the processes that have most likely occurred in her body.*
2. *What would you notice for clinical manifestations?*
3. *What diagnostic tests were used and what do these tell you?*
4. *What treatment measures would you anticipate?*

Log on to the Internet. Search for a relevant journal article or Web site (such as http://www.cancer.gov/cancertopics/types/endometrial/) that details endometrial cancer to confirm your predictions.

Practice Exam Questions

1. Your patient is complaining of menopausal hot flashes and other symptoms. Which of the following would you recommend as a nonpharmacologic method for the relief of these symptoms?
   a. Increase spicy foods
   b. Increase caffeine intake
   c. Use relaxation techniques
   d. Avoid soy products containing phytoestrogens

2. Your neighbor is taking an anatomy and physiology course and asks you what would happen if a person did not have ovarian interstitial cells. What would you say?
   a. The person would be lacking ovarian support structures
   b. The person would not be able to secrete estrogen
   c. The person would not have a place to house germ cells
   d. The person would have no difficulties as interstitial cells are not located in the ovaries

3. Your family is worried because your cousin has a testosterone deficiency. What would you notice for clinical manifestations?
   a. Increased skin thickness
   b. Clear skin, free of acne
   c. Excessive chest and facial hair
   d. Bulky skeletal muscle development

4. Your pregnant friend is complaining of nausea, headaches, constipation, indigestion, and swelling. What hormone is wrecking havoc in her body?
   a. Progesterone
   b. Estrogen
   c. Thyroid stimulating hormone
   d. Human chorionic gonadotropin hormone

5. Which of the following would be illustrative of a mobility impairment leading to infertility?
   a. Anovulation
   b. Presence of leiomyomas
   c. Low sperm production
   d. Menopause

6. Your 16-year-old niece confides in you that she has not had a period for 2 months. She does not think she is pregnant and denies having sexual intercourse. What is another likely explanation?
   a. Endometrial cancer
   b. Severe emotional stress
   c. Lack of physical activity
   d. FSH deficiency

7. Dave and his wife have been trying to conceive for the past 2 years. They go on a long awaited vacation and he wants to sit in the hot tub. Why is this not recommended for men who are trying to conceive?
   a. LH and FSH release are inhibited with exposure to chlorinated water
   b. Temperature does not make a difference; he can freely enjoy the hot tub
   c. Spermatogenesis requires a higher body temperature than that found with the core body temperature
   d. Spermatogenesis requires a cooler body temperature than that found with the core body temperature

8–15. Match the clinical model with the type of altered reproductive function:

8. Pelvic inflammatory disease
9. Ovarian cancer
10. Polycystic ovarian syndrome
11. Menopause
12. Erectile dysfunction
13. Benign prostatic hypertrophy
14. Prostate cancer
15. Testicular cancer

   a. Hormonal imbalance
   b. Motility problem
   c. Immune problem

Discussion and Application

1. What did I know about altered reproduction function prior to today?

2. What body processes are affected by altered reproduction function?

3. What are the potential etiologies for altered reproduction function? How does altered reproduction function develop?

4. Who is most at risk for developing altered reproduction function? How can altered reproduction function be prevented?

5. What are the human differences that affect the etiology, risk, or course of altered reproduction function?

6. What clinical manifestations are expected in the course of altered reproduction function?

7. What special diagnostic tests are useful in determining the diagnosis and course of altered reproduction function?

8. What are the goals of care for individuals with altered reproduction function?

9. How does the concept of altered reproduction function build on what I have learned in the previous chapters and in previous courses?

10. How can I use what I have learned?

RESOURCES

Resolve: The National Infertility Association:
http://www.resolve.org/site/PageServer

American Society for Reproductive Medicine (ASRM):
http://www.asrm.org

Center for Applied Reproductive Science (CARS):
http://www.ivf-et.com

REFERENCES

1. Yancik R. Ovarian cancer: age contrasts in incidence, histology, disease stage at diagnosis, and mortality. *Cancer.* 1993;71(2 suppl): 517–523.

2. American Cancer Society. *Cancer Facts and Figures 2009.* Atlanta: American Cancer Society; 2009. Available at: http://www.cancer.org/downloads/STT/500809web.pdf. Accessed June 30, 2010.

3. Rubin E, Gorstein F, Rubin R, et al. *Rubin's Pathology: Clinicopathologic Foundations of Medicine.* 4th ed. Baltimore: Lippincott Williams & Wilkins; 2005.

4. Reed SD, Newton KM, Lacroix AZ. Indications for hormone therapy: the post-Women's Health Initiative era. *Endocrinol Metab Clin North Am.* 2004;33(4):691–715.

5. Schmidt JB. Perspectives of estrogen treatment in skin aging. *Exp Dermatol.* 2005;14(2):156.

6. Fouad MN, Corbie-Amith G, Curb D, et al. Special populations recruitment for the Women's Health Initiative: successes and limitations. *Control Clin Trials.* 2004;25(4):335–352.

7. Parmet S, Lynm C, Glass R. Male sexual dysfunction. *JAMA.* 2004;291:3076.

8. Morgentaler A. A 66-year-old man with sexual dysfunction. *JAMA.* 2004;291:2994–3004.

9. Esposito K, Giugliano F, DiPalo C, et al. Effect of lifestyle changes on erectile dysfunction in obese men: a randomized control trial. *JAMA.* 2004;291:2978–2987.

10. National Kidney and Urologic Diseases Clearinghouse (NKUDIC). Prostate enlargement: benign prostatic hyperplasia. NIH Publication No. 04-3012; 2009. Available at: http://www.kidney. niddk.nih.gov/kudiseases/pubs/prostateenlargement/. Accessed January 8, 2010.

11. Garnick M. Prostate cancer: screening, diagnosis, and management. *Ann Intern Med.* 1993;118:804–818.

12. National Cancer Institute. Genetics of prostate cancer. 2005. Available at: http://www.cancer.gov/cancertopics/pdq/genetics/prostate/health-professional. Accessed January 13, 2006.

13. Bosl G, Bajorin D, Sheinfeld J, et al. Cancer of the testis. In: Devita B, Hellman S, Rosenberg S, eds. *Principles and Practice of Oncology.* 7th ed. Philadelphia: Lippincott Williams & Wilkins; 2005.

Chapter 13

Altered Ventilation and Diffusion

LEARNING OBJECTIVES

1. Define and use the key terms listed in this chapter.
2. Explain the role of ventilation and diffusion in oxygen/carbon dioxide gas exchange.
3. Describe the processes that can impair ventilation and diffusion.
4. Recognize the effects of impaired ventilation and diffusion.
5. Identify the common signs and symptoms of altered ventilation and diffusion.
6. Describe diagnostic tests and treatment strategies relevant to disordered ventilation and diffusion.
7. Apply the concepts of altered ventilation and diffusion to select clinical models.

INTRODUCTION

Take a deep breath. Exhale. Oxygen from the air goes in, carbon dioxide goes out. When you breathe four major processes are occurring as your chest rises and falls: ventilation, diffusion, perfusion, and respiration. **Ventilation** is the process of moving air into and out of the trachea, bronchi, and lungs. **Diffusion** is the process of moving and exchanging the oxygen acquired during ventilation and carbon dioxide waste across the alveolar capillary membranes. **Perfusion** is a process of supplying oxygenated blood to the lungs and organ systems via the blood vessels (Chapter 14). **Respiration** is a process in which cells throughout the body use oxygen aerobically to make energy. As a health care provider, it is critically important to recognize problems associated with altered ventilation and diffusion.

Module **1**

Pulmonary Structure and Function

The pulmonary, or respiratory, system is responsible for ventilation and diffusion. The major function is the exchange of gases between the environment and the blood. The pulmonary system is composed of the lungs, airways, chest wall, and pulmonary circulation (Fig. 13.1). The structural path of the pulmonary system is often divided into the upper and lower airways. The upper airway is composed of the nose or mouth, nasopharynx, and oropharynx. The laryngeal pharynx connects the upper and lower airways. The lower airway is composed of the trachea, bronchi, and bronchioles. The branching anatomic structure of the pulmonary system is ideal for maximizing surface area to allow for optimal gas diffusion, or movement of gases across the alveoli.

Because the pulmonary system is an exogenous conduit to the body, defense mechanisms are needed to protect the lungs from environmental injury. These defense mechanisms are highly effective and include:

- *Protective structures,* such as hairs and turbinates (shell-shaped structures) in the nose and cilia in the upper and lower airways, which trap and remove foreign particles from the air
- *Mucosal lining* of the upper and lower airways, which warms and humidifies air
- *Irritant receptors* throughout the nose and airways, which recognize injurious agents and respond by triggering a sneeze or cough reflex to remove foreign particles
- *Immune protections,* such as an immune coating in the respiratory tract mucosa and macrophages in the alveoli, which ingest and remove bacteria and other foreign materials via phagocytosis

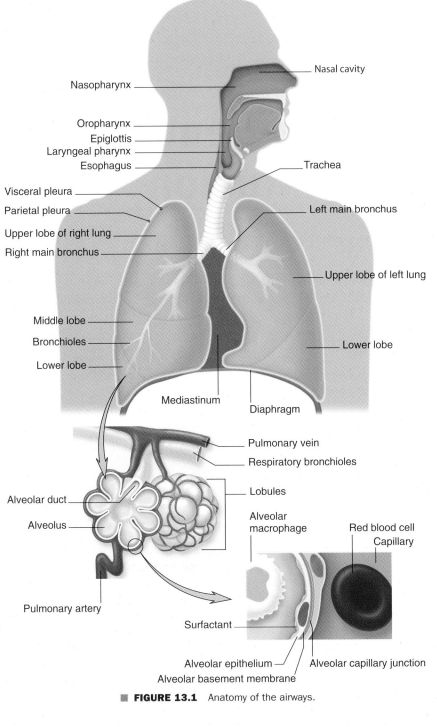

FIGURE 13.1 Anatomy of the airways.

● **STOP** *and Consider*

How are defense mechanisms and the body protections affected in the person who is a mouth breather?

Intercostal muscles, ribs, and skin surround the lungs and provide protection against injury. The muscles of the chest cavity and the diaphragm perform the muscular work of breathing. Two major membrane layers line the lungs and chest cavity: the (outer) parietal pleura and (inner) visceral pleura. These layers are separated by a pleural space, which is filled with a lubricating fluid, secreted by the pleura, that allows the two layers to slide over each other with minimal friction.

The pulmonary circulation is responsible for the delivery of oxygen and other nutrients to the lung tissues. It is also responsible for the filtration of clots, air, or other foreign materials from the circulation. The capillaries of the lungs near the alveoli facilitate the exchange of oxygen and carbon dioxide. The pulmonary circulation is discussed further in Chapter 14.

Ventilation

The process of ventilation involves both acquiring oxygen (inspiration) and removing carbon dioxide (expiration) from the blood. The transport of oxygen through the lungs is the *only* mechanism for acquiring oxygen. Oxygen is necessary for cellular metabolism, which means that for the cell to expend energy efficiently and perform its designated function, there must be oxygen present. The release of carbon dioxide is equally as important. Optimal cell functioning occurs within a very narrow pH range. The release and retention of carbon dioxide is one mechanism for maintaining this balance.

The rate and volume of ventilation is regulated by the following components:

- A functioning respiratory control center in the brain
- Lung receptors
- Chemoreceptors

The drive to ventilate is stimulated by the respiratory control center in the brainstem in response to chemical messages in the body. The respiratory control center is composed of neurons in the pons and medulla. It sends neuronal impulses to the diaphragm, intercostal muscles, sternocleidomastoid muscles, and other accessory muscles and causes them to contract or relax. The autonomic nervous system (ANS) also innervates the lungs and acts on the smooth muscles of the conducting airways to promote airway constriction (parasympathetic division) or dilation (sympathetic division). The activity of the ANS will increase or decrease the diameter of the airways and affect the amount of air that is able to get in and out of the lungs.

Neuronal impulses are directed by lung receptors that map the current state of breathing and lung function. Lung receptors are located in the epithelium and smooth muscle of the airways, and they are near the alveolar capillary junctions. Specific lung receptors have particular roles. For example, lung receptors located in the epithelium of the conducting airways are responsible for sensing irritants in the lungs and stimulating the cough reflex. Lung receptors in the smooth muscles of the airways are activated to promote expiration in order to prevent excessive lung inflation. Lung receptors in the capillaries detect increases in capillary pressure and stimulate a reduction in this pressure.

Chemoreceptors detect gas exchange needs based on the PaO_2, $PaCO_2$, and pH levels in the blood and cerebrospinal fluid (CSF). Central chemoreceptors are located near the respiratory control center and respond to pH changes in the CSF. Because CO_2 diffuses across the blood–brain barrier until both the arterial $PaCO_2$ and CSF $PaCO_2$ are equal, the CO_2 levels detected by the central chemoreceptors reflect that in the blood. The central chemoreceptors then alter the rate of breathing to adapt to the higher or lower levels of CO_2 in the body. Recall that carbon dioxide is acidic. If the blood is more acidic, the respiratory center increases the rate and depth of breathing to release or "blow off" excess carbon dioxide. If the blood is more alkaline, the respiratory center decreases the rate and depth of breathing to retain carbon dioxide. Peripheral chemoreceptors, which are most sensitive to oxygen levels in the arterial blood (PaO_2), are located in the aorta and carotid arteries. Peripheral chemoreceptors trigger an increase in ventilation in response to low oxygen levels in the blood. Cervical and thoracic nerves are then stimulated accordingly to conduct the specified breathing adaptation.

STOP *and Consider*

How does your breathing change when you exercise? Why do you think this happens?

The messages sent by the lung and chemoreceptors are ultimately sent to the cervical and thoracic nerves, which act on the pulmonary system to adapt the breathing pattern to maintain homeostasis. The work of breathing is improved with functional and strong muscles of ventilation, such as the intercostal muscles, diaphragm, and sternocleidomastoid muscles, along with proper lung compliance (allows maximal inspiration), elastic recoil (promotes expiration), and low airway resistance. **Compliance** is the expected distensibility, or expandability, of the lung tissue and chest wall. Airway resistance is based on the area of the inner lumen of the airway and on properties, such as viscosity and velocity, of the gas moving through that airway.

INSPIRATION

Inspiration is the process of breathing in to acquire oxygen. Similar to inflating a balloon, movement of air is always unidirectional and travels from an area of high pressure to low pressure. In this example, the pressure inside the balloon (the "lungs") is lower than that of the person blowing air into the balloon (the "atmosphere"). A major difference is that the *chest cavity changes size to alter the pressure gradient*, thereby drawing air into the lungs, as opposed to the air moving in and changing the size, as you would see with a balloon. Neuronal stimulation and the movement of the diaphragm downward and external intercostal muscles outward allows this increase in chest cavity size, reduces pressure inside the lungs, and pulls air into the lungs.

EXPIRATION

Expiration, the process of removing carbon dioxide out of the body through the lungs, is also regulated within the respiratory center of the brain. In expiration, the diaphragm and external intercostal muscles relax. The chest wall moves inward and the diaphragm moves upward. The intrathoracic (inside the thoracic cavity) pressure becomes greater than the atmospheric pressure. This stimulates air to flow passively out into the atmosphere. Exhalation can also be forced if the abdominal and intercostal muscles are contracted voluntarily, thereby increasing pressure to move the diaphragm upward and pull the ribs inward. The idea is to compress the lungs and increase the pressure inside the airways. Air then moves from higher to lower pressure, or, in this example, from the lungs to the atmosphere.

MEASUREMENT OF VENTILATION

The measurement of lung volumes can determine the effectiveness of inspiration and expiration. Measurements are completed by breathing in or out through a spirometer where measurement of air volume occur. Changes in lung volumes or pulmonary function can be an early sign of impaired ventilation. Predicted values (the measurement readings that are expected) vary based on age, height, and gender. The following are examples of major measurements of ventilatory capacity:

- **Tidal volume (TV)** is the amount of air that is exhaled after passive inspiration; this is the volume of air going in and out of the lungs at rest; in adults, this volume is approximately 500 mL.
- **Vital capacity (VC)** is the maximal amount of air that can be moved in and out of the lungs with forced inhalation and exhalation.

- **Forced vital capacity (FVC)** is the maximal amount of air that is exhaled from the lungs during a forced exhalation.
- **Forced expiratory volume in 1 second (FEV$_1$)** is the maximal amount of air that can be expired from the lungs in 1 second.
- **Residual volume (RV)** is the volume of air that remains in the lungs after maximal expiration.
- **Total lung capacity (TLC)** is the total amount of air in the lungs when they are maximally expanded and is the sum of the vital capacity and RV.

Diffusion

Oxygen and carbon dioxide are exchanged at the alveolar capillary junctions in the process of diffusion. The alveolar capillary junction is a thin membrane composed of a layer of alveolar epithelial cells with a basement membrane and the capillary epithelium with a basement membrane. These are separated by a narrow interstitial space and are supported by connective tissue. Between the alveolus and capillary, oxygen moves in to the circulation and carbon dioxide moves out to the atmosphere. Figure 13.1 depicts the proximity of the alveolus and capillary. The alveoli that compose the alveolar portion of this junction are commonly designated type I alveolar cells (those that provide structure and air exchange) or type II (those that are active in secreting **surfactant**, a lipoprotein lubricant that coats the inner portion of the alveolus, promotes ease of expansion, and repels fluid accumulation). Surfactant is essential to maintain the integrity, air exchange, and diffusion function of the pulmonary system. Without surfactant, inflation of the alveoli would be almost impossible and would make breathing difficult.

During diffusion, two major processes are occurring simultaneously: (1) oxygen is trying to get to all cells; and (2) carbon dioxide is trying to escape the body through the lungs. The effectiveness of this transaction depends upon:

- *Pressure:* the amount of partial pressure of the oxygen or carbon dioxide in the blood
- *Solubility:* carbon dioxide is much more soluble than oxygen; therefore, carbon dioxide is able to diffuse at a greater rate than oxygen
- *Membranes:* the thickness and surface areas of the alveolar and capillary membranes

PARTIAL PRESSURE

Oxygen and carbon dioxide are composed of countless particles in constant collision. The force of these collisions results in the formation of pressure. With oxygen, approximately 1% to 13% is carried in the circulation as a dissolved gas in the plasma. This portion creates a pressure in the plasma, which is referred to as the **partial pressure** and is reported in mm Hg. The symbol for the partial pressure of oxygen in the arterial blood is **PaO_2**. PaO_2 is measured as part of the arterial blood gas panel by drawing blood from a small artery. Because there is no direct method to measure oxygen concentrations in the body, the PaO_2 gives a reasonable estimate of the presence of oxygen in the blood based on the pressure exerted by this gas. PaO_2 is influenced by several factors, such as the presence and concentration of oxygen, altitude, or even aging. Similar to oxygen, the dissolved CO_2 in the plasma forms a partial pressure. The symbol for the partial pressure of carbon dioxide in arterial blood is **$PaCO_2$**. $PaCO_2$ is also part of the arterial blood gas panel. It is measured through an arterial blood sample and is reported in mm Hg.

OXYGEN DIFFUSION AND TRANSPORT

After inspiration and diffusion across the alveolar capillary junction occurs, oxygen dissolves in the plasma, forming a partial pressure (PaO_2). As the PaO_2 increases, oxygen dissociates from the plasma and connects with hemoglobin molecules on red blood cells (RBCs). The oxygen–hemoglobin combination is now called **oxyhemoglobin (HbO_2)**. The connection to hemoglobin is based on oxygen's attraction to iron. Iron is the magnet that pulls oxygen onto the hemoglobin molecule. The oxygen then circulates throughout the body. When the oxygen is on the hemoglobin, it is *not* accessible to the cell.

● STOP *and Consider*

What happens to your oxygen-attracting ability if you eat a diet low in iron?

This binding by attraction to hemoglobin continues until the hemoglobin molecules are completely saturated with oxygen. **Oxygen saturation (SaO_2)** refers to the amount of oxyhemoglobin; that is, the amount of hemoglobin that is combined, or saturated, with oxygen. Four oxygen molecules can ride on each hemoglobin vehicle. When all four seats are filled, the hemoglobin is termed **fully saturated** or 100% saturated. Less than this amount indicates a reduction in the presence of oxygen or carrying capacity of the hemoglobin vehicle. SaO_2 is *not* affected by blood volume or hemoglobin level. The SaO_2 is simply saying that for the hemoglobin present, this percent is saturated with oxygen. Feasibly,

an individual could have a severe hemorrhage and still measure an SaO_2 of 100%.

Once saturation has been achieved, oxygen continues to diffuse and dissolve in the plasma until the partial pressure in the arteries is equal to that of the partial pressure of the oxygen in the alveoli. Diffusion across the alveoli ceases until the need for oxygen is again detected by changes in the PaO_2. The dissolved oxygen in the plasma is diffused into and used by the cells for cellular metabolism. Oxygen is much less soluble than carbon dioxide; therefore, at any time, approximately 87% to 99% of the oxygen is combined with hemoglobin; the remainder is found dissolved in the plasma of the blood.

CARBON DIOXIDE DIFFUSION AND TRANSPORT

A major waste product of cellular function and respiration is carbon dioxide. If the cell is forced into anaerobic respiration, acidic metabolic wastes are produced in addition to CO_2. One mechanism for ridding the body of this excess acid is to free the CO_2 into the circulation, where it then travels to the alveoli and through the lungs for exhalation. Carbon dioxide diffuses much more readily than oxygen and moves easily across the alveolar capillary junctions. Once released from the cells, carbon dioxide is transported through the circulation similar to oxygen in that it is:

- *Dissolved* in the plasma (approximately 10% of the CO_2)
- *Bound* to hemoglobin (approximately 20% to 30% of the CO_2)
- *Diffused* into the RBC as bicarbonate (approximately 60% to 70% of the CO_2)

● STOP *and Consider*

What happens to oxygen and carbon dioxide transport if there is a lack of RBCs, as in the case of severe hemorrhaging?

The major portion of the CO_2 found diffused into the RBC is converted through the buffering systems to either carbonic acid or bicarbonate ions. Next, the carbonic acid or bicarbonate continues in the plasma to help regulate blood pH. Excess CO_2 is released easily from the hemoglobin, diffuses readily through alveolar capillary junction, and is exhaled through the lungs. Conditions that can decrease expiratory efficiency, such as fibrosis and air trapping in the alveoli, greatly affect CO_2 transport. The CO_2 will not be able to cross the alveolar membrane, will be retained in the body, and will lead to acidosis.

From the Lab

Oxygen saturation (oxyhemoglobin) (SaO$_2$) is often measured using pulse oximetry, a noninvasive method of determining hypoxemia even before clinical signs and symptoms are noted. The principle of pulse oximetry is based on red (600 to 750 nm wavelength) and infrared (850 to 1,000 nm wavelength) light absorption levels for oxygenated and deoxygenated hemoglobin. Oxygenated hemoglobin absorbs more *infrared* light and allows more red light to pass through. Deoxygenated hemoglobin absorbs more *red* light and allows more infrared light to pass through. A sensor is placed on the finger, toe, nose, earlobe, or forehead. Both red and infrared lights are transmitted to a photo detector. The sensor measures the amount of red and infrared light absorbed by hemoglobin. The expected range of SaO$_2$ is generally 95% to 100%. An SaO$_2$ below 70% may be life-threatening.

A fingertip oximeter sensor (adult). (Image from Evans-Smith P. *Taylor's Clinical Nursing Skills*. Philadelphia: Lippincott Williams & Wilkins; 2004, with permission.)

tatively. The **diffusing capacity** is defined as a measurement of carbon monoxide (CO), oxygen, or nitric oxide transfer from inspired gas to pulmonary capillary blood and reflects the volume of a gas that diffuses through the alveolar capillary membrane each minute. This volume is determined most commonly by comparing how much CO at nontoxic levels is taken up by the blood and dividing this by the pressure across the alveolar capillary membrane. Individuals with alveolar fibrosis or obstruction would be appropriate candidates for undergoing an analysis of diffusing capacity. During the test, the individual breathes in a gas containing CO and one or more tracer gases to allow determination of the gas exchanging capability of the lungs. For example, the oxygen-diffusing capacity in a state of rest averages about 21 mL/min/ mm Hg. If the average pressure difference between the alveoli and arterial blood is 11 mm Hg, the amount of oxygen that diffuses per minute would average $21 \times 11 = 230$ mL.

DIFFUSING CAPACITY

The ability of the alveolar capillary junction to exchange oxygen and carbon dioxide between the atmosphere and the blood can be measured quanti-

● STOP *and Consider*

Based on what you know about why and how SaO$_2$, PaO$_2$, and PaCO$_2$ are measured, what factors do you think would affect these readings?

Module 2

Impaired Ventilation

Impaired ventilation is a problem of blocking airflow in and out of the lungs, thereby restricting oxygen intake and carbon dioxide removal from the body. Two major mechanisms are implicated: (1) compression or narrowing of the airways; or (2) disruption of the neuronal transmissions needed to stimulate the mechanics of breathing. Compression or narrowing of the airways anywhere from the nose or mouth to alveoli increases airway resistance and leads to difficulties with airway clearance. This occlusion can be partial or complete. Examples of processes that

contribute to ineffective airway clearance include inflammation, edema, and exudate accumulation from an infectious process, a structural narrowing of the passageway, strangulation, or the presence of a foreign body. In these cases, air is restricted from moving in and out of the body.

Disruption of neuronal transmission to the lungs also alters ventilatory capacity by ignoring the messages sent by chemoreceptors and lung receptors and interrupting the mechanics of breathing. Oversedation during a surgical procedure or a drug overdose can promote a loss of neurologic stimulation on the respiratory center. Damage to the respiratory center of the brain, cervical nerves, or thoracic nerves leads to an unresponsive or ineffective breathing pattern that does not adapt to oxygen intake needs and carbon dioxide removal needs of the body. For example, severing the cervical nerves results in cessation of spontaneous lung function and requires external mechanical ventilation. Table 13.1 highlights effective and ineffective breathing patterns related to select physiologic and pathophysiologic processes. When a person's breathing pattern is responsive, the rate, depth, and rhythmic pattern of breathing adapt to physiologic changes occurring in the body. Breathing patterns become ineffective when these qualities (rate, depth, and rhythm) do not successfully maintain homeostasis, particularly in maintaining acid–base balance. All of the clinical models in this chapter demonstrate some level of ineffective airway clearance and modification in breathing patterns related to obstructive, restrictive, or altered neuronal processes.

STOP *and Consider*

How long can you hold your breath? How do you feel while you are holding your breath? When you cannot hold your breath any longer and you start to breathe, how does your body respond?

Impaired Ventilation–Perfusion Matching

A second mechanism for impairing gas exchange is termed ventilation–perfusion (V/Q) mismatching. This means either that areas of the lung are ventilated but not perfused or that the lung is perfused but not ventilated. Examples of problems that can impair ventilation are described in the previous section. With impaired ventilation, inadequate oxygen comes into the lungs even though the blood flow is ready and able to carry the oxygen that is present. If the perfusion aspect is impaired, the blood flow to the lungs is restricted in one or more areas. Oxygen may be coming into the body but there is no blood flow to carry this away to other body cells. A more complete discussion of V/Q mismatching is reserved for Chapter 14.

Impaired Diffusion

Impaired diffusion is a process of restricting the transfer of oxygen or carbon dioxide across the alveolar capillary junction. Because the rate of diffusion depends on the solubility and partial pressure of the gas, *and* on surface area and thickness of the membrane,

impaired gas exchange can occur with changes in any of these properties. All of the clinical models in this chapter demonstrate some level of impaired gas exchange related to a decrease in the functional alveolar capillary junction surface area.

Partial pressure is increased when more molecules are packed into a space, when the temperature increases (promoting an increase in particle collisions), and when the barometric pressure increases. A loss of partial pressure, and subsequent decrease in oxygen presence, can occur during a state of oxygen deprivation, during hypothermia, or when the body is responding to changes in atmospheric pressure (high altitude). The partial pressure of oxygen generally increases during the administration of high concentrations of oxygen and potentially during a fever. The partial pressure of carbon dioxide is increased during states of greater tissue metabolism, as it occurs with fever or strenuous exercise. This results in higher levels of carbon dioxide in the blood.

Changes in the alveolar capillary membrane also impair diffusion. Damage to the alveoli or capillaries limits the accessible and usable surface area and restricts oxygen and carbon dioxide transport. Many disease processes, such as pneumonia, pulmonary edema, and acute respiratory distress syndrome, fill the alveolar capillary junction with the products of inflammation or infection. This obstructs the passage of gases needed for cell function and for the maintenance of optimal pH in the blood. Chronic injury to the alveoli, such as with emphysema, can lead to fibrosis, or thickening of the alveolar capillary membrane, and can also impair gas exchange.

The Effects of Impaired Ventilation and Diffusion

Many conditions, even diseases outside of the "respiratory" system, can challenge the ventilatory and diffusion capabilities of the body. Any situation that presents a demand for higher levels of oxygen or an increase in cellular metabolism requires pulmonary adaptation to maintain homeostasis. For example, strenuous exercise requires extensive adaptation to provide adequate oxygen to cells and to remove the excess carbon dioxide (as a byproduct of cellular metabolism). When the body is unable to keep up with the demands, either because the demands are too great or the ventilation or diffusion capabilities are restricted, this can lead to:

1. Hypoxemia
2. Hypoxia
3. Hypercapnia

These three effects directly result from decreased oxygen presence or utilization, or the retention of carbon dioxide. Basically, the body is unable to take

Table 13.1 Adaptations in Breathing Patterns

Type of Breathing Pattern	Description of Pattern	Diagram of Pattern	Reason for Occurrence
Eupnea	The expected pattern of breathing characterized by a rate between 10 and 20 breaths per minute in adults, 500 and 800 mL in depth and a regular rhythm		Effective and responsive gas exchange
Tachypnea	Rapid, shallow breathing characterized by a rate of breathing above 24 breaths per minute in adults		The body needs to release excess carbon dioxide and responds by increasing the rate of breathing. This is an expected response to fever, fear, or exercise; can also occur with respiratory insufficiency pneumonia, or injury to respiratory center
Apnea	Cessation of breathing for 10 seconds or longer, usually interspersed with another breathing pattern described in this table		Can result from brain injury, premature birth, or as an obstructive process during sleep
Hyperpnea (Kussmaul's respirations), hyperventilation	Increase in the rate and the depth of breathing. Hyperpnea is responsive to PaO_2/$PaCO_2$ requirements; hyperventilation occurs in excess of what is needed to maintain $PaCO_2$		Excess carbon dioxide needs to be released. This can occur with extreme exertion, fear, or anxiety, or with diabetes ketoacidosis, aspirin overdose, or brain injury. Hyperventilation blows off excessive CO_2, causing a decreased level in the blood
Bradypnea, hypoventilation	Slow breathing with regular depth and rate. Hypoventilation refers to decreased and inadequate ventilation		Drug-induced depression of the respiratory center, increased intracranial pressure, diabetic coma
Cheyne–Stokes	A breathing pattern that alternates hyperpnea in a crescendo–decrescendo pattern and periods of apnea		Increased intracranial pressure, breathing bilateral damage to cerebral hemispheres or diencephalons, drug-induced respiratory depression, heart failure, uremia
Ataxic breathing	A breathing pattern of unpredictable irregularity. Can combine any or all breathing patterns above		Severe head trauma and damage to respiratory center, brain abscess, heat stroke, spinal meningitis, encephalitis
Obstructive breathing	Prolonged and incomplete expiration to overcome increased airway resistance and air trapping		Chronic obstructive lung disease, asthma, chronic bronchitis

Images of eupnea, tachypnea, apnea, bradypnea, and Cheyne–Stokes from *Nursing Procedures*. 4th ed. Ambler: Lippincott Williams & Wilkins; 2004, with permission. Images of hyperpnea, ataxic breathing, and obstructive breathing from Bickley LS, Szilagyi P. *Bates' Guide to Physical Examination and History Taking*. 8th ed. Philadelphia: Lippincott Williams & Wilkins; 2003, with permission.

in enough oxygen or is unable to release enough carbon dioxide. These basic effects directly apply to the selected clinical models in this chapter and all other conditions that affect ventilation and diffusion.

HYPOXEMIA AND HYPOXIA

Hypoxemia is decreased oxygen in the arterial blood leading to a decrease in the partial pressure of oxygen (PaO_2). The major causes of hypoxemia include oxygen deprivation, hypoventilation, problems with adequate diffusion, and inadequate uptake of oxygen in the blood. Hypoxemia can range from mild to severe and becomes problematic when cells are deprived of adequate oxygen, a condition referred to as **hypoxia**. When hypoxemia leads to hypoxia, the effects are widespread. All cells that depend on oxygen for efficient cellular metabolism are vulnerable, particularly cells within the vital organs (the brain, heart, and lungs). The brain has an incredibly high demand for oxygen and has minimal storage capacity. Oxygen deprivation throughout the body results in reduced cell metabolism and function. This, in turn, forces the cell to use anaerobic metabolism. Anaerobic metabolism leads to the rapid development of metabolic acidosis. The body needs to maintain a relatively constant pH for optimal cell functioning. Cellular death results from extreme or prolonged hypoxia. The cerebral effects of chronic hypoxia can range from restlessness (an early sign, particularly in children) to lethargy, coma, and eventually death.

Although hypoxemia can lead to hypoxia, hypoxia can result even when there is adequate arterial oxygen. For example, a reduction in circulation caused by an arterial blockage can deprive the cells distal to the blockage of oxygen even though the total amount of circulating oxygen is adequate. In this case, cell death results only in those cells deprived of oxygen.

HYPERCAPNIA

Hypercapnia refers to a state of increased carbon dioxide in the blood. Carbon dioxide is much more easily diffused than oxygen; therefore, hypercapnia presents only in cases of severe alveolar hypoventilation and subsequent hypoxia. Conditions that inhibit ventilation or promote trapping of air in the alveoli contribute to the development of hypercapnia. The major effect is respiratory acidosis caused by CO_2 retention. This can lead to electrolyte disturbances, which can alter cardiac conduction (see Chapter 14) and brain function, resulting in an ineffective heart rhythm, coma, and death. The determination of the level of hypercapnia requires measurement of arterial blood gases. Figure 13.2 summarizes the processes from ventilation and diffusion to hypoxemia, hypoxia, and hypercapnia.

STOP *and Consider*

How does the body respond to low oxygen or increased carbon dioxide in the blood or tissues?

General Manifestations of Impaired Ventilation and Diffusion

Although some subtle variations in manifestations exist across conditions, the local and systemic clinical manifestations of altered ventilation and diffusion have many commonalities. Local manifestations (those triggered in the airways and lung tissues) are most often related to inflammatory processes in response to injury. The injury triggers vasodilation, increased capillary permeability, exudate formation, and pain in the affected region of the airways, lungs,

or chest cavity. Potent chemical mediators regulate these inflammatory processes and are responsible for many of the local and systemic manifestations.

The following are potential local manifestations:

- Cough
- Excess mucus production
- Hemoptysis
- Dyspnea
- Use of accessory muscles
- Chest pain
- Barrel chest

A cough with or without excessive sputum production is a common clinical manifestation of altered ventilation and diffusion. The cough reflex is a protective mechanism that is triggered to rid the airways of an irritating agent. An acute cough typically lasts less than 3 to 8 weeks and is commonly associated with viral infections, seasonal allergies, **aspiration** (inhaling a foreign substance into the lungs), or pulmonary embolus (a blockage that occludes a pulmonary blood vessel). A chronic cough is one that extends beyond 8 weeks and is commonly associated with asthma, gastroesophageal reflux (gastric contents back up into the esophagus and stimulate the cough reflex), or chronic postnasal drainage. In smokers, chronic cough is a common manifestation of chronic bronchitis or lung cancer.

Excess mucus production of the airways is related to the inflammatory response. This mucus is often the irritating agent that triggers the cough reflex and often provides clues to the offending agent or process. This condition can be observed by having the individual **expectorate**, or spit out, the mucus that is ejected during the cough. **Sputum** refers to this expectorated material. **Phlegm** is a term that describes large amounts of sputum expectorated from the oropharynx. Specific pathogens may produce sputum with a distinct color or odor. For example, bacterial infections are often characterized by thick, purulent sputum. Pneumococcal pneumonia may lead to a rust-colored, dark sputum. Typically, the onset of a viral acute upper respiratory infection (a common cold) begins with clear, thin mucus. As phagocytes move into the area of inflammation to ward off any infection, these cells then die and are shed off as yellow or green mucus. **Hemoptysis** (coughing up blood from the respiratory tract) is defined by the presence of RBCs in the sputum. Blood in the sputum is often significant and can be caused by heavy exertion during coughing (blood streaking within the mucus) or from **tuberculosis (TB)**, a tumor, or more severe trauma. When combined with edema in the lung tissues (pulmonary edema), the sputum often becomes not only blood-tinged but also frothy or foamy.

Difficulty breathing is a common report in individuals with altered ventilation or diffusion. **Dyspnea** is the subjective feeling of shortness of breath or the

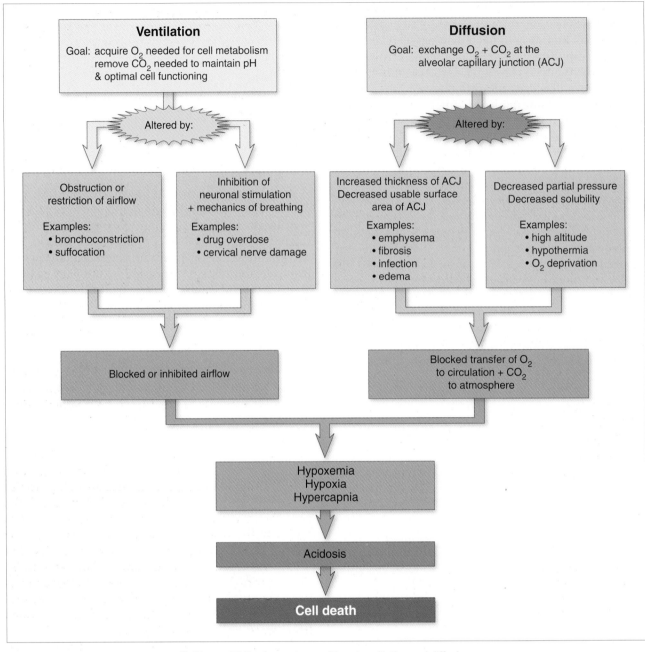

Figure 13.2 Concept map. Altered ventilation and diffusion.

inability to get enough air. The stimulus is based on the presence of hypoxemia, hypercapnia, and the subsequent reduction in pH; however, the exact mechanism is often unknown. One theory is that lung receptors or chemoreceptors act on the brain and muscles active in breathing to stimulate this sensation. Dyspnea often leads to certain physical and emotional responses, such as the physical need to sit in an upright or standing position, a condition called **orthopnea**, to maximize lung expansion. An individual may also use accessory muscles and demonstrate nasal flaring to promote the work of breathing. **Retractions** are the pulling in of accessory muscles usually in the intercostal, substernal, and supraclavicular spaces to promote more effective inspiration.

Along with position and effort changes, individuals experiencing air trapping may perform **pursed lip breathing**, a process of holding the lips puckered tightly together while slowly exhaling, to maintain positive airway pressure in the alveoli to minimize air trapping and promote expiration of carbon dioxide. Emotional manifestations of dyspnea include anxiety, a sense of panic, frustration, and anger.

Chest pain can originate in the visceral and parietal pleura, the airways, or the chest wall. Inflammatory processes within the pleura often lead to pleural pain, which increases with deep inspiration, and is often described as sharp or stabbing pain. **Auscultation** (listening with a stethoscope) will reveal a grating, scratching sound (called a pleural friction rub) with inspiration. Costochondritis, inflammation of one or more costal cartilages, is also characterized by pain in the anterior chest wall and may be triggered by coughing. Similarly, inflammation of the airways, intercostal muscles, or accessory muscles can also present as localized pain and be triggered by coughing. Chest pain, although frequently of pulmonary origin, must be differentiated from cardiac pain because of the possibility of the individual experiencing a myocardial infarction (heart attack).

Changes in the shape of the chest wall, known as barrel chest, can also occur with chronic lung disease. Typically, the chest wall shape is an oval, in which the anterior–posterior (AP) plane is narrower than the transverse (T) plane (an AP:T ratio of approximately 1:2). Chronic dilation and distention of the alveoli, as seen in emphysema, often results in a barrel chest appearance, in which the AP:T ratio becomes 1:1 (Fig. 13.3).

Changes in breathing patterns (see Table 13.1) and in the characteristics of breath sounds are also common local manifestations of altered ventilation

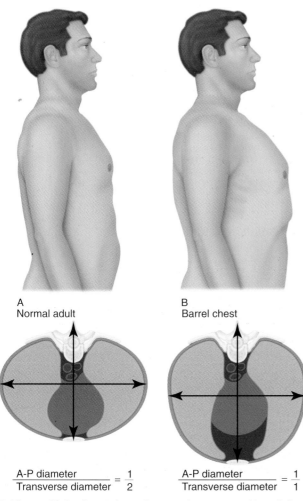

A
Normal adult

B
Barrel chest

$$\frac{\text{A-P diameter}}{\text{Transverse diameter}} = \frac{1}{2}$$ $$\frac{\text{A-P diameter}}{\text{Transverse diameter}} = \frac{1}{1}$$

Figure 13.3 Comparison of expected anatomy and barrel chest alteration that occurs with emphysema. **A:** The expected chest cross-section. **B:** The barrel chest.

Box 13.1 Adventitious Breath Sounds

Crackles are snapping, popping, or bubbling sounds emitted during inspiration and expiration and caused by fluid accumulation in the airways; fine crackles are higher pitched with a shorter duration and signify fluid in smaller airways; coarse crackles are louder and lower pitched and signify fluid in the larger airways.

Rales is a previously used term to describe fine crackles from fluid secretions in the airways; the term rales has been replaced with crackles.

Wheezing is a continuous, high-pitched, whistling sound; it is significant for obstruction or tightness in the small airways.

Rhonchi is a term used to describe both low-pitched wheezing sounds with a snoring quality (sonorous wheezing) when the airway narrowing is in the larger airways, and high-pitched wheezing sounds with a squeaking quality (sibilant wheezing) when the airway narrowing is in the smaller airways. Rhonchi occur when thick mucus partially blocks the airways.

Stridor is a harsh, high-pitched, creaking sound, which is significant for obstruction in the upper airway, especially of the trachea or larynx.

Diminished breath sounds is a term used to describe quieter breath sounds that are barely audible; this is significant for complete obstruction in one or more airways.

Absent breath sounds signifies no air movement through the lungs.

and diffusion. The sounds emitted by the lungs during inspiration and expiration also give clues to the presence and extent of altered ventilation and diffusion. **Adventitious**, or altered, breath sounds are typically the result of either airway constriction or fluid accumulation (Box 13.1). Airway constriction results in wheezing breath sounds. Fluid accumulation leads to fine or course crackles. The characteristics of these sounds vary based on anatomic location (larger vs. smaller airways) or type of secretions (thin, watery vs. thicker mucous).

Systemic manifestations of altered ventilation are caused by the effects of hypoxemia, hypoxia, and hypercapnia. In the presence of inflammation, systemic manifestations, such as fever, malaise, leukocytosis, and higher levels of circulating plasma proteins, can apply to problems of altered ventilation and diffusion. The intensity of the hypoxic or hypercapnic response is variable depending on the extent of oxygen deprivation and carbon dioxide retention. Responses may include:

- Dusky or cyanotic mucous membrane color
- Changes in arterial blood gases
- Mental status changes
- Finger clubbing

Changes in arterial blood gases, pH, PaO_2, and $PaCO_2$, and mental status changes are discussed above as effects of hypoxemia, hypoxia, and hypercapnia.

Changes in skin and mucous membrane color can also result from severe hypoxemia. **Cyanosis** is caused by a greater proportion of desaturated hemoglobin in the blood, which gives the blood a bluish hue. Central cyanosis, a problem of low oxygen saturation in the arterial blood, often presents as color changes in the skin and mucous membranes. In individuals with dark skin, the skin color change is often described as ashen or dusky. In light skin, the color is often described as pale or bluish. Because skin color varies among individuals, the most reliable indicator of central cyanosis on examination is the finding of a bluish color of the mucous membranes. Individuals with peripheral cyanosis, a problem of sluggish blood flow in the fingers and toes, often present with sluggish capillary refill (demonstrated by a slow return of blood when the nail bed is compressed and then released) and a pale or bluish hue in the nail beds (see Chapter 14).

Chronic problems with ventilation and diffusion may result in clubbing of the fingers. **Clubbing** is a painless enlargement and flattening of the tips of fingers or toes caused by chronic hypoxia (Fig. 13.4). Although the exact mechanism is unknown, clubbing is consistently associated with chronic conditions that disturb oxygenation, such as prolonged obstruction or fibrosis of the airways.

■ **Figure 13.4** Clubbing of the fingers. (Image from Crapo JD, Glassroth J, Karlinsky JB, et al. *Baum's Textbook of Pulmonary Diseases*. 7th ed. Philadelphia: Lippincott Williams & Wilkins; 2004, with permission.)

▨ Laboratory and Diagnostic Tests

Detection of altered ventilation and diffusion is based on a thorough patient history and physical examination supported by relevant diagnostic and laboratory tests. Table 13.2 presents common laboratory and diagnostic tests performed when an individual has a suspected alteration in ventilation and diffusion.

Table 13.2 Laboratory and Diagnostic Tests Performed to Determine Altered Ventilation and Diffusion

Lab or Diagnostic Test	Purpose of the Test
PFTs	Broad range of noninvasive tests including spirometry, lung volume measurements, and diffusion capacity that involve breathing into a tube that measures the pressure exerted during ventilation. Spirometry is useful in detecting obstructive lung disease by monitoring how well the lungs exhale
ABGs	Determines presence of acid–base imbalances and degree of hypoxemia and hypercapnia from an arterial blood sample
Pulse oximetry	Noninvasive test that measures oxygen saturation (see From the Lab)
Bronchoscopy	Direct visualization of bronchioles; can be used to take biopsy, take sputum samples, or remove foreign objects from airway
Radiograph, CT, MRI	Used to detect structural problems, presence of consolidation, obstruction, or cavitation in the airways and lung tissue
Nuclear (V/Q) lung scan[a]	Detects pulmonary embolism (lung blockage) and lung disease, such as emphysema and chronic obstructive pulmonary disease, by using a nuclear medicine camera and computer imaging to visualize the amount and distribution of minute amounts of radioactive materials inspired into the lungs (V) or injected into a vein (Q) that then flows to and perfuses the lung
Culture and sensitivity tests	Determines presence and type of microorganisms in the blood and/or sputum; the results dictate the appropriate antibiotic treatment if indicated
Thoracentesis	Determines the presence of a pleural effusion (excess fluid in the pleural space) by inserting a needle from the chest or back into the lung pleural space; the fluid is examined to determine the cellular and chemical composition, the presence of malignant cells, and the presence of microorganisms

[a]V = ventilation (airflow in and out of the lungs); Q = perfusion (blood flow to the lungs).
PFTs, Pulmonary function tests; ABGs, Arterial blood gases; CT, computed tomography; MRI, magnetic resonance imaging.

Table 13.3 Altered Ventilation and Diffusion Treatment Principles

Treatment	Mechanism of Action	Appropriate Uses
Anti-inflammatory medications	Reduces inflammatory response by acting on chemical mediators to decrease excess blood flow, swelling, heat, redness, and pain to the affected area	Inflammation that impinges on ventilatory function such as with asthma
Humidification	Moistens and liquefies secretions to aid in expectoration	Use in the presence of excessive, thick, or sticky mucus
Decongestants	Decreases nasal congestion through vascular vasoconstriction, which decreases blood flow, reduces exudate, and shrinks swollen mucous membranes	Use in the presence of excessive, thick, or sticky mucus
Antitussives	Suppresses cough by inhibiting cough receptors in the medulla (some have local effects as well)	Use when cough is excessive and interferes with sleep
Bronchodilators	Opens airways by relaxing bronchial smooth muscles	Conditions that cause bronchoconstriction: asthma, COPD
Chest physiotherapy	Using a pounding motion or vibration on the chest to physically loosen thick secretions	Conditions that result in thick, tenacious secretions such as in cystic fibrosis
Antimicrobials	Antibiotics have a range of mechanisms focused on destroying or reducing impact of bacteria; antivirals may also be prescribed as appropriate	Bacterial infection (antibiotics) such as bacterial pneumonia
Oxygen therapy	Provides direct oxygen supplementation	Hypoxia
Mechanical ventilation	Life support measure that provides the work of breathing	Respiratory failure
Surgery	Surgical removal of abnormal tissues or structures within the chest (thoracotomy)	Multiple uses, including confirmation of the diagnosis of lung disease, repair of the lung, removal of lung tumors, or removal of pus from pleural space (empyema)

COPD, chronic obstructive pulmonary disease.

Treating Impaired Ventilation and Diffusion

The treatment of any health condition is based on determining the cause. Occasionally, in conditions of altered ventilation and diffusion, the cause cannot be reversed. The principles that guide improving ventilation are based on:

1. Removing obstructions (i.e., foreign body, tumor, edema)
2. Restoring the integrity of the chest wall, lungs, and other respiratory structures
3. Decreasing inflammation
4. Decreasing, thinning, and moving mucus out of the airway
5. Opening and maintaining integrity of the airways
6. Supplementing oxygen
7. Controlling infectious processes
8. Using mechanical ventilation, as indicated

Table 13.3 outlines common treatment modalities for impaired ventilation and diffusion.

Module 3
Clinical Models

The following clinical models have been selected to aid in the understanding and application of altered ventilation and diffusion processes and effects. Commonalities and unique features of each clinical model should be noted when reading this section.

Pneumonia

Pneumonia is selected as a clinical model to demonstrate the impact of a common acute infectious process on ventilation and diffusion. **Pneumonia** refers to inflammation of the lungs occurring commonly in the bronchioles, interstitial lung tissue, or the alveoli. The elderly, the very young, and those individuals who smoke or are immunosuppressed are most at risk for developing pneumonia.

Pneumonia is the sixth leading cause of death in the United States. The incidence appears greater in men than in women. A major risk factor is exposure to the health care system, including hospitalization and outpatient visits. In one study of hospitals in Italy, 362 patients were diagnosed with pneumonia. Of these, 62% were community-acquired, 25% were hospital-acquired, and 13% were ventilator-associated. Associated mortality rates were as high as 8%, 18%, and 18%, respectively.[1]

PATHOPHYSIOLOGY

The injurious agent is most often a microorganism, including bacteria, viruses, and fungi, but pneumonia can also result from a noninfectious inhaled irritant. The spread most commonly occurs through respiratory droplets. Pneumonias are often distinguished as either community acquired or hospital acquired (nosocomial) depending on where the disease was contracted. Nosocomial pneumonias, particularly in the immunosuppressed individual, tend to be more severe and lead to a less favorable prognosis than community-acquired pneumonias. Typical community-acquired pneumonia is most commonly caused by *Streptococcus pneumoniae, Haemophilus influenzae,* and *Staphylococcus* species. Atypical forms of community-acquired pneumonia are caused by *Mycoplasma pneumoniae, Legionella,* and *Chlamydia* species. The influenza virus is the most common viral pathogen known to cause pneumonia. Nosocomial, or hospital-acquired, pneumonia is most commonly caused by infection with *Pseudomonas aeruginosa* or *Staphylococcus aureus.* Infection with an opportunistic fungal infection in the lungs, such as with *Candida albicans* or *Pneumocystis carinii,* indicates immunosuppression or immunodeficiency. Characteristics of these pathogens are further described in Chapter 5. Aspiration pneumonia results from breathing in items not intended for the lungs, such as foods, fluids, and stomach contents.

In many cases, the defense mechanisms in the nasopharynx and oropharynx of the upper respiratory tract effectively trap and expel microorganisms before causing infection. For pathogens that happen to escape the cough reflex and mucociliary blanket, macrophages located in the alveoli are often adequate to engulf and destroy the offending microorganism. When these defense mechanisms are inadequate, the inflammatory and immune responses are triggered, particularly in the interstitial lung tissue and alveoli. The inflamed alveoli fill with

■ **Figure 13.5** Chest radiograph in a 50-year-old patient with pneumonia shows opacity characteristic of lung consolidation. (Image from Crapo JD, Glassroth J, Karlinsky JB, et al. *Baum's Textbook of Pulmonary Diseases.* 7th ed. Philadelphia: Lippincott Williams & Wilkins; 2004, with permission.)

exudate. Other products of inflammation (RBCs, white blood cells [WBCs], and fibrin) accumulate as well and cause **consolidation**, or a solid mass in the lung tissue. These areas of consolidation are evident on radiograph and are often the key diagnostic features of typical pneumonia (Fig. 13.5).

With typical pneumonia, the presence of another viral infection, such as influenza, promotes attachment of the pneumococcal bacteria to the receptors on the respiratory epithelium. The bacteria can then infect the type II alveolar cells. The pneumococci multiply along the alveolus and penetrate the alveolar epithelium, thereby moving across to infect adjacent alveoli. In contrast, atypical pneumonia causes damage often through immune-mediated mechanisms rather than direct damage caused by the bacteria. The spread of infection with atypical pneumonia is more likely to spread beyond the lobar boundaries and is often bilateral.

Histologic changes in the lungs during the progression of pneumonia can be categorized in three stages:

1. Recent infection shows rapid filling of the alveolar capillaries with a frothy, serous, and blood-tinged fluid.
2. A "red hepatization" stage follows and is marked by the filling of alveoli with fibrinous exudates, which appear as areas of dry, granular, dark-red lung tissue.
3. Within 72 hours, the "gray hepatization" stage occurs marked by WBCs packing into the

small and the host has a competent immune system, the bacilli can be successfully ingested, contained, and killed. If the immune system is compromised, the containment and destruction of the bacilli is less likely, and larger areas of necrosis can develop. The infection can then more easily spread through the lymph nodes to other organs in the body.

The initial containment and destruction of the bacilli occurs through a granulomatous inflammatory response. The formation of a granuloma, or walled-off area of bacteria, is referred to as a **Ghon focus**. The Ghon focus is considered the primary lung lesion. Often, particularly when the number of infecting bacilli is large, the center of the granuloma develops a distinct type of necrosis, termed **caseous necrosis**, which is pasty, yellow, and cheeselike. The *M. tuberculosis* within the Ghon focus drain along lymph channels to lymph nodes in the lungs and form further granulomas. The Ghon focus and the additional granulomas that develop through the lymph channels are referred to as the **Ghon complex** (Fig. 13.6). An intact inflammatory and immune response eventually results in the formation of scar tissue and calcification of these Ghon complex lesions. However, small numbers of dormant bacteria can survive within these calcifications for years.

Tuberculosis is often distinguished as either primary or secondary TB. Primary infection is the initial exposure and growth of the bacilli in an individual with or without symptoms. Individuals *with* symptoms are believed to have an aggressive and destructive disease, termed active infection. Individuals *without* symptoms often have an effective inflammatory and immune response, and a healed Ghon complex eventually forms, surrounding dormant bacilli. If the immune system becomes compromised and the bacteria are allowed to again proliferate, the infection becomes active and progresses to secondary TB. Secondary TB is characterized by reactivation of the primary infection after a long period of dormancy or by reinfection with the pathogens known to cause TB. Secondary TB, which can spread to other organs, is marked by aggressive, destructive cavitations of the lung tissue. **Cavitations** are areas of necrosis that erode surrounding structures of the lungs, including the bronchioles, bronchi, and surrounding blood vessels. If untreated, secondary TB can continue to spread, destroying tissues throughout the body. The pathogenesis of TB is depicted in Figure 13.7.

STOP *and* **Consider**

How does the development of granulomas, fibrosis, and calcification in TB compare with other chronic inflammatory conditions, such as rheumatoid arthritis?

The impact of TB on ventilation and diffusion is based on the stage of infection (primary asymptomatic infection versus progressive active infection, or reinfection). In early phases of Ghon focus and Ghon complex development, the level of impact is based on the extent of damage. The potential damage is ideally minimized through the efforts of cellular immunity and containment of the bacteria. Most often, there is no noticeable impact on ventilation or diffusion. Only during the stage of cavitation and destruction of lung structures does evidence of hypoxemia and eventually hypoxia emerge. The impact on pulmonary volumes is most evident in reduced vital capacity (the amount of air moving in and out of the lungs) and in increased **dead space** (areas where gas exchange cannot take place). Both of these changes are related to lung tissue and alveolar damage from the invading bacteria.

CLINICAL MANIFESTATIONS

Most (90%) of individuals infected with primary TB are asymptomatic. In those individuals with progressive primary TB (10%), clinical manifestations may resemble those of chronic inflammation, such as malaise, weight loss, fatigue, anorexia, low-grade fever, and possibly night sweats. Ongoing destruction of lung tissue results in a severe chronic

■ **Figure 13.6** Tuberculosis showing a healed Ghon complex. (Image from Rubin E, Farber JL. *Pathology*. 4th ed. Philadelphia: Lippincott Williams & Wilkins; 2005, with permission.)

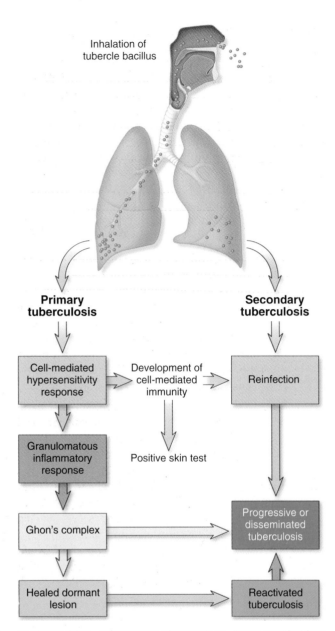

Inhalation of
tubercle bacillus

Primary
tuberculosis

Secondary
tuberculosis

| Cell-mediated hypersensitivity response | Development of cell-mediated immunity | Reinfection |

Granulomatous inflammatory response

Positive skin test

Ghon's complex

Progressive or disseminated tuberculosis

Healed dormant lesion

Reactivated tuberculosis

■ **Figure 13.7** Pathogenesis of tuberculosis. (Image modified from Porth CM. *Pathophysiology: Concepts of Altered Health States*. 7th ed. Philadelphia: Lippincott Williams & Wilkins; 2004, with permission.)

productive cough with hemoptysis. The bacteria readily reside in sputum and can be transmitted to others. Because secondary TB infection can reside in other organs of the body, clinical manifestations may extend outside of the pulmonary system. For example, TB found in the meninges of the brain will present with headache and mental status changes that may progress to coma over a period of days to weeks after infection.

DIAGNOSTIC CRITERIA

Active infection with TB is diagnosed through tuberculin skin tests (see From the Lab), chest radiograph, sputum culture, and sputum nucleic acid

amplification. A chest radiograph in primary TB often shows patchy or nodular infiltrates or pleural effusion. The upper lobe of the lung is most commonly affected. Advanced infection is noted by the presence of cavitation. Inactive "old" disease is noted by the presence of calcification. A CT scan may be needed if the results of the chest radiograph are unclear or inconclusive.

Sputum specimens should be collected in the early morning of three consecutive days. Fiberoptic bronchoscopy with transbronchial biopsy and bronchial washings may be needed to obtain sputum and tissue specimens for further analysis, particularly in those patients who are unable to expectorate sufficient sputum. The advantage to using nucleic acid amplification over sputum culture is that these newer technologies identify TB within 24 hours compared to a week or more with sputum cultures.

TREATMENT

Treatment is achieved through the use of multiple antimicrobial drugs over several months. The treatment protocol should include directly observed therapy (DOT). This means that the patient must be observed taking the medications at each administration by the health professional or designated personnel. DOT is required to promote complete eradication of the bacteria through improved patient compliance with the prolonged treatment regimen. Typically, treatment involves the use of four antimicrobial drugs: isoniazid, rifampin, pyrazinamide, and either ethambutol or streptomycin. Multiple drug resistance is a major treatment issue related to TB. Resistance to the prescribed antimicrobials is suspected if the patient shows no improvement within 1 to 2 weeks after starting the four first-line drugs. Those individuals with multiple drug-resistant TB are prescribed medications for which the bacteria are susceptible. To prevent transmission to others, hospitalized patients with suspected or diagnosed TB must be placed in isolation. This includes a private room with negative pressure and adequate air exchange mechanisms. Persons entering the room must wear masks or respirators capable of filtering droplet nuclei.

Bacillus Calmette–Guérin (BCG) is a vaccine for TB that is used in many countries with a high prevalence of TB to prevent childhood tuberculous meningitis or miliary (disseminated in the blood) tuberculosis. It is not widely recommended in North America because of the relatively low risk of infection and variable effectiveness against adult pulmonary TB. Individuals who have been vaccinated with BCG will have a positive tuberculin reaction when the PPD is administered; therefore, the tuberculin skin test is not an effective screening tool to detect TB exposure in those individuals vaccinated with BCG.

CHRONIC OBSTRUCTIVE PULMONARY DISEASE

Chronic obstructive pulmonary disease (COPD) is a generic term that describes all chronic obstructive lung problems, including asthma, emphysema, and chronic bronchitis, separately or in combination. COPD is one of the leading causes of death worldwide. A common misconception is that COPD is more common in men. However, in 2000, for the first time in US recorded history, more women than men died from COPD.[4]

COPD is primarily used to denote the presence of both emphysema and chronic bronchitis (and, to some extent, asthma). Inflammatory processes in both the alveoli and in the bronchi/bronchioles characterize COPD. The disease is progressive, unremitting, and irreversible, although progression can be slowed if treatment is implemented early in the course of the disease.[5] Although smoking has been implicated in the development of COPD, approximately 10% to 20% of those affected have never smoked.[6] Because of significant lung reserves, symptoms may only become apparent when lung function is at or below 50%. In this section, emphysema, chronic bronchitis, and asthma are discussed separately.

Emphysema

Emphysema is an irreversible enlargement of the air spaces beyond the terminal bronchioles, most notably in the alveoli, resulting in destruction of the alveolar walls and obstruction of airflow. The most notable cause of emphysema is chronic smoking, although in nonsmokers, development of emphysema is often due to the genetically inherited deficiency of alpha$_1$-antitrypsin (AAT). Less commonly, pulmonary vascular damage from the insoluble fillers (e.g., cornstarch or cotton fibers) found in intravenous drugs (such as methadone or cocaine), immune deficiency syndromes, or connective tissue disorders (such as Marfan syndrome) can lead to the development of emphysema.

PATHOPHYSIOLOGY

In early or mild emphysema, the primary source of obstruction is the development of inflammation in the small airways distal to the respiratory bronchioles. If diagnosed early, the inflammation in the small airways can be reduced, thereby providing some relief from airway obstruction. In moderate to severe disease, the loss of elastic recoil in the alveoli is the primary mechanism of airflow obstruction. This is not reversible. Vascular changes in the lungs develop simultaneously along with the airway obstruction. The inner lining of the arteries and

arterioles that perfuse the lungs become thicker and fibrotic. This further contributes to alveolar and capillary destruction. Patterns of alveolar destruction can occur in the respiratory bronchioles and spread peripherally, termed *centriacinar*, or uniformly destroy the entire alveolus, termed *panacinar*. Centriacinar emphysema is typically associated with chronic smoking and primarily affects the upper half of the lungs, whereas panacinar emphysema occurs in those with AAT deficiency.

Chronic smoking impairs alveolar function through the following cascade of events:

1. Inhalation of smoke triggers the inflammatory response.
2. Neutrophils and later macrophages are activated and retained in the lung tissue.
3. Neutrophils and macrophages release proteolytic enzymes, such as proteinases and elastases, that destroy components of the extracellular matrix, such as elastin, in the lungs.
4. The elasticity of the lung is significantly reduced leading to the inability of the alveoli to recoil and release CO_2 into the atmosphere.

Elasticity is essential in the alveoli. Loss of elasticity affects the ability of the alveoli to contract and move air back out of the body. The airspaces become enlarged and ineffective. If the alveolar walls collapse, air remains trapped in the alveoli (Fig. 13.8). **Air trapping** decreases effective O_2 intake and especially CO_2 release. The experience of air trapping is demonstrated through taking a full breath and releasing half of the air and then again taking a full deep breath and releasing half of the air. When a person takes a deep breath and releases only half of the air, hyperinflation occurs in the lungs. The alveoli

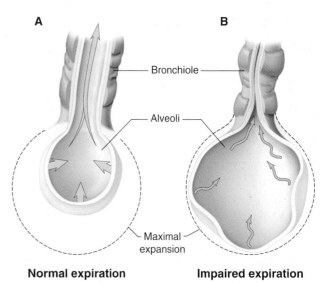

Normal expiration   **Impaired expiration**

■ **Figure 13.8**   Elastic recoil in the alveoli. **A:** Unaffected alveolus. **B:** Air trapping seen in emphysema caused by the loss of alveolar elastic recoil.

become further stretched and continue to lose elasticity. CO_2 is retained and blood pH is reduced.

The lungs require protection against the destruction imposed by proteolytic enzymes. This is the primary role of antiprotease enzymes, particularly AAT, an enzyme that is synthesized by cells in the lungs. This enzyme works to combat the destructive enzymes from digesting structural proteins and helps to maintain the integrity of the lungs. With emphysema, an imbalance of the destructive (proteolytic) and protective (antiproteolytic) enzymes exists, favoring the destructive. In smokers, lung destruction is a manifestation of excess proteinase release and a loss of antiproteinase defenses within the lungs.

The development of emphysema in nonsmokers is most often related to the manifestation of a genetic disorder attributed to a reduction or absence of antiprotease enzymes. In AAT deficiency, the affected individual has inherited an autosomal-codominant disorder located on the long arm of chromosome 14 (see Chapter 6). In codominant disorders, the phenotype is expressed in the individual who has inherited two equally dominant genes. This genetic defect causes an acceleration of the breakdown of cells and tissues in the lungs with the early onset of panacinar emphysema.

CLINICAL MANIFESTATIONS

Clinical manifestations are related to obstruction of the small airways and alveoli, chronic hypoxemia, and hypercapnia. Most patients with emphysema have smoked heavily for 20 or more years and present with a chronic productive cough, most notable upon waking in the morning. Dyspnea and wheezing may occur with minimal exertion. As the disease progresses, a barrel chest develops because of chronic hyperinflation of the airways. Patients with emphysema commonly perform pursed lip breathing to increase the pressure in the airways, to prevent alveolar wall collapse, and to allow the air to escape the alveoli. In severe disease, simple activities, such as brushing one's teeth, can cause tachypnea and respiratory distress.

DIAGNOSTIC CRITERIA

Diagnosis of emphysema is based on a thorough patient history and physical examination, noting a significant smoking history and characteristic clinical manifestations. Expiratory airflow should be measured using pulmonary function tests. In nonsmokers who have suspected emphysema, AAT levels can be measured and will be found to be well below the expected range. In general, individuals

with AAT deficiency and an increased risk for the development of emphysema will have 10% to 15% of the expected AAT level. Physical examination includes auscultation of lung sounds and observation of expiratory effort with simple activities. The respiratory rate tends to increase in proportion to disease severity. Cyanosis and peripheral edema may also be observed. Chest radiograph will show signs of hyperinflation.

Pulmonary function tests are critical in the diagnosis of emphysema and the level of airflow obstruction. Spirometry allows a determination of disease progression and the response to treatment. FEV_1 is the most common test to determine airflow obstruction; a prolonged forced expiratory time (FET) greater than 6 seconds indicates severe disease. Hypercapnia, measured in the arterial blood gas panel, is commonly observed when the FEV_1 falls below 30% of the predicted volume. For example, if a patient (based on age, gender, and height) is expected to forcefully exhale 4 L of air per second, hypercapnia will present when forced exhalation expels less than 1.2 L of air per second. This indicates severe outflow obstruction. Hypoxemia is often present in early disease and continues throughout the disease progression; however, hypercapnia predominates as the disease progresses.

TREATMENT

Because emphysema is irreversible, the goals of treatment are to maintain optimal lung function in order to allow the individual to perform the desired activities of daily living. Treatment begins with smoking cessation and may also include drug therapy (with danazol or tamoxifen) to increase production of AAT by the liver or by administering exogenous AAT via intravenous infusion or inhalation. Bronchodilators, steroid anti-inflammatory drugs, mucolytic agents (to reduce thickness and promote clearance of sputum), and antibiotics are the mainstays of therapy for individuals with emphysema. Supplemental oxygen is often required. Lung volume reduction or lung transplant are possible surgical treatment measures.

Chronic Bronchitis

Chronic bronchitis is defined by the presence of a persistent, productive cough with excessive mucus production that lasts for 3 months or longer for two or more consecutive years. The chronic bronchitis label is applied only after all other potential causes of chronic cough are excluded. The cause of chronic bronchitis is most commonly chronic smoking or exposure to environmental pollutants that irritate the airways.

PATHOPHYSIOLOGY

Chronic bronchitis results from several changes in the bronchi and bronchioles of the lungs in response to chronic injury including:

- Chronic inflammation and edema of the airways
- Hyperplasia of the bronchial mucous glands and smooth muscles
- Destruction of cilia
- Squamous cell metaplasia
- Bronchial wall thickening and development of fibrosis

The chronic inflammatory process, metaplasia, fibrosis, and mucous gland hyperplasia cause airway deformities and obstruct airflow by narrowing the airway lumen and further occluding this narrowed lumen through overproducing mucus. This is particularly problematic in the smaller airways and accounts for most airway obstructions. The loss of ciliated epithelium allows fine particles to enter the airway easily and predispose the individual to infection.

CLINICAL MANIFESTATIONS

The clinical manifestations of chronic bronchitis are often similar to that of emphysema because the two conditions often occur simultaneously. A chronic productive cough, often with purulent sputum, is frequent. Dyspnea occurs with minimal exertion. Chronic bronchitis leads to a prolonged expiratory phase along with wheezing and crackles upon auscultation of the lungs. Hypoxemia, hypercapnia, and cyanosis are more commonly found in those with chronic bronchitis compared with individuals with emphysema because of the presence of excessive bronchial mucus and obstructed ventilation.

DIAGNOSTIC CRITERIA

The diagnosis of chronic bronchitis is based on the clinical presentation of a persistent, productive cough over a period of 3 months or more within two consecutive years. A history of smoking is often present along with recurrent upper and lower respiratory infections. Arterial blood gases may be significant for hypoxemia and hypercapnia. Laboratory tests may indicate polycythemia (the overproduction of RBCs) as a compensatory measure to combat chronic hypoxemia. As with emphysema, pulmonary function tests are performed and demonstrate a reduction in FEV_1 and prolonged FET. Sputum specimens are often examined and tested for the presence of pathogens.

TREATMENT

As with emphysema, treatment of chronic bronchitis is aimed at alleviating symptoms, improving airway and lung function, slowing the progression of the disease, and improving overall quality of life. Treatment strategies are most effective when implemented early in the course of the disease. Smoking cessation is a critical component of success, as are pulmonary rehabilitation, bronchodilator therapy, steroid anti-inflammatory drugs, mucolytic agents, supplemental oxygen when indicated, and antibiotic therapy and immunizations to treat and protect against infection.

Asthma

Asthma is a chronic inflammatory disorder of the airways that results in intermittent or persistent airway obstruction because of bronchial hyperresponsiveness, inflammation, bronchoconstriction, and excess mucous production. The development of asthma often occurs in childhood, but the condition can emerge at any point in the lifespan. Overall, around 7% of adults have been told by a health professional that they have asthma. It is more common in women, those in poverty, and multiracial persons.[7] Individuals most likely to develop asthma include those considered **atopic**, or a genetic predisposition to developing hypersensitivities.

PATHOPHYSIOLOGY

Although the exact cause is unknown, asthma is increased in individuals who are frequently exposed to environmental allergens, such as cigarette smoke or dust mites. This discussion of asthma combines what is known about hypersensitivity reactions and the inflammatory process, because both of these concepts play a major role.

The inflammatory and immune response is often stimulated through exposure to an allergen. This allergen varies based on the individual and is often referred to as the asthma "trigger." Common environmental exposures that are known to result in hypersensitivity reactions and trigger the inflammatory response include smoke, dust, dust mites, mold, or animal hair. Other common triggers that can result in bronchospasm include exercise, temperature extremes, illness, and anxiety. Exercise-induced asthma (EIA) is a condition in which exercise or vigorous physical activity triggers acute bronchospasm, coughing, and wheezing in susceptible persons.

After an individual is exposed to the trigger, an IgE-mediated hypersensitivity reaction is immediate (Fig. 13.9A). IgE mast cells are stimulated to release chemical mediators. These chemical mediators

■ **Figure 13.9**   Asthma. **A:** Pathogenesis. (Image modified from Porth CM. *Pathophysiology: Concepts of Altered Health States.* 7th ed. Philadelphia: Lippincott Williams & Wilkins; 2004, with permission.) **B:** Narrowed bronchiole.

A

B   **Unaffected bronchiole**   **Obstructed bronchiole**

promote increased edema and subsequent bronchoconstriction in the airways. Further products of inflammation then move into the area. Mast cells call forth additional chemical mediators, such as histamine and prostaglandins. Hours later, leukot-rienes are released. These chemical mediators stimulate further bronchospasm, swelling, and excessive mucus production in the airways (Fig. 13.9B). The late inflammatory response occurs approximately 6 to 24 hours after exposure to the trigger and is marked by airway edema and the formation of mucus plugs from exudate and cell debris in the airways. The mucus plugs can take weeks to resolve. Over time, the cells of chronic inflammation, along with eosinophils, infiltrate the airways and cause destruction of the respiratory epithelium, smooth muscle hyperplasia, and narrowing of the airways. These structural changes, called airway remodeling, strongly affect the irreversibility of the condition.

CLINICAL MANIFESTATIONS

Clinical manifestations depend on the state of airway hyperreactivity and inflammation. In periods of remission, the individual is symptom free. As an exacerbation is emerging, the individual may not notice any symptoms, although pulmonary function tests begin to decline. In times of exacerbation, hyperreactivity and inflammation in the airways cause wheezing, breathlessness, chest tightness, excessive sputum production, and coughing, particularly at night or in the early morning. During an asthma episode, the individual may exhibit anxiety, tachypnea, and the use of accessory muscles. Hyperventilation initially leads to respiratory alkalosis; however, compensation is usually temporary, and acidosis develops because of ineffective expiration. Even with a partial airway obstruction, hypoxia quickly results.

STOP and Consider

Based on the basic pathophysiologic processes, construct a treatment plan for a person with asthma. What environmental modifications would you make? What would be the goals of pharmacologic therapy?

DIAGNOSTIC CRITERIA

The patient may request an evaluation for asthma during a time of remission or may present to the health professional in acute distress. The diagnosis includes evaluating signs and symptoms and determining the triggers to determine the likelihood that the manifestations are actually attributable to asthma. The patient history is often significant for atopy or asthma in the family. The patient may or may not be currently experiencing the characteristic clinical manifestations. Physical findings indicative of asthma include:

- Evidence of respiratory distress
- Pulsus paradoxus, an exaggerated decrease in systolic blood pressure during inspiration
- Wheezing breath sounds
- A prolonged expiratory phase
- Atopic dermatitis, eczema, or other allergic skin conditions that may indicate hypersensitivities

Laboratory findings may reveal eosinophilia (indicating allergy) and arterial blood gases indicative of hypoxemia and hypercapnia. Pulse oximetry is useful in screening for hypoxemia and may be used to grade asthma severity. Spirometry is used to determine the effectiveness of airflow. The peak expiratory flow rate (PEFR) is a common measure used to track forced expiration. The peak flow meter is a convenient, portable, inexpensive tool. Measurements over time can provide information about the patient's response to therapy and can indicate the emergence of an asthma exacerbation. Chest radiograph may demonstrate hyperinflation or infiltrates of the lung fields and can be used to rule out other sources of pleuritic chest pain, such as pneumonia or **pneumothorax** (the presence of air in the pleural space that causes the lung to collapse). Once diagnosed, asthma can then be classified based on severity, frequency, and duration of disease. The classification guides and treatment measures are found in Box 13.3.

TREATMENT

The treatment of asthma is composed of four major components:

1. Monitoring lung function through peak flow testing
2. Controlling environmental triggers
3. Pharmacologic therapy to reverse inflammation, bronchoconstriction, and mucus secretion
4. Patient education to facilitate adherence to the treatment plan

Research Notes

Alternative and complementary therapies have been implemented as possible treatments for conditions of altered ventilation and diffusion. One group of researchers explored the effectiveness of acupressure in promoting relaxation, decreasing anxiety, and alleviating dyspnea in patients with COPD. In this randomized clinical trial, patients were either provided true acupoint acupressure or a sham treatment. Those patients undergoing true acupoint acupressure demonstrated significant improvements in pulmonary function, dyspnea scores, 6-minute walking distance measurements, and state anxiety scale scores.[8]

A written action plan is an essential aspect of care for the individual with asthma. The action plan outlines methods for avoiding triggers and describes what to do when an asthma exacerbation is occurring.

Box 13.3 Asthma Classification and Treatment Based on Severity

- Mild intermittent
  - Intermittent symptoms occurring less than once a week with brief exacerbations
  - Nocturnal (nighttime) symptoms occurring less than twice a month
  - Asymptomatic with normal lung function between exacerbations
  - No daily medication needed
- FEV_1 or PEFR greater than 80%, with less than 20% variability
  - Mild persistent
  - Symptoms occurring more than once a week but less than once a day
  - Exacerbations affect activity and sleep
  - Nocturnal symptoms occurring more than twice a month
  - Low-dose inhaled anti-inflammatory one to four times per day and inhaled bronchodilator as needed
  - FEV_1 or PEFR greater than 80% predicted, with variability of 20% to 30%
- Moderate persistent
  - Daily symptoms
  - Exacerbations affect activity and sleep
  - Nocturnal symptoms occurring more than once a week
  - Medium-dose inhaled anti-inflammatory one to four times per day, a long-acting bronchodilator, especially for nighttime symptoms, and short-acting bronchodilator as needed
  - FEV_1 or PEFR 60% to 80% of predicted, with variability greater than 30%
- Severe persistent
  - Continuous symptoms with frequent exacerbations, nocturnal asthma symptoms
  - Physical activities limited by asthma symptoms
  - High-dose inhaled and oral anti-inflammatory, a long-acting bronchodilator, and short-acting bronchodilator as needed
  - FEV1 or PEFR less than 60%, with variability greater than 30%

The plan is based on the measurement of the PEFR using a peak flow meter. The individual determines his or her highest PEFR, or "personal best," over a symptom-free period of 1 to 3 weeks. The inability to expire at or above 80% of the personal best requires attention because an asthma exacerbation may be occurring.

Pharmacologic treatments are prescribed based on the classification of asthma severity. Medications used to treat asthma are divided into two major categories: bronchodilators and anti-inflammatory drugs. Inhaled β_2-adrenergic agonists (bronchodilators), such as albuterol, provide quick relief of bronchoconstriction and can prevent exercise-induced asthma. Anticholinergics and methylxanthines are

other drug categories used to promote bronchodilation. These medications relax the smooth muscles of the airway but do not effectively reduce airway inflammation. Long-term control medications, such as glucocorticoids, cromolyn, and leukotriene modifiers, are needed to prevent the frequency and severity of the inflammatory component of asthma. These medications also prevent chronic damage to the airways. For example, inhaled glucocorticoids suppress the activation of mast cells and other components active in inflammation and decrease airway hyperreactivity.

Asthma, although most often reversible, can lead to total airway obstruction if the inflammation is severe. In **status asthmaticus**, or intractable asthma, bronchospasm is not reversed by the patient's medications or other measures. Obstruction leads to decreased expiration, air trapping, hypoxemia, hypercapnia, and acidosis. Absent lung sounds and significant elevations in the $PaCO_2$ (above 70 mm Hg) indicate a poor prognosis. Status asthmaticus is life threatening and requires immediate emergency treatment.

Cystic Fibrosis

Cystic fibrosis (CF) is an autosomal recessive disorder of electrolytes and subsequently water transport that affects certain epithelial cells, such as those lining respiratory, digestive, and reproductive tracts. CF most commonly affects Caucasians of European descent and is the most common lethal inherited disease in that group. Incidence appears greatest in homogenous populations. This disorder leads to the production of excessive and thick exocrine secretions (e.g., mucus) leading to obstruction, inflammation, and infection. CF is also associated with impaired local immune defenses in the lungs as well as pancreatic insufficiency. Most affected individuals are diagnosed by 1 year of age. A small percentage of individuals exhibit a mild presentation and are not diagnosed until after 10 years of age. End-stage lung disease is the most common cause of death.

PATHOPHYSIOLOGY

Cystis fibrosis is caused by a mutation of the CF (also called the cystic fibrosis transmembrane conductance regulator, or CFTCR) gene located on the long arm of chromosome 7. Because CF is an autosomal recessive disease, a deleterious mutation is required on both inherited CFTCR alleles for the development of the disease. More than 1,000 possible CFTCR mutations, if found on both alleles in any combination, have been identified. Consistent with autosomal recessive inheritance, those with one mutated allele and one nonmutated allele are considered carriers and have no symptoms of the disease.

The CFTCR mutation leads to impaired electrolyte transportation across epithelial cells on mucosal surfaces. For example, the effective functioning of chloride ion channels depends on CFTCR, which encodes for a protein that serves as a chloride channel and is regulated by cyclic adenosine monophosphate (cAMP). Mutations in the gene for CFTCR lead to impairment in the cAMP-regulated chloride transport across many different types of epithelial cells on mucosal surfaces, such as those found lining the respiratory tract, pancreas, bile ducts, sweat ducts, and vas deferens. The inability of these epithelial cells to conduct chloride and therefore transport water across the mucosal surfaces leads to thick secretions and obstruction in the respiratory tract, pancreas, gastrointestinal tract, sweat glands, and other exocrine tissues. Although the manifestations appear mostly related to impaired transport of electrolytes, the complete mechanism of disease, particularly those leading to the complications associated with the lungs, is unknown.

CF is most strongly associated with mucus plugging, inflammation, and infection in the lungs with respiratory failure as the most common cause of death. Mucus plugging is a result of:

- A greater volume of mucus produced by a larger number of mucus-secreting cells in the airways
- Airway dehydration and thickened mucus caused by impaired chloride secretion, excessive sodium absorption, and decreased water content in the airway tissues
- Adherence of the mucus to the epithelium with impaired ciliary action required to clear the mucus from the airways

Mucus plugging, the formation of tenacious secretions, and a reduced ability to clear the secretions are optimal conditions for the growth and retention of bacteria. Progressive lung disease often begins shortly after birth with the emergence of a persistent respiratory infection. Impairment of local immune function leads to failure of opsonization and phagocytosis and contributes to this persistent lung infection with distinctive bacteria, such as *S. aureus* and *P. aeruginosa*. The progression from bronchitis to bronchiolitis, to bronchiectasis, and eventually to permanent lung damage largely depends on an intense, chronic inflammatory response dominated by neutrophils. The significance of the excessive presence of neutrophils is the release of proteases by these cells. Proteases promote an intense inflammatory response, cause destruction of lung tissue, inhibit destruction or neutralization of bacteria, and promote additional mucus production. Over time, the airways and lung tissue in CF are characterized by air trapping, hyperinflation, abscess formation, lung tissue consolidation, persis-

tent pneumonia, lung tissue fibrosis, and cyst formation, hence the name CF. Erosion of lung tissues and nearby bronchial arteries can lead to hemoptysis. Eventually, pulmonary involvement can lead to right-sided heart failure (cor pulmonale) and end-stage lung disease.

CF also has effects that go beyond ventilation and diffusion. Reduced chloride secretion and restricted water into the intestinal tract (along with inflammation, scarring, and strictures) leads to obstruction of intestinal contents. Along with intestinal motility problems, most individuals with CF (90% to 95%) have pancreatic insufficiency. Pancreatic insufficiency decreases digestion and the absorption of intestinal contents. The role of pancreatic enzymes, digestion, and absorption is described in detail in Chapter 15. The liver may also be affected in CF because the mutation of CFTCR leads to impairment of passive transport of chloride and water across the epithelial cells that line the biliary ductules. This leads to an increased viscosity of bile. Biliary obstruction can lead to obstructive cirrhosis.

CLINICAL MANIFESTATIONS

The presenting clinical manifestations, age at diagnosis, symptom severity, and rate of disease progression vary widely among individuals with CF. Clinical manifestations are associated with tenacious (thick) secretions leading to respiratory and gastrointestinal impairment. Recurrent respiratory infections, along with a chronic cough often accompanied by mucoid or purulent sputum, are common manifestations of CF. Coughing can be forceful and can lead to vomiting. Other respiratory manifestations include tachypnea, recurrent wheezing or crackles, hemoptysis, dyspnea on exertion, chest pain, and respiratory distress with chest retractions, cyanosis, barrel chest, recurrent sinusitis, and the development of nasal polyps. Finger clubbing can also be caused by chronic hypoxia.

Newborns may present with intestinal obstruction (a meconium ileus) at birth with a delayed or absent passage of meconium stool. Infants and children most commonly demonstrate increased frequency of large, greasy, malodorous stools, which indicate fat malabsorption. This condition can be accompanied by recurrent abdominal pain, distention, and poor absorption of fat-soluble vitamins. Weight loss or poor weight gain is common. Additional clinical manifestations include sweat abnormalities and excessive salt depletion. A child, when kissed by a caregiver, may have a salty taste to the skin. Jaundice, gastrointestinal bleeding, and rectal prolapse may occur.

Males with CF are frequently sterile because of the absence of vas deferens. The male child may also have undescended testicles or hydrocele. Secondary sexual development is often delayed in females with CF, although fertility is maintained or somewhat decreased.

DIAGNOSTIC CRITERIA

The diagnosis of CF is based on a thorough patient history and physical examination, noting the characteristic clinical manifestations. The diagnosis can be confirmed by a sweat test, which will reveal a sweat chloride concentration of 60 mEq/L or greater. Values of 40 to 60 mEq/L are considered borderline, and the test must be repeated because values in this range can be inconsistent with the diagnosis in some patients with typical features. Genetic testing may be performed to detect certain CFTCR mutations. The identification of two CFTCR mutations with associated clinical symptoms is diagnostic; however, negative results on genotype analysis do not exclude the diagnosis. The ability to sequence the entire gene will enable clinicians to detect all known mutations in any given individual and will have greater reliability in diagnosing CF. Other diagnostic tests, such as chest and sinus radiography and sputum analysis, can also contribute to the diagnosis. Chest radiography will reveal hyperinflation and peribronchial thickening. Sinusitis throughout all sinuses is uncommon in children and young adults, and its presence strongly suggests CF. The fluid obtained from a bronchoalveolar lavage usually shows a high percentage of neutrophils and the detection of *P. aeruginosa* supports the diagnosis of CF in an individual without the typical presentation. Because the early detection and treatment is critical in the course and prognosis of the disease, newborn screening has been recommended in many developed countries.

TREATMENT

Treatment goals for CF involve maximizing ventilation, diffusion, and nutrition through:

- Liquefying and clearing the airways of mucus
- Avoiding and controlling respiratory infections
- Reducing inflammation and promoting bronchodilation in the airways
- Providing or encouraging optimal nutrition through the use of enzyme supplements to reduce malabsorption, multivitamin and mineral supplements, and a high-calorie diet
- Managing disease complications, such as diabetes mellitus, bowel obstruction, fatty liver, biliary cirrhosis, and portal hypertension

Individuals with end-stage lung disease may consider lung transplantation. Currently, the median age of survival is 30 years; males survive significantly longer than females, although many individuals with CF are living into their 40s and 50s.

Acute Respiratory Distress Syndrome

Acute respiratory distress syndrome (ARDS) is a condition of severe acute inflammation and pulmonary edema without evidence of fluid overload or impaired cardiac function (Fig. 13.10). This condition was previously referred to as adult respiratory distress syndrome, but ARDS does occur in children.

PATHOPHYSIOLOGY

Damage to the alveolar epithelium and vascular endothelium triggers the onset of severe inflammation. Injury can result from inhalation of excessive smoke or toxic chemicals, overwhelming lung infections, aspiration of gastric contents into the lungs, lung trauma, anaphylaxis, lack of pulmonary blood flow, and other conditions that impair the alveoli. The presence of sepsis (bacterial infection in the blood) and the systemic inflammatory response syndrome (SIRS) are clinical conditions associated with the development of ARDS. In ARDS, the time from lung injury to respiratory distress is about 24 to 48 hours.

The inflammatory response is consistent with the process discussed in Chapter 3. Chemical mediators promote vasodilation and increased capillary permeability in the lungs. Inflammatory cells, proteins, and fluids escape the intravascular space and leak into the interstitium (lung tissues) and alveolar space, resulting in pulmonary edema, which damages the alveolar capillary junction. Damage to type II alveolar cells, increased protein, and fluid accumulation disrupts the production of surfactant resulting in **atelectasis** (alveolar nonaeration and collapse). Other potential causes of atelectasis are summarized in Box 13.4. Initially, oxygen diffusion is greatly impaired, but CO_2 is still able to cross the alveolar capillary junction to be expired. As the process of alveolar impairment advances, a hyaline membrane forms, and CO_2 release is also interrupted. The hyaline membrane is a thin, clear-basement membrane that is impervious to gases. This leads to a state of impaired ventilation and diffusion marked by poor lung expansion, hypoxemia, hypercapnia, and acidosis.

ARDS can be reversed if the symptoms are identified early. Healing involves reabsorption of the alveolar edema, regeneration of the epithelial cells and type II alveolar cells, and structural remodeling of the airway. In some cases, the patient has an uncomplicated acute inflammatory response with rapid

Phase 1. Injury reduces blood flow to the lungs. Platelets aggregate and release histamine (H), serotonin (S), and bradykinin (B).

Phase 2. Those substances, especially histamine, inflame and damage the alveolocapillary membrane, increasing capillary permeability. Fluids then shift into the interstitial space.

Phase 3. As capillary permeability increases, proteins and fluids leak out, increasing interstitial osmotic pressure and causing pulmonary edema.

Phase 4. Decreased blood flow and fluids in the alveoli damage surfactant and impair the cell's ability to produce more. As a result, alveoli collapse, impeding gas exchange and decreasing lung compliance.

Phase 5. Sufficient oxygen can't cross the alveolocapillary membrane, but carbon dioxide (CO_2) can and is lost with every exhalation. Oxygen (O_2) and CO_2 levels decrease in the blood.

Phase 6. Pulmonary edema worsens, inflammation leads to fibrosis, and gas exchange is further impeded.

■ **Figure 13.10**   Phases of acute respiratory distress syndrome. (Assets provided by Anatomical Chart Company.)

resolution. Other patients experience a permanent loss of lung volume and function attributed to lung tissue edema, necrosis, and alveolar fibrosis in affected areas. If untreated, death can ensue within 48 hours. The mortality rate, as a result of multisystem organ failure, is approximately 30% to 40%.

CLINICAL MANIFESTATIONS

Early clinical manifestations include tachypnea, dyspnea, retractions, crackles caused by fluid accumulation, and restlessness. Some patients may present in the course of disease without any signs or symptoms except for mild tachypnea. Within 48 hours, severe respiratory distress becomes apparent.

DIAGNOSTIC CRITERIA

The diagnosis of ARDS is based on a careful patient history, physical examination, laboratory, and imaging studies. A high index of suspicion is required when encountering any individual who has lung injury. Arterial blood gases often depict hypoxemia with early respiratory alkalosis quickly progressing to hypercapnia and respiratory alkalosis. Blood cultures may be needed to detect sepsis, the most common cause of ARDS. Chest radiograph is often normal early in the course of the disease, but then reveals bilateral diffuse infiltrates advancing to total opacity as the disease progresses.

From the Lab

Arterial blood gas analyses are the method of measuring arterial blood and determining levels of pH, PaO_2, and $PaCO_2$. In respiratory failure, pH falls below 7.3, PaO_2 falls below 50 mm Hg (the expected range is 80 to 100 mm Hg), and $PaCO_2$ rises above 50 mm Hg (the expected range is 35 to 45 mm Hg).

TREATMENT

Treatment strategies are supportive and focused on removing the causative factors triggering the inflammatory response. Administration of 100% oxygen is often warranted to keep oxygen saturations above 90%. If the oxygen saturations remain below this level and the patient becomes fatigued or acidotic, intubation with mechanical ventilation may be necessary. If mechanical ventilation is ineffective in maintaining oxygen saturations above 90%, positive end-expiratory pressure (PEEP) is instituted to maintain pressure in the airways during expiration and promote reinflation of alveoli. In patients with ARDS, maintenance of adequate alveolar ventilation is an important marker for survival.

Summary

- The process of ventilation involves both acquiring oxygen (inspiration) and removing carbon dioxide (expiration) from the blood.
- The transport of oxygen through the lungs is the *only* mechanism for acquiring oxygen.
- Oxygen is necessary for cellular metabolism, which means that for the cell to expend energy efficiently and perform its designated function, oxygen must be present.
- Optimal cell functioning occurs within a narrow pH range, and the release and retention of carbon dioxide is one mechanism for maintaining this balance.
- Oxygen and carbon dioxide are exchanged at the alveolar capillary junctions in the process of diffusion.
- Impaired ventilation is a problem of blocking airflow in and out of the lungs, thereby restricting oxygen intake and carbon dioxide removal from the body. Two major mechanisms are implicated: (1) compression or narrowing of the airways or (2) disruption of the neuronal transmissions needed to stimulate the mechanics of breathing.
- Impaired diffusion is a process of restricting the transfer of oxygen or carbon dioxide across the alveolar capillary junction. Because the rate of diffusion depends on the solubility and partial pressure of the gas, *and* surface area and thickness of the membrane, impaired gas exchange can occur with changes in any of these properties.
- Any situation that presents a demand for higher levels of oxygen or an increase in cellular metabolism requires pulmonary adaptation to maintain homeostasis, because oxygen deprivation and carbon dioxide retention affect all cells in the body.

- The major implications of altered ventilation and diffusion include hypoxemia, hypoxia, hypercapnia, and acidosis.
- Local manifestations of impaired ventilation and diffusion include cough, mucus production, sputum changes, dyspnea, use of accessory muscles, adventitious lung sounds, chest pain, barrel chest, and pursed lip breathing.
- Systemic manifestations of altered ventilation are caused by the effects of inflammation, hypoxemia, hypoxia, and hypercapnia. These manifestations include fever, malaise, leukocytosis, cyanosis, changes in arterial blood gases, mental status changes, and finger clubbing.

Case Study 13.1

A 6-month-old child has an acute respiratory syncytial virus (RSV) infection, which is an acute viral infection in the lungs. Think about which clinical model discussed in this chapter is most related to this process. From your reading and experience regarding infectious processes and now altered ventilation, answer the following questions:

1. *What process is most likely occurring in this child's body?*
2. *What are the probable ventilation and diffusion effects of exposure to this virus?*
3. *What would you expect for clinical manifestations?*
4. *What diagnostic tests could be used?*
5. *What treatment measures would you anticipate?*

Log on to the Internet. Search for a relevant journal article or Web site (such as http://www.emedicine. Com) that details RSV to confirm your predictions.

Case Study 13.2

Joan accompanies her husband Dan to the clinic and reports to the nurse that Dan's snoring seems to be getting worse over the past year. She has resorted to sleeping in a nearby bedroom with earplugs. Dan states that when he wakes up he doesn't feel that he has rested, although he does refer to himself as a "good sleeper" and states he is "able to fall asleep easily." Dan undergoes a sleep study and is diagnosed with obstructive sleep apnea. Think about which clinical model discussed in this chapter is most related to this process. From your reading and experience regarding obstructed ventilation, answer the following questions:

1. *What process is most likely occurring in this man's body?*
2. *What are the probable ventilation and diffusion effects from obstructive sleep apnea?*
3. *What would you expect for clinical manifestations?*
4. *What diagnostic tests could be used?*
5. *What treatment measures would you anticipate?*

Log on to the Internet. Search for a relevant journal article or Web site (such as http://emedicine.medscape.com/article/295807-overview) that details obstructive sleep apnea and confirm your predictions.

Practice Exam Questions

1. Which of the following does *not* affect diffusing capacity?
   a. The partial pressure of oxygen and carbon dioxide
   b. The alveolar surface area
   c. The density of the alveolar membrane
   d. The volume of air in the atmosphere

2. *Total* obstruction of the airway by aspirated material is manifested by:
   a. Hoarse cough
   b. Rapid loss of consciousness
   c. Dyspnea
   d. Inflammation of the mucosa

3. A reduced number of erythrocytes (RBCs) in the blood results in the following change in the oxygen saturation (SaO_2) of the blood:
   a. The SaO_2 would increase
   b. The SaO_2 would decrease
   c. The number of RBCs will not affect the SaO_2
   d. There will be a decrease only if the osmotic pressure of the blood is also decreased

4. Which is a major cause of respiratory failure?
   a. Aspiration
   b. Atelectasis
   c. Sepsis
   d. All of these

5. Emphysema differs from chronic bronchitis in that emphysema:
   a. Is characterized by mucus production and inflammation
   b. Obstructs the large airways
   c. Obstructs the alveoli
   d. There are no differences between the two conditions

6. You have admitted a 20-year-old male to the emergency room with a history of asthma. He is having an acute asthma attack and is wheezing, fighting for air, hypoxic, and afraid. What is causing these acute symptoms?
   a. Relaxation of bronchial smooth muscle with dry mucous membranes
   b. Constriction of the bronchial smooth muscle and air trapping
   c. Acute destruction of lung tissue
   d. Contraction of the elastic fibers of the lung

7. Which of the following clinical manifestations are related to hypoxemia?
   a. Cyanosis
   b. Cough
   c. Chest pain
   d. Hemoptysis

8. How would you know you have hypoxemia?
   a. Radiograph
   b. Measure the partial pressure of oxygen in blood
   c. Measure the partial pressure of carbon dioxide in blood
   d. All of these detect hypoxemia

9. Which of the following can trigger acute respiratory distress syndrome?
   a. Severe lung infection
   b. Inhaling toxic fumes
   c. Aspirating stomach contents into the lungs
   d. All of these

10. What is the major problem in cystic fibrosis
    a. Formation of cysts in fibrotic tissues
    b. Pancreatitis
    c. Lung injury
    d. Electrolyte and water transport

Discussion and Application

1. What did I know about altered ventilation and diffusion prior to today?

2. What body processes are affected by altered ventilation and diffusion? What are the expected functions of those processes? How does altered ventilation and diffusion affect those processes?

3. What are the potential etiologies for altered ventilation and diffusion? How does altered ventilation and diffusion develop?

4. Who is most at risk for developing altered ventilation and diffusion? How can altered ventilation and diffusion be prevented?

5. What are the human differences that affect the etiology, risk, or course of altered ventilation and diffusion?

6. What clinical manifestations are expected in the course of altered ventilation and diffusion?

7. What special diagnostic tests help determine the diagnosis and course of altered ventilation and diffusion?

8. What are the goals of care for individuals with altered ventilation and diffusion?

9. How does the concept of altered ventilation and diffusion build on what I have learned in the previous chapters and in previous courses?

10. How can I use what I have learned?

RESOURCES

The American Lung Association is an important source of information related to several types of lung diseases and includes current research updates at:
http://www.lungusa.org.

The Global Initiative for Asthma provides guidelines, reports, and other resources about asthma at:
http://www.ginasthma.org/GuidelinesResources.asp?l1=2&l2=0

Emedicine.com provides research-based authored articles related to many health conditions and can be accessed at:
http://www.emedicine.com.

The Foundation for Better Health Care (FBHC) provides information about a wide range of disease conditions including asthma, COPD, pneumonia, and TB, and can be found at:
http://www.fbhc.org.

MEDLINE Plus offers helpful tutorials that review basic physiology and pathophysiology of asthma and COPD at:
http://www.nlm.nih.gov/medlineplus/tutorials.html.

REFERENCES

1. Venditti M, Falcone M, Corrao S, et al. Outcome of patients hospitalized with community-acquired, health-care associated, and hospital-acquired pneumonia. *Ann Intern Med.* 2009;150:19–25.
2. Wolfson M, Schaffer T. Liquid ventilation: an adjunct for respiratory management. *Paediatr Anaesth.* 2004;14(1):15–23.
3. World Health Organization. Global tuberculosis database 2009. Available at: http://apps.who.int/globalatlas/dataQuery/default.asp. Accessed January 15, 2010
4. Mannino D, Homa D, Akinbami L, et al. Chronic obstructive pulmonary disease surveillance—United States, 1971–2000. *MMWR Surveill Summ.* 2002;51:1–16.
5. Doherty D, Gross N, Briggs D. Today's approach to the diagnosis and management of COPD. *Clin Rev.* 2004;14(1):97–105.
6. Global Initiative for Chronic Obstructive Lung Disease. Global strategy for the diagnosis, management, and prevention of chronic obstructive pulmonary disease. Medical Communication Resource, Inc; 2007. Available at: http://www.goldcopd.com/Guidelineitem.asp?l1=2&l2=1&intId=996. Accessed August 10, 2010.
7. Center for Disease Control National Center for Health Statistics. FastStat Health Statistics 2008. Available at: http://www.cdc.gov/nchs/fastats/asthma.htm. Accessed January 15, 2010.
8. Wu H, Wu S, Lin J, et al. Effectiveness of acupressure in improving dyspnea in chronic obstructive pulmonary disease. *J Adv Nurs.* 2004;45(3):252–259.

Chapter 14

Altered Perfusion

LEARNING OBJECTIVES

1. Define and use the key terms listed in this chapter.
2. Explain the role of perfusion in maintaining health.
3. Identify the key requirements for effective perfusion.
4. Determine processes that can alter perfusion.
5. Identify the common signs and symptoms of altered perfusion.
6. Describe diagnostic tests and treatment strategies relevant to altered perfusion.
7. Apply concepts of altered tissue perfusion to select clinical models.

INTRODUCTION

Think for a moment about the magnitude of a beating heart. Your heart beats about 70 times a minute, every minute, every day, of every year, of every decade of your life. Without fail, the heart beats, for without it we would die. What is it about the beating heart that keeps us alive? What other factors play a role in perfusing the body? What effect does reduction in perfusion have on the body? This chapter takes a careful look at these questions.

Module **1**

Perfusion

Perfusion is the process of forcing blood or other fluid to flow through a vessel and into the vascular bed of a tissue to provide oxygen and other nutrients. Requirements for effective perfusion include:

- *Adequate ventilation and diffusion:* The ability to breathe in and transport oxygen across the capillaries is mandatory for effective distribution of oxygen to the tissues.
- *Intact pulmonary circulation:* Pulmonary circulation is required for the uptake of oxygen from inspired air.
- *Adequate blood volume and components:* An expected blood volume is required to carry oxygen (on hemoglobin) and maintain blood pressure. The role of hemoglobin and oxygen saturation in the blood is discussed in Chapter 13.
- *Adequate cardiac output:* An optimal stroke volume, an optimal heart rate, and an efficient heart rhythm are needed to maximize perfusion to the tissues.
- *Intact cardiac control center in the medulla of the brain:* The cardiac control center is needed to regulate heart rate and force of cardiac contractions, and to detect and respond to changes in blood pressure.
- *Intact receptors:* Receptors play a major role in sensing changes in cardiac function and blood pressure, and they provide feedback to the cardiac control center in the brain.
- *Intact parasympathetic and sympathetic nervous systems:* The autonomic nervous system (ANS) is responsible for mediating changes in the cardiovascular system based on demands.

- *Intact cardiac conduction:* Conduction of impulses is essential in stimulating cardiac contractility.
- *Intact coronary circulation:* Coronary circulation maintains perfusion to cardiac structures, enabling the heart to distribute oxygenated blood to the remainder of the body.
- *Intact systemic circulation:* The coronary and systemic circulation is designed to distribute oxygenated blood to tissues and organs.
- *Adequate tissue uptake of oxygen:* Oxygen-dependent cells and tissues must be receptive to oxygen and nutrients to survive.

From Ventilation to Perfusion

Adequate ventilation and diffusion are required for intake and transport of oxygen and the removal of carbon dioxide. Perfusion with oxygenated blood cannot occur without the inhalation and diffusion of oxygen. Once oxygen enters the lungs and moves across the alveolar–capillary junction, the pulmonary circulation is crucial in taking up and distributing the oxygen. Therefore, effective gas exchange relies on a reasonably equal intake of oxygen (ventilation) and the movement of this oxygen (perfusion) from all areas of the lungs to the blood (Fig. 14.1).

The relationship between ventilation and perfusion is expressed as the **ventilation–perfusion ratio**, which is typically 0.8:0.9. This means that the rate of ventilation is usually slightly less than the rate of perfusion. The largest volume of ventilation

Arterial capillary · Bronchial tube · Venous capillary · Alveolus

Perfusion without ventilation · Optimal · Ventilation without perfusion

Figure 14.1 Matching ventilation and perfusion. **Center:** Optimal matching of ventilation and perfusion. **Left:** Perfusion without ventilation. **Right:** Ventilation without perfusion.

and perfusion is performed in the lower lobes of the lungs. In the lower lobes:

1. Ventilation is optimal because the surface tension for the alveoli is lowest and the lungs are most easily inflated.
2. Perfusion is optimal as the blood pressure through the lower lobes allows maximal blood flow.

Ventilation–perfusion is also affected by gravity. The lung tissues that are most dependent, or closest to the ground, are the most ventilated and perfused.

● STOP *and Consider*

Given that ventilation–perfusion is gravity dependent, how does your body position affect where the greatest volume of ventilation–perfusion occurs?

▨ Circulation

For effective perfusion, blood vessels must deliver oxygen and nutrients to tissues and remove waste. These steps occur through a process of circulation. In this chapter, circulation is discussed based on three critical, but interconnected, pathways:

- The pulmonary circulation, where circulation through the lungs provides the ability to transfer oxygen from the atmosphere into the body
- The cardiac circulation, where blood flow to the heart muscle supports the heart's work in pumping oxygenated blood to the body
- The systemic circulation, where oxygen and nutrients are distributed to other body tissues

Effective circulation depends on the patency of blood vessels and on the adjustment of the microcirculation to meet the demands of tissues. Arteries transport oxygenated and nutrient-rich blood to tissues; veins transport deoxygenated blood and waste products away from tissues for removal out of the body. Arterioles, capillaries, and venules form the microcirculation and are the primary locale for exchange of nutrients at the cellular level. A large network of capillaries in a tissue or organ increases the surface area for exchange of nutrients and wastes and allows for increased perfusion. For example, the heart, an organ that requires high levels of oxygen, has an extensive capillary network. When demands on the heart increase, vasodilation occurs and more blood flow is channeled to this organ. Similarly, oxygen transport to other organs adjusts related to demands, such as skeletal muscles during exercise. Cellular demands, measured by increased cell metabolism or energy expenditure, increase perfusion to the cells. This process involves a complex interaction of chemical mediators, metabolic waste products, and nucleotides that act on the blood, endothelial cells of the vessels, smooth muscle cells, and the extracellular matrix to open and widen capillary channels.

PULMONARY CIRCULATION

The pulmonary circulation forms the conduit by which oxygen and carbon dioxide can be exchanged between the atmosphere and the body. The pulmonary circulation is comprised of the right side of the heart and the pulmonary artery, capillaries, and veins. Note that the pulmonary artery carries deoxygenated blood to the lungs and that the pulmonary veins carry oxygenated blood to the left side of the heart. This portion of the circulation functions at a much lower pressure than the systemic circulation. Blood moves slowly past the lungs to allow maximum gas exchange.

● STOP *and Consider*

How would an ineffective right ventricle affect the pulmonary and systemic circulation?

SYSTEMIC CIRCULATION

The systemic circulation is comprised of all arteries, capillaries, and veins except those of the pulmonary circulation. The systemic circulation functions at a much higher pressure than the pulmonary circulation because blood must work against resistance to get to peripheral tissues. The systemic circulation is motored by the left side of the heart, particularly the left ventricle, which is the strongest pumping chamber.

CORONARY CIRCULATION

The coronary circulation is considered part of the systemic circulatory network, but it is singled out primarily because the heart is the pump that pushes oxygenated blood to the rest of the body. The heart is therefore considered a vital organ, and perfusion of this organ is essential for life. Cardiac muscle cells require a constant supply of oxygen and nutrients; these cells have little storage capacity. Perfusing the heart, by continuously providing oxygen and nutrients, occurs via the coronary circulation. Two major vessels, the right and left coronary artery, branch directly off the aorta to perfuse the right and left side of the myocardium (muscle) of the heart. The heart is also perfused by extensive collateral circulation (accessory arterial and venous branches) stemming from these major vessels. Additional

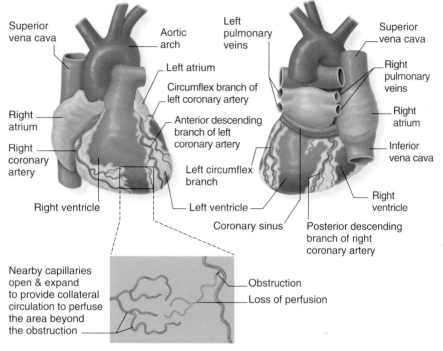

■ **Figure 14.2**   Coronary circulation and the development of collateral circulation.

collateral circulation develops when an increased need exists for blood flow to a specific area of the heart, such as with greater cardiac demands or obstruction of blood flow to heart tissues (Fig. 14.2).

● **STOP** *and* **Consider**

How would moderate to heavy aerobic exercise affect the development of collateral circulation of the heart?

Movement of Blood through the Circulation

The unique structural design of the heart promotes the movement of blood through the arteries to the capillaries (Fig. 14.3). The heart has three distinct layers:

● **Pericardium**: The outer covering of the heart, which holds the heart in place in the chest cavity, contains receptors that assist with the regulation of blood pressure and heart rate, and forms a first line of defense against infection and inflammation. Pericardial fluid is found between the layers of the pericardium, providing a cushion and lubricant to minimize friction as the heart beats.

● **Myocardium**: The thick muscular layer of the heart. The thickness of the myocardium varies depending on the location. The left ventricle often has the thickest myocardial area because this ventricle works harder than other heart

chambers to overcome the resistance of pumping blood to the aorta and to the systemic circulation. The myocardium undergoes hypertrophy if the heart workload increases.

● **Endocardium**: The inner lining of the heart that forms a continuous layer of endothelium

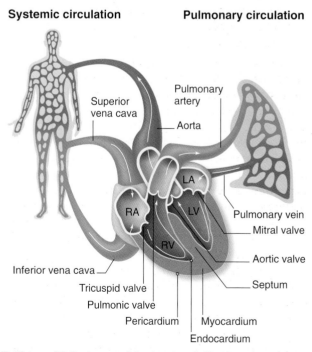

■ **Figure 14.3**   Layers of the heart and direction of continuous blood flow through the valves and heart chambers. LA, left atrium; LV, left ventricle; RA, right atrium; RV, right ventricle.

that joins the arteries and veins to the heart, forming a closed circulatory system.

● **STOP** *and Consider*

What is pericarditis? What would be the problem with this condition? What clinical manifestations do you think would be present?

The heart has four chambers: a right and left atrium and a right and left ventricle. The left and right sides of the heart are separated by a septum. Blood passes through valves that separate the atria from the ventricles, and the ventricles from the pulmonary artery and the aorta. The locations and characteristics of heart valves are depicted in Figures 14.3 and 14.4. These one-way valves are needed to promote forward movement of blood.

The movement of blood follows a predictable, continuous path. This discussion starts with the return of venous blood to the heart, which depends on skeletal muscle contractions and one-way valves within the veins that prevent backflow of blood. Blood that is returned from the head and arms travels through the superior vena cava, and blood that is returned from the trunk and legs travels through the inferior vena cava. Both paths lead to the right atrium. From here, the blood goes through the tricuspid valve to the right ventricle through the pulmonic valve to the pulmonary artery to the lungs. This deoxygenated blood becomes oxygenated through

the ventilation–perfusion exchange. The blood returns to the heart via the pulmonary vein to the left atrium through the bicuspid (mitral) valve, to the left ventricle through the aortic valve, to the aorta, to the systemic circulation, and again returning via venous return to the right side of the heart.

CARDIAC CYCLE

The myocardium of the heart contracts and relaxes, forming the pumping action of the heart that promotes perfusion. The **cardiac cycle** refers to one contraction and one relaxation phase. Contractions, called **systole**, forcefully move blood out of the ventricles. Relaxation, referred to as **diastole**, allows blood to fill the ventricles. After the ventricles fill, systole begins with the closure of atrioventricular (AV) valves. The AV valves are the bicuspid (mitral) valve and the tricuspid valve. AV valve closures correspond to the first heart sound. Traditionally, heart sounds are described as "lub dub." AV valve closures are the first part ("lub") of this description. The first heart sound is also referred to as S_1.

After AV valve closure, the ventricles contract, and pressure in the ventricles then becomes greater than that in the aorta and pulmonary artery. The semilunar valves, comprised of the aortic and pulmonic valves, open to eject blood from the ventricles. Once the blood is ejected at the end of systole, the ventricles relax. Pressure is now greater in the aorta and pulmonary artery. The valves prevent blood from flowing back into the ventricles. Rapid closure of the aortic and pulmonic valves prevents backflow of blood. Closure of these valves corresponds to the second heart sound ("dub" of lub dub). This second heart sound is also referred to as S_2.

During diastole, pressure again directs the valves. The ventricles are now relaxed and empty. Blood flow is accumulating and pressure becomes greater in the atria. The AV valves open and the blood moves into the ventricles. Additional heart sounds can sometimes be heard during this time. S_3 might be heard if there is rapid filling of the ventricle and the ventricle is weak, distended, or otherwise impaired. S_4 may be heard during atrial contraction.

CONDUCTION OF IMPULSES

Cardiac contractions rely on the passage of ions and electrical impulses from one myocardial cell to another. These impulses are generated and conducted as a weak electrical current within the heart itself. This process is generated through action potentials, or electrical currents moving charged ions (specifically, sodium, calcium, and potassium) along the cell

■ **Figure 14.4**   Superior view of the heart. Characteristics of semilunar versus atrioventricular valves.

Pulmonic (semilunar) valve

Aortic (semilunar) valve

Mitral (atrioventricular) valve

Tricuspid (atrioventricular) valve

membrane through channels. General action potentials and conduction are discussed in Chapter 9. In the cardiac cycle, two major types of action potentials (slow or fast responses) stimulate cardiac contraction and relaxation. These types of action potentials work in an organized manner to induce:

1. Rapid depolarization
2. Early repolarization
3. Plateau
4. Rapid repolarization
5. A resting phase

The cell membrane is typically found to have a positive net charge on its outer surface and negative charge on its inner surface. Depolarization is a change in polarity, in which ions shift, resulting in a sudden change in voltage. In depolarization, fast sodium channels open, allowing a rapid influx of sodium (positively charged) ions into the cell. As the cell voltage peaks, the fast sodium channel closes and the cell moves into the early stage of repolarization. This early repolarization is followed by a plateau phase, in which calcium and sodium ions slowly enter the cell through slow calcium and sodium channels. This calcium influx facilitates the prolonged contraction of cardiac muscle fibers. The cell then moves into rapid repolarization. Repolarization is basically a regrouping phase, in which the cell membrane becomes polarized again with a positive charge on the outer and a negative charge on the inner surface of the cell membrane. In the case of cardiac myocytes, the sodium and calcium channels close and sodium and calcium no longer move into the cell. To re-establish the polarity within the cell, the cell membrane becomes more permeable to potassium. This positively charged ion (K^+) exits the cell. This process is repeated again and again to produce cardiac contraction and relaxation that is characteristic of the heart.

The electrical activity imposed by ions on cardiac cells can be measured by using an electrocardiogram (ECG, also referred to as an EKG). Electrodes are placed on the body in designated areas and the electrical activity is transmitted to a screen. Figure 14.5 illustrates the ECG output and how this measurement corresponds to the action potential. It also demonstrates how the letters P, Q, R, S, and T represent certain points on the ECG. These letters correspond to the following aspects of the action potential:

- P wave = the depolarization of the atria via the sinoatrial node
- P-Q interval = the depolarization of the AV node and bundle fibers
- QRS = depolarization of the ventricles
- T = repolarization of the ventricles
- U = repolarization of Purkinje fibers

An important parallel process to the formation of action potentials is the orderly conduction of

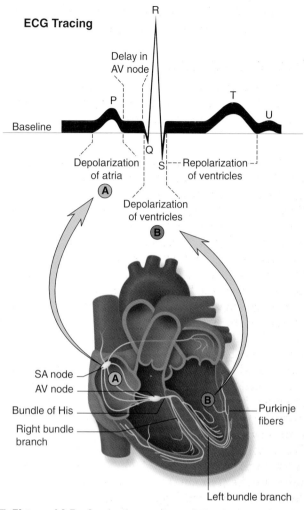

Figure 14.5 Conduction system of the heart and action potentials represented in the electrocardiogram (ECG) tracing. **A:** Depolarization of the atria. **B:** Depolarization of the ventricles. AV, atrioventricular; SA, sinoatrial.

impulses through the heart. The conduction system involves specialized myocardial cells in the **sinoatrial (SA) node**, or pacemaker, which generate a rhythmic impulse in the atria (see Fig. 14.5). As mentioned previously, action potentials consist of two types of responses: fast and slow. The SA node is stimulated by the slow response that occurs when the calcium and sodium channels open. As stated previously, this was where stimulation of a prolonged contraction phase of the heart was generated. The electrical message to contract then passes along the myocardial cell pathway to the **atrioventricular (AV) node**. The AV node, as its name suggests, connects the conduction of impulses between the atria and ventricles. The impulse is slowed upon reaching the AV node to allow the atria to empty blood completely into the ventricles before stimulating the ventricles to contract. The AV node generates the impulse that travels along specialized fibers, known as the AV bundle at the bundle of His, forming the left and right bundle branches and culminating into Purkinje fibers. These fibers conduct electrical impulses that stimulate the ventricle to contract. Blood is then ejected from the ventricles.

STOP *and Consider*

What would happen if the AV node conduction was blocked? What would happen if the bundle branch conduction was blocked?

CARDIAC OUTPUT

Measurement of the heart's efficiency to pump optimal amounts of blood is referred to as cardiac output. **Cardiac output (CO)** depends on stroke volume (SV) and heart rate (HR) and is expressed as: CO = SV × HR. **Stroke volume** is the amount of blood pumped out of one ventricle of the heart in a single beat. **Heart rate** is the number of heartbeats that occur in one minute. Cardiac output varies with age, body size, and metabolic needs of body tissues. The average cardiac output in adults is about 3.5 to 8.0 L/min. This means that every minute, up to 8 L of blood moves through the heart. During exercise, when metabolic needs increase, cardiac output can increase fourfold. Responsive cardiac output is based on five major factors, outlined in Box 14.1.

STOP *and Consider*

What happens to preload when venous return is sluggish? What happens to preload when venous return is excessive and cardiac muscle fibers get stretched too far?

BLOOD PRESSURE

Blood pressure is the pressure or tension of the blood within the systemic arteries. Blood pressure is needed to continuously perfuse vital organs. Pressure in the arteries is maintained by:

1. Contraction of the left ventricle
2. Peripheral vascular resistance
3. Elasticity of the arterial walls
4. Viscosity and volume of the blood

In other words, blood pressure is a product of cardiac output and the amount of resistance in the arteries.

STOP *and Consider*

What would your body need to do to maintain optimal blood pressure if you had increased peripheral vascular resistance as may occur with arteriosclerosis (a condition of stiffening of the arteries)?

Box 14.1 Major Factors Affecting Cardiac Output

- Preload
  - Work imposed on the heart just before contraction
  - Also called ventricular end-diastolic volume because it represents the pressure in the ventricles just before systole
  - Optimal preload depends on adequate venous return to fill the heart with blood and adequate cardiac muscle stretching to promote a strong contraction
  - An indicator of the filling and muscle stretching needed to eject an optimal amount of blood from the ventricles
- Cardiac contractility
  - The ability of the heart to increase the force of the contraction without changing the diastolic, or resting, pressure
  - Affected by calcium ions that aid in muscle contractions
- Afterload
  - The amount of pressure in the ventricle toward the end of the cardiac contraction
  - The cardiac muscle fibers are shortened and contracted and the ventricles have been emptied
  - Squeezing pressure against the resistance of blood trying to back up into the ventricles
  - Affected by increased resistance from the aorta and pulmonary artery
  - Increases when valves are impaired
- Heart rate
  - Part of the equation that predicts cardiac output
  - Must also respond to changes in demands to maximize perfusion
  - Slower heart rate equals greater diastolic filling
  - Excessively rapid heart rate can move blood quickly but does not allow maximal amounts of blood to be moved with each contraction
- Blood volume
  - Quantity and quality of blood affect the workload on the heart
  - Excessive blood increases pressure; deficient blood lowers pressure
  - Increased blood viscosity (thickness) increases pressure; thinner blood viscosity lowers vascular resistance and blood pressure
  - The heart must adjust to these pressures to maintain an optimal stroke volume

Blood pressure is measured in millimeters of mercury (mm Hg). The average blood pressure for adults is about 120/80. The first number (120 in the example) is called the systolic blood pressure. The second number (80 in the example) is called the diastolic blood pressure. Figure 14.6 illustrates the factors involved in blood pressure. **Systolic blood**

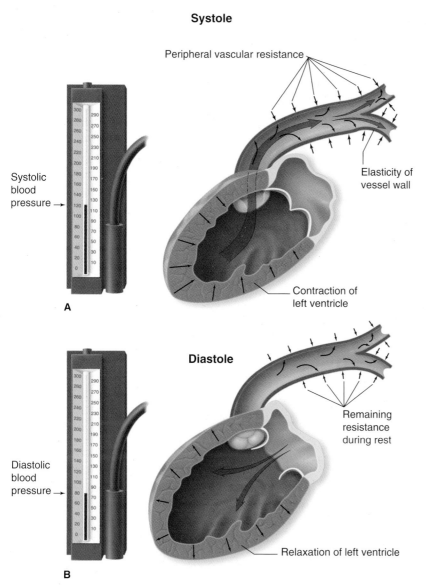

Systole

Peripheral vascular resistance

Systolic
blood
pressure →

Elasticity of
vessel wall

Contraction of
left ventricle

A

Diastole

Diastolic
blood
pressure →

Remaining
resistance
during rest

Relaxation of left ventricle

B

■ **Figure 14.6** Factors involved with systolic and diastolic blood pressure. **A:** Systolic blood pressure represents the ejection of blood into the aorta during systole, or contraction of the left ventricle. **B:** Diastolic blood pressure represents the pressure in the arterial system during diastole, or resting of the left ventricle.

pressure is the amount of pressure exerted during contraction of the left ventricle and ejection of blood into the aorta. The stroke volume, heart rate, and resistance in the aorta affect systolic blood pressure. Specific activities that can elevate systolic blood pressure include exercise, smoking, cardiovascular disease (CVD), and stress. **Diastolic blood pressure** is the amount of pressure that remains in the aorta during the resting phase of the cardiac cycle. Elevations in diastolic blood pressure may indicate that the arteries are not allowed to appropriately rest between cardiac contractions. Depressions in diastolic blood pressure are related to either lack of adequate resistance in the aorta or backflow of blood (and subsequently a loss of baseline pressure) through the aortic valve. The difference between the systolic and diastolic blood pressure is called the **pulse pressure**. Convergence, or narrowing, of the systolic and diastolic pressure often reflects a loss of systolic pressure rather than an elevation in diastolic pressure. For

example, extensive blood loss decreases systolic pressure while diastolic pressure remains unchanged. The **mean arterial pressure**, considered an adequate measure of *systemic* tissue perfusion, is one-third the pulse pressure plus diastolic pressure.

● **STOP** *and Consider*

Do you think that it is more problematic to have persistent elevations in systolic or diastolic blood pressure?

NEURONAL CONTROL OF BLOOD PRESSURE AND CARDIOVASCULAR ADAPTATION

How does the cardiovascular system adjust to the variable perfusion demands of the cells and tissues? Regulation and adaptation of cardiac and vascular function are controlled by neurons in the medulla and pons, which act on the ANS. The sympathetic division of the ANS stimulates the heart and blood vessels to increase heart rate, cardiac contractility, and the tension or resistance of blood vessels. The parasympathetic division of the ANS also acts on the heart to decrease heart rate. All of these adaptations are in response to multiple sources in the brain and cardiovascular system.

Blood pressure regulation requires adjustment in cardiac output (the pushing pressure) and peripheral vascular resistance (the resisting pressure) primarily through neuronal and hormonal mechanisms (Fig. 14.7). Similar to regulation of cardiac conduction, the ANS adjusts blood pressure. The sympathetic nervous branch increases heart rate and cardiac contractility and can selectively produce artery and arteriole vasoconstriction to increase peripheral vascular resistance. Changes in blood pressure occur in response to:

1. Baroreceptors and chemoreceptors in the arteries
2. The renin–angiotensin system
3. The kidneys

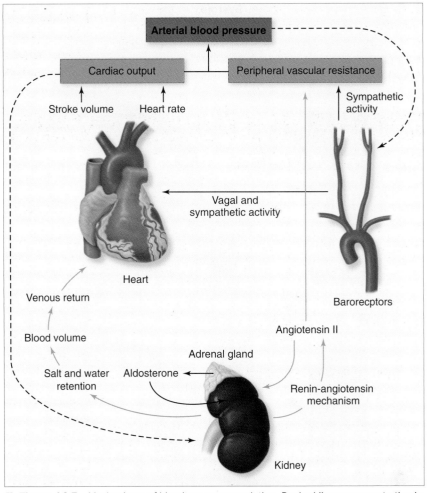

Figure 14.7 Mechanisms of blood pressure regulation. Dashed lines represent stimulation of blood pressure regulation. Solid lines represent response to stimulation of kidneys and baroreceptors. (Image from Porth CM. *Essentials of Pathophysiology: Concepts of Altered Health States.* Philadelphia: Lippincott Williams & Wilkins; 2003, with permission.)

Baroreceptors, located throughout the blood vessels and the heart, sense pressure changes in the arteries. For example, when the resistance, or stretch, of the artery decreases (the blood pressure is sensed as low), the baroreceptors alert the cardiac control center in the brain stem. The brain stem acts on the sympathetic nervous system to stimulate β_1 receptors in the heart. β_1 receptors increase cardiac output. Simultaneously, α_1 receptors in the blood vessels are stimulated, causing vasoconstriction. These receptors are mentioned because they are major targets of pharmacologic treatment with hypertension. Blocking these receptors reduces cardiac output and reduces vascular vasoconstriction. When optimal blood pressure is achieved, sympathetic stimulation by the baroreceptors subsides. Chemoreceptors in the aorta and carotid arteries also play a vital role in blood pressure regulation by detecting changes in oxygen, carbon dioxide, and pH of the blood. Chemoreceptors

then provide feedback to alter ventilation and promote vasoconstriction as needed to maximize oxygenation of vital organs.

Circulating enzymes, hormones, plasma proteins, and neurotransmitters also affect blood pressure regulation. Renin, an enzyme produced and secreted from the kidneys, converts the plasma protein angiotensinogen to angiotensin I. Angiotensin I is converted to angiotensin II by an enzyme in the lungs. Angiotensin II is a potent circulating vasoconstrictor. Angiotensin II therefore works to promote an increase in blood pressure when acting on the arteries and arterioles. Angiotensin II also stimulates the adrenal cortex to increase production and secretion of aldosterone (see Chapter 11). Aldosterone increases salt and water retention by the kidneys and can contribute to expanding blood volume. Antidiuretic hormone (vasopressin) also plays a role in blood pressure regulation. In high doses, antidiuretic hormone, secreted from the posterior pituitary, is a potent vasoconstrictor.

Antidiuretic hormone also promotes retention of fluids, which can enhance blood volume. Epinephrine, a neurotransmitter, acts to promote blood pressure directly by stimulating heart rate and cardiac contractility and promoting tension in the vessels.

● **STOP** *and Consider*

Think back to the last time that you felt dizzy when you stood up too fast. Why do you think this occurred? How did the baroreceptors respond?

Module 2

Altered Perfusion

Altered perfusion is defined as the inability to adequately oxygenate tissues at the capillary level (Fig. 14.8). This inability could be the result of low oxygen presence or poor utilization of oxygen.

Many factors can alter perfusion, including:

* Ventilation–perfusion mismatching
* Impaired circulation
* Inadequate cardiac output
* Excessive perfusion demands

▨ Ventilation–Perfusion Mismatching

Problem with the ventilation–perfusion ratio is the most common cause of hypoxemia. A ventilation–perfusion mismatch can occur because of the following conditions:

* Inadequate ventilation in well-perfused areas of the lungs. This occurs with conditions such as asthma, pneumonia, and pulmonary edema.
* Inadequate perfusion in well-ventilated areas of the lungs. This occurs with vascular obstructive processes in the lung, such as with a pulmonary embolus.

▨ Impaired Circulation

Problems with circulation lead to inadequate or excess blood flow to tissues or organs. Impaired circulatory patency and functioning can result from injury to the vessels, obstructive processes, inadequate movement of blood, or inadequate blood volume. Injury to the vessels leads to loss of integrity and hemorrhage. **Hemorrhage**, the loss of blood through the vessel wall, is most commonly caused by vascular injury often due to trauma. Hemorrhage can also occur because of aneurysms, coagulation disorders, and degradation of the vessel by neoplasms.

Obstruction within the vessel also contributes to altered perfusion by blocking free movement of blood through the circulatory system. Occluded arteries do not allow oxygenated blood to reach peripheral tissues. For example, applying a tourniquet or otherwise compressing a vessel will disallow blood flow to the peripheral tissues. Occluded veins restrict venous return and lead to circulatory congestion. Obstruction commonly occurs through the development of a thrombus, or blood clot. Remember that the formation of a blood clot, or **thrombosis**,

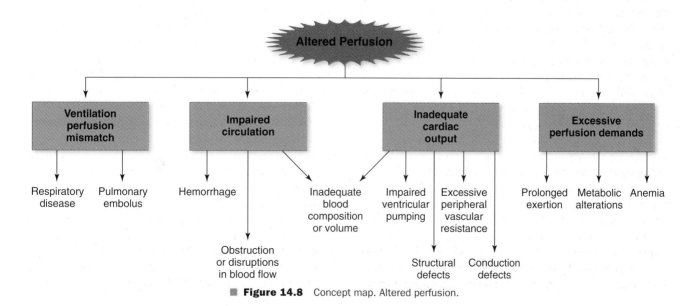

■ Figure 14.8   Concept map. Altered perfusion.

occurs in response to injury and is essential during the wound healing process. Undesired thrombi can also form in either arteries or veins and subsequently occlude blood flow.

In both arteries and veins, three major factors are responsible for thrombus formation. These factors, listed below, are collectively known as **Virchow's triad**:

1. Vessel wall damage
2. Excessive clotting
3. Alterations in blood flow, such as turbulence or sluggish blood movement

Injury to vessel endothelium, followed by the formation of atherosclerosis, is the most common cause of thrombus formation in arteries and also contributes to venous thrombosis.

Atherosclerosis is a condition of irregularly distributed lipid deposits in the inner lining, or intima, of large or medium arteries. The onset of atherosclerosis is theorized to begin as a process of injury to the intima (inner lining of the vessel), perhaps from hypertension, smoking, or environmental exposures. Low-density lipoprotein (LDL) filters into the lining of the artery and becomes trapped along the injured intima. The lipoprotein becomes oxidized and engulfed by macrophages, producing foam cells. Foam cells accumulate and combine with additional lipids to form fatty streaks. These fatty streaks gradually become fibrous plaques. Fibrous plaques accumulate at the sites of injury covered by platelet caps that continue to expand. These areas of atherosclerosis may eventually occlude the artery.

Turbulent or stagnant blood flow also contributes to thrombus formation. Bifurcations, aneurysms, and areas of venous stasis are common sites of altered blood flow. **Bifurcations** are regions wherein a vessel branches. Blood flow slows or backs up in an effort to negotiate the narrowed pathway. Arterial **aneurysms** are local outpouchings caused by weakness in the vessel wall (Fig. 14.9). Damage to the vessel wall, as may occur with atherosclerosis, promotes the development of aneurysms. The loss of vessel wall pressure allows slower transit of blood. **Venous stasis** occurs in veins with reduced venous return. Situations that promote venous stasis include heart failure, varicose veins, or prolonged bed rest or immobilization. Venous stasis is most commonly found in the legs, where blood pools in the extremities. These three situations (bifurcations, aneurysms, and venous stasis) all impede forward movement of blood. This allows the accumulation of clotting factors needed to form thrombi.

⬤ **STOP** *and* **Consider**

What is the mechanism for development of venous thrombi formation in an individual on bed rest?

▨ **Figure 14.9** Bifurcation, aneurysm, and atherosclerosis. These conditions cause turbulent blood flow.

Disorders of excess clotting allow unregulated formation of thrombi throughout the body. Hypercoagulability can be congenital or acquired. Genetic mutations can result in excess coagulant factors or deficient anticoagulant mechanisms. Acquired causes of hypercoagulability include:

- Autoimmune mechanisms that activate platelets and alter coagulation factors
- Certain types of cancer, or myeloproliferative disorders, such as **thrombocythemia** (excess platelets)
- Sickle cell anemia
- Polycythemia vera
- Use of oral contraceptives
- Vascular changes in the late stage of pregnancy

The following outcomes may potentially occur with thrombus formation:

1. The thrombus continues to grow and occlude the vessel completely.
2. The thrombus is degraded by enzymes and decreases in size.
3. All or part of the thrombus breaks off and travels through the circulation (Fig. 14.10).

Once a thrombus breaks off and travels, it is referred to as a **thromboembolus**, or simply an embolus. An **embolus** is any plug of material, such as thrombi, air, neoplasms, microorganisms, or

■ Figure 14.10 Potential outcomes of thrombus formation. **A:** Partial or total occlusion of the vessel. **B:** Enzymes degrade thrombus. **C:** The thrombus dislodges, forming an embolus, which travels within the vessels and occludes a smaller blood vessel at a distant site.

amniotic fluid, that travels in the circulation and can obstruct the lumen of a vessel.

● **STOP** *and* **Consider**

When preparing an intravenous fluid or medication, all air must be removed from the tubing or syringe. Describe the consequence of being careless in air removal.

When a vessel becomes obstructed, it can result in an infarct. An **infarct** is an area of necrosis resulting from a sudden insufficiency of arterial or venous blood supply. The process of obstructing the vessel is referred to as an **infarction**. Loss of blood supply and necrosis formation results in loss of function of the affected tissue. The severity of the infarction depends on the size and location of the emboli. Small emboli result in small and less significant areas of necrosis. Areas with extensive collateral

circulation are capable of perfusing tissue around the obstructed vessel. Larger emboli can lodge into larger vessels, occlude the large vessel and all of the large vessel's tributaries, and cause sudden death. Venous thromboemboli most often originate in the deep veins of the legs, break off, travel along the vein, and lodge in the pulmonary arteries where the vessels narrow and bifurcate. Arterial thromboemboli most often originate in the heart as atherosclerotic plaques, and they can travel to the brain, intestines, lower extremities, or kidneys. Myocardial infarction (MI) and stroke are two clinical models that are presented in this chapter to illustrate the impact of infarction on vital organs.

▧ Inadequate Cardiac Output

Cardiac output is inadequate when the heart is unable to successfully eject the necessary amount of blood to the pulmonary and systemic circulation. Major categories of problems leading to inadequate cardiac output include:

- Changes in blood volume, composition, or viscosity
- Impaired ventricular pumping
- Structural heart defects, such as valve defects that allow leaking or regurgitation of blood
- Conduction defects that lead to an unresponsive heart rate and rhythm
- Excessive or significantly reduced peripheral vascular resistance

Changes in blood volume, composition, or viscosity can affect cardiac output and result in altered perfusion. Blood volume and viscosity is altered with such conditions as hypercoagulation, dehydration, or hemorrhage. Disseminated intravascular coagulation (DIC) is a clinical model in this chapter used to illustrate the impact of coagulation disorders and hemorrhage on cardiac output and perfusion. Basically, blood outside of the circulation is not accessible to tissues. Blood composition, particularly with anemia, alters oxygen transport. In anemia, in which there aren't enough red blood cells to carry oxygen, the heart tries to move the small number of cells at a faster heart rate and becomes overtaxed.

Impaired ventricular pumping is a second major category of problems that lead to impaired cardiac output. The heart is a muscle. Loss of muscle activity leads to the inability to move blood effectively forward through the arterial circulation. This leads to congestion of venous blood and impaired venous return. Heart failure is a clinical model selected to further illustrate problems with impaired ventricular pumping and venous insufficiency.

Structural heart defects are a third category of problems leading to impaired cardiac output.

Several potential structural heart defects exist that can affect cardiac output. Structural heart defects basically impair the smooth, directional flow of blood through the heart chambers (Fig. 14.11). Heart defects can involve:

- Openings between the chamber septa, such as with an atrial septal defect (ASD) or ventricular septal defect (VSD)
- Transposition or coarctation (narrowing) of the great vessels
- Lack of closure of the ductus arteriosis at or shortly after birth
- Valve defects such as stenosis, regurgitation, or prolapse

Openings between the atria and ventricles allow blood to move between the right and left side of the heart. ASD is an opening between the left and right atria. VSD is an opening between the left and right ventricle. Two major problems with septal defects are (1) the comingling of oxygenated and deoxygenated blood within the heart chambers and (2) changes in blood flow volume and subsequent cardiac output.

Blood movement across the chambers is referred to as **shunting**. The direction of blood movement across chambers will go from the area of greater to lesser pressure. A left-to-right shunt is the movement of blood from the left side (oxygenated) of the heart to the right side (deoxygenated). The pressure on the right side of the heart and in the pulmonary circulation becomes greater. Larger defects allow greater volumes of blood to move left to right, leading to excessive pressure in the right ventricle and pulmonary edema. Cardiac output from the left ventricle to the systemic circulation is compromised because of loss of blood from the left side of the heart through the defect. A right-to-left shunt is the movement of blood from the right side (deoxygenated) of the heart to the left side (oxygenated). Movement of blood from right to left causes deoxygenated blood to be pumped into the systemic circulation. Small defects can be asymptomatic. Larger defects can lead to an overtaxed left ventricle and severe hypoxemia.

● STOP *and Consider*

Based on the pressure differential between the right and left sides of the heart, do you think it is more common to have a left-to-right or right-to-left shunt? Which one would most likely result in cyanosis?

Valvular defects are congenital or acquired. The bicuspid (mitral) and aortic valves are most often affected. Acquired causes of these defects include infection, inflammation, trauma, and degeneration. Such problems cause the valve to open or close improperly. **Stenosis** is a problem in which narrowing of the valve occurs, making the valve unable to open adequately. This narrowing causes increased resistance and turbulence as the blood moves past the valve. The heart ventricle must work harder to pump blood past the stenotic valve. **Regurgitation** is a problem of incompetence of the valve, in which it is unable to properly close, allowing reflux of blood. Again, the heart chambers must work harder against the constant backflow of blood.

A fourth problem of cardiac output, conduction defects alter an optimal heart rate and rhythm. **Cardiac dysrhythmias** are indicative of problems with maintaining an efficient heart rhythm. Dysrhythmias can stem from problems with the SA node, AV node, cardiac cells that join the SA and AV nodes, or conduction systems in the atria or ventricles. Without a regular, productive, efficient heart rhythm, the heart is unable to perfuse body tissues adequately. The most problematic dysrhythmias are found with the ventricular conduction system, which restricts the heart's ability to pump blood to the aorta or pulmonary artery. One example is ventricular **fibrillation**, which is a problem of the heart ventricle vibrating instead of effectively pumping. This problem can also occur in the atria and is then referred to as atrial fibrillation. A defibrillator uses an electrical current to shock the heart in an attempt to re-establish the efficient heart rhythm. Another potential problem that results in dysrhythmias is obstruction of cardiac conduction, often at the AV node, a condition referred to as **heart block**. Without coordination of the atria and ventricles, the movement of blood through the heart is uncoordinated and inefficient.

Excessive Perfusion Demands

Altered, or excessive, tissue metabolism can lead to altered perfusion from lack of meeting this excessive demand. Even though all other aspects of ventilation and diffusion are functioning optimally, the tissues are asking too much. This can result from extreme and prolonged exertion or metabolic alterations, as with hyperthyroidism (see Chapter 11).

General Manifestations of Altered Perfusion

The general manifestations of altered perfusion depend on the cause. The effects of chronic hypoxia have been discussed in Chapter 13. Impaired cardiac output produces clinical manifestations, such

■ **Figure 14.11**   Examples of structural heart defects. **A:** Atrial septal defect. Blood is shunted from the higher pressure left atria to the lower pressure right atria. **B:** Ventricular septal defect. Blood is shunted from the higher pressure left ventricle to the lower pressure right ventricle. **C:** Transposition of the great vessels. The pulmonary artery is attached to the left side of the heart and the aorta to the right side. **D:** Coarctation (narrowing) of the aorta. **E:** Patent ductus arteriosis. The high pressure blood of the aorta is shunted back to the pulmonary artery. **F:** Thickened and stenotic valve leaflets. **G:** Regurgitant valve that does not completely close.

as cyanosis, edema, shortness of breath, impaired growth, tachycardia, tachypnea, and fatigue. Changes in blood volume or peripheral vascular resistance can lead to hypotension or hypertension. Obstructive processes, such as myocardial or cerebral infarction, generally result in loss of function of that organ because of ischemia, along with pain and edema. The formation of deep vein thrombosis, also an obstructive process, may manifest as tenderness in the calf, especially with dorsiflexion of the foot, called **Homans sign**. Total occlusion of veins leads to edema, coolness, pallor, and cyanosis of the lower extremity. Hemorrhage also leads to altered perfusion. Skin manifestations of hemorrhage are **ecchymoses**, bruises from superficial bleeding into the skin, **petechiae**, pinpoint hemorrhages, or **purpura**, diffuse hemorrhages of the skin or mucous membranes. Larger accumulations of blood in the tissue form a **hematoma**. Heart murmurs are a diagnostic clue to the presence of valve or septal defects.

Diagnosing and Treating Altered Perfusion

Multiple diagnostic aids are available to identify altered perfusion. Treatment measures are aimed at improving cardiac output and maintaining the integrity of circulation. Tables 14.1 and 14.2 illustrate select diagnostic tools and treatment measures indicated in altered perfusion.

Table 14.1 Select Diagnostic Aids to Detect Altered Perfusion

Diagnostic Test	Type of Test	Rationale for Use
Echocardiography (cardiac ultrasound)	Ultrasound picture of cardiac structures and great vessels	Detects cardiovascular and valvular lesions, changes in heart size, changes in heart position, and wall motion abnormalities; transesophageal echocardiography provides a clearer view of heart and great vessel structures with a probe that is positioned in the esophagus
Cardiac catheterization	Insertion of a catheter (small tube) that is passed into the heart from a vein or artery	Used to withdraw blood samples, measure pressures, or inject contrast media to detect functional and structural defects (coronary angiography); also used to surgically correct certain cardiac defects
Chest radiograph	Radiographic picture of chest	Shows heart borders; detects changes in heart size and position; detects pulmonary congestion and pleural effusion
Electrocardiography (ECG)	Measurement of electrical impulses in the heart	Detects disturbances in cardiac conduction and increases in chamber size, the presence of ischemia, or myocardial infarction; a Holter monitor is a portable device that records 24-hour ECG activity as a patient performs his or her usual daily activities
Pressure measurements	Sphygmomanometry is an indirect, noninvasive measurement of systolic and diastolic blood pressure using a blood pressure cuff and sphygmomanometer; invasive pressure measurements involve directly threading a catheter (often from the femoral artery) into the structure of interest	Determines hypotension or hypertension; cardiac catheterization measures pressure in the arteries, veins, and heart chambers
Stress test	Treadmill or bicycle exercise is used in conjunction with ECG, blood pressure monitoring, or other imaging studies; stress can also be induced through pharmacologic agents and is typically used in combination with imaging studies, such as radionucleotide imaging and echocardiography	Determines elicitation of chest pain, ECG, or imaging study changes significant for myocardial ischemia
Cardiac nuclear scanning	Uses intravenous radioactive compounds, which collect in the heart, and a gamma camera to produce diagnostic images; myocardial perfusion scanning allows the visualization of blood flow patterns to the myocardium; cardiac gating synchronizes images of the heart with cardiac conduction based on the ECG output	Indicated for individuals with unexplained or exercise-induced chest pain to permit the early detection of heart disease or to determine the effective revascularization of the heart after PTCA or bypass surgery; detects myocardial activity and blood flow; may be used in combination with a stress test
Doppler ultrasonography	A noninvasive form of ultrasound that measures the changes in sound frequencies to detect movement, most commonly of red blood cells	Measures aortic and other blood vessel flow velocities; can be used to augment echocardiography to determine flow velocities within the echocardiographic image; Doppler color flow uses computer-generated images to depict different directions of flow (represented by different colors)

PTCA, percutaneous transluminal coronary angioplasty.

Module 3

Clinical Models

The following clinical models have been selected to aid in the understanding and application of altered perfusion processes and effects. We are in the midst of a true cardiovascular pandemic. Heart disease is not only the leading cause of death, disability, and health care expense in the United States, but also the leading

cause of death worldwide. CVD is the leading cause of mortality in every region of the world except sub-Saharan Africa, and it is anticipated that CVD will eclipse infectious disease there within the next few years. All of the issues that contribute to the continued impact of CVD in the United States—access to

Table 14.2 Treatment Measures Related to Altered Perfusion

Treatment Strategy	Rationale for Use
Surgery	Surgery has multiple applications to relieve altered perfusion: • Coronary artery bypass grafting is a procedure used to bypass an obstructed coronary artery • Percutaneous transluminal coronary angioplasty is performed during cardiac catheterization to compress fatty deposits in the coronary arteries and relieve the occlusion • Laser angioplasty vaporizes fatty deposits with a hot-tip laser device • Surgery is also used to repair valve defects, remove varicose veins, and drain excess fluid from the pericardial cavity
Pharmacologic	• ASA (aspirin) therapy may be instituted to reduce platelet aggregation and clot formation therapies • Medications may be prescribed to dilate blood vessels, reduce or increase blood pressure, control the heart rate/rhythm, increase myocardial contractility, reduce myocardial workload, or improve cardiac output • Thrombolytic agents may be needed to break through an obstruction and revascularize myocardial tissue • Pain medications are often needed for acute myocardial infarction • Oxygen therapy is frequently indicated to reduce hypoxemia
Intravenous	Fluid volume or blood replacement with severe hemorrhage or dehydration administration of blood or fluids
Pacemaker placement	A pacemaker may be placed to mechanically control heart rate and rhythm
Lifestyle	Reduction of risks or modification of lifestyle after a diagnosis related to altered perfusion modifications should include weight reduction, blood pressure management, stress reduction, smoking cessation, exercise, healthy nutrition, and diabetes management

care, quality of care, aging of the population, explosion in the prevalence of obesity and diabetes, tobacco consumption, and physical inactivity—have profound global implications.

Hypertension

Hypertension is a progressive cardiovascular syndrome detected by an elevation in blood pressure (systolic pressure above 140 mm Hg or a diastolic pressure above 90 mm Hg) or by the presence of organ damage due to persistent blood pressure elevations. Most individuals with hypertension remain untreated or uncontrolled. If the systolic blood pressure is elevated without an elevation in the diastolic blood pressure, this is referred to as **isolated systolic hypertension**. Systolic hypertension is highly significant. In individuals older than 50 years of age, persistent systolic blood pressure greater than 140 mm Hg is a stronger predictor of CVD than an elevation in diastolic blood pressure.[1]

PATHOPHYSIOLOGY

The prevalence of hypertension reaches about 50% by the age of 65 years in most populations. The majority of individuals with hypertension (90% to 95%) are diagnosed as having primary hypertension, also called essential hypertension. Secondary hypertension is high blood pressure that is a manifestation of another condition, such as a narrowing of the aorta (coarctation) or kidney disease. The specific cause of primary hypertension is often

Research Notes

Globally, there have been significant advances in genetic determinants of disease. This has not been the case thus far with hypertension. Since African Americans in the United States are disproportionately hypertensive, the researchers sought to discover genetic variants and pathways most strongly associated with blood pressure regulation. They conducted a genome-wide association scan using over 800,000 genetic markers in an African American sample of 1,017 adults in Washington, D.C. Evidence was found to suggest that genetic variants in several genes, including PMS1, SLC24A4, YWHA7, IPO7, and CACANA1H, are significantly associated with systolic BP levels. No clear association was found for diastolic levels. The findings advance our understanding of the genetic factors that influence BP with the hope that these insights will eventually translate to new and better treatment options for hypertension in African Americans and other global populations.[2]

unknown. It is considered a multifactorial disease resulting from a complex interaction of genetic and environmental triggers. Certain risk factors for the development of primary hypertension have been identified and include:

- Family history of hypertension
- Aging
- Diabetes mellitus
- Excessive dietary sodium intake
- Obesity
- Sedentary lifestyle
- Excessive alcohol intake
- Smoking

Hypertension is a manifestation of increased cardiac output or peripheral resistance and is characterized by structural and functional changes in the heart and vascular system. Cardiac output is elevated by conditions that increase stroke volume or heart rate. Peripheral resistance is elevated by conditions that restrict peripheral blood flow, such as increased blood viscosity or vasoconstriction. Recall the mechanisms for regulating blood pressure. Autoregulatory systems are designed to adjust to changes in cardiovascular demand. Impairments in these regulatory mechanisms can increase peripheral vascular resistance and promote the development of hypertension:

- Sympathetic nervous system overstimulation (systemic vasoconstriction)
- Renin–angiotensin–aldosterone overstimulation (systemic vasoconstriction, salt and water retention by kidneys, increased blood volume)
- Impaired sodium excretion by the kidneys (salt and water retention, increased blood volume)

Chronic hypertension damages the blood vessel walls through direct injury to the intima (inner lining) from prolonged vasoconstriction and high pressures. The inflammatory response increases systemic capillary permeability and further damages the vessel wall. The vessel walls adapt through hypertrophy and hyperplasia to withstand this stress. The vessel lumen permanently narrows.

Three major body systems are affected by hypertension: the central nervous system (CNS), cardiovascular system, and renal system. In severe hypertension, the CNS is affected because the elevated BP overwhelms the cerebral blood flow. Usually, as the blood pressure increases and cerebral arterioles vasoconstrict, cerebral blood flow remains constant. During a hypertensive crisis (a rapid and severe elevation in blood pressure), the hypertension overwhelms arteriolar control over vasoconstriction. Pressurized fluid leaks across the capillaries and into the brain tissue and other brain structures. Arterioles are damaged during this process. Intracranial pressure increases, oxygen transport is impaired, and brain function is reduced.

Hypertension also affects the cardiovascular system. Hypertension was previously mentioned as a factor in the development of atherosclerosis and can contribute to obstruction in arteries. Pressure in the small arterioles, or microvasculature, can lead to altered function of the target organ. The small vessels in the kidneys, eyes, brain, and heart are particularly vulnerable. Hypertensive pressure is also a strain on the heart, which must continue to work against this pressure to perfuse the body. The left ventricle is most affected by the pressure resistance. The left ventricle becomes hypertrophic. Ineffective left ventricle pumping impairs venous return and systemic perfusion. This leads to pulmonary edema, myocardial ischemia, and peripheral hypoxemia.

Prolonged pressure in the kidney arterioles promotes chronic injury and inflammation. This leads to nephrosclerosis, which is basically an overgrowth and hardening of the connective tissues of the kidney. Hypertension is perpetuated as renin and aldosterone secretion is stimulated by reduced blood flow to the kidneys. Blood volume expands and increases blood pressure.

CLINICAL MANIFESTATIONS

Primary hypertension is often asymptomatic and may be detected only through a series of blood pressure screenings. When clinical manifestations *are* present, this often reflects years of undetected hypertension. CNS manifestations include headache, new-onset blurred vision, nausea, vomiting, weakness, fatigue, confusion, and mental status changes. Rupture of cerebral vessels due to hypertension leads to stroke. Cardiovascular manifestations may include the signs and symptoms of pulmonary edema and other manifestations of heart failure (see Heart Failure below). Renal insufficiency manifests as poor urinary output, hematuria, proteinuria, and problems with eliminating urinary waste.

From the Lab

The preferred investigation for plasma lipids and lipoproteins is one that measures total cholesterol, triglycerides, high-density lipoprotein (HDL) cholesterol, and LDL cholesterol after a 14-hour fast (water permitted). Levels that would cause concern are a total cholesterol level over 180 mg/dL, an LDL cholesterol level over 135 mg/dL, an HDL cholesterol level below 35 mg/dL, and a triglyceride level over 150 mg/dL. Other coronary heart disease (CHD) risk factors that are now measured in many laboratories include fibrinogen, C-reactive protein (CRP) (an inflammatory marker), and homocysteine.

DIAGNOSTIC CRITERIA

Because hypertension is associated with elevated risks of CVDs (especially stroke, MI, and cardiovascular death), early recognition is critical to prevent such complications. Diagnosis is based on a careful patient history, physical examination, and laboratory and diagnostic tests. The patient history should include identifying hypertensive family members and other risk factors described previously. Physical examination must include the noninvasive auscultatory-method measurement of blood pressure as well as a focus on detecting target organ damage and CVD.

Diagnosis of hypertension is *not* based on an isolated elevation in blood pressure. Rather, a series of properly performed blood pressure measurements (usually three) over a 3- to 6-month period is needed to confirm the presence of primary hypertension. Once a persistent elevation in blood pressure is identified, the level of hypertension can be classified according to severity:[1]

- *Prehypertension:* systolic BP 120 to 139 mm Hg, diastolic BP 80 to 89 mm Hg
- *Stage 1:* systolic BP 140 to 159 mm Hg, diastolic BP 90 to 99 mm Hg
- *Stage 2:* systolic BP greater than 159 mm Hg, diastolic BP greater than 99 mm Hg

Even before an elevated blood pressure is noticed, some individuals are at risk for the development of CVD. For example, an individual with a blood pressure of 130/80 mm Hg may have signs of damage to their heart, kidneys, or eyes caused by blood pressure, whereas another individual with the same blood pressure reading may have no such organ damage and therefore be at lower risk for a heart attack or stroke. The point is that the diagnosis of hypertension is supported by elevations in blood pressure, but the emphasis should be on evaluating the person's overall risk for CVD.

Relevant laboratory studies that contribute to this evaluation include electrolyte levels, urinalysis, blood urea nitrogen (BUN), and creatinine, which detect evidence of renal impairment. A lipid profile is useful to detect hypercholesterolemia. Blood glucose testing is needed to detect diabetes. In a hypertensive crisis, a chest radiograph may be needed to determine congestive heart failure, pulmonary edema, or coarctation of the aorta. A computed tomography (CT) scan of the brain may be needed to determine intracranial bleeding, edema, or infarction. An ECG may also be useful to assess for cardiac ischemia or infarction.

TREATMENT

Treatment of hypertension includes consideration of pharmacologic and nonpharmacologic interventions. The following measures are appropriate in all persons with hypertension: weight reduction; decreased alcohol, salt, and saturated fat intake; increased aerobic physical activity and fruit and vegetable (potassium) intake; and smoking cessation. Pharmacologic treatments, when indicated, work to decrease fluid volume (diuretics), decrease cardiac contractility or cardiac output (β-blockers, α-blockers, calcium channel blockers), or decrease peripheral vascular resistance (angiotensin-converting enzyme [ACE] inhibitors, angiotensin II receptor antagonists, and vasodilators). The overall goal of pharmacologic therapy is to decrease peripheral vascular resistance and reduce the workload of the heart by reducing arterial pressure below 140/90. In individuals with diabetes or renal disease, this goal is even lower; that is, less than 130/80 mm Hg.[1] Most individuals with hypertension require two or more antihypertensive drugs to achieve this goal. Pharmacotherapy is not curative, but it reduces both the symptoms and the risk for long-term complications. Table 14.3 provides more detail on pharmacologic options.

Shock

Shock is a condition of circulatory failure and impaired perfusion of vital organs. Shock is often equated with **hypotension**, or reduced blood pressure, although this is considered a late sign and signals ineffective compensation.

PATHOPHYSIOLOGY

Effective blood circulation depends on cardiac output (including an optimal blood volume) and on peripheral vascular resistance. Shock represents a deficit in one or more of these requisites and is often classified accordingly:

- Ineffective cardiac pumping: *cardiogenic shock*
- Decreased blood volume: *hypovolemic shock*
- Massive systemic vasodilation:
  - From severe infection: *septic shock*
  - From brain or spinal cord injury: *neurogenic shock*
  - From severe immunoglobulin E (IgE)–mediated hypersensitivity reaction: *anaphylactic shock*

Cardiogenic shock results from inadequate or ineffective cardiac pumping. The most common cause is MI, although any cardiac condition that reduces heart efficiency can lead to cardiogenic shock. The basic problem is that impaired pumping leads to reduced cardiac output, low blood pressure, and restricted movement of oxygenated blood through the circulation. This leads to systemic hypotension or pulmonary edema. The mortality rate is approximately 70% for patients who do not undergo rapid

Table 14.3 Select Pharmacologic Options for Treatment of Hypertension

Type of Drug (Example)	Site of Action	Action	Rationale for Use
Centrally acting α_2 agonist (clonidine)	Brain stem	Suppresses sympathetic outflow to the heart and blood vessels, causing a decrease in cardiac output and vasodilation	Decreases cardiac output and peripheral vascular resistance
Diuretics (furosemide)	Renal tubules of the kidneys	Decrease vascular volume by action on renal reabsorption of sodium and promoting sodium and water excretion	Decrease cardiac output and fluid volume overload with an eventual reduction in peripheral vascular resistance
β Blockers (propranolol)	Cardiac β_1 receptors	Decreases heart rate and contractile force	Decreases myocardial oxygen demand
α Blockers (prazosin)	Vascular α_1 receptors	Stimulates vasodilation of blood vessels	Decreases peripheral vascular resistance
ACE inhibitors (captopril)	Angiotensin-converting enzyme (ACE)	Inhibits the conversion of angiotensin I to angiotensin II, thereby preventing vasoconstriction and decreasing aldosterone levels	Decreases peripheral vascular resistance
Angiotensin II blockers (losartan)	Angiotensin II receptors	Blocks the actions of angiotensin II, preventing angiotensin II–mediated vasoconstriction and aldosterone-mediated fluid retention	Decreases peripheral vascular resistance and decreases fluid volume to reduce cardiac output
Calcium channel blockers (verapamil)	Vascular and cardiac muscle cells	Blocks the movement of calcium into the arterial smooth muscle cells, thereby decreasing vasoconstriction	Decreases peripheral vascular resistance

revascularization to promote myocardial blood flow. For those treated with angioplasty, stent placements in the obstructed coronary artery, or thrombolytic therapy, the mortality rate is reduced to approximately 30% to 50%.[3]

Hypovolemic shock is the result of inadequate blood/plasma volume and typically occurs when this volume is reduced by 15% to 20%. This type of shock can result from severe hemorrhage, burns, diarrhea, or polyuria, as occurs with diabetes insipidus. The problem is that blood and fluid losses in the vascular space lead to deficient venous return and reduced circulation. Reduction in the volume of red blood cells also reduces oxygen transport through the circulation. Without correcting the underlying cause, inadequate perfusion leads to multiple organ failure.

Septic shock is the result of overwhelming systemic infection where about half are caused by gram-positive microorganisms, followed closely by gram-negative microorganisms, although in some cases the exact pathogen is unknown. Gram-negative microorganisms contain endotoxin that can produce a massive inflammatory response by releasing potent chemical mediators. These chemical mediators induce widespread tissue injury. Endothelial cells that line blood vessels vasodilate and become permeable. Injury to these endothelial cells not only allows fluid to escape the intravascular compartment but also damages these cells, directly causing vascular collapse. Septic shock is considered a grave condition that has a mortality rate of approximately 30% to 50%.

Neurogenic shock is a result of brain or spinal cord injury, the depressant actions of certain drugs, general anesthesia, hypoglycemia, or hypoxia. Altered neuronal transmission leads to a loss of sympathetic control of tension in the blood vessels. This loss of tension allows unregulated vasodilation. Vasodilation decreases peripheral vascular resistance, blood pressure is reduced, and perfusion to vital organs is reduced. Neurogenic shock is the rarest cause of shock, is readily treatable, and generally responds well to medical therapy.

Anaphylactic shock is the result of a massive immune (type 1 or IgE-mediated) hypersensitivity response (see Chapter 4). Similar to septic shock, anaphylaxis leads to massive vasodilation and increased vascular permeability. Peripheral vascular resistance is reduced significantly, fluid is allowed to move outside of the vascular space, blood pressure is reduced, and circulation is impaired.

All types of shocks deprive the cells of oxygen and nutrients and thus impair cellular metabolism, resulting in acidosis. Initially, hypoxia and acidosis are met with compensatory mechanisms that involve:

- *Stimulating the sympathetic nervous system:* The sympathetic nervous system is stimulated to increase heart rate and cardiac contractility and to alter blood vessel tone. Regulation of vessel tone promotes (1) vasodilation of vessels leading to the heart and brain, and (2) vasoconstriction to other less vital areas of the body.
- *Stimulating the renin–angiotensin–aldosterone mechanism:* Renin and angiotensin promote

compensatory vasoconstriction. These hormones also promote sodium and water reabsorption to increase intravascular volume.

The general goals of compensation are to (1) shunt blood to the heart and brain; and (2) promote cardiac output by increasing intravascular volume, heart rate, and cardiac contractility. Sometimes these compensatory mechanisms are adequate to reverse shock. Unfortunately, in many cases, these compensations are temporary. A downward spiral from prolonged reliance on compensatory mechanisms leads to increasing hypoxia marked by:

1. Endothelial (vessel lining) injury, allowing further loss of intravascular fluids
2. Fluid deprivation in the vessel, promoting further difficulties with cardiac output
3. Continued reduction in perfusion, promoting cellular injury, anaerobic metabolism, and metabolic acidosis

All cells become deprived of oxygen and other nutrients and convert to inefficient anaerobic metabolism. Eventually, cellular metabolism is unable to generate enough energy to maintain cellular homeostasis. This leads to impairment of the cell membrane ion pump, accumulation of intracellular sodium, and the loss of intracellular potassium. The cell swells, ruptures, and dies. In 50% of those experiencing severe shock, multiple organ failure, particularly of the heart, brain, kidneys, lungs, and skeletal muscle, leads to somatic death.

CLINICAL MANIFESTATIONS

Early clinical manifestations of shock are related to the triggering event. Because the primary cause of cardiogenic shock is MI, early clinical manifestations may include chest pain, shortness of breath, labored breathing, diaphoresis, nausea, or vomiting. In hypovolemic shock, manifestations are related to the extent of blood or plasma loss. Infection leading to septic shock promotes fever and flushed, warm skin. Anaphylactic shock triggers generalized skin flushing and may lead to airway obstruction.

Clinical manifestations consistent across the potential etiologies are those indicative of circulatory impairment and collapse and include marked tachycardia, tachypnea, cool and clammy extremities, poor peripheral pulses, decreased arterial blood pressure (a late sign indicative of decompensation), cyanosis, pallor, restlessness, apprehension, decreased mental function, and poor urinary output. Because shock reduces perfusion throughout the body, multiple manifestations are possible related to general organ dysfunction.

DIAGNOSTIC CRITERIA

No one test is completely specific or sensitive for shock. The diagnosis of shock is based on a thorough patient history, physical examination, and laboratory and diagnostic tests. The patient history reveals a triggering event, such as MI, massive hemorrhage, systemic infection, spinal cord injury, or anaphylaxis. Physical assessment includes observation of skin color, temperature, pulses, capillary refill, heart rate, blood pressure, urine output, and mental status. Laboratory studies vary and are directed at the potential cause. For example, in cardiogenic shock, laboratory tests include cardiac enzymes (creatine kinase, troponin, myoglobin), a complete blood count, electrolytes, arterial blood gases, and blood coagulation tests. An ECG and echocardiogram are used to detect the pattern and location of heart injury.

TREATMENT

Shock is considered a medical emergency and requires attention to the patient's airway, breathing, and circulation. Unless contraindicated, hypovolemic patients should be placed in a supine position with legs elevated to maximize cerebral blood flow. The use of blankets is often needed to keep the patient warm. Treatment is focused on removing or reducing the underlying cause. In cardiogenic shock, treatment involves surgically revascularizing the heart at the point of obstruction (see treatment of MI below). Medical treatment is aimed at improving cardiac output, reducing the workload on the heart, providing oxygen therapy, and regulating fluid volumes in the body. With cardiogenic shock caused by MI, thrombolytic therapy may be used if surgical options are not available.

In hypovolemic shock, treatment is focused on improving tissue perfusion through intravenous fluid/blood replacement. Sources of bleeding or fluid loss must be identified and corrected. Oxygen may be administered depending on the level of hypoxemia. Inotropic medications increase myocardial contractility. Various drugs in this group have either vasoconstricting (epinephrine, norepinephrine) or vasodilating (dobutamine) effects on peripheral vascular resistance. Dopamine is a drug that, at low doses, has a vasodilatory effect but at higher doses causes peripheral and central vasoconstriction. The choice of action on the peripheral vessels depends on the shock etiology, fluid volume, and contractile ability of the heart.

Septic shock treatment is aimed at treating the source of infection and supporting circulation. Pharmacologic treatment includes broad-spectrum antimicrobial drugs that provide coverage for possible pathogens and vasopressor drugs that promote vasoconstriction. Corticosteroids are often needed in anaphylactic shock to decrease the systemic inflammatory response. Neurogenic shock treatment is aimed at identifying and correcting the cause if possible and supporting vasoconstriction with inotropic medications. Frequent monitoring of vital organ function and hemodynamic status is required for all patients with shock.

Myocardial Infarction

CHD is a term used to identify any problem of impaired coronary circulation. Atherosclerosis is primarily implicated in the development of CHD. Consequences of CHD range from compensation through the development of collateral circulation to the myocardial cells to sudden death from myocardial anoxia. Because multiple processes are at work during cardiac perfusion, the loss of coronary circulation can lead to a spectrum of problems, including impaired conduction, impaired myocardial pumping, and heart failure.

Research Notes

The completion of the Human Genome Project has sparked an intensive interest in the genetic variants that underlie susceptibility to MI. Although many genes have been implicated in increasing MI risk, evidence for gender differences related to these genetic variants and the development of CVD has been inconclusive. One study examined the role of estrogen and protection against MI.[4] Even though estrogen is believed to have a protective effect, administration of exogenous estrogen has shown a lack of benefit in protecting against CVD. Others have examined the role of estrogen receptors and have found a twofold increase in MI events in women who had a specific haplotype.[5] Therefore, the types of receptors may have a more conclusive role in predicting MI risk than the presence of estrogen.

PATHOPHYSIOLOGY

Myocardial infarction is the total occlusion of one or more coronary arteries resulting in ischemia and death of myocardial tissues (Fig. 14.12). Consistent with CHD, the most common cause is atherosclerosis. Atherosclerotic accumulations can either directly obstruct the artery, or break off, causing platelets to aggregate at the site of injury and form a thrombus that occludes the artery. Major risk factors for the development of atherosclerosis and subsequent MI include:

- *Family history:* Individuals with a family history of atherosclerosis and MI are at greater risk, particularly those with a father or other male first-degree relative who experienced an MI or sudden death from a coronary event prior to 55 years of age; or a mother or other female

first-degree relative experiencing the same prior to 65 years of age.

- *Hypertension and smoking:* Hypertension and smoking injure the endothelial lining, promoting the development of atherosclerosis. Systolic blood pressure above 160 mm Hg is associated with a threefold increase in risk of developing CHD. Diastolic elevations are significant contributors as well.
- *Blood cholesterol levels:* The amount of cholesterol, particularly high LDL, in the blood is related to dietary intake of saturated fat and promotes lipid accumulation in the vessels.
- *Concurrent diabetes mellitus:* Type 2 diabetes is associated with elevations in blood lipid levels. The role of diabetes mellitus in the development of atherosclerosis is further discussed in Chapter 18.
- *High-sensitivity C-reactive protein:* CRP is a nonspecific acute phase protein that is produced by the liver in response to tissue injury and is considered a sensitive marker of inflammation. Elevated CRP is an emerging indicator of risk for the development of MI because inflammation has been linked with the pathogenesis of atherosclerosis.
- *Hyperhomocysteinemia:* Homocysteine is one of many potential risk factors for the development of MI. Homocysteine is derived primarily from a dietary amino acid found in animal protein. Homocysteine plays a role in coagulation. High levels of circulating homocysteine are toxic to endothelial cells and may promote excessive blood coagulation and thrombus formation. About half of those experiencing an acute MI or stroke have hyperhomocysteinemia.

The size, location, duration of occlusion, and presence of collateral circulation dictate the major effects of the MI. Larger arteries, when obstructed, result in more widespread damage to the myocardium. Location of occlusion also dictates major effects. The left coronary artery supplies blood to the left side of the heart. The left coronary artery branches into the anterior descending left coronary artery, which perfuses primarily the left ventricle, and the circumflex left coronary artery, which perfuses primarily the left atrium and portions of the left ventricle. Obstruction impairs the left ventricle and affects the ability of the heart to pump blood systemically. Ventricular fibrillation is a major cause of sudden death from MI. The right

A

B

Figure 14.12 Myocardial infarction. **A:** Left coronary artery obstruction shows zones of necrosis and ischemia. **B:** A cross-section of the left ventricle reveals a sharply circumscribed, soft, yellow area of necrosis. (Image from Rubin E, Farber JL. *Pathology.* 4th ed. Philadelphia: Lippincott Williams & Wilkins; 2005, with permission.)

Labels on image A: Obstruction, Ischemia, Necrosis

coronary artery and branches perfuse the right side of the heart, most notably the SA and AV nodes. Obstruction impacts cardiac conduction of impulses and can lead to irregularities in heart rhythm. Right heart failure also impedes the ability to manage venous return effectively. The myocardium can withstand oxygen deprivation for approximately 20 minutes. Beyond this, myocardial cell death is irreversible. Myocardial cells are replaced by nonfunctional scar tissue.

⬤ **STOP** *and* *Consider*

Low-dose daily aspirin is commonly used to prevent MI. Aspirin reduces platelet aggregation. How would this medication help to prevent MI?

CLINICAL MANIFESTATIONS

The clinical manifestations of MI are variable but may include: chest pain or a crushing pressure, often radiating to the left arm, shoulder, or jaw. Dizziness, sweating, indigestion (heartburn) pain, nausea, vomiting, fatigue, weakness, anxiety, cool, moist skin, pallor, or shortness of breath may also be reported. It is common for the individual to deny the chest pain as related to an MI. Women are particularly vulnerable because clinical manifestations

are considered atypical or subtle (fatigue, syncope, or weakness), and may be ignored. **Angina pectoris** is a term used to describe chest pain or pressure that is intermittent and associated with myocardial ischemia, a reduction in blood flow to the coronary arteries caused atherosclerosis that is often accompanied by vasospasm. The presence of ischemia and subsequent angina are exacerbated with increased cardiac workload, such as with exercise, and are typically reduced with rest. With MI, rest or nitroglycerine tablets do not alleviate the presence of angina.

DIAGNOSTIC CRITERIA

Diagnosis of MI is based on presenting symptoms (if any), ECG findings, and cardiac protein and enzyme measurements (see From the Lab below). Depending on the location of the MI, ECG tracings may demonstrate ST segment (see Fig. 14.5) elevations, indicating problems with ventricular repolarization. In larger infarcts, the Q wave may also be prolonged. Angiography in the cardiac catheterization laboratory determines the location and extent of obstruction. Echocardiography will reveal wall motion abnormalities and ventricular function. A chest radiograph may be used to detect complications of acute MI, particularly congestive heart failure and pulmonary edema.

TREATMENT

Rapid treatment (within 90 minutes) is preferred to re-establish coronary perfusion and to salvage the myocardium as much as possible. Before the patient arrives at the emergency department, ambulance personnel should obtain intravenous access, provide supplemental oxygen, and administer oral aspirin. Nitroglycerine (vasodilator) and morphine (analgesic) should be administered for active chest pain. Emergency treatment involves medical or surgical interventions. Percutaneous coronary intervention (PCI) is the treatment of choice for many patients with MI. PCI is a group of techniques capable of relieving coronary artery narrowing. One example is percutaneous transluminal coronary angioplasty (PTCA), a procedure that involves inserting a thin wire into the coronary artery from a distant access point via cardiac catheterization, inflating a balloon within this wire at the site of obstruction, and pushing open the stenotic vessel. This procedure often includes placement of a stent to keep the vessel open and patent. Some patients require coronary artery bypass surgery when other medical or surgical interventions have been ineffective (Fig. 14.13). Thrombolytic agents, combined with a potent platelet inhibitor, are recommended when PCI is not available within a 90-minute time frame. These drugs break though thromboses and reduce platelet aggregation at the site. Oxygen, nitroglycerin, analgesics, and aspirin therapies are continued while the patient is under emergency care. Long-term treatment is aimed at supporting cardiac conduction, output, and blood pressure through medication therapy (often with aspirin, β-blockers, ACE inhibitors, or angiotensin receptor blockers) and prescribed rest, exercise, and modification of risk factors (i.e., no smoking, reduced alcohol intake, nutritious diet, and weight loss).

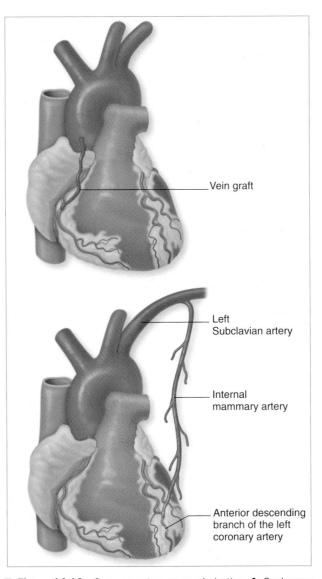

■ **Figure 14.13**   Coronary artery revascularization. **A:** Saphenous vein bypass graft. The vein segment is sutured to the ascending aorta and the right coronary artery at a point distal to the occlusion. **B:** Mammary artery bypass. The mammary artery is connected to the anterior descending left coronary artery at a point distal to the occlusion.

From the Lab

Creatine kinase (CK) is an important enzyme that is elevated in MI. CK is found in muscle cells and is needed to convert ADP to ATP. Four to eight hours after myocardial injury, CK, along with the myocardial band (MB) isoenzyme (CK-MB), is increased. These gradually decline and reach preinjury levels at between 48 and 72 hours. Myoglobin is a sensitive marker of acute myocardial necrosis. A third indicator of MI is elevations in troponin, a complex of three proteins (troponin-C, troponin-I, and troponin-T) present in striated muscle. These proteins regulate muscle contractions. Troponin-T is specific for cardiac muscle; blood levels rise within 4 hours and remain elevated for 10 to 14 days after MI.

Heart Failure

Heart failure reflects an inadequacy of heart pumping, so that the heart fails to maintain the circulation of blood. The basis for the development of altered perfusion of tissues is a result of *impaired cardiac functioning* or *excessive workload demands* that cannot be met by the heart. Heart failure occurs secondary to other conditions that perpetuate impaired cardiac functioning or workload. Examples of conditions that result in impaired cardiac functioning include MI, structural defects of the heart, or infection and inflammation of the heart tissue layers. Examples of conditions that create excessive work demands on the heart include hypertension, fluid volume overload, or anemia.

PATHOPHYSIOLOGY

Because forward movement of blood is restricted, the result is congestion and edema in pulmonary or peripheral tissues. In those with heart failure, cardiac reserve (the ability to increase output during increased activity) is expended during rest. Simple tasks become exceedingly taxing to the heart.

Left Heart Failure

Traditionally, heart failure is discussed based on the location of origin, either the left or right side of the heart. Despite isolating left and right, remember that these are both part of a continuous system. Therefore, impaired pumping and excessive peripheral vascular resistance eventually compromise both the left and the right sides of the heart.

In left heart failure, the left ventricle is unable to effectively meet cardiovascular demands, forward movement of blood through the circulation is inhibited, and fluid accumulates in the lung tissues. Loss of contractile ability, called **systolic failure**, results

in the heart being unable to pump enough blood into the circulation. Stiffness of the ventricle and loss of relaxation ability, called **diastolic failure**, impairs the ability to optimally fill with blood between cardiac contractions.

STOP and Consider

How do you think pharmacologic interventions differ between systolic and diastolic left ventricular failure?

Recall that the left ventricle receives blood from the pulmonary vein and left atrium. When the left ventricle is ineffective, blood backs up into the pulmonary vein, and subsequently into the lung tissues, resulting in pulmonary edema. **Congestive heart failure** is another term used to describe left heart failure. Causes of left heart failure include any condition that (1) impairs left ventricular pumping, such as what occurs with MI; or (2) increases the workload on the left ventricle, such as valvular disorders (aortic and bicuspid), in which the left ventricle must pump harder to compensate for stenosis or regurgitation (Fig. 14.14).

Right Heart Failure

Right heart failure begins on the right side of the heart. This impairs the heart's ability to move deoxygenated blood forward to the pulmonary circulation. The result is congestion of blood backward into the systemic circulation. The systemic congestion produces peripheral edema. The development of edema

Figure 14.14 Congestive heart failure. **A:** An unaffected heart. **B:** Notable enlargement of the heart related to chronic heart failure secondary to ischemic injury.

Research Notes

Researchers have found that overweight or obese people without obvious heart disease have changes in heart muscle structure and function that increase the likelihood of developing heart failure. The study included 73 women and 69 men who had an average age of 44 years. None had existing heart disease, high blood pressure, diabetes, or known symptoms of congestive heart failure. When compared with the left ventricles of people of normal weight, the left ventricles of severely obese participants had both a significantly weakened ability to contract (systolic dysfunction) and a reduced ability to fully relax to allow the ventricle to be refilled with blood during the rest period between heartbeats (diastolic dysfunction). Researchers found smaller but still significant impairments of left ventricle function in overweight or mildly obese volunteers and suggested a metabolic effect of obesity on the heart muscle.[6]

has been discussed in Chapter 8. Dependent areas of the body (i.e., extremities or areas closest to the ground) become swollen. The lower extremities are most commonly affected. The liver, spleen, gastrointestinal tract, and peritoneum can become engorged with fluid as blood backs up into the hepatic veins and portal circulation.

Causes of right heart failure include any process that restricts blood flow into the lungs. **Cor pulmonale** is an alteration in the structure and function of

the right ventricle caused by a primary disorder of the respiratory system. Lung injury, infections, inflammation, and pulmonary edema are most often implicated. The resulting pulmonary hypertension is the common link between these lung injuries and the development of cor pulmonale. Because left heart failure results in pulmonary edema, right heart failure can be a consequence of left heart failure. However, only primary lung conditions are termed cor pulmonale. Valvular defects of the tricuspid and pulmonic valves can also put a strain on the right ventricle and contribute to the development of right heart failure.

The tissues need oxygen. With both left and right heart failure, the heart is unable to keep up with the demand. Compensatory mechanisms are needed to maintain as much oxygenation as possible (Fig. 14.15). The goals are to help to ease congestion and improve cardiac pumping strength and efficiency. The mechanisms for achieving these goals focus on:

■ **Figure 14.15** Compensatory mechanisms in heart failure. (Image modified from Porth CM. *Essentials of Pathophysiology: Concepts of Altered Health States.* Philadelphia: Lippincott Williams & Wilkins; 2003, with permission.)

- *Improving venous return:* The tension in the veins increases, allowing improved movement of blood forward. This increases preload and improves cardiac output by increasing the amount of blood that fills the ventricles at the end of diastole. Diuretics may be used to support this compensatory mechanism by decreasing fluid volume and relieving peripheral vascular resistance.
- *Stimulating the sympathetic nervous system:* The sympathetic nervous system is stimulated to increase heart rate, cardiac contractility, and vessel tone to perfuse vital organs.
- *Stimulating the renin–angiotensin mechanism:* The kidneys increase renin secretion, resulting in elevations of angiotensin. This promotes compensatory vasoconstriction.
- *Enlarging the heart muscle:* Hypertrophy of the heart muscle occurs in response to workload demands of the ventricles. Compensatory hypertrophy initially improves cardiac contractility.

⬤ **STOP** and *Consider*

How are compensatory mechanisms similar between shock and heart failure? How are these different?

These compensatory mechanisms become ineffective with severe, prolonged heart failure. Although venous return is initially improved, prolonged venous congestion is too overwhelming for compensatory mechanisms. Sympathetic stimulation promotes perfusion to vital organs. Over time, this mechanism can trigger dysrhythmias and deprive "nonvital" organs (i.e., skin, muscle, and kidneys) of oxygen. Most notably, poor renal perfusion leads to increased sodium and water retention, thereby further taxing venous return. Another factor contributing to sodium and water retention is the stimulation of aldosterone production by angiotensin II. Myocardial hypertrophy can initially contribute to contractility but eventually impairs diastole and promotes oxygen deprivation to the myocardium. The myocardium becomes noncompliant, or tense, and the heart chamber size is reduced. These compensatory mechanisms are helpful in the early stages of heart failure, but over time may cause more harm than good.

CLINICAL MANIFESTATIONS

Figure 14.16 compares the clinical manifestations between right and left heart failure. In right heart failure, the clinical manifestations are related to congestion in peripheral tissues from the ineffective right ventricle. Early clinical manifestations in left heart failure can be absent. When present, clinical manifestations specific to left heart failure are related to decreased cardiac output and pulmonary congestion from a failing left ventricle, which leads to poor tissue and organ perfusion. Fluid congestion in the lungs leads to shortness of breath, coughing, and lung crackles with auscultation. Poor tissue and organ perfusion leads to many potential indicators, including cyanosis, exercise intolerance, poor urinary output, fluid and sodium retention, anorexia, and fatigue.

Likewise, early clinical manifestations in right heart failure can be absent or subtle, such as fatigue, exertional dyspnea, or syncope with exertion. Although these early manifestations are often attributed to the underlying pulmonary disease, the symptoms reflect the relative inability to increase cardiac output and a decrease in systemic arterial pressure with exertion. Ischemia of the right ventricle and pulmonary artery stretching can cause chest pain with exertion. In advanced stages, anorexia, weight loss, gastric and right upper quadrant pain, and jaundice can result from fluid congestion in the gastrointestinal tract and liver. Swelling in the extremities is also related to systemic edema.

DIAGNOSTIC CRITERIA

The diagnosis of heart failure is established based on a thorough patient history and physical examination, during which the presence of clinical manifestations listed above are noted. Chest radiography can detect pulmonary congestion, whereas two-dimensional echocardiography detects the heart's pumping ability, chamber size and thickness, the presence of valvular abnormalities, and measurements of various heart pressures. ECG supplies information on conduction impairments. Cardiac catheterization may be needed to visualize structural defects or to determine pressure levels in the heart chambers. Severity is based on the level of activity restriction imposed by the heart failure.

TREATMENT

Treatment of heart failure is focused on correcting the cause if possible. Surgically replacing defective valves, treating an underlying respiratory infection, or treating anemia are examples of correcting a heart failure cause. In many cases, the cause cannot be reversed. Treatment then focuses on providing supplemental oxygen, improving cardiac output, and reducing peripheral vascular resistance (see Hypertension) with an overall goal of improving quality of life. Heart failure is often a progressive, chronic problem with a poor prognosis. The 5-year survival rate is approximately 50%.

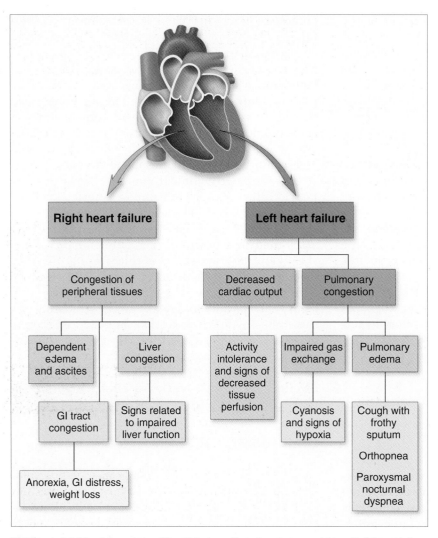

■ **Figure 14.16** Comparison of the clinical manifestations between right and left heart failure. GI, gastrointestinal. (Image modified from Porth CM. *Essentials of Pathophysiology: Concepts of Altered Health States.* Philadelphia: Lippincott Williams & Wilkins; 2003, with permission.)

distribution of cerebral infarcts and areas of necrosis. The process is similar to the development of MI. **Transient ischemic attack (TIA)** is a term used to describe a brief period of inadequate cerebral perfusion that causes a sudden focal loss of neurologic function. Full recovery of function usually occurs within 24 hours. TIAs may be the result of intermittent obstruction by platelets accumulating at the site of thrombosis or from temporary vasospasm. A completed stroke, however, causes permanent neurologic deficits. Embolic stroke similarly causes obstruction but results from emboli that dislodge from distant sites, travel to the brain, and occlude small arteries. Stroke from cerebral hemorrhage can be caused by trauma or defects in the cerebral vessels. Persistent hypertension and neoplasia can lead to cerebral vessel weakness, erosion, and rupture. The bleeding vessel fills and compresses adjacent brain tissue and brain ventricles.

On the cellular level, any process that disrupts blood flow to a portion of the brain unleashes a cascade of events typical of ischemia and inflammation, leading to the death of neurons. Within seconds to minutes of the loss of perfusion to a portion of the brain, the ischemic neuron becomes depolarized. ATP is depleted and membrane ion-transport systems fail. Neurotransmitters are released through the influx of calcium, and excitatory receptors on other neurons are activated. These neurons then become depolarized, causing further calcium influx, further neuronal excitation, and expanded ischemia. Neuronal damage is exacerbated by the excessive calcium influx, which releases destructive enzymes, the release of free radicals, and the presence of potent chemical mediators. This ischemic area coalesces into an infracted core within hours of the onset of the stroke.

Stroke

Stroke is defined as any clinical event, such as shock, cerebral hemorrhage, ischemia, or infarction, that leads to the impairment of cerebral circulation. Stroke is often referred to as a cerebrovascular accident. Major risk factors include hypertension, smoking, and diabetes.

PATHOPHYSIOLOGY

Stroke is often differentiated as thrombotic, embolic, or hemorrhagic to distinguish the process leading to altered cerebral perfusion. Thrombotic strokes are caused by occlusions of cerebral arteries, often from atherosclerosis. The most common site for atherosclerosis formation is in the common carotid artery where the artery bifurcates. Figure 14.17 illustrates the

CLINICAL MANIFESTATIONS

Stroke typically results in the abrupt onset of clinical manifestations characteristic of a focal brain injury. The level of cerebral edema varies based on the extent of cellular injury. Loss of function is based

■ **Figure 14.17** Cerebral infarction. **A:** Distribution of cerebral infarcts and areas of necrosis. **B:** A horizontal section of the brain depicting expansion and softening in the cortex from an occluded middle cerebral artery. (Image from Rubin E, Farber JL. *Pathology.* 4th ed. Philadelphia: Lippincott Williams & Wilkins; 2005, with permission.)

Occlusion of trifurcation of middle cerebral artery and area of necrosis

Occlusion of striate artery with infarction and area of necrosis

Occlusion of internal carotid artery

External carotid artery

Common carotid artery

A

B

on the part of the brain that is ischemic or compressed by the accumulation of blood. For example, hemorrhage of vessels leading to the medulla affects vital respiratory and cardiac centers and will result in sudden death. Cerebellar stroke impairs coordination. Common symptoms of stroke include the abrupt onset of hemiparesis (weakness on one side of the body), vision loss, visual field deficits, diplopia (double vision), dizziness, ataxia (lack of coordinated movement), aphasia (language impairment), or a sudden decrease in the level of consciousness.

In the cerebrum, hemorrhage or occlusion on one side of the brain results in hemiparesis or hemiplegia (paralysis) on the opposite side of the body. Therefore, if the stroke manifests as left-sided weakness, the obstruction or hemorrhage most likely exists on the right side of the cerebrum. Other possible manifestations of stroke include severe headache, sensory deficits, and vomiting. Again, the clinical presentation is extent and site dependent as ischemic brain tissue becomes necrotic and nonfunctional.

DIAGNOSTIC CRITERIA

The diagnosis of stroke is based on a careful patient history and physical examination, as well as laboratory and diagnostic studies. If the patient is aphasic, the history must include observer reports of time of

onset and progression of symptoms, if possible. Essential components of the physical examination include the neurologic evaluation of mental status and the level of consciousness, cranial nerves, motor function, sensory function, cerebellar function, gait, and deep tendon reflexes. This examination can be guided and quantified by published stroke scales to determine stroke severity and progress. Laboratory tests, including a complete blood count, blood chemistry panel, coagulation studies, and cardiac enzymes, may be needed to determine the cause of stroke or to rule out other health problems that can mimic a stroke. The primary diagnostic tool is CT scan, which can be used to distinguish the type and location of infarction. The CT scan is critical for determining the most appropriate treatment pathway; patients with thrombotic stroke may receive thrombolytic therapy, whereas individuals with a brain hemorrhage do not.

TREATMENT

Treatment is based on the cause. Efforts are initially aimed at reducing cerebral edema and the resulting increased intracranial pressure. Thrombotic or embolic stroke may be treated with thrombolytic or anticoagulant therapy. Hemorrhagic stroke will require prevention of further bleeding, and aspiration of accumulated blood may be indicated. Treatment is often focused on rehabilitation in an effort to adapt to reduced function and maximize independence.

Disseminated Intravascular Coagulation

Disseminated intravascular coagulation (DIC) is a condition of uncontrolled activation of clotting factors that results in widespread thrombi formation, followed by depletion of coagulation factors and platelets leading to massive hemorrhage. DIC is initiated by endothelial or tissue injury, such as that occurs with trauma, surgery, burns, malignant neoplasms, infections, or shock. Obstetric complications during labor and delivery are also commonly cited as a trigger for DIC.

PATHOPHYSIOLOGY

With DIC, injury triggers an imbalance between clotting and **fibrinolysis**, the dissolution of clots. Clotting factors, thrombin, and platelets accumulate throughout the cardiovascular system. This is particularly problematic in the microvessels, where the clots cause widespread tissue ischemia. The imbalance of clotting and clot dissolution is demonstrated, as blood-clotting mechanisms can then become depleted or clot-dissolving mechanisms increased. This allows massive systemic hemorrhage. DIC is a serious condition that requires immediate recognition and treatment.

CLINICAL MANIFESTATIONS

The effects of DIC are variable and depend on the presence of excessive clotting or hemorrhage. DIC can manifest as an acute hemorrhagic disorder caused by widespread clot dissolution from excess plasmin formation. This development is most commonly caused by infection, acute tissue injury, or obstetric complications and leads to bruising, petechiae, and epistaxis. Blood may be found in the sputum, stool, emesis, and urine. Severe bleeding and hemorrhage can lead to hypovolemic shock. Alternatively, DIC can manifest as a chronic or subacute state characterized by excess clotting (thrombin) formation. This occurs more commonly with malignancy, chronic renal disease, venous thrombosis, and certain connective tissue disorders. Widespread clotting can lead to multiple manifestations, depending on the location of thromboses. In the brain, it can lead to headache, weakness, seizures, and even coma. Within the kidneys, thromboses are manifested as poor urine output, which can progress to renal failure. In the heart and lungs, manifestations include cough, shortness of breath, respiratory distress, or chest pain. Vascular occlusions in larger vessels lead to the manifestations of infarction in the affected organ.

DIAGNOSTIC CRITERIA

Identification of the underlying problem leading to DIC is critical. A thorough patient history and physical examination are needed to identify this underlying cause, such as infection, malignancy, major traumatic injury, labor and delivery complications, or recent surgery. Screening laboratory tests include prothrombin time (PT), activated partial thromboplastin time (aPTT), platelet count, and fibrinogen level. The D-dimer test measures the degradation of fibrin products, which is significant for both thrombus formation and breakdown, and detects the simultaneous formation of both thrombin and plasmin. This is considered a confirmatory test that strongly suggests the presence of DIC.

TREATMENT

Treatment is focused on correcting the underlying cause, and it depends on the presence of hemorrhage versus thromboses. The goal is to replace the missing blood components. Massive clotting

From the Lab

Coagulation results from a sequence of events involving proteins (coagulation factors) produced by the liver and secreted into the bloodstream. PT, aPTT, and fibrinogen levels are screening tests for DIC. PT is used to evaluate the adequacy of the extrinsic clotting system (clotting that is triggered by the release of tissue thromboplastin), including factors I (fibrinogen), II (prothrombin), V, VII, and X. PT is measured in seconds, the expected range is usually approximately 11 to 14 seconds, and a prolonged PT indicates a deficiency in one or more of these factors. aPTT (also referred to as PTT) detects clotting factor deficiencies in the intrinsic clotting system (those factors already present in the plasma) and is a broader screening test for deficiencies in factors I, II, V, VIII, IX, X, XII, and XII. aPTT is measured in seconds; the expected range is approximately 22 to 34 seconds and is significant when prolonged. Typically, when a prolonged PT or aPTT is noted, more specific tests are needed to identify the affected coagulation factor. Fibrinogen levels screen specifically for the presence of factor I. The most common cause for a reduced fibrinogen level is DIC.

requires anticoagulation therapy. Massive hemorrhage requires exogenous administration of clotting factors and platelets to replace what was lost. Treatment of DIC is a careful balancing act focused on restoring the body's ability to coagulate appropriately.

Summary

- Perfusion is the process of forcing blood or other fluid to flow through a vessel and into the vascular bed of a tissue to provide oxygen and other nutrients.
- Effective perfusion is a complex interaction of ventilation, responsive neuronal control of cardiac impulses, cardiac muscle contraction, and circulation.
- Altered perfusion impairs tissue oxygenation and can stem from altered ventilation, diffusion, or circulation.
- Examples of situations that can impair circulation include brain injury at the cardiac control center in the medulla, blockage of the conduction system of the heart, structural defects, overtaxing, or necrosis of the heart (which reduces cardiac output), and obstruction and hemorrhage in the arteries and veins.
- General manifestations of altered perfusion depend on the process but may include tachycardia, tachypnea, fatigue, heart murmurs, ECG changes, pallor or erythema, cyanosis, edema, shortness of breath, impaired growth, hypotension or hypertension, hemorrhage, and pain.
- Multiple diagnostic tests are used to detect problems with perfusion, including blood tests for hypercholesterolemia, anemia, and hypoxemia. Visualization, through the use of echocardiography, nuclear scanning, and radiography, allows detection of structural and functional problems with the heart's pumping capabilities and blood flow. ECG is frequently used to determine conduction problems with the heart.

Case Study 14.1

James is a 55-year-old male who presents in the Emergency Department (ED) with sudden swelling in his left leg. He is complaining of a dull ache in his calf that increases when he is walking. He states, "My left leg feels really tight and hot." He works as a truck driver and has just finished a long route that lasted 10 days. He does admit to an injury to his lower leg about 2 weeks ago, but he thought that the injury was resolved. He does not exercise regularly. He is a smoker. He reports no other significant health history. After physical examination, he undergoes a Doppler compression ultrasound, and a deep vein thrombosis is detected.

1. *Outline the process that is most likely occurring in this man's body.*
2. *What would you expect for clinical manifestations?*
3. *What diagnostic tests could be used?*
4. *What treatment measures and complications would you anticipate?*

Log on to the Internet. Search for a relevant journal article or Web site (such as http://www.emedicine.com/med/topic2785.htm) that details deep vein thrombosis to confirm your predictions.

Case Study 14.2

Jamie is a 15-year-old female who has concerns about excessive bleeding with her last menstrual period. She has noticed recently that she bruises easily and bleeds readily, particularly with her gums while brushing her teeth. She also has had nosebleeds recently. She comes into your clinic for examination. You note nonpalpable petechiae of her legs and arms, purpura, and gingival bleeding. Her platelet count is less than $20,000/mm^3$. She is diagnosed with idiopathic thrombocytopenic purpura.

1. *Outline the process that is most likely occurring in this adolescent's body.*
2. *What would you expect for clinical manifestations?*
3. *What diagnostic tests could be used?*
4. *What treatment measures and complications would you anticipate?*

Log on to the Internet. Search for a relevant journal article or Web site (such as http://emedicine.medscape.com/article/779545-overview) that details idiopathic thrombocytopenic purpura to confirm your predictions.

Practice Exam Questions

1. In evaluating modifiable cardiovascular risk factors for your patient, which one is NOT considered modifiable?
   a. Poorly controlled diabetes mellitus
   b. Hyperlipidemia
   c. Hypertension
   d. Female gender

2. Your patient is experiencing peripheral edema, hepatomegaly, ascites, and splenomegaly. Which of the following conditions would be consistent with the patient's findings?
   a. Endocarditis
   b. Myocardial infarction
   c. Right-sided heart failure
   d. Left-sided heart failure

3. It is a very hot summer day. Your neighbor stops at your house after jogging 5 miles. She is sweating and tells you she feels dizzy and thirsty and can't make it home. You check her blood pressure and find it to be LOW. What could you do right in your home to raise her blood pressure?
   a. Place a cold washcloth on her head
   b. Have her drink a large glass of cool water
   c. Have her take a shower with warm water
   d. Encourage her to take slow, deep breaths

4. Your neighbor again comes to your door (see previous question). She has been running in the snow and it is very cold outside. She has a headache and her heart is pounding. Again you check her blood pressure and find it to be HIGH. What could you do this time right in your home to decrease her blood pressure?
   a. Have her drink some hot chocolate
   b. Have her lay down on your couch
   c. Let her take a hot shower
   d. Give her something really salty to eat

5. Which of the following situations of altered perfusion could be triggered by chronic obstructive pulmonary disease?
   a. Impaired cardiac output
   b. Impaired circulation
   c. Ventilation–perfusion mismatching
   d. Excessive cardiac demand

6. Which mechanism increases peripheral vascular resistance and contributes to the development of hypertension?
   a. Impaired sodium excretion by the kidneys
   b. Parasympathetic nervous system overstimulation
   c. Reduced renin–angiotensin–aldosterone secretion
   d. None of these

7. Which is not a requirement for effective perfusion?
   a. Absence of chronic disease
   b. Adequate blood volume
   c. Functional systemic circulation
   d. An open airway

8. Your neighbor tells you that she was in the hospital and they told her she had a bundle branch block. What does this mean?
   a. She cannot conduct electrical impulses to stimulate the heart ventricle to contract
   b. She has had a cardiac arrest
   c. She is experiencing obstructed P wave depolarization of the atria
   d. She has an excessive calcium influx causing prolonged myocardial contraction

9. You are listening to your lab partners heart in skills lab and you hear the "lub dub" sound. What are you hearing?
   a. The sodium ions rapidly influxing into the cells
   b. The closure of the heart valves
   c. The contraction of the left ventricle
   d. Blood forcing its way through the aorta

10. At what point in the cardiac cycle do you measure preload?
    a. Just after systole
    b. Just before systole
    c. During systole
    d. It is not possible to measure preload

Discussion and Application

1. What did I know about altered perfusion prior to today?

2. What body processes are affected by altered perfusion? What are the expected functions of those processes? How does altered perfusion affect those processes?

3. What are the potential etiologies for altered perfusion? How does altered perfusion develop?

4. Who is most at risk for developing altered perfusion? How can altered perfusion be prevented?

5. What are the human differences that affect the etiology, risk, or course of altered perfusion?

6. What clinical manifestations are expected in the course of altered perfusion?

7. What special diagnostic tests help determine the diagnosis and course of altered perfusion?

8. What are the goals of care for individuals with altered perfusion?

9. How does the concept of altered perfusion build on what I have learned in the previous chapters and in previous courses?

10. How can I use what I have learned?

RESOURCES

American Heart Association Web site:
http://www.americanheart.org

A Medline Plus tutorial on Congestive Heart Failure:
http://www.nlm.nih.gov/medlineplus/tutorials/congestiveheart-
    failure/htm/index.htm

Current research involving clinical trials and results:
http://www.clinicaltrials.gov

**The Stanford Stroke Center at the Stanford School of
    Medicine has a listing of stroke scales designed to guide
    the neurologic quantification of stroke manifestations:**
http://strokecenter.stanford.edu/scales/

REFERENCES

1. The U.S. Department of Health and Human Services. The Seventh Report of the Joint National Committee on Detection, Evaluation, and Treatment of High Blood Pressure. 2003. Available at: http://www.nhlbi.nih.gov/guidelines/hypertension/express.pdf. Accessed January 30, 2010. The Eighth Report is available Summer 2010.

2. Adeyemo A, Gerry N, Chen G, et al. A genome-wide association study of hypertension and blood pressure in African Americans. *PLoS Genet.* 2009. Available online at: http://www.plosgenetics.org/article/info%3Adoi%2F10.1371%2Fjournal.pgen.1000564.Accessed June 29, 2010

3. Hostetler M. Cardiogenic shock. 2010. Available at: http://www.emedicine.com/emerg/topic530.htm. Accessed January 30, 2010.

4. Anderson G, Limacher M, Assaf A, et al. Effects of conjugated equine estrogen in postmenopausal women with hysterectomy: the Women's Health Initiative randomized control trial. *JAMA.* 2004;291:1701–1712.

5. Schuit S, Oie H, Witteman J, et al. Estrogen receptor [alpha] gene polymorphisms and risk of myocardial infarction. *JAMA.* 2004;291: 2969–2977.

6. Wong C, O'Moore Sullivan T, Leano R, et al. Alterations of left ventricular myocardial characteristics associated with obesity. *Circulation.* 2004;110:3081–3087.

Chapter 15

Altered Nutrition

LEARNING OBJECTIVES

1. Define and use the key terms listed in this chapter.
2. Explain the role of nutrition in maintaining health.
3. Identify the processes that can alter nutrition.
4. Identify common signs and symptoms related to altered nutrition.
5. Describe diagnostic tests and treatment strategies relevant to altered nutrition.
6. Apply concepts of altered nutrition to select clinical models.

INTRODUCTION

What did you eat for breakfast? How did that food contribute to your health? Every day we put nutrients into our bodies with little consideration of exactly what those nutrients are doing to maintain homeostasis. Adequate nutrition relies on optimal intake, digestion, absorption, and transportation of nutrients, as well as the excretion of waste products. We choose to eat a variety of foods because they are appealing to us in one way or another. Once the food goes through the process of digestion, the extracted nutrients are made suitable for absorption and transportation. The nutrients in their simplest form are then used for a predictable purpose. This chapter takes a closer look at essential food-derived nutrients and the role these nutrients play in facilitating basic physiologic processes. Clinical models are selected to illustrate the effects of nutrient deficiencies or excesses on healthy functioning.

Nutrition

Nutrition is the process of ingestion and utilization of nutrients for energy. Ultimately, we obtain nutrition and **energy**, or the capacity to do work, from the sun via organisms and plants that undergo photosynthesis. Energy from ingested nutrients is released when food is metabolized. Metabolism allows chemical reactions that (1) produce heat to maintain body temperature, (2) conduct neuronal impulses, and (3) contract muscles. Nutrition also provides the substances needed for growth, repair, and maintenance of cells.

A **nutrient** is a food or liquid that supplies the body with the chemicals needed for metabolism. Nutrients are frequently categorized as macronutrients, micronutrients, and water. **Macronutrients** are proteins, carbohydrates, and fats. **Micronutrients** are vitamins and minerals. The body is capable of synthesizing certain nutrients from other products (e.g., the synthesis of glucose from amino acids and glycerol). Many nutrients, however, must be consumed regularly in the diet, because the body is unable to synthesize the nutrient in quantities sufficient to meet its needs. These are called **essential nutrients**.

Water

Water is the largest single component of the body and is essential for all body functions, including digestion, absorption, transportation, and excretion. Specifically, water functions to:

- Serve as a solvent promoting availability of solutes to the cell
- Promote and maintain fluid balance
- Provide a transport medium for nutrients and waste products
- Serve as a lubricant
- Contribute to the regulation of body temperature
- Provide the foundation for metabolic reactions
- Contribute to the structure of the cells and circulatory system

Because the body is unable to store water, regular intake of water is required to offset that lost through perspiration or other mechanisms. Although individuals can survive several weeks without food, adults (in moderate weather) can survive only 10 days without water and children can survive only 5 days.[1] Metabolically active cells, such as muscle cells, have the highest concentrations of water and are most devastated by deficiencies. Chapter 8 further details the clinical effects of water imbalance. The major point is that water is an essential nutrient; a reduction in total body water of 20% or greater may cause death.

Macronutrients: Proteins, Lipids, and Carbohydrates

The major macronutrients that are converted to usable sources of energy are proteins, lipids, and carbohydrates. Protein is composed of linear chains of amino acids that are linked as directed by DNA coding. During digestion, proteins are broken down into amino acids and absorbed into the circulation. The body contains 20 different types of amino acids. Of these, nine are considered essential and therefore must be consumed within the diet. From amino acids, body proteins are synthesized. Protein is needed to build and maintain structural body tissues such as muscle, bone matrix, and connective tissue. It also composes blood, cell membranes, immune

From the Lab

Unique to macronutrients, protein contains nitrogen. Nitrogen balance is a biochemical technique used to determine protein status. Nitrogen balance is calculated based on daily protein intake and the amount of nitrogen excretion in the urine. A correction is added for insensible losses of nitrogen, such as through the skin and gastrointestinal (GI) tract. In healthy adults, the nitrogen balance should equate to zero. If the person has a positive nitrogen balance, this individual is taking in more protein than is being excreted, which should occur in times of growth, pregnancy, and healing. If the person has a negative nitrogen balance, this individual is excreting more protein than is being consumed, as occurs in a state of tissue destruction, such as with burns, infection, or other tissue trauma.

factors, enzymes, and hormones. Proteins transport other substances across membranes and throughout the body and can combine with other substances to form new substances. For example, proteins can combine with nucleic acids to form DNA and RNA, carbohydrates to form glycoproteins, lipids to form lipoproteins, and metals to form hemoglobin.

Lipids are also considered macronutrients and are a group of substances that are insoluble in water. Lipids are categorized as:

1. Simple lipids or fats: fatty acids and glycerol
2. Compound lipids or lipoids: phospholipids, lipoproteins, and glycolipids
3. Sterols: cholesterol and bile salts

Triglycerides, a fatty acid and glycerol complex, are a form of simple lipids readily found in dietary fat. **Saturated fatty acids** are fatty acids that have no double bonds and elevate blood cholesterol levels. These fatty acids are found in animal sources and are solid at room temperature. **Unsaturated fatty acids** have one or more double bonds and are not known to elevate blood cholesterol levels. These are usually found in plant sources and are often liquid at room temperature.

Lipids provide a rich source of energy. Most dietary fat is stored in the body within adipose cells, also called adipocytes. Adipose cells contain storage fats, which accumulate around tissues and within body cavities and are used when energy is needed. Adipose cells can sustain the body's energy provision for weeks. The accumulation of storage fats is considered a health epidemic, particularly for those consuming a Western diet. Obesity is selected as a clinical model within this chapter to illustrate the health effects of excessive storage fat. A small amount of lipids can be stored in other locations, such as within liver cells. An accumulation of fat in liver cells inhibits liver cell function.

Structural fat is a type of fat that is not accessed for energy; rather, it provides support and protection to body organs and nerves. Structural fats are found inside cell structures of the brain, liver, kidney, lung, heart, spleen, muscle, and other cells, and they are essential for survival. The subcutaneous fat layer provides insulation and maintenance of body temperature.

Aside from being a rich source of energy, lipids facilitate numerous processes after ingestion and absorption into the body. Dietary fat supports digestion by decreasing gastric motility and secretions. Along with this function, dietary fat stimulates pancreatic and bile secretion and facilitates the digestion, absorption, and transportation of fat-soluble vitamins. The brain, central nervous system (CNS), and cell membranes throughout the body require essential fatty acids to function optimally. Essential fatty acids influence cell membrane fluidity, receptor function, enzyme activity, and cytokine production. Linoleic acid, an omega-3 fatty acid derived from fish and plant oils, is considered an essential fatty acid and has been demonstrated to reduce many disease states, including heart disease. This substance acts by (1) reducing fibrinogen and other clotting proteins and decreasing the likelihood that a clot will form and (2) stimulating endothelial cells to produce substances that promote vascular relaxation. Phospholipids, a form of complex lipid, are an important structural component of cell membranes. Lipids are also an integral aspect of hormones that mediate multiple body processes.

Carbohydrates are also considered macronutrients. The three categories of carbohydrates are:

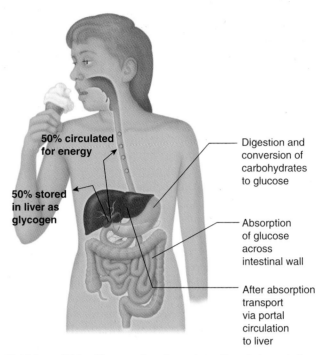

■ Figure 15.1 Glucose digestion, absorption, transportation, storage, and utilization.

1. Monosaccharides: glucose or fructose
2. Disaccharides and oligosaccharides: sucrose or lactose
3. Polysaccharides: starches and fiber

Dietary carbohydrates are digested and converted primarily into glucose. Once digested, the glucose is absorbed across the intestinal wall and transported to the liver via the portal circulation, where about 50% is used for oxidation or stored as glycogen. The remaining glucose exits the liver and is circulated throughout the body to be used by cells for energy (Fig. 15.1). The role of insulin and the uptake of glucose are discussed in detail in Chapter 18.

The major role of carbohydrates is to provide energy. Interestingly, carbohydrates are not considered essential. Glucose is important and the brain is the largest consumer; however, lipids and proteins can provide this energy source. Glucose can be synthesized by converting amino acids and glycerol from triglycerides into glucose. This is not the most efficient way of achieving an adequate glucose level (see Malnutrition discussed below under Altered Nutrition); therefore, carbohydrates should compose the largest proportion of daily food intake. Complex carbohydrates are preferred over simple sugars because these food sources provide other nutrients, such as vitamins and minerals. Fiber, a nondigestible carbohydrate, is important in the reduction of serum cholesterol levels and works primarily by binding to bile acids, a source of cholesterol, and by preventing cholesterol absorption. Fiber also plays a key role in gastric motility.

Table 15.1 Vitamins and Their Major Physiologic Functions

Vitamin	Functions This Vitamin Plays a Key Role in:
Vitamin A	• Maintenance of visual pigment and photoreception • Maintenance of epithelial cells and mucous membranes • Cellular growth and differentiation by contributing to glycoprotein (cell-surface regulator) synthesis • Synthesis of collagen and bone • Regulation of gene expression • Reproduction and immune function
Vitamin D	• Absorption and metabolism of calcium and phosphorus • Regulation of gene expression • Stimulation of differentiation of intestinal epithelial cells and osteoblasts
Vitamin E	• Protection against oxidative degradation from reactive oxygen species (free radicals)
Vitamin K	• Coagulation of blood • Formation of bone
Ascorbic acid (vitamin C)	• Synthesis of collagen and mucous membrane integrity • Protection against oxidative degradation from reactive oxygen species (free radicals) • Facilitation of iron absorption • Maintenance of lung function • Metabolism of amino acids • Synthesis of steroid hormones • Promotion of resistance to infection
Thiamin (vitamin B$_1$)	• Carbohydrate metabolism—serves as a coenzyme in the process of energy metabolism • Regulation of neuronal function, although the mechanism is unclear
Riboflavin (vitamin B$_2$)	• Carbohydrate, amino acid, and fatty acid metabolism • Support for antioxidant properties
Niacin	• Carbohydrate, amino acid, and fatty acid metabolism
Pyridoxine (vitamin B$_6$)	• Amino acid metabolism • Release of glucose from glycogen • Biosynthesizing neurotransmitters and histamine • Biosynthesizing myelin sheaths of nerve cells • Modulation of steroid hormone receptors • Critical for the production of antibodies
Folate	• Amino acid and nucleotide metabolism • DNA/RNA synthesis • Embryogenesis • Formation of red and white blood cells in the bone marrow • Reduction of homocysteine levels (see Chapter 14)
Biotin	• Carbohydrate, amino acid, and fatty acid metabolism
Pantothenic acid	• Carbohydrate, amino acid, and fatty acid metabolism
Cobalamin (vitamin B$_{12}$)	• Amino acid metabolism • Essential for metabolism of all cells, particularly those of the gastrointestinal tract, bone marrow, and nervous tissue • Reduction of homocysteine levels

Micronutrients: Vitamins and Minerals

Vitamins are organic substances that the body is unable to manufacture and therefore must consume. Vitamins are often classified according to solubility (fat or water soluble) or by metabolic function.

Fat-soluble vitamins include vitamins A, D, E, and K. *Water-soluble vitamins* are ascorbic acid (vitamin C), thiamin (B$_1$), riboflavin (B$_2$), niacin, pyridoxine (B$_6$), biotin, pantothenic acid, folate, and cobalamin (B$_{12}$). The physiologic impact of each of the vitamins is depicted in Table 15.1. As is evident in this table, many vitamins play a critical role in the metabolism of carbohydrates, amino acids, and fatty acids. The metabolic value of vitamins includes categories such as:

1. Membrane stabilizers (such as with antioxidants)
2. Hydrogen and electron donors and acceptors
3. Hormones
4. Coenzymes

Basically, vitamins are part of enzyme systems that release energy from macronutrients. Other major roles of vitamins are to help develop genetic materials, red blood cells, hormones, collagen, and nervous system tissue.

Research Notes

Researchers, through a multitude of studies, have attempted to determine the effects of antioxidants on health. A search of ClinicalTrials.gov revealed almost 400 studies in progress related to antioxidant use to treat a variety of conditions. Completed studies have focused on the impact of antioxidants on everything from reducing pregnancy-induced hypertension to Alzheimer disease (AD). As with many studies on antioxidants, a meta-analysis of AD antioxidant revealed conflicting findings. A few of the studies found a positive health benefit with antioxidant use for the prevention of AD. However, most studies in the meta-analysis discovered that vitamin E supplementation actually contributed to mortality and should not be recommended for the prevention of AD.[2] A large-scale randomized clinical trial was recommended to further clarify these conflicting findings.

STOP *and Consider*

How do you think vitamin A and C deficiencies affect wound healing?

Minerals are inorganic substances critical to the regulation of hundreds of cellular processes. Minerals constitute bone, hemoglobin, enzymes, hormones, and chemical mediators. Charged (ionic) minerals mediate impulse conduction within the nervous system. Minerals maintain water balance, acid-base balance, and osmotic pressure. Minerals are critical for muscle contraction and form the structural components of bones and teeth.

Minerals are subcategorized as macrominerals or microminerals. The macrominerals include sodium, potassium, calcium, phosphorus, magnesium, and sulfur. These substances are primarily ions and therefore exist in a charged state. The role of electrolytes was discussed in Chapter 8. The microminerals include iron, zinc, fluoride, and copper. Microminerals do not exist in blood, tissues, and cellular fluids in a free ionic state; rather, these substances are bound to proteins. Microminerals are often referred to as trace metals. These metals act on enzymes and hormones to elicit a specific response. They also interact with DNA to regulate the transcription of proteins. In this way, microminerals, or metals, affect the whole body. Microminerals can be further subdivided

as ultratrace minerals, in which extremely minute amounts are required. The ultratrace minerals are iodine, selenium, manganese, molybdenum, cobalt, boron, and chromium. The specific contributions of select minerals are presented in Table 15.2.

Nutritional Intake Requirements

Nutritional intake requirements, such as the Recommended Daily Allowances (RDAs), have been published to designate the recommended intake for most nutrients. The goal of adhering to the RDAs is to minimize the health effects that can occur with overnutrition or undernutrition. Caloric requirements are determined based on the kcal/kg needed to maintain body weight. Caloric intake requirements depend on age, gender, activity level, current weight, pregnancy, and lactation. During times of growth, caloric requirements are higher. For example, caloric requirements are 115 kcal/kg at birth. This requirement decreases to 80 kcal/kg between ages 1 and 10 years and is about half of that (30 to 40 kcal/kg) in adulthood. Pregnancy demands add an additional 300 kcal/day. Lactation (breastfeeding) increases the requirement by 500 kcal/day.

STOP *and Consider*

What is your approximate caloric requirement per day to maintain your body weight?

Micronutrient requirements are expressed primarily in micrograms (μg) or milligrams (mg) per day. For example, the RDA for vitamin A for adults is 700 μg/day for women and 900 μg/day for men. Macronutrient intake recommendations are based on percentage of calories consumed:

- Carbohydrates: 50% to 60%
- Proteins: 10% to 20%
- Fats: 30% or less

The United States Department of Agriculture introduced the "MyPyramid" campaign (Fig. 15.2) to promote healthy food choices and physical activity. Similarly, Canada's Office of Nutrition Policy and Promotion sponsors Canada's Food Guide to Healthy Eating (see Resources). Both the MyPyramid Guide and Canada's Food Guide are useful basic assessment and nutritional teaching tools that can be adapted to individual food preferences.

Table 15.2 Physiologic Contributions of Select Minerals

Mineral	Function
Calcium	Calcium is the most abundant mineral in the body and is essential for bone and teeth formation, muscle contraction, blood coagulation, transmission of nervous impulses, cell membrane permeability, and enzyme activation
Phosphorus	Phosphorus is the second most abundant mineral in the body and is an essential component of DNA and RNA, cellular energy (the P of ATP), membrane receptors, cell membranes, acid-base buffer systems (phosphate system), bones, and teeth.
Iron	Iron is essential for multiple processes, including red blood cell function, transportation of oxygen, myoglobin function, and modulation of enzyme activity involved in cellular respiration and energy (ATP) production. Iron supports immune function and may play a role in promoting cognitive performance
Zinc	Zinc is an intracellular ion that modulates the effects of numerous enzymes; the major roles are in metabolism of macronutrients and nucleic acids, as a component of protein structure, gene expression, cell division, osteoblastic activity, immune function, and neuron function
Fluoride	Fluoride supports tooth enamel and has antibacterial properties leading to resistance against dental caries
Copper	Copper is a component of numerous enzymes and therefore plays a role in numerous processes, such as the synthesis of energy, catecholamines, collagen, elastin, and melanin. Copper also protects against reactive oxygen species and promotes iron oxidation
Iodine	Iodine is needed for the synthesis of thyroid hormones
Selenium	Selenium has antioxidant properties and plays a role in lipid metabolism and thyroid hormone production, and it may reduce cancer risk
Manganese	Manganese is a component of numerous enzymes. It plays a role in carbohydrate and lipid metabolism, growth, reproduction, and formation of connective tissues and bone
Chromium	Chromium is active in macronutrient metabolism and gene expression
Molybdenum	Molybdenum is active in multiple enzymatic reactions
Boron	Boron is a component of cell membranes and plays a role in modulating enzymatic reactions, most notably supporting brain and bone function
Cobalt	Cobalt is a component of B_{12}; its primary role is red blood cell maturation. Cobalt also supports the function of all other cells and promotes enzymes active in DNA to RNA transcription

Intake and Storage of Nutrients

Maintenance of body weight and composition requires a balance of energy intake and expenditure. During times of growth, energy requirements increase to offset the evident growth expenditures. Energy intake is regulated by numerous factors, including hunger, **satiety**, or a feeling of fullness, food availability, and emotional and physical health. Hunger and satiety are regulated in the brain by the hypothalamus, based on feedback from the digestive tract on the quantity and quality of food in the stomach and intestines. Some examples of feedback messages from GI tract and nutrient storage sites to the hypothalamus include:

- The presence of low blood glucose or a lack of food in the GI tract induces hunger.
- The presence of food in the GI tract triggers stretch receptors and insulin secretion and subsequently reduces appetite.
- The presence of fat stimulates cholecystokinin, a GI hormone that contributes to satiety.
- Increases in fat stores stimulate the release of leptin, a hormone with the ability to suppress appetite, increase energy expenditures, and ultimately increase metabolism.

The hypothalamus responds by secreting hormones that contribute to energy intake, expenditure, and metabolism. In response, the short-term desire to eat is reduced or stimulated. Over a longer period, body weight and composition are maintained.

Storage of nutrients is also critical to health. Adipocytes (fat cells) store lipids as a key energy source when the need arises. The liver stores certain vitamins and minerals, such as vitamins A, B_{12}, D, E, K, iron, and copper, and then releases these in times of need. The liver also stores glycogen, and when glycogen stores are exhausted, the liver then converts amino acids and glycerol to glucose.

Digestion

The digestive system is essential for (1) digesting and extracting macronutrients, (2) absorbing nutrients, and (3) forming a physiologic and chemical barrier against microorganisms and other foreign materials introduced during food ingestion. Stomach acid forms a first line of defense by destroying many types of microorganisms and other harmful substances on contact. Figure 15.3 illustrates the digestive system, composed of the GI tract and accessory organs.

Anatomy of MyPyramid

USDA
U.S. Department of Agriculture
Center for Nutrition Policy and Promotion
April 2005
CNPP-16

One size doesn't fit all

USDA's new MyPyramid symbolizes a personalized approach to healthy eating and physical activity. The symbol has been designed to be simple. It has been developed to remind consumers to make healthy food choices and to be active every day. The different parts of the symbol are described below.

Activity

Activity is represented by the steps and the person climbing them, as a reminder of the importance of daily physical activity.

Moderation

Moderation is represented by the narrowing of each food group from bottom to top. The wider base stands for foods with little or no solid fats or added sugars. These should be selected more often. The narrower top area stands for foods containing more added sugars and solid fats. The more active you are, the more of these foods can fit into your diet.

Personalization

Personalization is shown by the person on the steps, the slogan, and the URL. Find the kinds and amounts of food to eat each day at MyPyramid.gov.

MyPyramid.gov
STEPS TO A HEALTHIER YOU

Proportionality

Proportionality is shown by the different widths of the food group bands. The widths suggest how much food a person should choose from each group. The widths are just a general guide, not exact proportions. Check the web site for how much is right for you.

Variety

Variety is symbolized by the 6 color bands representing the 5 food groups of the Pyramid and oils. This illustrates that foods from all groups are needed each day for good health.

Gradual Improvement

Gradual improvement is encouraged by the slogan. It suggests that individuals can benefit from taking small steps to improve their diet and lifestyle each day.

GRAINS	VEGETABLES	FRUITS	MILK	MEAT & BEANS
Make half your grains whole	Vary your veggies	Focus on fruits	Get your calcium-rich foods	Go lean with protein
Eat at least 3 oz. of whole-grain cereals, breads, crackers, rice, or pasta every day

1 oz. is about 1 slice of bread, about 1 cup of breakfast cereal, or ½ cup of cooked rice, cereal, or pasta | Eat more dark-green veggies like broccoli, spinach, and other dark leafy greens

Eat more orange vegetables like carrots and sweet potatoes

Eat more dry beans and peas like pinto beans, kidney beans, and lentils | Eat a variety of fruit

Choose fresh, frozen, canned, or dried fruit

Go easy on fruit juices | Go low-fat or fat-free when you choose milk, yogurt, and other milk products

If you don't or can't consume milk, choose lactose-free products or other calcium sources such as fortified foods and beverages | Choose low-fat or lean meats and poultry

Bake it, broil it, or grill it

Vary your protein routine- choose more fish, beans, peas, nuts, and seeds |

For a 2,000-calorie diet, you need the amounts below from each food group. To find the amounts that are right for you, go to MyPyramid.gov.

Eat 6 oz. every day	Eat 2½ cups every day	Eat 2 cups every day	Get 3 cups every day; for kids aged 2 to 8, it's 2	Eat 5½ oz every day

Find your balance between food and physical activity

- Be sure to stay within your daily calorie needs.
- Be physically active for at least 30 minutes most days of the week.
- About 60 minutes a day of physical activity may be needed to prevent weight gain.
- For sustaining weight loss, at least 60 to 90 minutes a day of physical activity may be required.
- Children and teenagers should be physically active for 60 minutes every, or most days.

Know the limits on fats, sugars, and salt (sodium)

- Make most of your fat sources from fish, nuts, and vegetable oils.
- Limit solid fats like butter, stick margarine, shortening, and lard, as well as foods that contain these.
- Check the Nutrition Facts label to keep saturated fats, *trans* fats, and sodium low.
- Choose food and beverages low in added sugars. Added sugars contribute calories with few, if any, nutrients.

■ **Figure 15.2**   Food Guide. United States Department of Agriculture: MyPyramid.

Figure 15.3 The digestive system.

Digestion is the process by which food is broken down mechanically and chemically in the GI tract and converted into absorbable components. The mouth, stomach, and small intestine each have a significant role in mechanical and chemical digestive processes. Mechanical digestion is the process of physically breaking down and moving substances through the digestive tract. Chewing food is a major mechanism for mechanical digestion. Continued mechanical churning of food occurs in the stomach.

Chemical digestion is the work of digestive enzymes and bile, which convert ingested substances into absorbable components. Accessory organs, most notably the salivary glands, pancreas, and liver are critical in producing and secreting digestive enzymes and bile into the GI tract. Chemical digestion is stimulated by chewing and begins in the mouth as food

mixes with saliva, a substance consisting mostly of water, bicarbonate, chloride, potassium, and salivary amylase. Salivary amylase, from salivary glands, is an enzyme responsible for initiating carbohydrate digestion.

In the stomach, food is mixed with hydrochloric acid, pepsin, and other digestive enzymes. Four major secretory cells are found in the stomach:

- *Mucous cells*, which secrete alkaline mucus and protect the epithelium from stress and acid contact
- *Parietal cells*, which secrete both hydrochloric acid, a strong acid, needed to activate pepsinogen and destroy pathogens and intrinsic factor, a glycoprotein needed for intestinal absorption of vitamin B_{12}

- *Chief cells*, which secrete pepsin, a proteolytic enzyme, critical to protein digestion
- *G cells*, which secrete gastrin, a hormone responsible for controlling acid secretion and stimulating gastric motility

Gastric epithelial cells are also stimulated to secrete other enzymes, such as lipase and gelatinase. The most important digestive contribution of the stomach is the initiation of protein digestion.

The final stages of chemical digestion occur through small intestinal villi, the functional units of the small intestine, which are lined with columnar and mucus-secreting epithelial cells. Villi are capable of both enzyme secretion and absorption of nutrients. Microvilli, located on the columnar epithelium, are referred to as the "brush border" and serve to greatly increase the surface area of the small intestine. Intestinal mucosal folds slow the passage of food to provide adequate time for digestion. As the nutrients move into the small intestine, they are met with bile salts from the liver (critical for fat digestion), bicarbonate from the pancreas (needed to neutralize hydrochloric acid), and enzymes also from the pancreas (critical for digestion of fats, proteins, and carbohydrates). Within the small intestine, nutrients are mixed with bile and the pancreatic enzymes. The specific locations and roles of select digestive enzymes are discussed in Table 15.3. Emulsifying agents, critical for fat digestion, are discussed below to illustrate the absorption of fatty acids and glycerol.

The regulation of digestion, with the exception of chewing, swallowing, and defecation, is directed through hormone feedback mechanisms and the autonomic nervous system. Both the sympathetic and parasympathetic branches of the autonomic nervous system act on the walls of the GI tract to promote digestion. The walls of the GI tract contain four basic layers (the inner mucosa, submucosa, muscularis, and serosa). The inner mucosa, which lines the lumen and is in direct contact with nutrients, varies in structure and function depending on the location within the GI tract. The epithelial cells that compose the mucosa are capable of secretion, absorption, and the production of hormones. In addition to other immune protections, Peyer's patches (lymphoid follicles) and lymphocytes (primarily IgA-secreting B cells) are also located within the mucosa and extend into the submucosa. Peyer's patches are needed to house lymphocytes and ultimately protect the GI tract against pathogens.

The submucosa is a connective tissue layer. It contains blood and lymphatic vessels and the submucous plexus (nerve branches), which provide local and autonomic nervous system stimuli to the GI tract. The muscularis layer, composed primarily of two thick layers of smooth muscle, promotes mechanical movement of nutrients through the lumen and, similar to the submucosa, also contains a myenteric plexus to allow neuronal stimulation. The serosa is the outermost covering of the GI tract. Within the abdominal cavity, the mesentery, a suspensory structure, connects to the serosa and supports the digestive tract and provides pathways for vascular and neuronal stimulation.

Glands and ducts within the mucosa and submucosa allow the secretion of digestive substances into the GI lumen. Gastrin and motilin are two hormones that act on the GI tract to *stimulate* gastric emptying. Gastrin stimulates gastric glands to secrete pepsinogen (a proenzyme that later converts to pepsin) and hydrochloric acid. Secretin, gastric inhibitory

Table 15.3 Enzymes Active in the Chemical Digestive Process

Enzyme	Location	Function
Salivary amylase (ptyalin)	Mouth and stomach	Initiates carbohydrate digestion
Pepsin	Stomach	Breaks down protein and forms polypeptides in the stomach
Pancreatic amylase	Pancreas	Promotes conversion of oligosaccharides and dextrins (carbohydrates) into lactose, maltose, and sucrose
Lactase, maltase, sucrase ("brush-border enzymes")	Small intestine	Convert disaccharides (lactose, maltose, and sucrose) into monosaccharides (galactose, glucose, and fructose)
Trypsin, chymotrypsin, and carboxypeptidase (pancreatic enzymes)	Pancreas	Convert protein polypeptides into smaller protein units
Aminopeptidases and dipeptidases ("brush-border enzymes")	Small intestine	Convert protein polypeptides and dipeptides into amino acids
Pancreatic lipases	Pancreas	Convert fats into monoglycerides, glycerol, and fatty acids
Intestinal lipase	Small intestine	Converts fatty acids into glycerol

peptide, and cholecystokinin, from the duodenum, are three hormones that *inhibit* gastric emptying. Secretin is responsible for triggering the release of bicarbonate from the pancreas and bile from the liver. Gastric inhibitory peptide decreases stomach churning. Cholecystokinin stimulates the release of digestive enzymes in the pancreas and the emptying of bile from the gall bladder.

The overall goal of digestion is to prepare nutrients for absorption by:

1. Converting carbohydrates to monosaccharides
2. Converting proteins into amino acids
3. Converting fats to fatty acids and glycerol
4. Unleashing vitamins and minerals from macronutrients
5. Separating water from nutrients to promote water absorption

Figure 15.4 illustrates the conversion of nutrients into absorbable components and should be referred to frequently during the discussion of absorption below.

Absorption

Absorption is a complex process of taking in nutrients and moving these to the circulation to be used by cells. Certain locations within the digestive system are better equipped to absorb specific nutrients. Figure 15.5 details the major sites of absorption for specific nutrients along the GI tract. Recognition of these major sites of absorption allows the ability to anticipate nutrition problems that can occur with inadequate absorption at certain locations within the GI tract.

The small intestine is an ideal site for absorption of nutrients because of the extensive surface area and absorptive fluid layer along the brush border. Also unique to the small intestine is the presence of **lacteals**, or lymphatic channels within each villus, which are critical to the absorption of fat molecules. Some substances, such as water, are absorbed primarily in the large intestine and stomach. Vitamin D can be absorbed through the skin.

After absorption and traveling within the circulation, the liver receives the nutrients that were once in the intestinal lumen. Once in the liver, the nutrients are metabolized, converted, or synthesized into other nutrients, or they are stored for later use. The liver then releases the nutrients back into the circulation to be used by body cells.

GLUCOSE AND FRUCTOSE ABSORPTION

Carbohydrates represent the largest proportion of nutrients absorbed within the digestive tract. Monosaccharides (glucose or fructose) are rarely consumed in a typical diet. Therefore, more complex carbohydrates (sucrose, lactose, and starches) must

be degraded by enzymes and reduced to monosaccharides for absorption. The following list outlines key aspects of carbohydrate absorption:

- Pancreatic amylase acts on dietary carbohydrates to begin the reduction into simple sugars (primarily starches into maltose).
- The final enzymatic digestion, which liberates more complex carbohydrates into monosaccharides (primarily glucose, also fructose and galactose), is the work of brush-border enzymes (disaccharidases, such as sucrase and lactase, and oligosaccharidase, such as maltase) secreted from the small intestine.
- Glucose requires the cotransport of sodium to be absorbed into the lumen of the small intestine.

Glucose and galactose are absorbed into the enterocyte (intestinal cell) *with sodium* via active transport. **Active transport** is a process that uses *energy* to move nutrients across a pressure gradient (Fig. 15.6). The source of this energy is adenosine triphosphate (ATP), which is the product of a chemical reaction between oxygen and nutrient products (see Chapter 2). Energy is required for the transport of glucose and sodium because the concentration of sodium outside the cell is far greater than inside the cell. In fact, many nutrients, including galactose, calcium, iron, amino acids, potassium, fatty acids, and magnesium, require energy-dependent transport pumps to be absorbed across the mucosa.

For glucose transport, two sodium ions bind to the transporter. A change in the transporter then occurs, allowing glucose to bind to the transporter, and only then can these molecules move into the cell. The energy stored in the membrane gradient drives glucose through the enterocyte. Glucose then diffuses down its concentration gradient into the capillaries within the villus of the small intestine.

Fructose enters the enterocyte through the process of passive facilitated diffusion through a transporter. **Passive diffusion**, which is the random migration of nutrients across the mucosa from areas of higher to lower concentration or pressure, can be a simple or facilitated process. *Simple diffusion* allows nutrients to move through or between channel proteins. *Facilitated diffusion* uses carrier proteins that move nutrients across the GI mucosa. Passive diffusion is also represented by the absorption of most vitamins and water, which pass unchanged from the GI tract to the circulation.

AMINO ACID AND SMALL PEPTIDE ABSORPTION

The facilitation of amino acid and small peptide (two or three linked amino acids) absorption is accomplished through the work of proteolytic enzymes, which degrade dietary proteins into smaller peptides

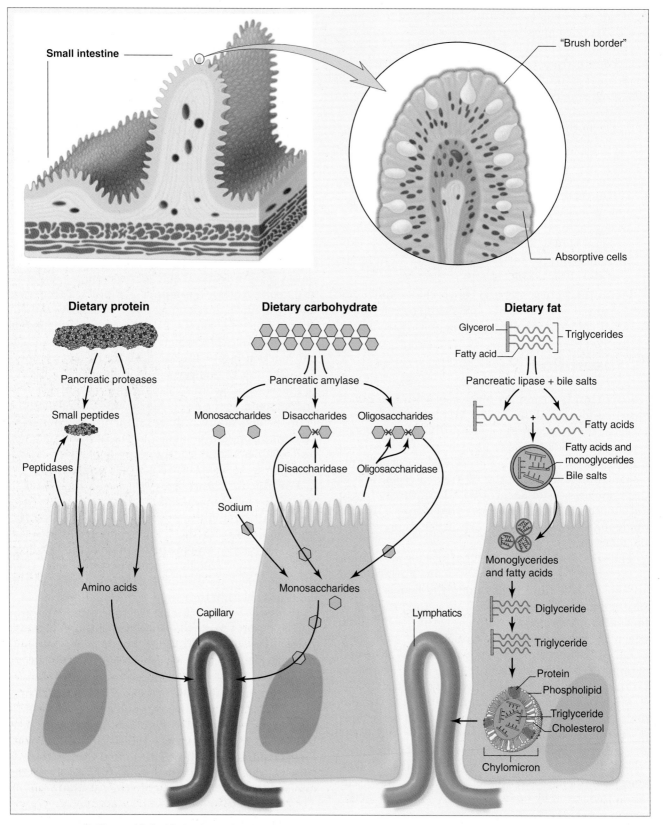

Figure 15.4 Mechanisms of nutrient digestion and absorption within the small intestine. (Image modified from Rubin E, Farber JL. *Pathology*. 4th ed. Philadelphia: Lippincott Williams & Wilkins; 2005, with permission.)

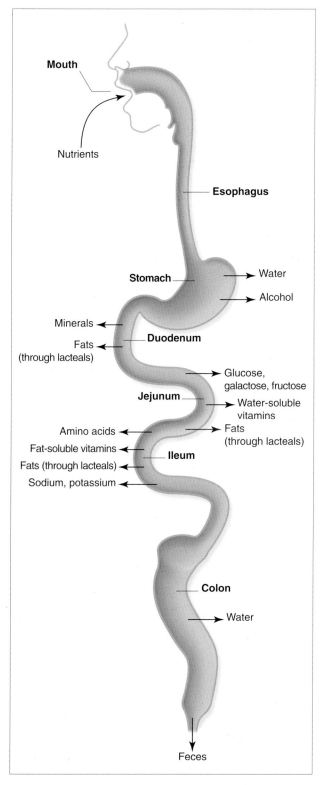

Figure 15.5 Major sites for absorption in the gastrointestinal tract. The gastrointestinal tract absorbs specific nutrients at specific locations.

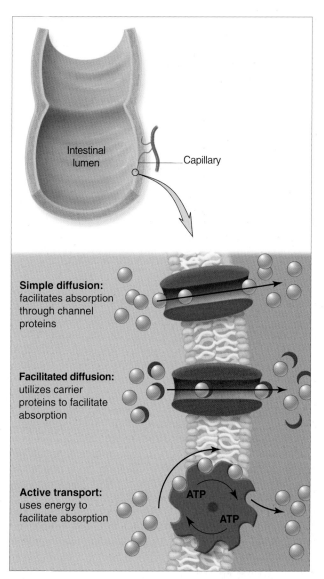

Figure 15.6 Passive diffusion and active transport mechanisms of absorption.

brush border. The mechanism for absorption of a single amino acid is essentially the same as monosaccharides. Sodium-dependent transporters are needed, using energy across an electrochemical gradient, to move amino acids into the intestinal epithelium. Interestingly, small peptides are absorbed without depending on sodium. Rather, these small-chain amino acids travel through a single transport molecule. Once in the enterocyte, small peptides are reduced to amino acids and move with other transport molecules into the circulation. This final stage of absorption for all amino acids does not rely on sodium cotransport and is not across an energy gradient.

FATTY ACID AND GLYCEROL ABSORPTION

The conversion of dietary fats into fatty acids and glycerol requires two major steps: emulsification

and then into amino acids. Three major sources of proteolytic enzymes include the (1) active protease pepsin (from the stomach), (2) pancreatic proteases (such as trypsin, chymotrypsin, and carboxypeptidases), and (3) peptidases found in the intestinal and enzymatic digestion. Emulsification promotes fat solubility and is accomplished via bile salts, which are synthesized in the liver and secreted from the gall bladder. Emulsification is a process of coating the lipid molecules with bile salts, which have both hydrophilic (water-attracting) and hydrophobic (water-repellent) components. Ultimately, the lipid molecules are broken down into smaller and smaller droplets, the hydrophobic end adheres to the lipid molecule and the hydrophilic end composes an outer soluble surface.

● STOP *and Consider*

What dietary recommendations would you make for the individual who is not able to effectively produce or utilize bile?

Research Notes

The obesity epidemic has triggered intense interest in the treatment of obesity through the use of digestive enzyme inhibitors. Xenical (orlistat 120 mg) is a pancreatic lipase inhibitor that acts by inhibiting the absorption of dietary fats. The overall goal of treatment with this drug is to reduce fat absorption and subsequently promote weight loss. After extensive research, the drug was FDA approved in 1999 for use with adults and in 2003 for use in adolescents. In clinical trials in adults, 60% of study participants had a 5% reduction in body weight, and an additional 27% of adults had a 10% reduction in body weight when combined with a nutritious, balanced diet and exercise.[3] More recently, Alli (orlistat 60 mg) was approved for over-the-counter (OTC) use for weight loss. A 2009 FDA report revealed liver-related adverse events in patients taking orlistat (both in the prescription form [Xenical] and the OTC form [Alli]). Between 1999 and October 2008, 32 reports of serious liver injury, including six cases of liver failure, in patients using orlistat were submitted to FDA's Adverse Event Reporting System. Consumers should consult their health care professional if they are experiencing symptoms possibly associated with the use of orlistat and development of liver injury, particularly weakness or fatigue, fever, jaundice, or brown urine. Other symptoms may include abdominal pain, nausea, vomiting, light-colored stools, itching, or loss of appetite.[4]

Once emulsified, pancreatic lipase (a water-soluble enzyme) acts on the surface of triglyceride droplets to further degrade triglycerides into free fatty acids, monoglycerides, and diglycerides. These substances form a complex with bile salts and other lipids called micelles. The micelles move along the brush border of the small intestine, where they can be absorbed through a process of simple diffusion (discussed below) or via a fatty acid transporter protein across the plasma membrane.

Two major differences characterize the absorption of fats as compared to amino acids and sugars:

1. Fatty acids and monoglycerides resynthesize back into triglycerides after moving across the plasma membrane.

2. Transport into the circulation occurs via lacteals, lymphatic vessels within each villus, rather than through the blood vessels.

After absorption in the enterocytes of the small intestinal mucosa, the triglycerides are resynthesized and made soluble again through the production of lipoprotein complexes (chylomicrons). Chylomicrons from the intestine are released into the blood through lacteals and are delivered to tissues or stored for the later production of energy through oxidation. Fatty acids are stored as triglycerides, primarily within adipocytes. These fatty acids can be mobilized when needed. The activation of mobilization occurs in response to hormones that bind cell-surface receptors. In a series of complex events, free fatty acids diffuse from adipocytes, combine with albumin, are transported to other tissues, and passively diffuse into cells.

Absorption is affected by several factors. Competition for carriers blocks absorption of certain nutrients. Saturation of carriers slows the absorption process. Absorption can be enhanced or inhibited when select substances coexist. For example, ascorbic acid (vitamin C), such as that found in orange juice, enhances the absorption of iron. Another example is the presence of dietary fat, which is needed for absorption of fat-soluble vitamins. Physiologic factors, such as gastric pH and motility, may affect bioavailability and subsequent absorption of minerals. **Bioavailability** indicates that the mineral is unbound and must remain unbound (also called an ionic state) to be absorbed, such as with calcium. Bound minerals are unused and are eliminated in the feces. Iron is one exception. Iron can be absorbed in a bound state. To add additional complexity, the structure and function of the intestinal cells regulate and promote maximal absorption and can also limit the potential for nutrient toxicity.

● STOP *and Consider*

What will happen to nutrient absorption in Crohn disease when large portions of the small intestine are inflamed?

Module 2

Altered Nutrition

Altered nutrition, or malnutrition, is a state of inadequate or excessive exposure to nutrients (Fig. 15.7). This exposure can include intake, digestion, absorption, or metabolism of nutrients. Altered nutrition has multiple potential causes, including:

- Genetic defects that impact metabolism or absorption of nutrients
- Malformation or damage to the GI mucosa
- Inadequate or excessive dietary intake of required nutrients
- Excessive nutrient losses, such as through vomiting, diarrhea, or laxative use
- Hypermetabolic states that exert excessive demands, such as with hyperthyroidism, cancer, burns, fever, or severe infection
- Malabsorptive syndromes
- Ingestion of unsafe food and water sources

Inherited Metabolic Disorders

Inherited metabolic disorders, most often related to errors in amino acid and lipid metabolism, commonly result from a genetically based defect in enzyme activity. These are also called inborn errors of metabolism. Nutritional genomics is a field of science that considers the role of nutrients on gene expression. For example, in phenylketonuria (PKU), phenylalanine hydroxylase deficiency causes an inability to convert phenylalanine, an essential amino acid, to tyrosine. Tyrosine is needed for the synthesis of protein, thyroxine, catecholamines, and melanin. Accumulations of phenylalanine, without the necessary conversion to tyrosine, result in impaired CNS development, impaired myelination, and brain degeneration. Dietary modifications are needed to restrict phenylalanine consumption.

A second major category of inherited metabolic disorders is lysosomal storage diseases. These diseases are defects of lipid metabolism as a result of a missing lysosomal enzyme. An example is Tay–Sachs disease, which is inherited as an autosomal-recessive disorder and found most commonly in those of Ashkenazi Jewish and Eastern European descent. In Tay–Sachs disease, a deficiency of beta-hexosaminidase A (an enzyme) results in the impaired catabolism and accumulation of fatty substances, called G_{M2} gangliosides, inside neuronal lysosomes in the brain. This leads to severe neurologic impairment marked by developmental delays, neurodegeneration, blindness, deafness, muscle atrophy, paralysis, and death (often by 4 years of age). Presently, there is no treatment. The major problem with inherited metabolic disorders is the accumulation of substances within the cells of the body, leading to cell death.

Undernutrition

Undernutrition is a lack of intake of nutrients most often related to inadequate calorie consumption, inadequate intake of essential vitamins and

Figure 15.7   Concept map. Altered nutrition. PKU, phenylketonuria.

minerals, or problems with digestion, absorption, or distribution of nutrients in the body. Protein, iron, and vitamins are the most common nutrients that are inadequately consumed or in great demand in those presenting with undernutrition. Excess use of muscle mass and adipose stores for energy results in weight loss and muscle wasting. In severe or prolonged illness, loss of muscle mass and function is not limited to the skeletal muscle and can affect cardiac and respiratory functioning. The elderly, particularly those in nursing homes, are at particular risk for undernutrition due to poor appetite, alterations in the sense of taste, problems with eating or swallowing, limited income, inadequate social support, and physical mobility limitations.

Research Notes

In a randomized, double-blind, placebo-controlled study of multivitamin and mineral supplementation, those who took a daily multivitamin and mineral supplement were less likely (43% taking supplement versus 73% of those not taking supplement) to report having one or more infections over the 1-year study. This was particularly true in those participants with diabetes, in which 93% of those not taking the supplement reported one or more infections compared with 17% of those taking the multivitamin and mineral supplement.[5]

VITAMIN AND MINERAL DEFICIENCIES

Vitamin and mineral deficiencies can result from the inadequate intake or malabsorption of dietary sources. Mineral bioavailability also affects mineral absorption. Because fat intake is critical for fat-soluble vitamin absorption, lack of dietary fat impairs the cellular availability of vitamins A, D, E, and K. Table 15.4 compares the problems associated with select vitamin and mineral deficits.

PROTEIN-ENERGY MALNUTRITION

Protein-energy malnutrition is related to either (1) deprivation of all food, a condition of starvation that leads to **marasmus** or (2) protein deprivation in persons consuming adequate carbohydrates, a condition called **kwashiorkor**. Glucose is a major energy source for body tissues. In marasmus, dietary glucose is unavailable for glucose-dependent tissues, such as the brain and muscle tissue. The body attempts to manufacture glucose in a process called gluconeogenesis by breaking down muscle proteins. The muscle then releases acidic byproducts, promoting metabolic acidosis (Chapter 8).

Protective mechanisms are needed at this point because continued gluconeogenesis produces significant muscle wasting, destruction of vital organs, and death. Whether the body effectively adapts, or

preserves, muscle tissue during the state of starvation depends on insulin. Insulin is a hormone that promotes glucose production and uptake by cells *and* inhibits the use of fat stores for energy. If the body is to adapt to starvation effectively, insulin production must be suppressed to inhibit glucose uptake and gluconeogenesis, and another energy source must be used at a greater level than glucose. This is accomplished through a compensatory increase in glucagon, cortisone, epinephrine, and growth hormone. These hormones all have anti-insulin effects and also stimulate enzymes on the adipocytes to release fatty acids for energy. The fatty acids travel to the liver and are converted to ketones. Ketones are the replacement energy source that allows sparing of muscle catabolism. The brain and other glucose-dependent tissues prefer glucose but will use ketones for energy as an adaptive response. When ketones are used for energy, protein losses are minimized and muscle tissue is spared.

A state of starvation can be maintained for approximately 1 month in someone who maintains water intake. Unfortunately, adipose stores eventually become depleted. The body must again turn to glucose, leading to increased muscle catabolism for gluconeogenesis. Vital organs that rely on muscle, including the heart and lungs, are impaired and the individual will die.

STOP *and Consider*

Inflammation, particularly that occurs with infection, stimulates the release of chemical mediators that promote insulin secretion. Insulin presence promotes the use of glucose for energy. How do you think this affects the adaptation to starvation?

Kwashiorkor, a condition of protein deficit, leads to problems with protein synthesis, repair and healing, fluid balance, and energy. In kwashiorkor, the continued intake of carbohydrates stimulates insulin production, which encourages glucose uptake for energy. This means that when an individual is still eating carbohydrates and not taking in proteins, the body does *not* effectively spare muscle tissue and access fat stores for energy. Stimulation of insulin production also limits the body's ability to synthesize new proteins from those already present in muscle tissue and also limits ATP (energy) production. The lack of protein intake, coupled with the inability to synthesize new proteins within the body, leads to severe edema. The protuberant abdomen characteristic of kwashiorkor is related to liver enlargement, weak abdominal

Table 15.4 Clinical Manifestations and Health Conditions Resulting from Select Vitamin and Mineral Deficits and Excesses

Vitamin	Causes of Deficiency	Clinical Manifestations and Health Problems Related to Deficiency	Causes of Excess	Clinical Manifestations and Health Problems Related to Excess
A	Inadequate intake or malabsorption, insufficient dietary fat, liver or pancreatic disease, protein-energy malnutrition, zinc deficiency	Impaired vision, impaired embryonic development, anemia, poor growth, impaired immunity, impaired osteoclast activity (bone accumulation), keratinization of mucous membranes, dry/scaly/rough skin	Excessive dietary or supplement intake; also found in retinoic acid (accutane), a potent antiacne medication, which affects fetal growth and development in pregnant women who are taking this drug	Vitamin A intoxication leads to liver disease, dry mucous membranes, dryness, erythema, scaling, or peeling of skin, hair, and nails, headache, nausea, vomiting, and bone fractures
D	Inadequate intake of vitamin D, lipid malabsorption, prolonged breastfeeding in infants without sunlight exposure, deficiencies of calcium and phosphorus, and long-term anticonvulsant therapy	Vitamin D deficiency is manifested as rickets in children and osteomalacia in adults. Rickets involves impaired mineralization of growing bones resulting in structural abnormalities, bone pain, and muscle tenderness. Osteomalacia involves generalized reductions in bone density, muscle weakness, bone tenderness, and fractures	Excessive intake	Vitamin D intoxication leads to hypercalcemia and hyperphosphatemia, calcification of soft tissues of kidneys, lungs, heart, and tympanic membrane, headache, nausea, bone fragility, and retarded growth
Thiamin	Inadequate intake or malabsorption; subclinical thiamin deficiency may result in people with alcoholism because of inadequate intake and impaired absorption	Thiamin deficiency results in beriberi, a condition manifested by anorexia, weight loss, confusion, muscular wasting, edema, peripheral neuropathy, tachycardia, and cardiomegaly	Excessive intake	Excessive thiamin results in headache, seizures, muscle weakness, cardiac dysrhythmias, and allergic reactions; massive doses result in respiratory depression and death
Niacin	Inadequate intake or absorption	Early manifestations are muscle weakness, anorexia, indigestion, and skin lesions; pellagra is a condition of severe niacin deficiency characterized by dermatitis, dementia, diarrhea, tremors, inflammation of mucous membranes; can lead to death	Excessive intake is rare, although niacin has been used in high doses to treat hypercholesterolemia, and toxicity may result in these individuals	Niacin excess promotes histamine release, which results in flushing; high-dose niacin is also toxic to the liver
B12	Inadequate intake or malabsorption	DNA synthesis is impaired leading to problems with cell division; clinical manifestations include anemia, neuropathy characterized by numbness, tingling, and burning in extremities, and generalized weakness, stomatitis, and skin lesions; all rapidly dividing cells are affected; pernicious anemia is a condition of B12 malabsorption caused by a lack of intrinsic factor in the stomach from atrophic parietal cells (Chapter 3: Inflammation and Tissue Repair)	Not applicable	Vitamin B12 is not known to result in severe toxicity[1]
Folate	Inadequate intake or malabsorption.	Impaired synthesis of DNA and RNA, cell division is reduced; homocysteine levels increase; clinical manifestations include anemia, impaired skin integrity, impaired immunity, weakness, depression, neuropathy, and poor growth; embryonic development is impaired in pregnant women deficient in folate resulting in neural tube defects.	Excessive intake.	No major adverse effects have been documented that are directly related to folate excess.[1]

(Continued)

Table 15.4 Clinical Manifestations and Health Conditions Resulting from Select Vitamin and Mineral Deficits and Excesses *(Continued)*

Vitamin	Causes of Deficiency	Clinical Manifestations and Health Problems Related to Deficiency	Causes of Excess	Clinical Manifestations and Health Problems Related to Excess
C	Inadequate intake or malabsorption	Scurvy is a condition of vitamin C deficiency resulting in skin lesions, impaired wound healing, lethargy, atrophy, edema, bleeding, impaired bone, cartilage, tooth, and connective tissue development	Excessive intake	Vitamin C excess results in gastric upset and diarrhea and may contribute to the development of renal calculi
Calcium	Inadequate intake, bioavailability, or absorption	Contributes to reduced bone mass, weakness, and osteomalacia; may impact the development of colon cancer and hypertension	Excessive intake	Excessive intake can lead to hypercalcemia and lead to calcification in soft tissues; interferes with absorption of other minerals; can impair cardiac conduction
Phosphorus	Deficiencies are rare because of wide availability of dietary sources	Phosphorus deficit has lethal consequences; clinical manifestations are related to loss of ATP synthesis and can include problems with the nervous system, bones, blood cells, skin, kidneys, heart, and lungs because of abnormalities in all energy-dependent cells	Chronic consumption of a low-calcium and high-phosphorus diet	Toxicity can lead to frequent bone fractures throughout the skeleton
Zinc	Inadequate intake, malabsorption, or excessive losses through urine or other secretions	Zinc deficiency was previously common but has declined because of the fortification in cereal products; clinical manifestations include impaired growth, delayed sexual maturation, hair loss, delayed wound healing, skin lesions, anorexia, impaired immune function, visual disturbances, and impaired taste	Toxicity is rare but can occur with excessive intake	Manifestations of toxicity include anemia, fever, vomiting, diarrhea, and impaired central nervous system function
Copper	Inadequate intake, malabsorption, or excessive losses	Copper deficiency leads to anemia, neutropenia, bone demineralization and osteoporosis, changes in skin pigment, impaired collagen and elastin production, growth impairment, and brain tissue degeneration	Excessive copper supplement intake and chronic liver disease can lead to copper toxicity. Copper is excreted in bile. Liver disease promotes bile retention and copper toxicity	Manifestations of toxicity are related to liver cirrhosis and red blood cell malformation

muscles, and ascites from inadequate protein (albumin) intake and synthesis (Fig. 15.8). The liver enlarges because of fat accumulation. This accumulation is a problem of suppressed use of fat stores for energy and a lack of proteins to transport the lipids out of the liver. Other manifestations are related to GI disturbances, impairment of neurologic, heart, and lung function, immunodeficiency, and death.

Overnutrition

Overnutrition is a state of excessive exposure to nutrients. Overnutrition is generally related to overconsumption of nutrients, including ingesting excessive calories or toxic levels of vitamins and minerals. The health effects of vitamin and mineral excesses

are detailed in Table 15.4. Obesity is a major health concern of epidemic proportions and is selected as one of the clinical models discussed in this chapter.

Malabsorption

Malabsorption indicates a lack of movement of specific nutrients across the GI mucosa. Malabsorption can affect one nutrient, such as lactose or vitamin B_{12}, or it can affect all nutrients at one segment or the entire length of the intestinal mucosa. The **malabsorption syndrome** is a condition in which several nutrients are not adequately absorbed. Fat and fat-soluble substances are almost always included in the malabsorption syndrome. Various causes of malabsorption are depicted in Figure 15.9 and may include:

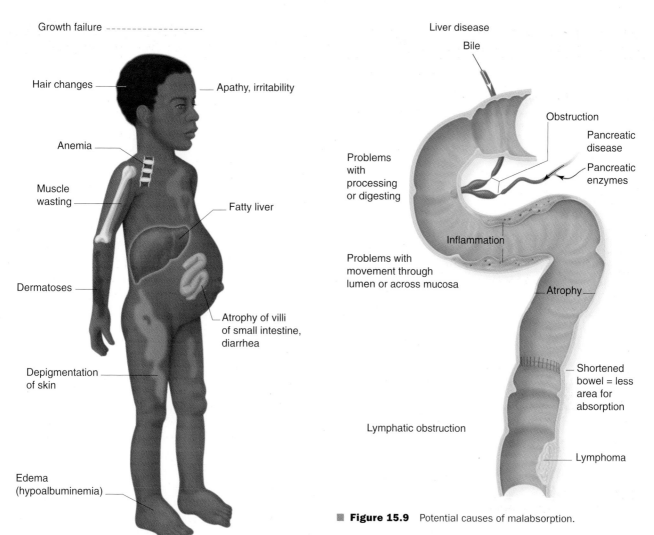

■ **Figure 15.8** Manifestations of kwashiorkor. (Image modified from Rubin E, Farber JL. *Pathology*. 4th ed. Philadelphia: Lippincott Williams & Wilkins; 2005, with permission.)

- Problems with processing or digesting nutrients: pancreatic dysfunction, enzyme deficiencies, or inadequate bile secretion
- Problems with moving substances across the mucosa: inflammatory conditions, GI atrophy, excessive ingestion of a nutrient, use of certain medications, or protein deficiencies
- Lymphatic obstruction: inhibits transport of nutrients once they have been absorbed across the mucosa and may occur with neoplasms or infectious processes

● **STOP** *and Consider*

Why would pancreatic dysfunction lead to problems with absorption?

Malabsorption of a specific vitamin or mineral presents clinically as a deficiency of that nutrient.

■ **Figure 15.9** Potential causes of malabsorption.

Exocrine pancreas insufficiency and impaired bile production are major problems that lead to fat malabsorption. These problems contribute to weight loss and to deficiencies in fat-soluble vitamins. As with fat malabsorption, pancreatic enzyme deficiency contributes to the development of protein malabsorption. The loss of protein in the stool, as may occur because of inflammation in the mucosa, can also contribute to protein deficiency.

Carbohydrate malabsorption is often the result of pancreatic enzyme deficiencies, absence or reduction of brush-border disaccharidases, congenital deficiency of the glucose-galactose transporter, or bacterial flora overgrowth in the intestine. Carbohydrate malabsorption results in an increase in fermentation, or breakdown, of carbohydrates by intestinal bacterial flora to convert these carbohydrates into short-chain fatty acids (for absorption) and gases. The short-chain fatty acids are needed to (1) maintain GI function, (2) recoup some of the energy that would be lost, and (3) facilitate sodium and water absorption in the large intestine. The undigested carbohydrates draw extensive fluid into the intestines. The process of fermentation leads to the clinical manifestations characteristic of carbohydrate malabsorption, including abdominal distention, bloating, pain, diarrhea, weight loss, and flatulence. Celiac disease is selected as a clinical model in this chapter to illustrate the problem of malabsorption.

General Manifestations of Altered Nutrition

The clinical manifestations of altered nutrition are reflective of the cause and pathophysiologic problems. Because cells and body tissues rely on adequate nutrition for optimal functioning, clinical manifestations are exhibited throughout the body. In general, malnutritive processes involving undernutrition can lead to weight loss, muscle wasting, muscle weakness, dehydration, fatigue, and evidence of vitamin and mineral deficiencies (Table 15.4). Rapidly dividing cells, such as those of the skin, are particularly vulnerable to malnourishment. Skin manifestations include poor wound healing, purpura, ulceration, dry skin, or pallor. Mucous membranes become inflamed and friable. Angular cheilitis, a problem with fissure development in the corners of the mouth, is often associated with riboflavin deficiency. The manifestations of malabsorption are often related to the rapid transit of nutrients through the intestinal lumen. As mentioned previously, problems with carbohydrate absorption typically manifest as weight loss, diarrhea, bloating, abdominal cramping, and excessive flatulence. Fat malabsorption leads to foul-smelling, greasy, diarrhea stools. Excessive nutrient intake leads to an increase in weight and body fatness. Toxicity of vitamins and minerals can also occur (Table 15.4).

Diagnostic and Treatment Strategies Related to Altered Nutrition

Diagnostic tests related to altered nutrition are used to determine the cause for the nutrition imbalance as well as the potential effects. A complete nutritional assessment is indicated, which includes a multiple-day dietary intake recall, to determine adequate or excessive nutrient intake, and measurement of height, weight, and body mass index. Laboratory evaluation is often helpful and may include a complete blood count with red blood cell indices and a peripheral smear, sedimentation rate (to detect inflammation), serum electrolytes, urinalysis, and urine culture. The evaluation may also include measures of protein status, including serum albumin, transferrin, creatinine, and blood urea nitrogen levels. Other serum tests are used to detect blood levels of specific nutrients, such as iron, B_{12}, or folate. Enzyme levels can also be measured to determine whether digestive or absorptive problems are present. Hormone levels may be investigated if metabolic regulation is impaired. Stool specimens may also be evaluated for the presence of pathogens that affect absorption. Direct visualization or biopsy of the GI tract may be required to determine a structural cause for the nutrition imbalance.

Treatment modalities are directed at eliminating the cause of the nutrition imbalance or reducing the harmful effects. This often includes specific dietary interventions, such as increasing intake of particular macronutrients, taking vitamin and mineral supplements, reducing overall caloric intake, or avoiding specific foods that exacerbate symptoms. Treatment may also include pharmacologic interventions, such as the administration of exogenous digestive enzymes, to support digestion and absorption. Diagnostic and treatment modalities are discussed in greater detail within the clinical models of this chapter.

Module 3

Clinical Models

The following clinical models have been selected to aid in the understanding and application of altered nutrition pathophysiology, manifestations, diagnosis, and treatment.

Iron-Deficiency Anemia

Anemia is the reduction in the mass of circulating blood cells and subsequently reduced hemoglobin levels. Anemia is typically not considered an

isolated disease; rather, it represents a manifestation of another problem. In Chapter 6, sickle cell anemia was presented as a clinical model related to a genetic defect that results in red blood cell destruction. The development of anemia can also result from severe hemorrhage, decreased red blood cell production, or vitamin and mineral deficiencies. The vitamins and minerals related to red blood cell and hemoglobin integrity include B_{12}, folate, and iron. The most common cause of all anemias is iron deficiency; it is also the most prevalent nutritional deficiency worldwide.

PATHOPHYSIOLOGY

Iron-deficiency anemia represents a problem of iron demand on red blood cell development that cannot be met with current iron stores. Iron is required for hemoglobin synthesis, oxygen and electron transport, and DNA synthesis. Iron is found within hemoglobin, myoglobin, and enzymes, and it is stored in transport proteins such as ferritin, hemosiderin, and transferrin. Iron balance is maintained through the careful regulation of iron absorption in the small intestine. Most iron is recycled in the body after release from dying red blood cells. Minute amounts are lost through defecation, sweating, and sloughing of skin cells.

The major causes of iron-deficiency anemia are inadequate iron intake, chronic hemorrhage, malabsorption, and high iron demands as occurs in infancy, adolescence, and with pregnancy or lactation. Chronic blood loss, as with a monthly menstruation, GI ulcers, cancer, or hemorrhoids, is a common cause of excessive loss of body iron. Certain medications, such as antacids, can bind with iron and impair absorption.

CLINICAL MANIFESTATIONS

Clinical manifestations usually present when hemoglobin content is less than that required to meet the oxygen-carrying demands of the body. Iron-deficiency anemia can develop slowly and therefore be asymptomatic. When present, clinical manifestations are related to decreased hemoglobin synthesis, altered blood composition, and subsequently poor oxygen-carrying capacity and hypoxia. These manifestations include pallor of the skin and mucous membranes, fatigue, weakness, lightheadedness, breathlessness, palpitations, headache, tachycardia, and syncope. Chronic hypoxia impairs cell functioning, particularly in epithelial cells, and leads to brittle hair and nails and mouth sores. **Pica** (pagophagia), the compulsion to eat ice or non-food substances such as dirt or clay, is another manifestation of iron-deficient anemia that is not clearly understood.

DIAGNOSTIC CRITERIA

Preliminary diagnosis of iron-deficiency anemia is based on a thorough patient history and physical examination. A higher index of suspicion is present in individuals who are vegetarian or who report mani-

Research Notes

Racial and ethnic differences in the prevalence of iron-deficiency anemia have been noted in the literature. In one study, Mexican-American females demonstrated a higher prevalence of iron-deficiency anemia (6.2%) than non-Hispanic White females (2.3%). After adjusting for many other factors, family household income was the most striking difference that may help explain the reason for this disparity.[6]

festations of chronic blood loss. In iron deficiency, laboratory tests may reveal reduced serum hemoglobin and hematocrit levels and reduced mean corpuscular volume (MCV) and mean corpuscular hemoglobin concentration (MCHC). MCV is an indicator of red blood cell size; therefore, a reduction in hemoglobin and hematocrit, along with a reduced MCV, indicates microcytic anemia. Overall, the number and quality of red blood cells are reduced; RBCs are **hypochromic** (pale) and **microcytic** (small) (Fig. 15.10). **Poikilocytosis** is a term used to describe the irregular shape of iron-deficient red blood cells.

If individuals are unresponsive to treatment, additional confirmatory tests are needed to distinguish iron deficiency from the other types of anemia,

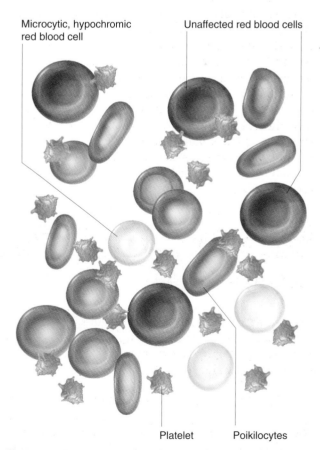

Microcytic, hypochromic red blood cell

Unaffected red blood cells

Platelet

Poikilocytes

■ **Figure 15.10** Peripheral blood smear in iron-deficiency anemia. (Asset provided by Anatomical Chart Company.)

Table 15.5 Differentiation of Various Types of Anemia Based on Laboratory Test Results

	Iron Deficiency	B₁₂ Deficiency	Folate Deficiency	Thalassemia	Anemia of Chronic Diseases
RBC size	Microcytic	Macrocytic	Macrocytic	Microcytic	Normocytic
Reticulocyte (immature RBC) count	Low	Low	Low	Normal	Low/normal
MCH	Low	Normal	Normal	Low	Normal
Serum iron	Low	High	High	Normal	Variable
Total iron-binding capacity	High	Normal	Normal	Normal	Normal
Ferritin level	Low	High	High	Normal	Normal
B₁₂ level	Normal	Low	Normal	Normal	Normal
Folate level	Normal	Normal	Low	Normal	Normal

MCH, mean corpuscular hemoglobin; RBC, red blood cell.

as depicted in Table 15.5. Confirmatory tests may include serum iron, total iron-binding capacity, transferrin saturation, and ferritin levels (see From the Lab, below). Additional tests may be needed to determine sources of acute or chronic blood loss.

The diagnosis of anemia must take into consideration that certain factors affect hemoglobin levels, such as:

- *Age:* Hemoglobin levels are typically much lower in adults than newborns.
- *Gender:* Males have a higher hemoglobin level than women.
- *Pregnancy status:* The physiologic demands of pregnancy and hemodilution result in lower hemoglobin levels in pregnancy.
- *Altitude:* Reduced oxygen exposure at high altitudes induces erythropoiesis and can affect hemoglobin levels.
- *Race or ethnicity:* African-American females have been found to have lower venous hemoglobin concentrations (mean = 13.0 g/dL) than White females (13.8 g/dL).[7] For all races, better information is needed to improve functional, meaningful definitions of iron-deficiency anemia and iron status.

diet, often taken with a source of ascorbic acid to increase absorption. Iron can also be administered parenterally if oral supplements are inadequate or not tolerated. Iron deficiency related to blood loss requires stopping the source of bleeding and may require a blood transfusion.

Anorexia Nervosa

Anorexia nervosa (AN) is an eating disorder characterized by:

1. A refusal to maintain a minimally healthy body weight
2. An intense fear of gaining weight
3. Body image distortion
4. Amenorrhea

The term anorexia designates a lack of appetite, although with AN, hunger is largely ignored. AN primarily affects adolescent and young adult women, particularly in developed countries that value a thin body type. The ratio of females to males affected 10–20 to 1. AN is selected as a clinical model to demonstrate the physiologic effects of malnutrition from restricted nutrient intake.

From the Lab

Serum ferritin is often used as a confirmatory test of iron deficiency. Ferritin is a protein that stores iron. When the iron supply increases, ferritin levels expand to store the additional iron. Ferritin levels can then be measured as an indicator of iron stores.

PATHOPHYSIOLOGY

The exact etiology of AN is unknown, but several forces (biologic, psychologic, genetic, familial, and cultural) may contribute to the development of this condition.[1]

Several theories have been suggested that lead to AN, including:

- An introverted, obsessive, and perfectionist personality with low self-esteem

TREATMENT

Treatment is focused on the cause. Poor iron intake is treated with iron supplements and an iron-rich

- Family dysfunction, such as enmeshment, over-protectiveness, or unresolved family conflict
- Concurrent mental health conditions, such as a personality, depressive, or anxiety disorder
- Cultural pressures to become thinner

AN links a severe mental health disorder with devastating physical health problems caused by self-starvation. The disturbance in body image contributes to malnutrition. Malnutrition encompasses both macronutrient and micronutrient deficiencies, although the use of supplements may protect against micronutrient deficiencies. Macronutrient, particularly caloric restriction, leads to mobilization of lipid stores, protein catabolism, and metabolic stress with a reduced metabolic rate. Malnutrition can then further exacerbate depression and psychologic deterioration.

All body systems are affected by malnutrition. Fluid and electrolyte levels become imbalanced. Skeletal muscle wasting and a loss of body fat are evident as macronutrient levels are inadequate; the body uses all available fat and protein stores for energy. The brain mass and CNS function are reduced. Seizures can develop, and tingling in the extremities is common. The heart size and function is reduced because of hypovolemia and hypotension. The heart rate slows, dysrhythmias and conduction defects can develop, and valves can become ineffective with a reduction in cardiac output. GI effects demonstrate reduced gastric emptying time with a structural functional loss of GI tract tone. Gallstones are more prevalent, and the liver can become necrotic. Liver dysfunction can lead to elevated cholesterol and blood lipid levels. Bones become porous and prone to fractures. The development of blood cells and clotting factors is impaired. This leads to problems with bleeding, anemia, and infection as the inflammatory and immune responses become compromised. Endocrine function is also affected: (1) antidiuretic hormone secretion is restricted, leading to the inability to concentrate urine, (2) reproductive hormone levels decline, and (3) cortisol levels increase because of the stress of malnutrition. The mortality rate is approximately 5% to 15%; most deaths are related to cardiovascular complications.

CLINICAL MANIFESTATIONS

Individuals with AN can exhibit many clinical manifestations related to restricted caloric (energy) and nutrient intake. Common physical characteristics are related to the pathophysiologic processes discussed previously and include an extremely thin stature, **lanugo** (a fine downy hair that covers the body), amenorrhea, brittle hair and nails, peripheral cyanosis, dry skin, bradycardia, hypotension, hypothermia, abdominal bloating, and constipation.

DIAGNOSTIC CRITERIA

The American Psychiatric Association has proposed the following revised criteria to diagnose AN for the 2011 DSM-V:[8]

1. Restriction of food intake relative to caloric requirements leading to the maintenance of a body weight less than a minimally normal weight for age and height (e.g., weight loss leading to maintenance of body weight less than 85% of that expected; or failure to make expected weight gain during period of growth, leading to body weight less than 85% of that expected)
2. Intense fear of gaining weight or becoming fat, even though underweight, or persistent behavior to avoid weight gain, even though underweight
3. Disturbance in the way in which one's body weight or shape is experienced, undue influence of body weight or shape on self-evaluation, or persistent lack of recognition of the seriousness of the current low body weight

A nutritional assessment often reveals restriction of caloric intake to less than 1,000 kcal/day. Laboratory studies can determine the resulting health effects and help to direct treatment strategies. Starvation may reveal normocytic, normochromic anemia and leukopenia from bone marrow suppression. Severe hypokalemia may be noted from laxative abuse or vomiting. Additional blood tests may reveal hypocalcemia, protein deficiency, reduced liver function, and significant electrolyte imbalance, including low sodium and chloride levels. Possible electrocardiogram changes include nonspecific ST- and T-segment abnormalities, atrial tachycardia, idioventricular conduction delay, heart block, and premature ventricular contractions (Chapter 14). The basis for cardiac conduction impairment is attributed to starvation, electrolyte imbalance, and neuroendocrine alterations.

TREATMENT

An interdisciplinary team treatment approach is recommended. This team should include the patient, the patient's family, psychotherapists, physicians, nurses, dieticians, and recreational and occupational therapists. The goals of treatment are stabilizing mental health and achieving and maintaining a healthy weight and nutritional intake. This includes a gradual refeeding process that induces a

1 to 2 pound weight gain per week. The health care team must monitor for complications of AN throughout the treatment and watch for GI, fluid, electrolyte, and cardiac disturbances. Although close monitoring, effective refeeding, and initiating of psychotherapy has shown a decrease in mortality rates among those with AN, two thirds or more will have ongoing food and weight preoccupations.

Celiac Disease (Gluten-Sensitive Enteropathy)

Celiac disease, also called gluten-sensitive enteropathy or celiac sprue, is a disorder of gluten malabsorption caused by a T-cell mediated hypersensitivity to gluten in persons who are genetically predisposed to developing this condition. The prevalence of the condition in first-degree relatives is approximately 10%.[9] Celiac disease is most prevalent in Western Europe and in places to which Europeans emigrated, such as North America and Australia. The disease is increasing in Africa and Asia.[9] **Glutens** are specific proteins found in wheat, rye, oats, and barley. Common foods that are made with glutens, which are ubiquitous to the human diet, are difficult to avoid. These include many types of cereals, breads, and pastas. The condition is most often detected between infancy and young adulthood.

PATHOPHYSIOLOGY

Although the exact cause of celiac disease is often unknown, a strong hereditary component exists. Exposure to gluten elicits a hypersensitivity response that results in chronic inflammation and atrophy of the mucosa of the small intestine. Damage to the intestinal mucosa inhibits digestion because of damage to the villi that produce and secrete digestive hormones and enzymes. Inadequate secretion of hormones and enzymes inhibits gallbladder and pancreatic function. This further restricts the digestive processes. Absorption is also impaired because these villi undergo atrophy, which disallows the effective passage of nutrients across the mucosa. Absorption is further disrupted with a loss of carrier substances needed to transport nutrients across the mucosa.

CLINICAL MANIFESTATIONS

Clinical manifestations are consistent with other malabsorption conditions and include weight loss, diarrhea, steatorrhea, malodorous stools, abdominal bloating, fatigue, and macronutrient, mineral, and vitamin deficiencies. Because the clinical manifestations are nonspecific and sometimes even nonexistent, the condition is frequently misdiagnosed and underdiagnosed.

DIAGNOSTIC CRITERIA

Diagnostic suspicion is raised in the presence of clinical manifestations. Laboratory screening may include serum detection of antibodies against (1) the endomysium or muscle fiber connective tissue, (2) gliadin, a class of protein related to wheat and rye gluten, or (3) IgA tissue transglutaminase, the autoantigen that triggers the immune response. Diagnostic confirmation is made with a small bowel biopsy demonstrating inflammatory and atrophic changes.

TREATMENT

Treatment is focused on permanently eliminating sources of gluten from the diet. Corn and rice do not contain glutens and form a major portion of grain intake for those with celiac disease. Symptoms usually improve within 1 to 2 months of eliminating gluten sources. In the absence of gluten in the diet, the intestinal mucosa sometimes resumes optimal structure and function. Anti-inflammatory and hypersensitivity-blocking medications may be needed if elimination of gluten is not completely effective. Vitamin and mineral supplementation is often warranted. Lack of treatment leads to chronic intestinal ulcerations and can possibly lead to malignancy of the bowel and lymph glands.

● **STOP** *and Consider*

You are providing nutritional counseling for a person with celiac disease. What specific foods would you recommend avoiding? What foods would you suggest as substitutions?

Obesity

An estimated 1 billion people across the world are now overweight or obese. The worldwide trend is caused in part due to the increasing westernization of many traditional diets—fruits, vegetables, and whole grains are being replaced by calorie-dense, easily accessible foods that are high in saturated fat, sugar, and refined carbohydrates. The WHO also estimates that 60% of the world population lacks adequate physical activity, a major contributor to obesity.[10]

Body weight is the composite of bone, muscle, organs, body fluids, and adipose tissue. Body fat is divided into essential fat, which is needed for physiologic functioning, and **storage fat**, which accumulates under the skin and around internal

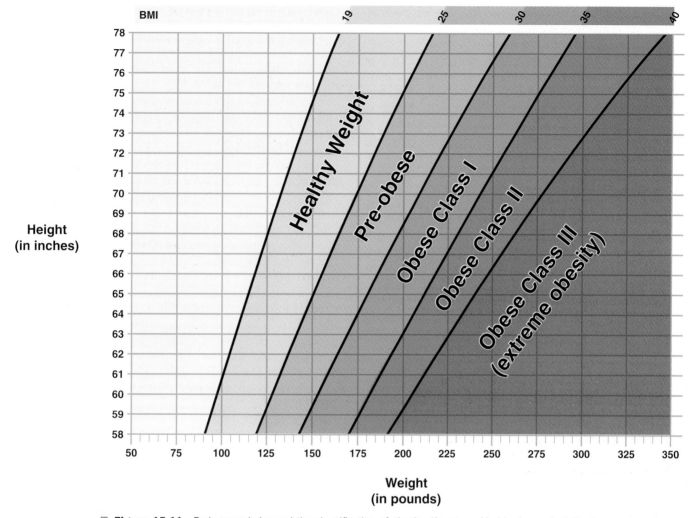

Figure 15.11 Body mass index and the classification of obesity. (Asset provided by Anatomical Chart Company and modified according to the WHO International Classification of Adult Obesity According to BMI, 2010.)

organs. Body fat is often determined using a mathematical calculation termed **body mass index (BMI)**. BMI is calculated by measuring weight in kilograms and dividing this by height in meters squared (BMI = kg/m^2). Preobese is defined as a BMI between 25 and 29.99 kg/m^2. **Obesity** is a state of excessive body fat (Fig. 15.11), in which the BMI is greater than 30 kg/m^2.

STOP *and Consider*

Take a minute to calculate your BMI. Do this by measuring your weight in pounds and converting this to kilograms (1 pound = 0.45 kilograms). Then, measure your height in inches and convert this to meters squared (multiply inches ×2.54 cm; divide this number by 100 cm/meter; multiply this final number × itself to get meters squared). Then, the final step is to take your weight in kilograms and divide it by your height in meters squared. What number did you get?

PATHOPHYSIOLOGY

Obesity is characterized by hypertrophy of adipose cells and excessive storage fat. Dietary lipids are removed from the blood after absorption and are transported across the capillary wall into the adipose cell. Enzymes and hormones mediate this process. Lipoprotein lipase is one enzyme that regulates fat absorption into the adipose cell. Lipoprotein lipase levels increase significantly during times of weight gain, thereby contributing to the development of obesity. Hormones also contribute to lipid deposits in adipose cells. For example, estrogen stimulates lipid movement into adipose cells in the hip and upper thigh regions. The same hormone restricts lipid movement into adipose cells in the abdominal region. Women with adequate estrogen levels therefore typically have broader hips and narrower waists. Once adipose cells have reached a maximum size, adipose cell hyperplasia can occur in those cells capable of division. Obesity is always induced by adipocyte hypertrophy and in some cases is accompanied by hyperplasia. In those with adipo-cyte hyperplasia, the additional adipose cells remain even in times of weight loss.

Maintaining body weight requires a balance of energy intake and expenditure mediated by a complex interaction of neurologic mechanisms, hormones, and other chemicals in the body. Many of these factors are genetically determined. Neurologic mechanisms, specifically neurotransmitters acting on the hypothalamus, stimulate and suppress hunger and satiety. Hunger and satiety messages, when altered, can lead to an increased intake of food followed by weight gain. Digestive chemicals are released during food consumption and also act on neurologic mechanisms to further signal satiety. Hormones, such as thyroid hormone, insulin, and leptin, contribute to body fat and weight. Insulin, secreted by the pancreas, acts on the CNS to inhibit food intake and is involved in synthesis and storage of fat. Leptin, a hormone secreted by adipose cells, is in higher concentrations in those with greater body fat.

The etiology of obesity involves both genetic and environmental factors, and is highly complex. Genetics is estimated to be responsible for about onethird of the individual's BMI. The number and size of adipose cells, distribution of body fat, and resting metabolic rate are genetically influenced with well over 200 genes involved in the process of obesity. Consumption of a diet with excessive calories combined with a sedentary lifestyle also contributes to the development of obesity. Put simply, weight increases are related to increased energy intake, reduced energy expenditure, hormone alterations, and health conditions that can cause stagnation of metabolism or energy usage. The complexity arises when one considers the myriad of factors that contribute to energy intake, energy expenditure, hormone regulation, digestion, absorption, and overall health status.

CLINICAL MANIFESTATIONS

Distribution of body fat in overweight and obese individuals generally follows one of two patterns: truncal-abdominal or gluteofemoral fat deposition. The first is manifested by excess fat from the shoulders to the hips and is more common in men. The second is manifested by increased fat deposits around the thighs and buttocks and is generally more common in women. Obesity carries a long list of health risks, including type 2 diabetes, heart disease, hypertension, hyperlipidemia, stroke, osteoarthritis, liver disease, gall stones, poor wound healing, sleep apnea, and certain cancers (Fig. 15.12).

DIAGNOSTIC CRITERIA

Diagnosis is based on physical examination, noting excess fat accumulation, along with the calculation of BMI. Other methods used to estimate body fat include measuring skinfold thickness and waist-hip circumference, and bioelectrical impedance. Skinfold thickness involves the use of calipers to measure grasped adipose tissue in certain areas of the body, such as the triceps, biceps, suprailiac, or subscapular areas. Waist-hip circumference compares the distance around the waist at the umbilicus and at the hip. Bioelectrical impedance relies on changes in body composition, measured by an extremely small and safe electrical current that passes between two electrodes, one placed on the wrist and the other on the ankle. The current moves easily across water and is impeded by fat tissue. Potential physiologic causes must be explored by laboratory evaluation of thyroid function, dyslipidemia associated with metabolic syndrome, and a 24-hour free urine cortisol to determine the presence of hypercortisolism. The diagnosis may also include a screening evaluation for additional health problems related to obesity, including blood glucose, serum cholesterol, and blood pressure.

TREATMENT

Treatment of obesity is lifelong and is focused on attaining and maintaining the best possible weight to improve overall health. Basic treatment principles focus on weight reduction and physical activity programs. Pharmacologic therapy or surgery may be indicated, but these do not replace lifestyle modifications. Pharmacologic therapies primarily aim to suppress appetite, increase metabolism, or interfere with fat absorption. Gastric surgery basically reduces the size of the stomach, thereby restricting food intake.

Summary

- Adequate nutrition relies on optimal intake, digestion, absorption, metabolism, and transportation of nutrients, as well as on the excretion of waste products.
- The major macronutrients that are converted to usable sources of energy are proteins, lipids, and carbohydrates. Micronutrients include vitamins and minerals. Macronutrients have multiple roles, including the provision of calories that are converted into energy. Proteins build and maintain structural body tissues, compose blood, cell membranes, immune factors, enzymes, and hormones, and transport substances across membranes.

Lipids are a rich source of energy and facilitate numerous processes, such as supporting digestion and absorption. They influence cell membrane fluidity, receptor function, hormone function, enzyme activity, and cytokine production. Structural fat provides support and protection to body organs. The major role of carbohydrates is to provide energy.

- Many vitamins play a critical role in metabolism of carbohydrates, amino acids, and fatty acids. Basically, vitamins are part of enzyme systems that release energy from macronutrients. The other major role of vitamins is to aid in the development of genetic materials, red blood cells, hormones, collagen, and nervous system tissue.

- Minerals regulate hundreds of cellular processes. Minerals constitute bone, hemoglobin, enzymes, hormones, and chemical mediators. Charged (ionic) minerals mediate impulse conduction within the nervous system. Minerals maintain water balance, acid-base balance, and osmotic pressure. Minerals are critical for muscle contraction and form the structural components of bones and teeth.

- The intake and storage of nutrients is critical to overall health and is regulated primarily by neuroendocrine systems. Digestion and absorption is a process involving mechanical and enzymatic degradation of nutrients into usable components that can be absorbed. The GI tract, most notably the small intestine, is a major site for digestion and absorption of nutrients.

- Altered nutrition, or malnutrition, is a state of inadequate or excessive exposure to nutrients. This can include intake, digestion, or absorption of nutrients. Protein-energy malnutrition is related to deprivation of all food (marasmus) or protein deprivation in individuals consuming adequate carbohydrates (kwashiorkor).

- Undernutrition is a lack of intake of nutrients most often related to inadequate calorie consumption, inadequate intake of essential vitamins and minerals, or problems with digestion, absorption, or distribution of nutrients in the body. Undernutrition can lead to weight loss, muscle wasting, muscle weakness, dehydration, fatigue, and evidence of vitamin and mineral deficiencies. Skin manifestations are often present and may include poor wound healing, purpura, ulceration, dry skin, or pallor. Mucous membranes become inflamed and friable.

- Malabsorption is a form of undernutrition in which specific nutrients do not move across the GI mucosa. Malabsorption typically manifests as weight loss, diarrhea, bloating, abdominal cramping, and excessive flatulence.
- Overnutrition is a state of excessive exposure to nutrients. Overnutrition is generally related to overconsumption of nutrients, including excessive calories or ingesting toxic levels of vitamins and minerals. Overnutrition leads to increases in weight and body fatness.
- Toxicity of vitamins or minerals can have varying clinical manifestations depending on the physiologic function of the specific nutrient and may include headache, seizures, nausea, vomiting, skin changes, liver disease, skeletal impairment, and cardiac dysrhythmias.
- Diagnostic and treatment strategies for altered nutrition are focused on determining the cause for the nutrition imbalance and the potential effects.

Case Study 15.1

Jill is a 14-year-old African-American girl who presents to the clinic complaining of intermittent diarrhea, bloating, abdominal pain, and gas about 30 minutes after eating some meals, particularly breakfast. Further history elicited that she eats a bowl of cereal with milk each morning. Others in her family have lactose intolerance. She thinks that when she avoids milk she doesn't have the symptoms. You suspect lactose intolerance in her as well.

1. *Outline the process that is most likely occurring in this person's body.*
2. *What would you expect for clinical manifestations?*
3. *What diagnostic tests could be used?*
4. *What treatment measures would you anticipate?*

Log on to the Internet. Search for a relevant journal article or Web site (such as http://digestive.niddk.nih.gov/ddiseases/pubs/lactoseintolerance/#whatis) that details lactose intolerance to confirm your predictions.

Case Study 15.2

Pam is a 40-year-old woman who has been seeing an eating disorder specialist for the past 6 months due to a prolonged binge-eating disorder. She is obese with a BMI of 34. Her eating disorder became problematic around age 18 when her weight continued to elevate over time. She binges about once per week now and it is usually triggered by family-related stress. She eats rapidly at all meals. She noticed though that she has been binging only when she is alone. After a binging episode Pam feels embarrassed but helpless. She is not able to stop the behavior.

1. *Outline the process that is most likely occurring in this person's body.*
2. *What would you expect for clinical manifestations?*
3. *What diagnostic tests could be used?*
4. *What treatment measures would you anticipate?*

Log on to the Internet. Search for a relevant journal article or Web site (such as http://www.mayo-clinic.com/health/binge-eating-disorder/DS00608) that details binge-eating disorder, to confirm your predictions.

Practice Exam Questions

1. You have inflammation of the large intestine, a condition called ulcerative colitis. What is the most probable reason that you would develop iron-deficiency anemia?
   a. You are experiencing chronic blood loss in your stools
   b. You have inadequate hydrochloric acid for absorption of iron
   c. You have lost usable surface area in the large intestine for absorption of iron
   d. You do not have an adequate iron intake in your diet

2. You are part of the health care team at a clinic for adolescents with anorexia nervosa. Which of the assessments that you perform is focused on recognizing the most common cause for mortality in those with AN?
   a. Lung assessment
   b. Cardiovascular assessment
   c. Skin assessment
   d. Neurologic assessment

3. Which dietary change would be recommended for the individual with celiac disease?
   a. Avoid milk or milk products
   b. Avoid wheat, barley, rye, and oats
   c. Avoid rice, soy, and nuts
   d. Avoid long-chain fatty acids

4. Which of the following affects the sensations of hunger and satiety and therefore plays a major role in the development of obesity?
   a. The hypothalamus
   b. The pituitary gland
   c. The thyroid gland
   d. The pancreas

5. Which of the following does not contribute as an energy source in the diet?
   a. Carbohydrates   c. Proteins
   b. Fats   d. Vitamins

6. You are caring for an individual with liver disease. What are you most concerned about with regard to nutrition?
   a. The patient may be unable to adequately store nutrients
   b. The patient may be unable to synthesize nutrients
   c. The patient may be unable to metabolize macronutrients
   d. All of these are major concerns

7. Your patient has gall bladder disease and is unable to store and release adequate bile to the small intestine. What dietary modifications do you suggest?
   a. Increase protein intake
   b. Decrease fat intake
   c. Increase complex carbohydrates
   d. No dietary changes are needed

8. You are working in the newborn nursery and are an advocate for breastfeeding. It is the winter in northern Minnesota and you are concerned about low sunlight exposure in infants who are breastfeeding as they may develop vitamin D deficiency. What is the major manifestation of vitamin D deficiency?
   a. Impaired mineralization in growing bones
   b. Impaired retinal development
   c. Impaired osteoclast activity
   d. Keratinization of mucous membranes

9. You are planning a nutritional in-service to your clinic's service area in California. What concept of altered nutrition should you focus your talk in order to address the largest nutritional problem in your area?
   a. Altered metabolism
   b. Undernutrition
   c. Overnutrition
   d. All of these are equally prevalent

10. What is known about glucose transport into the small intestine?
    a. Requires cotransport with sodium
    b. Occurs through active transport
    c. Must first be reduced as is rarely consumed in the typical diet
    d. All of these are true about glucose transport

Discussion and Application

1. What did I know about altered nutrition prior to today?

2. What body processes are affected by altered nutrition? What are the expected functions of those processes? How does altered nutrition affect those processes?

3. What are the potential etiologies for altered nutrition? How does altered nutrition develop?

4. Who is most at risk for developing altered nutrition? How can altered nutrition be prevented?

5. What are the human differences that affect the etiology, risk, or course of altered nutrition?

6. What clinical manifestations are expected in the course of altered nutrition?

7. What special diagnostic tests are useful in determining the diagnosis and course of altered nutrition?

8. What are the goals of care for individuals with altered nutrition?

9. How does the concept of altered perfusion build on what I have learned in the previous chapters and in previous courses?

10. How can I use what I have learned?

RESOURCES

American Obesity Organization:
http://www.obesity.org

Body Mass Index Calculator:
http://www.cdc.gov/healthyweight/assessing/index.html

American Dietetics Association:
http://www.eatright.org/HealthProfessionals/

United States Department of Agriculture (USDA) "MyPyramid: Steps to a Healthier You":
http://www.mypyramid.gov/

Canada's Food and Nutrition Website:
http://www.hc-sc.gc.ca/fn-an/index-eng.php

REFERENCES

1. Mahan L, Escott-Stump S. *Food, Nutrition, and Diet Therapy.* Philadelphia: Saunders; 2004.
2. Boothby L, Doering P. Vitamin C and vitamin E for Alzheimer's disease. *Ann Pharmacother.* 2005;39:2073–2079.
3. United States Food and Drug Administration. Orlistat FDA approval: executive summary; 2003. Available at: http://www. fda.gov/cder/foi/esum/2003/20766se5-018_Orlistat_ BPCA_CLINICAL_ltr.pdf. Accessed March 1, 2010.
4. United States Food and Drug Administration. Early communication about an ongoing safety review orlistat (marketed as Alli and Xenical); 2009. Available at: http://www.fda.gov/Drugs/DrugSafety/PostmarketDrugSafetyInformationforPatientsandProviders/DrugSafetyInformationforHeathcareProfessionals/ucm179166.htm. Accessed March 1, 2010.
5. Barringer T, Kirk J, Santaniello A, et al. Effect of a multivitamin and mineral supplement on infection and quality of life. *Ann Intern Med.* 2003;138:365–371.
6. Frith-Terhune A, Cogswell M, Khan L, et al. Iron deficiency anemia: higher prevalence in Mexican American than in non-Hispanic white females in the third National Health and Nutrition Examination Survey, 1988–1994. *Am J Clin Nutr.* 2000;72:963–968.
7. Pivarnik J, Braun M, Hergenroeder A, et al. Ethnicity affects aerobic fitness in U.S. adolescent girls. *Med Sci Sports Exerc.* 1995;27:1635–1638.
8. American Psychiatric Association. DSM-5 development: DSM-5 proposed diagnostic criteria for anorexia nervosa. Available at: http://www.dsm5.org/ProposedRevisions/Pages/proposedrevision .aspx?rid=24. Accessed March 1, 2010.
9. Klapproth J, Yang V. Celiac sprue. 2009. Available at: http://emedicine.medscape.com/article/171805-overview. Accessed March 1, 2010.
10. World Health Organization. Obesity and Overweight. 2010. Available at: http://www.who.int/dietphysicalactivity/publications/facts/obesity/en/. Accessed March 1, 2010.

Chapter 16

Altered Elimination

LEARNING OBJECTIVES

1. Define and use the key terms listed in this chapter.
2. Describe the processes of the production and elimination of urine and stool.
3. Identify the role of neural, motor, endocrine, and physical processes in altered elimination.
4. Outline the processes involved in altered elimination.
5. Characterize the clinical manifestations in altered urinary and gastrointestinal elimination.
6. Recognize health conditions that can precipitate impaired elimination.
7. Detail alterations in systemic organ systems as a response to altered elimination.
8. List the common diagnostic procedures used to identify altered urinary and bowel elimination.
9. Describe treatment modalities used in altered urinary and bowel elimination.
10. Apply concepts of altered elimination to select clinical models.

INTRODUCTION

As you have seen in the previous chapters, maintenance of homeostasis requires a delicate balance and careful coordination of many body systems. The same is true of the process of elimination. When you eat and drink in response to hunger and thirst, you feel satisfied. We often take for granted what happens to the food and drink after our needs are met. Once nutrients have been extracted from the foods and liquids we eat, the remaining contents must be eliminated. Urine and stool are the final waste products of what was once our favorite foods and drinks. For the body to function efficiently, the waste products that remain after energy and nutrients are absorbed must be excreted. Impairment of the ability to eliminate waste products results in the clinical manifestations and pathophysiologic alterations associated with the disease. In this chapter, the processes of altered urinary and gastrointestinal (GI) elimination and their clinical manifestations are described in Modules 1 and 2. The application of these altered processes is considered in Module 3, selected clinical models of altered elimination.

Module 1

Altered Urinary Elimination

Elimination processes require motility and patency of structures involved in the movement of waste for excretion. These processes are regulated by neuromuscular signaling and are influenced by transport functions and adequacy of perfusion. Regulation of body fluid and the balance between acids and bases are two of the primary roles of the kidney, as described in Chapter 8. Water and ion movement across the cell membranes of the renal tubules in close association with the vasculature of the kidneys is the mechanism that allows fluid and waste secretion in the form of urine.

Urine Production Process

Urine is produced by the kidney, is stored in the bladder, and is excreted through the urethra through a complex interplay between neural, motor, and hormonal mechanisms. The basic processes of the renal system include:

- Regulation of body fluid volume and composition
- Elimination of metabolic wastes
- Synthesis, release, or activation of hormones
  - Erythropoietin
  - Renin
  - Vitamin D
- Regulation of blood pressure

The renal system is illustrated in Figure 16.1, which provides a visual review of the urinary system location in relation to other anatomic structures in the body (Fig. 16.1A), an overview of the internal structures of the kidney (Fig. 16.1B), and a detailed view of the functional unit of the kidney, the nephron (Fig. 16.1C).

URINE PRODUCTION

The **nephron** is the functional unit of the kidney and is composed of the **glomerulus** (capillary network and Bowman's capsule), the proximal tubule, loop of Henle, distal tubule, and collecting duct. There are approximately 1 million nephrons in the cortex of each kidney. The role of the nephron is to:

- Filter water-soluble substances from the blood
- Reabsorb filtered nutrients, water, and electrolytes
- Secrete waste

The kidneys are responsible for processing 20% to 25% of the cardiac output, approximately 1000 mL of blood per minute. This allows the kidneys to be perfused with enough blood supply to meet the high oxygen and metabolic demands of the organ. Blood enters the kidney through the renal artery, dividing into interlobular arteries, arcuate arteries, afferent arterioles, and glomerular capillaries. Blood entering the glomerular capillaries via the afferent arteriole is filtered with the resulting fluid called filtrate. Filtrate enters Bowman's capsule, where it then enters the renal tubular system. The blood remaining in the glomerular capillaries exits the glomerulus via the efferent arteriole, which then branches into the peritubular capillaries. The peritubular capillaries surround the proximal and distal convoluted tubules. Additional capillaries, vasa recta, surround the loops of Henle deep within the medulla, serving an important role in the concentration of urine through exchange of water and solutes from the filtrate flowing in the opposite direction (**countercurrent exchanger**). Blood travels into the interlobular venules and veins and returns to the venous circulation via the renal vein.

Filtrate travels from Bowman's capsule to the proximal tubule, where the majority of sodium is reabsorbed back into the blood. Other reabsorbed substances include glucose, potassium, amino acids, HCO_3^-, PO_4^-, urea, and water. Hydrogen is secreted from the resulting isotonic fluid. Fluid moves down the loop of Henle where it is progressively more concentrated (**countercurrent multiplier**). Water is reabsorbed and sodium diffuses into the descending loop, with sodium actively reabsorbed in the ascending loop. The **countercurrent mechanism** involves the countercurrent exchanger and multiplier and is responsible for maintaining the vertical gradient in the interstitium (Fig. 16.2). In the distal tubule, sodium (through the actions of the hormone, aldosterone) and HCO_3^- are reabsorbed. Epithelial cells adjacent to the distal tubule, the macula densa, provide information about sodium content in the filtrate to the cells of the juxtaglomerular apparatus, regulating aldosterone release via the renin–angiotensin–aldosterone system (RAAS). Secretion of potassium, urea, hydrogen, and ammonia (NH_3) occurs; the remaining filtrate moves into the collecting duct. Here, additional water is reabsorbed in an ADH-dependent mechanism, in addition to sodium, hydrogen, potassium, and NH_3. The end product produced by the nephron is urine, which is transported via the ureters to the bladder, where it is stored until it is eliminated through the urethra.

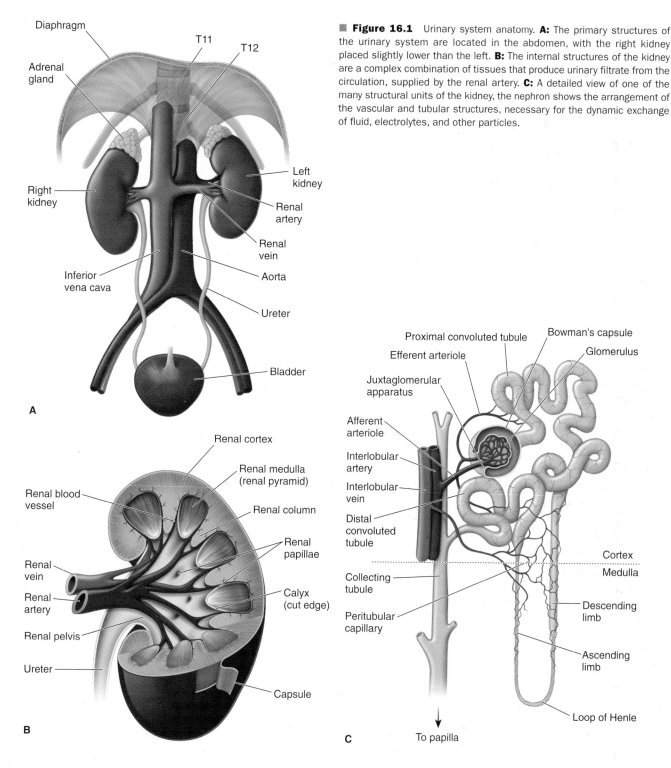

Figure 16.1 Urinary system anatomy. **A:** The primary structures of the urinary system are located in the abdomen, with the right kidney placed slightly lower than the left. **B:** The internal structures of the kidney are a complex combination of tissues that produce urinary filtrate from the circulation, supplied by the renal artery. **C:** A detailed view of one of the many structural units of the kidney, the nephron shows the arrangement of the vascular and tubular structures, necessary for the dynamic exchange of fluid, electrolytes, and other particles.

Table 16.1 describes the mechanisms of tubular transport for selected substances.

STOP *and Consider*

Why is it necessary for urine to become concentrated before it is excreted?

URINE REMOVAL

Urine enters the ureters via the renal pelvis, promoting flow out of the kidneys. Ureters are composed of smooth muscle fibers that propel the urine to the bladder by the process of peristalsis. Urine enters the bladder via the trigone. The **trigone** is a

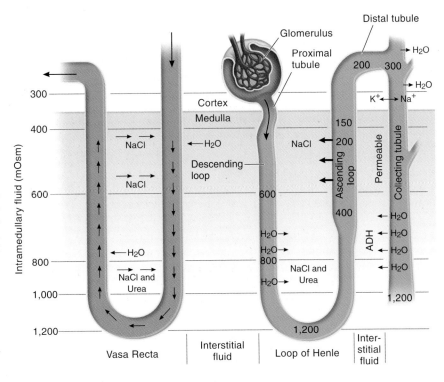

Figure 16.2 Urinary filtrate flow and concentration. Movement of water and solutes between the vasa recta and loops of Henle in the juxtamedullary nephrons promote concentration of urine. The flow of filtrate in the loop of Henle runs in the opposite direction of the flow of blood in the parallel vasa recta. This countercurrent design combined with the selective permeabilities of the loop of Henle contributes to the concentration of osmotically active particles in the medullary interstitium. In the collecting tubule, ADH allows water to move from filtrate into the interstitium, drawn by osmotic forces. Water then is reabsorbed into the blood to achieve optimal water balance. (Image modified from Premkumar K. *The Massage Connection: Anatomy and Physiology.* Baltimore: Lippincott Williams & Wilkins; 2004, with permission.)

Table 16.1 Tubular Transport

Substance	Mechanisms and Sites of Transport
Sodium	Filtered at the glomerulus
	Reabsorbed in the proximal tubule by facilitated diffusion and in the proximal tubule, thick ascending loop of Henle, and distal convoluted tubule by active transport
Potassium	Filtered at the glomerulus
	Reabsorbed passively in the proximal tubule and actively in the thick ascending loop of Henle
	Secreted or actively reabsorbed in the distal convoluted or collecting tubules; depends on blood potassium levels
Chloride	Filtered at the glomerulus
	Reabsorbed passively in the late proximal and distal convoluted tubule
	Reabsorbed actively in the proximal tubule, ascending loop of Henle, and distal convoluted tubule
Hydrogen	Secreted actively in the proximal, distal convoluted, and collecting tubules
	Reabsorbed by cation exchangers in the proximal convoluted tubules
Bicarbonate	Filtered at the glomerulus
	Reabsorbed passively in the proximal and distal convoluted tubules
Glucose	Filtered at the glomerulus
	Entirely reabsorbed by active mechanisms unless tubular maximum is exceeded
Urea	Filtered at the glomerulus
	Reabsorbed passively in the proximal, late distal tubules, and collecting duct
	Entry into the descending and thin ascending loops of Henle depends on concentration gradient in the surrounding interstitium
Calcium	Filtered at the glomerulus
	Reabsorbed passively in the proximal tubule and the thin loop of Henle
	Reabsorbed actively in the ascending thick loop of Henle and early distal convoluted tubule
Phosphate	Filtered at the glomerulus
	Reabsorbed actively in proximal tubule
Magnesium	Filtered at the glomerulus
	Reabsorbed actively and passively in the thick ascending loop of Henle
Uric acid	Filtered at the glomerulus
	Reabsorbed in the early and late proximal tubule
	Secreted in the midproximal tubule
Protein	Limited filtration at the glomerulus due to large size and negative charge
	Amino acids actively reabsorbed in the proximal distal tubule
	Large peptides reabsorbed by endocytosis for entry into lysozymes (metabolized into amino acids)

triangular, smooth area at the base of the bladder between the openings of the two ureters and the urethra, serving as a functional sphincter that prevents urine from moving in a retrograde manner back into the ureter from the bladder. The **bladder** is a muscular organ lined with transitional epithelium and innervated by the pelvic nerves. The body of the bladder is composed of the **detrusor muscle** (skeletal muscle). Filling of the bladder activates sensory stretch receptors, and the generated action potential is transmitted to the sacral region of the spinal cord. Contraction of the detrusor muscle is stimulated by parasympathetic cholinergic motor fibers. Relaxation of the muscle of the bladder neck, the **internal urethral sphincter** (composed of a ring of circular smooth muscle), promotes release of urine from the bladder (**micturition**). Somatic control of the **external urethral sphincter** muscle (skeletal muscle) innervated by the pudendal nerve allows for voluntary release of urine. Tonic contraction of the smooth muscle of the urethra prevents the leakage of urine until pressure in the bladder exceeds threshold. Urethral length differs between genders; the female urethra is much shorter than the male urethra, which spans the length of the penis. Figure 16.3 illustrates the structures of the bladder. A summary of the steps involved in the micturition reflex is highlighted in Box 16.1.

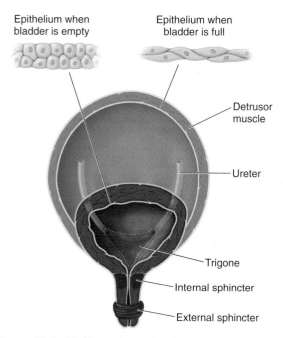

■ **Figure 16.3** Bladder structures in urinary excretion. The path of urine excretion through the ureters, trigone area, and internal and external sphincters is shown. Contraction of the detrusor muscle promotes passage of urine. The structural relationship of the epithelium lining the bladder cavity depends on bladder volume. (Image modified from Porth CM. *Pathophysiology: Concepts of Altered Health States.* 7th ed. Philadelphia: Lippincott Williams & Wilkins; 2004, with permission.)

Box 16.1 Micturition Reflex

Bladder filling stimulates the micturition reflex. The steps involved in the micturition reflex are primarily involuntary, but they may be modulated by the cerebral cortex, enabling conscious control. The micturition reflex involves four major steps:

1. Stimulation of stretch receptors in bladder walls transmits impulse to the sacral spinal cord.
2. Neural impulse ascends from the sacral cord segments to the micturition center in the pons of the brain.
3. Neural impulse descends from the micturition center, initiating contraction of the detrusor muscle and relaxation of the internal sphincter.
4. Voluntary relaxation of the external sphincter stimulates release of urine.

Urine Characteristics

Urine is a clear yellow fluid composed primarily of water, which contains a variety of water-soluble waste products. Total volume produced is approximately 750 to 2000 mL over a 24-hour period. Urine has a slight ammonia odor from the breakdown of urea. Variations in color, derived from urochrome pigments, indicate hydration status. Concentrated, dark, strong-smelling urine may indicate dehydration, whereas dilute, pale-colored urine may indicate increased fluid volume.

Urine samples can be collected to determine the specific characteristics. Methods of urine collection for analysis include:

- Random collection
  - May be taken at any time of the day
  - No special preparation required
- Clean-catch
  - Requires special cleansing of the external urethral meatus
  - Midstream urine collection (urine collected does not include fluid from the initial or final urinary stream)
- Bladder catheterization
  - Sterile insertion of a catheter through the urinary meatus into the bladder to collect urine sample
- Suprapubic aspiration
  - Insertion of a sterile needle transabdominally into the bladder for urine collection

STOP *and Consider*

Why would the indication for urine collection influence the method selection?

Urine Analysis

Urine is analyzed in two different ways: macroscopic and microscopic. **Macroscopic analysis** consists of the visual determination of color and clarity. In addition, biochemical analyses can be obtained by testing urine with a **urine dipstick**. Color changes indicate the absence or presence (including a gross estimate of quantity) of substances in urine. These substances provide information such as:

- pH
- Specific gravity
- Protein
- Glucose
- Ketones
- Nitrite
- Leukocyte esterase

Microscopic analysis is performed by using a specially prepared urine sample. A small sample (10 to 15 mL) of urine is centrifuged for approximately 10 minutes until the sediment forms at the bottom of the test tube. All but a small amount of fluid is removed and the sediment is resuspended in the remaining fluid. A sample is placed onto a glass slide with a coverslip for viewing under the microscope. Low-power examination can detect the presence of crystals, casts, squamous cells, and other large components. High-power examination can detect crystals, cells (white blood cells [WBCs] and red blood cells [RBCs]), and bacteria.

Urine should be free of protein, glucose, ketones, nitrite, bacteria, leukocyte esterase, crystals, and stones. **Casts**, structures consisting of a protein meshwork of entrapped cells formed in the distal collecting tubules and collecting ducts, are also absent in normal urine. Epithelial cells may be present in small numbers, but increased amounts detected in urine may indicate pathology. Identification of these abnormal findings provides evidence of clinical disease.

From the Lab

The number of specific sediment components seen under microscopic examination can be quantified. The degree of magnification is also indicated and is determined with low-power field (LPF) or high-power field (HPF). Several fields, or areas, are counted and then averaged to provide an accurate estimate.

ALTERED URINARY ELIMINATION

Elimination involves a complex interplay between neural, vascular, muscular, and hormonal influences. Additionally, the structures involved in the movement of urine from its production to its exit must be patent and functional.

Processes of Altered Urinary Elimination

Alteration in motility, neuromuscular function, vascular insufficiency, and obstruction are most commonly associated with altered urinary elimination. The following review of etiology and implications of altered motility, neuromuscular function, perfusion, and patency in the urinary system provides the essential content for concept application in Module 3, Clinical Models.

ALTERATION IN URINARY MOTILITY

Alteration in motility can promote stasis of filtrate in the renal tubules as well as stasis of urine in the bladder. Casts may form because of low flow rate, increased sodium concentration, and low pH, all factors favoring precipitation. Precipitation of urinary fluid components may contribute to blockage of essential renal structures. The specific type of cell trapped in the cast meshwork may provide information on the site of pathology. Trapping of RBCs within casts may indicate glomerulonephritis. Epithelial cells may indicate sloughing of tubular cells (**acute tubular necrosis**) (Fig. 16.4), whereas WBCs may indicate pyelonephritis (Fig. 16.5). Stasis of urine in the bladder may promote growth of bacteria, leading to local and ascending infection in the kidneys.

ALTERATION IN URINARY NEUROMUSCULAR FUNCTION

Alteration in neuromuscular function in urinary elimination may result in urinary retention or incontinence. Impaired neural control of urinary elimination may involve the neurons of the peripheral and central nervous systems, neurotransmitter production and availability, or coordination of neural impulses from initiation to action. From generation of an action potential to transduction of the nerve impulse (see Chapter 9), failure to provide an appropriate stimulus for the desired response will result in a limited or absent ability to eliminate urine. Exaggerated responses may prompt stimulation to prematurely release urine. Additionally, muscles must have the ability to respond to a generated nerve impulse to achieve the intended effect. Muscle function involved in urinary

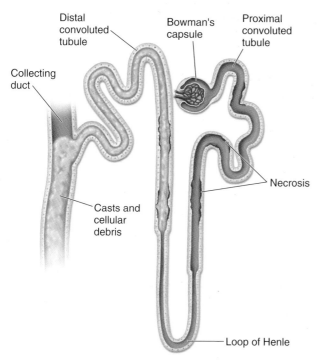

Figure 16.4 Acute tubular necrosis. Casts and cellular debris are sloughed into the tubular lumen in both ischemic necrosis and nephrotoxic injury.

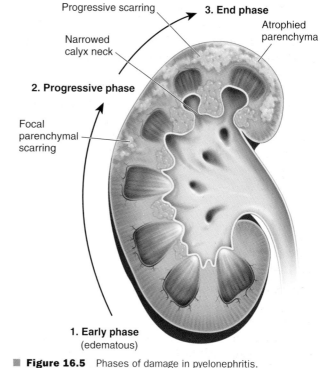

Figure 16.5 Phases of damage in pyelonephritis.

elimination includes peristalsis in the renal tubules, contraction or relaxation of smooth and skeletal muscles. Conscious control of the circumstances involving timing of urinary elimination may be impaired as a consequence of altered mobility and the resulting reduction in toileting independence.

ALTERATION IN URINARY PERFUSION

Inadequate arterial blood supply results in ischemia and infarction. Decreased oxygen delivery by the arterial blood supply may result in damage to renal structures because of inability to meet metabolic demands. Decreased perfusion leading to impaired oxygenation of tissue may be due to excessive constriction of arterioles, inadequate vascular volume, or obstructed patency of the arterial supply, as occurs with an embolism. Loss of functional tissue through necrosis leads to pain, bleeding, and obstruction of the branches of the venous system, draining the affected tissue. Conversely, enhanced perfusion represents additional workload and has the potential to stress the individual organ system. The general consequences of impaired perfusion are detailed in Chapter 2 and Chapter 14.

ALTERATION IN URINARY PATENCY

Blockage of structures involved in the passage of urine may result in obstruction.

The consequences of obstruction are influenced by the:

- Degree of the obstruction (complete or partial)
- Duration of the obstruction
- Acuity or chronicity of the condition

Obstructions are characterized by a buildup of pressure behind the blockage. Prolonged or severe pressure results in structural damage and impaired function. Ischemia and necrosis may result, adding to the consequences of perfusion impairment, because of mechanical obstruction of the arterial or venous system. Blockage may be caused by precipitation of substances in smaller lumen structures, or structural blockage resulting from endogenous or exogenous sources such as polyps or tumors. Mechanical obstructions may result from urine precipitation, scar tissue or adhesions, tumor, or inflammation.

Urine flow is impeded in the obstruction of the renal and urinary systems (Table 16.2). Dilation of the structures proximal to the obstruction causes dilation and stasis, leading to infection and structural damage. **Hydroureter**, accumulation of fluid in the urinary ureter, is a consequence of complete ureteral obstruction (Fig. 16.6). Increased hydrostatic pressure extends up to the renal pelvis and tubules, leading to hydronephrosis. The glomerular filtration rate (GFR) decreases, reflecting impairment of renal function. Fluid escapes from the tubules into the surrounding capillary system. Excretion of sodium, urea,

Table 16.2 Types of Obstructive Disease

Type of Obstruction	Pathology	Clinical Manifestations	Laboratory Findings	Sequelae If Left Untreated
Urinary	Stasis of urine behind the obstruction of renal structures, ureters, or urethra	Pain Pressure Frequency of urination Oliguria Abdominal distention	Bacteruria Hematuria	Hydronephrosis Renal failure Infection Hypertension Dehydration Hypovolemia
Intestine	Collection of gas and fluid behind the obstruction	Abdominal pain, nausea, vomiting Diaphragmatic pressure, ⇓ respiratory volume Edema caused by ⇑ capillary permeability Fever caused by release of toxins	⇑ Hematocrit (hemoconcentration) Ketosis, acidosis Hypokalemia, hypochloremia	Shock Pneumonia Peritonitis

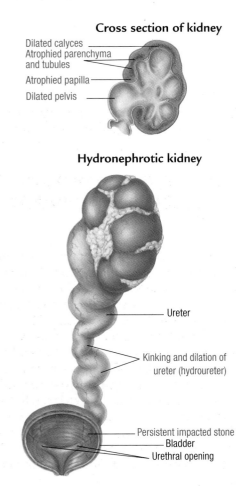

Cross section of kidney

Dilated calyces
Atrophied parenchyma and tubules
Atrophied papilla
Dilated pelvis

Hydronephrotic kidney

Ureter

Kinking and dilation of ureter (hydroureter)

Persistent impacted stone
Bladder
Urethral opening

■ **Figure 16.6** Hydronephrosis. Obstruction of the ureter causes pressure to build, resulting in hydroureter and hydronephrosis. (Images courtesy Anatomical Chart Company.)

and water is impaired. Local hormonal responses to promote renal perfusion are effective for a short time. Impaired perfusion develops within 24 hours, leading to ischemia, tubular atrophy, and damaged glomeruli if the condition is not corrected. Sequelae include infection, sepsis, and loss of renal function leading to renal failure.

General Manifestations of Altered Urinary Elimination

Impairment of the processes involved in urinary elimination result in a variety of clinical manifestations. Specific manifestations are related to the underlying pathology. Generally, manifestations include:

- Altered volume of excretion
- Altered excretion characteristics
- Bleeding
- Pain
- Distention
- Anorexia
- Nausea
- Vomiting
- Fever

Urinary volume may be increased or decreased. In the case of obstruction or damage to the renal structures themselves, oliguria (scanty urine production) or anuria (absent urine production) may be seen. Other conditions may be associated with increased urine output and are often the result of hormonal stimulation of a compensatory response or regulation of fluid balance. Urine composition may also be altered, reflecting the origin of the pathology. An analysis of urine associated with kidney disorders is detailed in Table 16.3.

Table 16.3 Pathologic Indications of Altered Urinary Elimination

Condition	Description of Condition	Laboratory Confirmation	Possible Etiologies
Proteinuria	Protein in urine	150 mg/24-hour sample	Renal failure
			Nephrotic syndrome Preeclampsia
			Renal artery/vein thrombosis
			Glomerular disease
			Tubulopathy
Glucosuria	Glucose in urine	>130 mg/24-hour sample	Diabetes mellitus
Ketonuria	Ketones in urine (acetone, acetoacetic acid, beta-hydroxybutyric acid)		Diabetes mellitus
			Ketoacidosis
Hematuria	RBCs in urine	>1 RBC/HPF	Starvation
			Glomerular damage
			Tumors
			Kidney trauma
			Urinary tract infection
			Acute tubular necrosis
Pyuria	WBCs in urine	2 WBC/HPF + leukocyte esterase >100,000 CFU	Urinary tract obstruction
			Upper and lower urinary tract infection
			Acute glomerulonephritis
Bacteruria	Bacteria in urine	+nitrites	Renal calculi
			Upper and lower urinary tract infection

CFU, colony-forming unit; HPF, high-power field; RBC, red blood cell; WBC, white blood cell.

Hematuria, evidenced by frank bleeding or clots, can be identified based on urine color. Small amounts of blood require microscopic detection.

Pain is a frequent symptom associated with altered renal and urinary function. Renal and ureteral nociceptors transmit pain impulses to the spinal cord between T10 and L1. The associated dermatomes include the lower abdomen anteriorly and posteriorly at the level of the **costovertebral angle (CVA)** or flank area. Most nociceptive receptors are located in the renal capsule rather than in the kidney itself and are stimulated by stretching and inflammation. Stretching induced by distention produces the sensation of dull, persistent pain. In contrast, many pain receptors are located in the remaining parts of the descending urinary system. The pain sensations from this region are usually intermittent and sharp.

Manifestations of infection promote feelings of general malaise, anorexia, and fever. Infection in the lower urinary tract is presented as a clinical model in Chapter 5 to illustrate the typical pathology, clinical manifestations, diagnosis, and treatment of this condition. Ascending infection of the pathogen through the ureters into the kidneys represents the potential for renal structural damage, significantly affecting the ability to produce urine. Nausea and vomiting may occur in ascending infection or systemic illness, such as pyelonephritis.

● **STOP** *and* **Consider**

What mechanisms of infection and inflammation may contribute to damage to renal structures?

DIAGNOSIS OF CONDITIONS OF THE RENAL AND URINARY SYSTEMS

Diagnosis of altered elimination processes is important to prevent further damage to involved organs. Both the cause and effect of altered elimination are critical to the effective management and treatment of individuals with these conditions. Microscopic and macroscopic urinalysis provides a useful resource in the diagnosis of conditions resulting in altered elimination. Normal values for urinary electrolytes are not standardized because the kidneys function dynamically to maintain electrolyte homeostasis in the plasma. Calculation of GFR and creatinine clearance indicates nephron function. Radiographic diagnostic testing useful in the determination of anatomic and functional anomalies includes:

- *Intravenous pyelogram (IVP):* Intravenous injection of a radiocontrast medium to allow radiographic visualization of the kidneys, ureters, and bladder.

- *Voiding cystourethrogram (VCUG):* X-ray examination of the bladder and urethra completed after insertion of contrast into bladder via a urinary catheter. Fluoroscopy is used to determine ureteral reflux and bladder/urethra configuration during voiding.
- *Renal angiogram:* Contrast injected into the renal artery via the aorta to diagnose renal artery stenosis or intrarenal vascular obstructions.
- *Renal ultrasound:* Noninvasive image produced by sound waves. Useful in the determination of kidney size, hydroureter, cysts, obstructions, or fluid collection. Renal artery flow can also be determined with Doppler ultrasound.

Treatment of Altered Urinary Elimination

Treatment of conditions contributing to altered urinary elimination is determined by the condition underlying the clinical manifestations. A thorough review of medical history, description of symptoms, physical examination, and diagnostic testing may be necessary to specify treatment. Altered urinary elimination is often associated with impaired regulation of fluid balance. Control of fluid balance through administration of supplemental fluids to correct body fluid deficit or the use of diuretics to correct body fluid excess may be indicated.

Module 2

Alteration in Stool Elimination

Processes of Stool Elimination

The process of stool elimination involves the organs of the GI system. From oral nutrient intake to the elimination of waste by the passage of stool, exchange and processing of the products is complex. This chapter describes the final processes of stool production and elimination by the large intestine, which occur after nutrient extraction detailed in Chapter 15.

The large intestine is a hollow organ surrounding the small intestine in the abdominal cavity. The **large intestine/colon** is composed of the cecum, appendix, colon, rectum, and anal canal. The colon can be divided further into the ascending, transverse, descending, and sigmoid portions. The ileocecal valve directs the flow of fecal matter from the ileum of the small intestine to the cecum of the large intestine. Composed of the cecum, colon (ascending, transverse, descending, sigmoid), and rectal segments, the large intestine begins at the end of the ileum of the small intestine and terminates at the anus. The appendix is a long, narrow blind pouch projecting from the cecum. Measuring approximately 1.5 m, the diameter of the large intestine reduces as it progresses towards the rectum. At the rectum, the colon dilates leading to increased capacity for stool. The superior and inferior mesenteric arteries are the origin for blood supply to the large intestine. The autonomic nervous system provides the primary neural control of the GI tract (Fig. 16.7).

STOOL ELIMINATION

Food ingestion begins the digestive processes and results in the excretion of stool. Bowel motility, perfusion, patency, and response to neural signals are critical to stool elimination.

Stool Production

Stool is a product of digestion, as detailed in Chapter 15. As digestive processes continue throughout the length of large intestine, fecal matter entering at the cecum via the ileocecal valve is propelled toward the rectum for excretion. Water and electrolytes are removed from the fecal matter as it moves through the large intestine. Continued processing of fecal matter as it exits the large intestine results in the final product, stool.

Large intestine functional responses are related to the rate of movement of contents, with more rapid movement allowing less time for intestinal processes and slower movement leading to extended time. While the greatest absorption of nutrients occurs in the small intestine, the large intestine provides the final opportunity for achievement of water and electrolyte balance. Of the 7 to 10 L of water entering the small intestine, only 1 to 1.5 L enters the large intestine on a daily basis. The final product of the large intestine, stool, includes approximately 100 to 200 mL of water. Absorption of water and electrolytes occurs in and around the epithelial cells that line the large intestine. The small intestine chyme is altered from a liquid to a

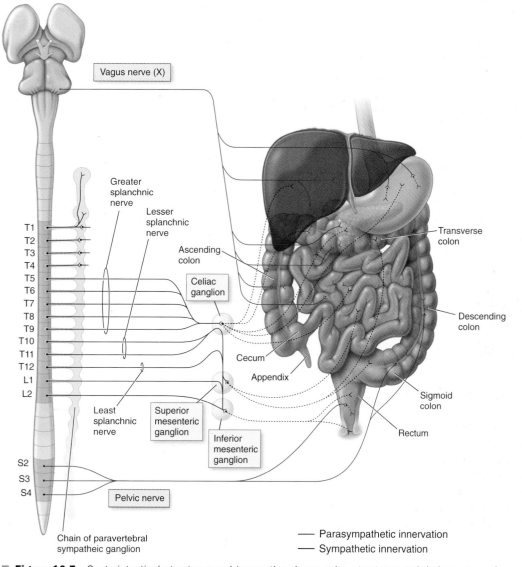

■ **Figure 16.7** Gastrointestinal structures and innervation. Large colon structures and their sources of innervation are labeled. (Image modified from Porth CM. *Pathophysiology: Concepts of Altered Health States.* 7th ed. Philadelphia: Lippincott Williams & Wilkins; 2004, with permission.)

semisolid form in the ascending and transverse large intestine segments. The intestinal contents retain indigestible carbohydrates, including dietary fiber, as well as remaining sodium, magnesium, and chloride. The time from dietary intake through elimination of remaining intestinal contents varies from 2 to 5 days, on average.

As the fecal matter progresses through the large intestine, the majority of water is reabsorbed along with several B complex vitamins and vitamin K, much of which is produced by intestinal bacteria. The remaining fecal matter combines with intestinal mucous and resident bacteria, known as **intestinal flora**, and becomes feces. The greatest concentration of GI bacterial resides in the large colon. The complex bacterial flora contains primarily anaerobic organisms, though composition among adults is variable and in large part dependent on diet. The food an individual eats provides sources of energy and carbon for intestinal bacteria, directing the persistence of particular types of bacteria. Intestinal bacteria break down some remaining dietary fiber, releasing byproducts including short chain fatty acids used by the epithelial cells of the colon. Resident intestinal flora protect the intestine from harmful pathogens through the maintenance of a local homeostatic balance.

Stool Evacuation

Stool is stored in the large intestine until the time of evacuation (**defecation**). It is estimated to take 18 hours for the contents of the intestine to pass from the proximal end of the large intestine to the distal end. The continuous inner layer of circular smooth muscle of the muscularis externa is surrounded by an outer, discontinuous layer of longitudinal smooth muscle. Contraction of smooth muscle occurs through the sliding filament mechanism. Along the length of the large intestine, the longitudinal muscle forms three distinct bands known as **teniae coli**. When contracted, **haustras** (pouches) are created. Smooth muscle contraction of the longitudinal and circular muscle layers of the large intestine provides the primary mechanism for the movement of stool, generating propulsive movements. The closeness of smooth muscle fibers to each another makes it easier for action potentials to be transmitted to adjacent fibers, propagating the nerve impulse along the length of the large intestine. The result is **peristalsis** caused by squeezing of circular fibers, which promotes a forward movement of intestine contents. Circular fiber contraction and relaxation occurs at different locations, producing the characteristic **segmental movement** of the large intestine. **Mass movements**, or strong peristaltic movements, occur three to four times a day, promoting the propulsion of stool.

STOP *and Consider*

Reduced peristalsis would slow the movement of stool through the large intestine. How might this affect water concentration in the stool?

Muscle fibers are innervated locally by the intrinsic **enteric nervous system**, including the **myenteric (Auerbach) plexus** found between the longitudinal and circular muscle layers and the **Meissner plexus**, located in the submucosa. Myenteric impulses promote control of GI movement, while the Meissner plexus transmits sensory impulses through stretch receptors. Both systems are involved in the reflexes necessary for stool movement and evaluation. Myenteric plexus stimulation provides increased tonic contractions as well as increased intensity, rate, and velocity of rhythmic contractions. It is induced via colon distention. The enteric nervous system is modulated by the autonomic nervous system. Sympathetic stimulation via the sacral nerves of the spinal cord has an inhibitory effect, whereas parasympathetic stimulation serves an excitatory function via the vagus nerve.

Two sphincters are involved in the process of defecation. The **internal rectal sphincter** is made up of a thick layer of smooth muscle and is tonically constricted because of sympathetic control. Movement of stool into the rectum stimulates the reflex to defecate, also known as the **rectal reflex**. Parasympathetic stimulation prompts relaxation of the internal anal sphincter. The skeletal muscle of

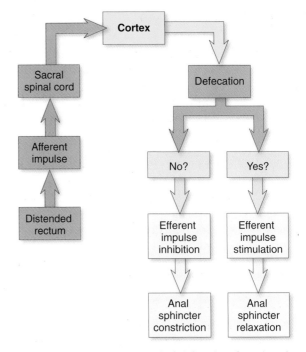

Figure 16.8 Voluntary control of defecation. Conscious intent provides voluntary control of defecation.

the **external anal sphincter** surrounds the internal rectal sphincter and is innervated by the pudendal nerve (somatic nervous system), providing voluntary control. The external sphincter can override the defecation reflex, allowing for voluntary control of defecation (Fig. 16.8). Straining through **Valsalva maneuvers**, the generation of intra-abdominal pressure through inhalation that forces the diaphragm and chest muscles against the glottis, stimulates the vagus nerve and assists in stool evacuation. A summary of the steps involved in the rectal reflex is highlighted in Box 16.2.

Box 16.2 Rectal Reflex

Distention or irritation of the rectal wall stimulates the rectal reflex. The steps involved in the rectal reflex are primarily involuntary, but they may be modulated by voluntary control suppression. If suppressed, the reflex is subsequently stimulated when rectal mass increases. The rectal reflex involves five major steps:

1. Stimulation of stretch receptors in the rectal wall transmits sensory impulse to the sacral spinal cord.
2. Sensory neurons synapse on parasympathetic nerves, promoting relaxation of the internal anal sphincter (smooth muscle).
3. Interneuron stimulation promotes contraction of abdominal muscles.
4. Motor signal from the cerebral cortex stimulates opening of the external anal sphincter (skeletal muscle).
5. Defecation assisted by voluntary contractions of the abdominal muscles.

Stool Characteristics

One of the main functions of the large intestine is compaction of feces. As water is absorbed as the fecal matter moves along the length of the large intestine, the solid matter in the feces becomes more compact. Approximately 400 to 800 mL of water, along with sodium, chloride, and bicarbonate are absorbed out of the large intestine and approximately 5 mEq potassium is secreted into the lumen of the large intestine daily. Constituents of stool include approximately 100 mL of water and 25 to 50 g of solids consisting of remaining unabsorbed nutrients, sloughed epithelial cells, bile pigments, bacteria (30%), fat (10% to 20%), undigested dietary fiber (30%), and inorganic solids (20%). Water composes approximately 75% of stool content.

Normal adult stool appears firm and moist. The characteristic brown color is derived from the bilirubin pigment in bile, **stercobilin**. Chemical reactions resulting in the breakdown of fecal components during digestion produce compounds, including hydrogen sulfide, that provide the characteristic odor of feces. Upon defecation, stool is soft, moist and semisolid. Formed in the shape of the rectum, stool averages approximately one inch in diameter and should be easy to pass. The amount and frequency of defecation is variable among individuals, though the average for adults is a 200 to 300 g stool once per day.

The characteristics of stools in newborns and infants are quite different from those of adults. Many of these differences can be explained by the major sources of oral intake during development. In utero, the fetus swallows amniotic fluid, which passes through the GI system. Peristalsis and stool production are typical findings in the developing fetus. Normally, the fetus does not pass stool in utero, but is expected to pass the first stool in the early newborn period after birth. This first stool, **meconium**, represents the digestion of amniotic fluid and is sterile, black, sticky, and odorless. Once feedings are begun, the stool transitions to reflect the newborn's main source of oral intake. Breastfed babies have stool that is soft, unformed, and yellow. The odor is mild and uncharacteristic of a normal fecal scent. Babies fed artificial milk, or formula, have light brown stools. Frequency of bowel movements is often increased in breastfed babies due to the efficient digestion of breast milk, compared to the less frequent stooling patterns characteristic of formula-fed babies. As table foods and supplemental liquids are introduced in late infancy, stool patterns alter to reflect the composition of these ingested foods.

Stool analysis is based upon elimination patterns and characteristics. Laboratory analysis of stool may include microscopic examination or chemical evaluation. Color, consistency, volume, shape, and odor should be consistent with characteristics described previously. Stool should be free of blood, mucous, pus, and harmful parasites. Stool pH should be 6 and it should contain less than 2 mg of reducing factors (i.e., sugars).

Altered Bowel Elimination

Impaired large intestine function may alter the final steps of retrieval of water and electrolytes from the fecal matter that enters the cecum from the small intestine. Absorption of vitamins produced by intestinal bacterial flora may also be altered if there is impaired function of the large intestine. Further, the social and personal concerns regarding alteration in bowel elimination have the potential to impact quality of life.

Stool elimination is a part of daily life for all individuals. Even though stooling is a common activity for all, the process is impacted by perceptions of social acceptability. The social norms and rules of stool elimination may represent a major source of stress in individuals. Many people are concerned about the public perception of stooling and the associated odor that accompanies the process. Concern may be so great that they may attempt to override the need to pass stool until a private opportunity is available. Some individuals have great anxiety if they are unable to toilet in their home, leading to restricted travel and activities outside of their home environment.

PROCESSES OF ALTERED BOWEL ELIMINATION

The forward movement of the fecal matter is essential, propelling the intestinal contents towards the anus, leaving the body as stool through the process of defecation. Impaired bowel elimination often results from alterations in bowel motility, neuromuscular function, perfusion, or patency.

Alteration in Bowel Motility

Motility of the large intestine determines the rate that fecal matter passes through for evacuation. Increased motility may impair nutrition, preventing adequate opportunity for nutrient and water absorption, and it may enhance loss of water and electrolytes. Decreased motility prolongs storage time in the large intestine, promoting an enhanced loss of fluid from fecal matter and potentially promoting the return of waste products to the circulation. The composition of forms of bacterial intestinal flora may also influence motility of the large intestine, with *Lactobacillus acidophilus* and *Bifidobacterium bifidum* promoting motility, and *Escherichia coli* inhibiting motility. Diarrhea and constipation are the most common clinical manifestations of altered motility of the large intestine.

Factors that alter the transit time of stool also present potential stressors to the process of stool elimination. Certain foods may serve as irritants to the intestine, enhancing the speed that the feces moves from the cecum to the anus. Shortened transit time limits water absorption, leading to stool that is less formed due to the increased water content. Such stools are often passed with more frequency and urgency. In contrast, some individuals respond to particular foods with a slowed transit time, leading to increased water movement out of the feces. The result is often hard, formed stools with reduced frequency in elimination.

Alteration in Bowel Neuromuscular Function

Coordination of neurologic and muscular functional components is essential to optimal bowel function. Any alteration in neural signal transduction or muscle responsiveness may result in altered bowel function. Impaired function associated with loss of propulsive activity may result from abdominal surgery or from electrolyte imbalances affecting contractile function, peritonitis, or spinal trauma. Impaired motility is often seen as a side effect of narcotic analgesia. Emotional stress may alter stool elimination processes due to the influence of the central nervous system in the integrative processes involved in bowel function.

Reduced activity may also impact the process of stool elimination. Walking, running, swimming, and other active movements enhance neuromuscular activity and coordination in the large intestine, promoting peristalsis and bowel elimination. Loss of mobility often serves as a stressor to bowel elimination, leading to reduced intestinal smooth muscle contractions. As the time that feces remains in the large intestine increases, more water is removed and stool becomes harder. Further, the products of digestion in the form of gas build up, leading to distention of the abdomen and pain if the passing of flatus is impaired.

● **STOP** *and Consider*

What are some common reasons that intestinal mobility can be reduced, leading to slowed intestinal smooth muscle contraction?

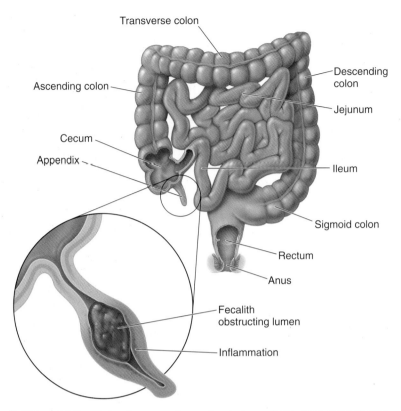

■ **Figure 16.9** Obstruction and inflammation in appendicitis. Fecal mass obstruction stimulates an inflammatory response, leading to appendicitis.

Alteration in Bowel Perfusion

A continous source of perfusion to the large intestine is essential for optimal cellular function. Disruption in perfusion may be the result of either focal or global etiologies (see Chapters 13 and 14). Perfusion can be reduced or absent to a portion of bowel as a result of obstructed flow from a variety of reasons, including a clot or pressure from a space-occupying mass. Erosion of blood vessels supplying perfusion to the intestine due to ulceration or trauma may also lead to impaired circulation. Ischemia resulting from impaired oxygenation is often manifested by pain and altered bowel function. If hypoxia persists, necrosis of cells and tissues may result.

Ventilation/perfusion mismatch, inadequate vascular volume, and inadequate cardiac output are common etiologies that may lead to global circulation deficits, denying perfusion to cells and tissues of the lower intestine. During times of circulatory challenge, blood is redistributed away from the digestive system to the vital organs. Altered perfusion may occur as a result of excessive perfusion demands, such as infection. A common infection of the GI system is appendicitis. Appendicitis is the result of trapped fecal material in the appendix of the colon (Fig. 16.9). The obstruction causes an inflammatory response, followed by infection. Once the obstruction is identified, surgical removal

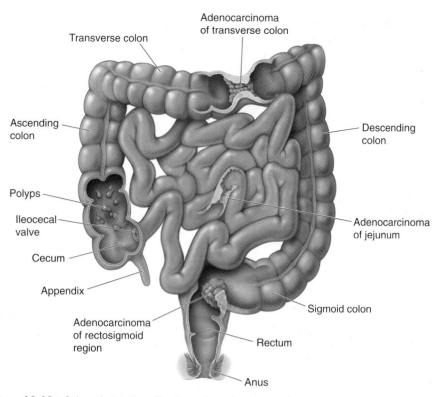

Transverse colon

Adenocarcinoma
of transverse colon

Ascending
colon

Descending
colon

Polyps

Ileocecal
valve

Cecum

Appendix

Adenocarcinoma
of jejunum

Adenocarcinoma
of rectosigmoid
region

Sigmoid colon

Rectum

Anus

■ **Figure 16.10**   Colon obstruction. The formation of polyps and tumors represents potential sites for obstruction along the length of the colon.

of the appendix is the method of treatment. Untreated, rupture of the appendix is likely to occur. Upon rupture, the bacterial flora escapes into the peritoneal cavity, resulting in peritonitis and septic shock. Reduced perfusion to all organ systems, especially the GI tract, results from septic shock.

Alteration in Bowel Patency

Bowel obstruction is due to a space-occupying lesion which blocks the intestinal lumen, either partially or totally. Common space-occupying lesions include tumors, polyps, and impacted feces (Fig. 16.10). Often associated with fluid and gas accumulation, bowel obstruction is manifested by abdominal distention and pain (see Table 16.2). When the space-occupying lesion impairs capacity for venous return, the development of edema in the wall of the large intestine leads to reducing the absorptive capacity. Edema promotes continued fluid and gas accumulation because of the movement of water and gas into the bowel lumen. Hydrostatic forces may increase so that fluid is forced through the bowel wall into the peritoneum. Further, bacteria may gain access to the circulation, promoting the development of sepsis. Perforation may result from pressure that exceeds the ability of the tissue to retain its structure.

General Manifestations of Altered Bowel Elimination

Identification of altered intestinal function can be accomplished by listening to bowel sounds. Bowel sounds are a reflection of intestinal smooth muscle contractions that are active intermittently. Bowel sounds can often be heard by the naked ear, but are more carefully evaluated through **auscultation**, or listening with a stethoscope. The quality, location, and frequency of bowel sounds provide an indication of peristaltic function.

The appearance of the abdomen is another indicator of bowel function. The abdomen should be soft when pressed or palpated and flat relative to body size. Abdominal size may increase due to the trapping of gas, leading to hardening and tightening of the abdomen. Typically, the gaseous byproducts of digestion, flatus, are passed, indicating bowel function. Often when stool transit is slowed due to slowed intestinal smooth muscle contraction and coordination, the gaseous products of digestion build and cause the abdomen to enlarge, or become distended.

The volume and characteristics of stool may be altered in conditions that affect the large intestine. Loose, watery stools are characteristic of diarrhea. Bowel inflammation, infection, and increased motility are often associated with diarrhea. Constipation, or absence of bowel movement, may be a consequence of impaired mobility or obstruction. In complete obstruction, fecal matter cannot pass beyond the obstruction. The characteristics of fecal matter passed in the presence of partial obstruction may provide clues as to the location of the obstruction. Obstructions occurring closest to the cecum may allow watery stool to pass because the water content of the stool is high. Partial obstructions located at the distal end of the colon may allow the passage of small quantities of harder, more solidly formed stool.

● STOP *and Consider*

Why would you expect stool in the ascending colon to have more water content than stool in the descending colon?

Stool may also have color changes characteristic of specific disease states. Bright red blood around stool or seen on toilet paper after defecation is generally caused by hemorrhoids. Hemorrhoids can be seen on the outside of the anus or they may be located internally. Larger amounts of frank red blood may indicate internal bleeding of a more serious nature, such as occurs in colon cancer. A darker pigment of red, or maroon, characterizes bleeding from a source in the midportion of the GI tract, such as that seen with diverticulitis (see clinical model, Diverticular Disease). Black stool (**melena**) also signifies a bleeding concern. The darkened color represents a source of bleeding higher up in the GI system. Blood in stools should be identified and a definitive cause determined because of the potential serious consequences of this sign.

● STOP *and Consider*

Why do bloody stools suggest the potential diagnosis of cancer?

Light-colored stools indicate the absence of bile pigments. This is a common finding associated with conditions of the accessory organs of the GI tract (pancreas, gall bladder, and liver). For example, the stool from a person infected with hepatitis may be white, gray, or yellow. Bile acids are absent in some malabsorption syndromes and are associated with large fat content, known as **steatorrhea**. Stools lacking bile pigments caused by obstruction of bile entry into the intestine may cause stools to have a "silver" color. Ampullary cancer is a pancreatic neoplasm that arises from the ampulla of Vater.[1] The ampulla of Vater is a small projection from the pancreas into the

duodenum, serving as the opening of the pancreatic and bile ducts. Obstruction of the ampulla of Vater blocks the entry of pancreatic and biliary secretions into the intestine. Manifestations of secretion blockage include jaundice caused by impaired bilirubin processing and elimination and light-colored "silver" stools caused by absence of bile in fecal matter.

Alterations in texture can provide information on a causative factor. These alterations include:

- Watery
  - Acute onset caused by gastroenteritis or anxiety
  - Chronic pattern linked to inflammatory conditions or a high-fiber diet; also caused by intolerance to particular foods or the effects of certain medications
- Hard
  - Water content low, resulting in a dry stool that is difficult to pass
  - May contribute to the development of hemorrhoids; linked to low-fiber diet, side effects of certain medications, or voluntary avoidance of stool evacuation
- Stringy
  - May be caused by parasitic infections
- Fatty
  - Caused by malabsorption of fat
  - Likely to float
- Foul odor
  - May be caused by steatorrhea, parasitic infection, or malabsorption syndromes

Pain is often a characteristic of intestinal disorders, although it seldom occurs without other symptoms. Origins of pain include mechanical, inflammatory, or ischemic causes. The biochemical mediators of pain (histamine, bradykinin, and serotonin) provide stimulation to nerve endings, resulting in the pain response (detailed in Chapter 10). Abdominal pain can be categorized into three main types:

1. Visceral
   - Characterized as diffuse, radiating, and generalized; difficult to determine precise location
   - Caused by stretching, distention, or inflammation, inducing edema and vascular congestion
2. Somatic (also known as parietal)
   - Described as sharp, intense, and localized to a specific site
   - Caused by injury to the abdominal wall or parietal peritoneum
3. Referred
   - Felt at a location different from origin of pain
   - Caused by the sharing of a common afferent pathway between origin of pain and referred location

Acute onset of pain is usually caused by a precipitating event, such as perforation. Persistent pain with a gradual onset is often associated with chronic conditions, such as ulcerative colitis.

Anorexia (loss of appetite) is often associated with nausea and vomiting. These symptoms are general and do not point to a specific condition. Abdominal distention often indicates increased pressure from fluid or feces in the bowel lumen, inflammation, and edema of the intestine, or increased production of gas. Fever is a common finding resulting from infection, such as **peritonitis** (inflammation of the peritoneal membrane).

Diagnosis of Bowel Conditions

Specific conditions can be identified by examination of stool. These conditions include allergy to a dietary substance (such as milk protein in infants), inflammation, infection, bleeding, or malabsorption. In cases of infection, stool can be examined to determine the specific organism involved. Many organisms are naturally found in the intestine (normal flora) and are important for specific GI functions. Harmful bacteria or parasites that infect the GI tract must be identified to determine the most effective treatment. Fat content can be determined to indicate the presence or absence of a disorder of malabsorption. These determinations may require either microscopic analysis or culture of stool. Determination of **occult** (too small to be seen) blood in stool can be made by placing a small sample on a collection card and applying a chemical solution. A color change indicates the presence or absence of blood. This test is commonly referred to as a *guaiac test.* Stool samples for microscopic analysis or culture should be collected in clean, dry, disposable containers. Immediate delivery to the laboratory provides the best conditions for analysis of the sample.

Mechanical obstructions resulting from growths extending into the colon lumen, including tumors or polyps, can be diagnosed using techniques that allow visualization of the colon lumen. Diagnostic tests for disorders of the colon include:

- *Barium enema:* Determination of colon and rectal anatomic abnormalities with the aid of contrast medium (barium) inserted via the anus. Visualization of the rectum and colon is completed by radiograph. Common conditions identified include diverticulitis, alterations in motility, obstruction, and colon dimensions.
- *Sigmoidoscopy:* Insertion of a flexible tube into the anus to visualize the rectum and the lower colon. This diagnostic test may be indicated for manifestations of bleeding, altered bowel habits, rectal pain, and diarrhea.
- *Colonoscopy:* Insertion of a flexible tube into the anus for observation of the entire colon, from the small intestine to the rectum. This test is often done in response to manifestations of abdominal pain, diarrhea, alteration in bowel habits, or as a follow-up to an abnormality found during another procedure, such as the barium enema or computed tomography scan.

Treatment of Altered Bowel Elimination

Similar to treatment of altered urinary elimination, treatment of conditions causing altered GI elimination is determined by the condition underlying the clinical manifestations. Diarrhea, a form of excessive GI elimination, may be associated with impaired regulation of fluid balance. Diarrhea may result from a variety of primary conditions, or it may represent an adverse effect of treatment. Pharmacotherapy may be used to diminish excessive fluid loss from diarrhea. Antidiarrheal drugs work by:

- Slowing the passage of stool through the intestine
  - Antimotility agents (Imodium)
    - Promotes water removal from fecal matter
    - Useful for chronic conditions
- Moving diarrhea-causing factors out of the stool
  - Adsorbents (Kaopectate)
    - May also pull out other essential products
- Decreasing secretion of fluid into intestine
  - Reduce inflammatory response to pathogens (antibiotics)
    - Decreases fluid movement into intestinal contents
- Using bulk-forming agents
  - Absorbs excess fluid (psyllium)
    - Firms stool

Constipation can be managed with exercise, high dietary fiber, adequate fluid intake, stool softeners, laxatives, and enemas. Bulk-forming laxatives absorb water from the intestine to make stool softer. Stimulants promote peristalsis, enhancing propulsion of fecal matter through the colon. Stool softeners promote moisture content in stool without the stimulant effect. Lubricants promote smoother passage and evacuation of fecal matter. Saline laxatives work by attracting water into the colon.

Table 16.4 Impact of Selected Intestinal Conditions on the Health of Individuals

Condition	Incidence/ Prevalence	Mortality	Hospitalizations	Ambulatory Care Visits (per year)	Disability (persons affected)
Hemorrhoids	8.5 million (prevalence)	18	168,000	1.9 million	38,000
Constipation	3.1 million (prevalence)	121	398,000	1.4 million	30,000
Infectious diarrhea	16 million (incidence)	2,481	375,000–777,000	8–12 million	Not reported
Irritable bowel syndrome	2.1 million (prevalence)	22	119,000	1.3 million	46,000
Abdominal wall hernia	4.5 million	1,143	322,000	3.3 million	467,000
Diverticular disease	2.5 million	3,324	576,000	1.2 million	86,000

Available at: http://digestive.niddk.nih.gov/statistics/statistics.htm#specific. Accessed on February 5, 2010.

Obstructive abnormalities may require surgical treatment for removal. Alterations in neuromuscular function may require assistive devices or bladder/bowel training programs for elimination of urine and stool.

Trends for selected conditions related to large intestine impairment are provided in Table 16.4, based on information from the National Institutes of Diabetes and Digestive and Kidney Diseases (NIDDK).

Clinical Models

The following clinical models have been selected to aid in the understanding and application of altered elimination. The student should pay attention to the commonalities and unique features of each condition when studying these models. Alterations in elimination often lead to physical and emotional distress and disruption of daily life. Processes leading to altered elimination are summarized in Figure 16.11.

Urolithiasis

Urolithiasis, commonly known as kidney stones, is the development of calculi in the renal system.[1] Renal calculi are solid masses, often composed of salts, and inorganic or organic acids, which precipitate out of urinary filtrate. The diagnosis of kidney stones represents one of the most prevalent conditions of the urinary tract system. The condition occurs more frequently in men compared to women, and in Caucasians compared to African Americans.[2] Recent trends link increasing rates among women to obesity, diabetes mellitus, and metabolic syndrome, decreasing the male to female ratio to 1.7:1.[3]

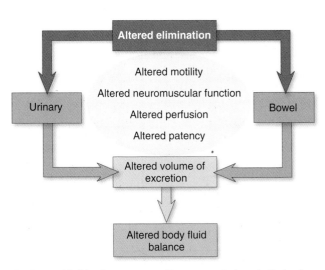

Figure 16.11 Concept map. Processes of altered elimination.

PATHOPHYSIOLOGY

Calcium (oxalate and phosphate) is the most common component of stones, which may also form because of magnesium ammonium phosphate (**struvite**), uric acid, or cystine. Elevated urinary levels

Figure 16.12   Common forms of renal calculi. **A:** Uric acid/urate stones. **B:** Magnesium ammonium phosphate (struvite) stones. **C:** Calcium oxalate/calcium phosphate stones. (Images courtesy Anatomical Chart Company.)

of these substances or stasis from urinary filtrate may promote development of calculi. As stones progress through the urinary system, from the renal tubules to the urethra, they often result in obstruction of these narrow lumen structures.

Individuals at risk for development of kidney stones include those with:

- Genetic predisposition
- Urinary tract infection
- Cystic kidney disease
- Hyperparathyroidism
- Hypercalciuria

● **STOP** and *Consider*

Why are people with hyperparathyroidism and hypercalciuria at risk for development of renal calculi?

CLINICAL MANIFESTATIONS

The most obvious clinical manifestation of kidney stones is pain. This pain is characterized as severe and shooting and is localized in the lateral aspect of the lower back (flank) at the CVA. Pain can be further described in two ways:

1. Colic
   - Caused by stretching of the collecting system or ureter from the obstructed flow
   - Characterized as acute, intermittent, radiating, and excruciating
2. Noncolic
   - Caused by distention of renal calices or pelvis
   - Characterized as dull and deep
   - Ranging in intensity from mild to severe

DIAGNOSTIC CRITERIA

Imaging of the renal calculi with computed tomography (CT), renal ultrasonogrphy, or IVP is the preferred approach for diagnosis. Diagnosis of renal

calculi can also be made using a routine radiograph because most stones are radiopaque. IVP may be used to obtain information about the collecting system and ureters because the contrast media is filtered by the glomerulus and can be tracked through the urinary system. Hydronephrosis can be detected using ultrasound to provide additional information about the consequences of the obstruction.

Determination of underlying causes contributing to stone development and the composition of the stone itself helps establish effective treatment. Individuals are often provided a device that strains the urine, collecting any stones that are excreted. The stones can then be analyzed to determine the content and infer cause. Types of calculi are shown in Figure 16.12 and include:

- Calcium oxalate and phosphate
   - Hypercalcemia/hypercalciuria
   - Immobility
   - Renal tubular acidosis
- Magnesium ammonium phosphate/struvite
   - Urinary tract infection
- Uric acid/urate
   - Precipitated in acidic urine (pH of 5.5 or less)
   - Diet high in purines
   - Gout

TREATMENT

Treatment of calculi involves supportive care, including pain control. Fluids may be encouraged to promote filtrate flow and movement of stone through the urinary system. If stones do not pass spontaneously, removal of calculi is often necessary to prevent damage to renal structures. The indications for surgical removal include:[4]

- Retaining the stone and constant pain over a reasonable period
- Stone size too large to pass
- Obstructing urine flow
- Causing ongoing urinary tract infection

- Causing damage to kidney or evidence of constant hematuria
- Continuing to grow in size

Surgical procedures to remove kidney stones are selected in consideration of the greatest effectiveness and lowest complication rate to achieve desired result.[5] **Extracorporeal shockwave lithotripsy (ESWL)** is the most common procedure for kidney stone removal. Large stones are localized by ultrasound or radiograph and then are broken down into small, sandlike bits using acoustic shock waves. The decreased size promotes spontaneous passage of the

- Beets
- Chocolate
- Coffee
- Cola
- Nuts
- Rhubarb
- Spinach
- Strawberries
- Tea
- Wheat bran

Combining calcium restriction with diuretic therapy promotes movement of filtrate through the renal system, reducing the likelihood of calculi development. Treatment and prevention of urinary tract infections may decrease the risk for struvite-based calculi. Management of primary conditions, such as gout and hyperparathyroidism, reduces the availability of the minerals and alters pH, reducing the risk of calculi formation.

From the Lab

Urinalysis in a person with renal calculi may show hematuria, infection, crystals, or altered urine pH. The urinalysis findings may provide clues about the cause of calculi formation, which is useful in directing treatment strategies.

stone in the urine. Passage is occasionally assisted by placing a stent (a small tube) through the bladder into the ureter. This procedure is useful when stones are located in the renal calyx, pelvis, and upper third of the ureter. **Percutaneous nephrolithotomy** is a surgical procedure used when the stone is too large for ESWL. The stone is located and removed using a nephroscope, inserted into the kidney through a small flank incision. Stones too large for removal are fragmented using an energy probe. The insertion of a nephrostomy tube assists in healing after the procedure. **Ureteroscopic stone removal** is used when stones are located in the mid or distal portions of the ureters. Calculi removal is accomplished through a ureteroscope placed into the ureter through the urethra and bladder. After localization, the stone is removed or fragmented with a shock wave device. Placement of a ureteral stent is often done along with this procedure.

Prevention strategies to avoid development and recurrence of calculi in high-risk individuals may be useful. Adequate fluid intake and alkalinization of urine are strategies that can be used in prevention of renal calculi as they reduce urine saturation and precipitation of calcium-forming salts.[6] Diet manipulation to increase fluid intake, reduce dietary oxalate, and limit sodium intake to 2 to 3 g/day may decrease risk for calculi development. Restriction of dietary calcium is not associated with reduced risk of calculi formation in most cases.[7] Foods high in oxalate should be avoided in persons with calcium oxalate-based stones. These foods include:

Urinary Incontinence

Urinary incontinence, or **enuresis**, is defined as the inability to voluntarily prevent the discharge of urine. A symptom rather than a diagnosis, urinary incontinence is often the manifestation of conditions that alter the structure or function of the urinary tract. Urinary incontinence is often considered a women's disease, although it is known to occur in 17% of an estimated 34 million men older than 60 years in the United States.[8] It is estimated that up to 75% of women in the United States report occasional urinary leakage, with 20% to 50% reporting more frequent leakage.[9,10]

PATHOPHYSIOLOGY

A variety of processes can impair voiding, including those involving muscular contraction, neural transmission, hormonal stimulation, or mechanical factors. In women, relaxation of pelvic structures may occur, especially after pregnancy. Male incontinence may be caused by mechanical obstruction by the prostate on the penile urethra. In both genders, neurologic diseases, including Parkinson disease, multiple sclerosis, spinal cord injury, and stroke, may contribute to voiding dysfunction. Advancing age and loss of mobility and dexterity may also contribute to functional incontinence.

A detailed history about the specific characteristics of the incontinence is critical to the determination of incontinence type, which also affects the choice of treatment modalities. The patient should keep a record, or voiding diary, on urinary frequency, leakage, voiding volumes, and fluid intake. This record should span at least 3 days, but 1 week is preferable to accurately identify patterns. Leakage can also be quantified by a pad count or weight, providing details of volume.

CLINICAL MANIFESTATIONS

Temporary incontinence may result from the use of certain medications or from illness, immobility, or constipation. Chronic types of incontinence can be classified into four different forms. **Stress incontinence** occurs because of an exertional stimulus. The stimulus may be as benign as coughing, sneezing, or laughing. Other exertional activities that prompt incontinence include exercise or lifting objects. Impaired sphincter function and control is often associated with stress incontinence. **Urge incontinence**, also known as **overactive bladder**, refers to urine leaking that is accompanied or immediately preceded by a strong urge to void (urgency), nocturia, and frequency.[11] This impulse is often so sudden that incontinence results before the individual can toilet. Overactivity of the detrusor muscle of the bladder is responsible for this type of incontinence. Often, individuals may have a mix of symptoms of both urge and stress incontinence. Incontinence may also result from urine volumes exceeding bladder capacity, known as **overflow incontinence**. **Functional incontinence** is characterized by normal bladder control coupled with an impaired ability to transport to toilet facilities, such as with impaired mobility. Incontinence can be classified further as nocturnal enuresis, continuous leakage, postvoid dribble, and extraurethral (urine loss through fistula) incontinence.

DIAGNOSTIC CRITERIA

Diagnosis is based on careful history in addition to physical examination and specialized testing. Urodynamic and endoscopic testing, in addition to the imaging studies previously described, may be used to establish an accurate diagnosis. The following are tests and diagnostic findings for incontinence:

- Post residual volume (PRV)
  - After voiding, residual urine in the bladder is measured
  - PRV of less than 50 mL indicates adequate bladder emptying
- Urodynamic testing
  - Cystometry
    - Measures anatomic and functional ability of the bladder and urethra
    - Measures capacity of the bladder, providing evaluation of the function of the detrusor muscle
  - Cystometrogram
    - Measures pressures of the total bladder, detrusor, and intraabdomen
  - Voiding cystometrogram
    - Identifies outlet obstruction during voiding
- Endoscopic tests
  - Cystoscopy
    - Visualizes bladder mucosa to identify the presence of lesions

TREATMENT

Treatment for incontinence reflects behavioral strategies, use of medication, and surgery. Assistance with toileting, **bladder training** (learning to hold urine for increasing intervals), intravaginal support devices, and strengthening of the pelvic muscles are common strategies used for functional and stress incontinence. Pelvic muscles can be strengthened by Kegel exercises, vaginal weights, and electrical stimulation. Anticholinergic medications help urge incontinence because they decrease the contractile force of the detrusor muscle. Improved urethral tone can be assisted by the use of α-adrenergic antagonist drugs to improve tone and contractile function.

In females, surgical correction for renewed anatomic support can be performed with an abdominal bladder suspension. Also known as the Burch or Marshall–Marchetti–Krantz (MMK) procedure, the bladder and urethra are returned to their normal position, promoting increased voluntary control of urine. This procedure can be done through an abdominal incision or it can be done laparoscopically. Another procedure, the sling procedure, places support material directly under the urethra and attaches to abdominal muscle connective tissue. One of the newest procedures, the tension-free vaginal tape procedure uses a thin strip of supporting tape to form a hammock under the urethra. This procedure, similar to the sling procedure, is performed through a small incision in the vagina. These procedures are intended to support the urethra during strain that would induce stress incontinence. Surgical techniques in males with incontinence are designed to remove mechanical obstruction of the urethra from an enlarged prostate.

Polycystic Kidney Disease

Polycystic kidney disease (PKD) is a condition characterized by growth of fluid-filled cysts in kidney tissue bilaterally, leading to progressive loss of renal nephrons. PKD may be inherited or acquired. The inherited form of PKD is the most common genetic cause of chronic kidney disease.[12] The progressive nature of PKD may result in increasing loss of renal function, leading to renal failure. Of the primary conditions associated with need for treatment of end-stage renal disease among over 500,000 US residents in 2006, PKD represented the fourth leading cause.[13]

PATHOPHYSIOLOGY

Cysts of increasing size and number replace functional tissue, leading to end-stage renal disease. Pressure on renal blood vessels obstructs perfusion, leading to tissue degeneration and obstructed tubular flow (Fig. 16.13). A variable pattern of cyst involvement exists in nephrons—cyst-affected nephrons are interspersed with normal, unaffected nephrons.

Three categories of PKD are known:

1. Genetic, autosomal dominant
2. Genetic, autosomal recessive
3. Acquired

The autosomal dominant form of PKD is the most common inherited form, accounting for 90% of PKD cases. Genetic mutations in the *PKD1* and *PKD2* genes lead to altered protein production of polycystin-1 and polycystin-2. The less common recessive form is the result of mutations in the *PKHD1* gene, encoding the fibrocystin protein. Clinical manifestations of kidney disease usually appear between the ages of 30 and 40 years in the autosomal dominant form, although individuals can have symptoms at a younger age. Symptoms appear early in the autosomal-recessive form of PKD, usually in the early infant period or even during fetal life. PKD can also be acquired, which is usually associated with other long-term kidney problems. Evidence of this form of PKD does not present until much later in life and is more frequent among the elderly.

Cysts begin to grow in the nephrons of the kidney, filling with glomerular filtrate, eventually growing larger and moving away into adjacent tissue. Kidney size increases in proportion to the size and number of cysts, which can number into the thousands (Fig. 16.14). One of the earliest manifestations of the disease is hypertension from compression of the renal vessels and subsequent

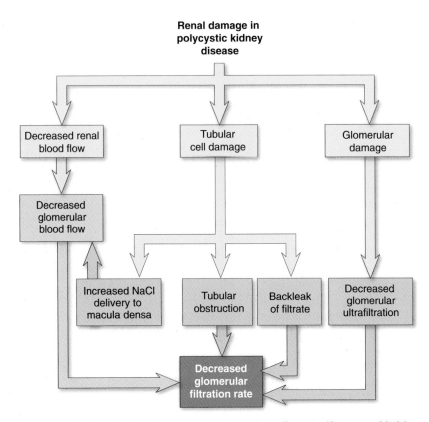

■ **Figure 16.13** Renal damage in polycystic kidney disease. (Asset provided by Anatomical Chart Company.)

activation of the RAAS (see Chapter 8). Other common symptoms include:

- Flank pain
- Headaches
- Nausea and anorexia
- Urinary tract infection
- Liver and pancreatic cysts
- Cardiac valvular disease
- Hypertension
- Renal calculi
- Cerebral aneurysms
- Diverticular disease

Accumulation of nitrogenous wastes, altered fluid/electrolyte balance, and impaired function in multiple organ systems become evident as renal function worsens.

DIAGNOSTIC CRITERIA

PKD diagnosis is confirmed by the presence of three or more kidney cysts verified by ultrasound. Family history of PKD and extrarenal cysts also suggest PKD. Progression of the disease may be slow, delaying onset of symptoms. Genetic testing may also be useful in detecting mutations in genes associated with the disease, such as *PKD1* (chromosome 16) and *PKD2* (chromosome 4). These

Cross section

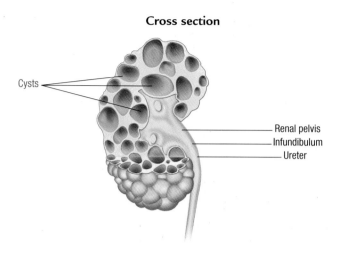

Cysts

Renal pelvis
Infundibulum
Ureter

■ **Figure 16.14** Polycystic kidney. Cysts in nephrons and in the renal cortex alter renal function. (Asset provided by Anatomical Chart Company.)

findings are limited to determining diagnosis but do not indicate prognosis.

TREATMENT

Treatment of PKD includes symptomatic care, strategies to promote renal function, and supportive care during end-stage renal disease. In autosomal dominant PKD, kidney transplantation is indicated.[14] Pain is controlled by analgesics. Urinary tract infections are treated with antibiotics, but they do present challenges because the pathogens can ascend more easily and are more difficult to treat (antibiotics have poor penetration into the cystic tissue). Control of blood pressure using angiotensin-converting enzyme inhibitor and angiotensin receptor blocker antihypertensive agents may slow the progression of the disease. Novel treatments in development target pathways that lead to cell proliferation, differentiation, and fluid secretion.[12]

The progression of disease over time may result in chronic renal failure (Fig. 16.15). End-stage renal disease requires dialysis or transplant for individuals to survive. Dialysis options include hemodialysis and peritoneal dialysis. **Hemodialysis** uses special filters through the mechanisms of diffusion, osmosis, and ultrafiltration to remove wastes that the kidneys no longer can remove on their own. This procedure requires access to the blood supply so that blood can travel through a set of tubes into a dialyzer, where waste products and excess water are removed. All

molecules with the exception of blood cells and plasma proteins can move freely between the semipermeable filter membrane between the blood and dialysis fluid. The purified blood is then returned through another set of tubes back into the body for circulation (Fig. 16.16). Treatments are scheduled for three times per week, each lasting 3 to 5 hours. Access to blood can be achieved by the surgical attachment of an artery to a vein, known as an **arteriovenous (AV) fistula**. The blood pressure from the artery enlarges the more passive vein, making it an ideal structure for repeated venipuncture (needle insertion). This procedure requires enough time for adequate enlargement of the vein, limiting its immediate use. Another method used to obtain access to the blood supply is a graft or **arteriovenous shunt**, connecting the artery to the vein using a synthetic tube. This method can be used more quickly, but it carries an increased risk for clot development and infection. Heparin, an anticoagulant, is used during dialysis to prevent the formation of clots during the procedure. Hemodialysis can be done either at a dialysis center or at home with proper patient training.

Peritoneal dialysis provides another option for treatment in renal failure. Waste and excess water is removed using the peritoneal membrane as the semipermeable "filter," with the same transport mechanisms used in hemodialysis. Solution designed to draw out wastes from small capillaries in the peritoneum is inserted into the abdomen via a tube, previously placed surgically. After several hours, this solution is drained and discarded along with the waste products, and water is removed. This cycle is considered an exchange. Risks include peritonitis, which is minimized with the use of sterile technique. The types of peritoneal dialysis include:

- Continuous ambulatory peritoneal dialysis (CAPD)
  - Most common type

From the Lab

Glomerular filtration can indicate the development and progression of renal failure. GFR normally ranges between 120 and 130 mL/min, with a GFR ≥ 90 mL/min considered within normal limits. Progressive decline in GFR is characteristic of decline in kidney function as follows:

- Mild disease, GFR 60 to 89 mL/min
- Moderate disease, GFR 30 to 59 mL/min
- Severe disease, GFR 15 to 29 mL/min
- Renal failure, GFR < 15 mL/min

Blood urea nitrogen, serum creatinine, and potassium levels become elevated. Decreased hemoglobin, arterial pH, and bicarbonate also indicate worsening renal function.

Chronic renal failure

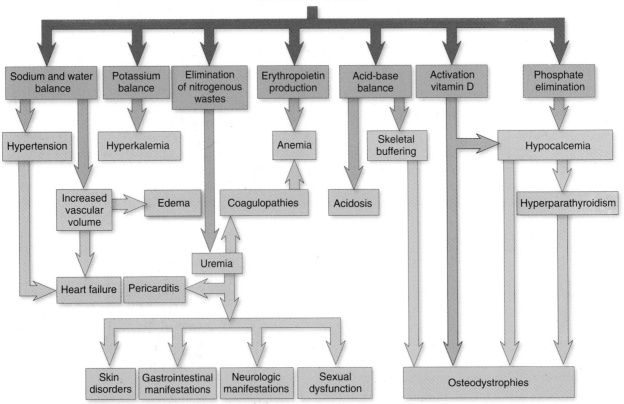

■ **Figure 16.15**   Pathophysiology of chronic renal failure. Clinical manifestations are present in multiple organ systems as a result of renal failure. (Image modified from Porth CM. *Pathophysiology: Concepts of Altered Health States.* 7th ed. Philadelphia: Lippincott Williams & Wilkins; 2004, with permission.)

■ Dialysis fluid is inserted into the abdomen, where it remains for 4 to 6 hours (dwell time), followed by drainage
■ Repeated with fresh dialysis solution up to four times a day on a daily basis
● Continuous cycler-assisted peritoneal dialysis (CCPD)
■ A special machine (cycler) fills and empties abdomen of dialysis fluid three to five times a night during sleep
■ Fluid is inserted in the morning with a dwell time lasting the entire day
● Combination CAPD and CCPD

Individuals who require dialysis should eat a diet low in products likely to produce harmful waste. Recommendations for diet include:

● Balanced amounts of protein (chicken, meat, and fish)
● Low potassium, sodium, and phosphorus
● Fluid restriction

Kidney transplant may be necessary in severe cases of PKD. The sources of the kidney can be from a family member (living, related donor), another person not related (living, unrelated donor), or from a person who recently died (deceased donor). One of the greatest risks in transplantation is that of rejection, as detailed in Chapter 4. Factors considered when determining a match or lower risk of rejection include:

● Blood type
■ Most important aspect
■ Must be compatible
● Human leukocyte antigens (HLAs)
■ A total of six HLAs exist
■ Risk of rejection is decreased with increased number of HLA matches
● Cross-matching antigens
■ Antigen–antibody reactions between donor and recipient blood
■ Risk of rejection is decreased in the absence of reaction (negative cross-match)

Figure 16.16 Hemodialysis. **A:** Hemodialysis uses special filters to remove wastes that the kidneys no longer can do on their own through the mechanisms of diffusion, osmosis, and ultrafiltration. **B:** Arteriovenous fistula. **C:** Arteriovenous shunt.

Immunosuppressant administration helps decrease rejection risk after surgery.

STOP *and Consider*

Why do individuals suffering from renal failure become anemic?

Diverticular Disease

Diverticular disease affects the large intestine. Processes that characterize diverticular disease include decreased motility, obstruction, and impaired perfusion.

PATHOPHYSIOLOGY

A **diverticulum** (small sac or outpouching) forms along the wall of the colon, most often in the ascending colon. Typically, diverticulum develops at a site of weakness in the intestinal wall. More than one diverticulum is called **diverticula**. The presence of diverticula is commonly referred to as the condition **diverticulosis**. Fecal matter caught in sacs may promote the development of infection, known as **diverticulitis**. Herniation of the diverticulum makes the blood vessels supplying the intestinal wall susceptible to trauma and bleeding.[15]

Chronic constipation is linked to the development of diverticular disease. Slow movement of fecal matter leads to increased, prolonged pressure on the walls of the large intestine, altering structure and function. Most people are unaware of the problem until it leads to bleeding, infection, obstruction, and ischemia of the affected area of the colon. Perforation resulting from these processes results in hemorrhage, abscess, sepsis, or peritonitis (Fig. 16.17).

CLINICAL MANIFESTATIONS

Clinical manifestations of diverticulitis mirror those described earlier under general manifestations and include abdominal pain, fever, nausea, and vomiting. Symptoms are often severe enough to prompt medical attention. Sudden onset of rectal bleeding may occur when blood vessels are injured.

DIAGNOSTIC CRITERIA

Acute diverticulitis is determined by examination of stool for blood, evaluation of blood samples for anemia and signs of active infection, or identification of inflamed or ruptured sacs using radiograph, ultrasound, or computed tomography scan. Once the acute infection has resolved, diverticula can be evaluated with a barium enema, flexible sigmoidoscopy, or colonoscopy.

TREATMENT

Immediate treatment goals include control of infection, resting of the bowel, and prevention of complications. Prevention involves dietary and lifestyle alterations designed to prevent constipation. These strategies include:

- Diet high in fiber and low in fat
- Avoidance of foods that may lead to constipation, such as bananas and rice
- Avoidance of foods more likely to be retained in diverticula, including nuts, seeds, and strawberries

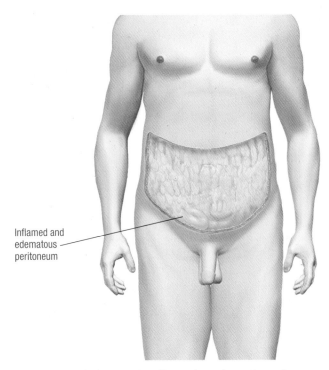

Inflamed and edematous peritoneum

■ **Figure 16.17** Peritonitis. The peritoneal membrane becomes edematous and inflamed in peritonitis. (Asset provided by Anatomical Chart Company.)

- Fluid intake, preferably water, of at least 2 L/day
- Daily exercise

Pharmacotherapy may include the use of bulk-forming laxatives and antispasmodic drugs for abdominal cramping. Surgical treatment may be required for emergencies, including perforation or infarction of diverticula. **Bowel resection**, or removal of a portion of the large intestine, may be required. A **colostomy** (establishment of an artificial opening of the large intestine externally on the abdomen) may be required as a temporary measure until the colon is healed, at which time it may be reconnected (reanastomosis). Oral intake is withheld after surgery because of the expected decrease in motility common after abdominal surgery. Oral intake slowly resumes after assurance of the return of bowel function, indicated by the presence of bowel sounds and the passing of flatus (gas passed through the anus). Introduction of food or fluid into the GI tract before this time may result in a **paralytic ileus**, a nonmechanical bowel obstruction characterized by a lack of peristalsis.

Encopresis

Encopresis is a condition of fecal incontinence characterized by inappropriate fecal soiling, frequently seen in the pediatric population. Fecal loss usually occurs while the child is dressed; it is therefore often captured in the underwear. Impaired defecation accounts for approximately 25% of visits to pediatric gastroenterologists[16] and 3% of pediatric outpatient visits.[17] Encopresis is four times more common among males compared to females.[18] Research on the topic of encopresis highlights the voluntary control mechanisms that can be used to impair stool elimination.

PATHOPHYSIOLOGY

Also known as **functional nonretentive soiling**, encopresis accounts for up to 20% of all cases of fecal incontinence.[19] Fecal soiling is usually accompanied by normal daily bowel movements; an organic cause is infrequent. Evacuation of stool is either voluntary or involuntary and occurs in the absence of an appropriate toileting situation. More often, nonretentive fecal soiling results from resistant behaviors in the child or ineffective toilet-training management strategies in the parents.[19] **Retentive incontinence** may be caused by withholding of feces from fear of pain on defecation, resulting in constipation and overflow soiling.[18]

CLINICAL MANIFESTATIONS

Symptom-based diagnostic classifications, known as the Rome II criteria, were developed to help recognize and treat defecation and other GI disorders.[20] Criteria for diagnosis of functional nonretentive encopresis have been developed based on clinical manifestations and stool patterns. The Rome II diagnostic classifications include age of more than 4 years and incontinence occurring at least once per week.[17] In addition, there should be a history of the following:

- Defecation at a time or place that is socially inappropriate
- Absence of organic disease
- Absence of retentive posturing (purposeful avoidance of defecation by voluntary contraction of the pelvic floor and buttocks)

DIAGNOSTIC CRITERIA

It is important to determine the cause of encopresis and characteristics of incontinence. Identification of a potential medical, developmental, or behavioral pathology is the first step in finding a specific diagnosis. A history of incontinence is examined, including stool pattern (size, consistency, and interval), evidence of constipation, factors related to soiling episodes (age of onset, type, and amount), diet history, associated pain, current medications, associated urinary symptoms (enuresis, infection),

family history of constipation, and emotional stress. Developmental readiness for toileting is also important to evaluate. Physical examination, including neurologic examination, may point to an anatomic or functional condition. Most cases of retentive encopresis are caused by functional constipation, whereas nonretentive encopresis is usually caused by nonorganic factors. Consideration must be given to the presence of neurogenic, neuromuscular, endocrine, or anatomic conditions to make these determinations.

TREATMENT

Behaviors contributing to toilet-refusal behavior should be addressed, and strategies should be used to promote positive, more enjoyable toileting experiences. Methods promoting soft stool minimize discomfort during defecation, helping individuals to overcome the fear of pain-associated bowel movements. Another effective strategy includes having scheduled time on the toilet and creating a relaxed atmosphere that promotes bowel training and effective toileting skills. Incentives for positive experiences may motivate the child and promote eventual self-initiation of bowel movements. Mental health analysis to explore roots of oppositional and defiant behaviors must also be considered.

● **STOP** and *Consider*

Why is the diagnosis of nonretentive encopresis limited to children at least 4 years of age?

▨ Summary

- Alterations in elimination can develop because of the processes regulating production or elimination of urine and stool, causing symptoms ranging from inconvenient to life threatening.
- Urine is a product of the renal system, composed of water and water-soluble waste products filtered from the circulation. Characteristics can provide evidence of altered elimination processes.
- Transport processes throughout the nephron contribute to the characteristics of urine filtrate.
- The renal system is important in the regulation of body fluid volume and composition, elimination of metabolic wastes, regulation of blood pressure and the synthesis, and release or activation of hormones.
- Stool is the waste product eliminated by the GI tract. Stool characteristics and patterns provide evidence of altered processes of GI elimination.
- Urinary and stool elimination may be impaired because of alterations in motility, neuromuscular function, perfusion, and patency. Manifestations

can include altered volume and color, bleeding, pain, distention, and anorexia.

- Diagnostic strategies include analysis of urine and stool content and testing for structural anomalies.
- Impaired elimination can be the cause of other body system alterations, and it can contribute to the development of impairment in other systems as well. A thorough understanding of these altered processes helps to rapidly identify and effectively manage related conditions.

■ Case Study 16.1

A female neonate was born 8 weeks premature at 32 weeks' gestation. She is currently 3 weeks of age and has recently advanced to oral feedings with artificial infant formula as her sole source of nutrition. She developed symptoms that suggest that she is developing necrotizing enterocolitis (NEC). From your reading on NEC, answer the following questions:

1. *What anatomical problem would most likely lead to the symptoms associated with NEC?*
2. *What causes the underlying pathology associated with NEC?*
3. *What are the risk factors for this neonate that would suggest NEC?*
4. *What are the clinical manifestations you would expect with NEC?*
5. *What diagnostic tests might be used to identify NEC?*
6. *How would you manage an infant with NEC?*

Log onto the Internet. Search for a relevant journal article or Web site that details NEC to confirm your predictions.

Practice Exam Questions

1. Which of the following provides the most objective measurement of renal dysfunction?
   a. White blood cell count
   b. Glomerular filtration rate
   c. Altered urinary electrolytes
   d. Presence of nitrites in urine

2. A characteristic change in stool that may indicate the presence of blood includes which one of the following?
   a. Melena   c. Floating
   b. Hematuria   d. Gray-like color

3. Which of the following diagnostic procedures allows analysis of the entire large colon?
   a. Barium enema
   b. Flexible sigmoidoscopy
   c. Flexible gastroscopy
   d. Colonoscopy

4. Which of the following foods should be avoided in people with renal calculi?
   a. Grape juice   c. Strawberries
   b. Ground beef   d. Cinnamon

5. Which of the following foods should be avoided in people with diverticular disease?
   a. Grape juice   c. Strawberries
   b. Ground beef   d. Cinnamon

6. Which type of urinary incontinence can be attributed to muscle overactivity?

   a. Stress incontinence
   b. Urge incontinence
   c. Overflow incontinence
   d. Functional incontinence

7. The enteric nervous system component located between the circular and longitudinal muscle layers of the large intestine:
   a. Myenteric plexus   c. Meissner Plexus
   b. Submucosal plexus   d. Solar Plexus

8. The area of the large intestine that absorbs the majority of water is the:
   a. Ileum   c. Descending colon
   b. Ascending colon   d. Rectum

9. The process by which fecal contents enters the rectum is known as:
   a. Peristalsis
   b. Segmental contractions
   c. Mass movement
   d. Tetany

10. The average volume of urine eliminated each day totals:
    a. 200 mL   c. 1500 mL
    b. 800 mL   d. 3000 mL

11. The_____ sphincter is made of skeletal muscle and is under voluntary control.
    a. Internal   c. Anterior
    b. External   d. Posterior

12. Urine specific gravity of 1:030 indicates:
    a. Concentrated urine
    b. Dilute urine
    c. Urine high in bacteria
    d. Casts in urine

13. Which of the following diagnostic criteria is consistent with the diagnosis of encopresis?
    a. Age of 1 year
    b. Age of 3 years
    c. Age of 5 years
    d. All of the above

14. A GFR of 95 mL/min indicates
    a. Normal renal function
    b. Mild renal disease
    c. Moderate renal disease
    d. Severe renal disease

15. Which of the following increases the risk for renal calculi?
    a. Running 5 miles
    b. Drinking 32 ounces of milk per day
    c. Sedentary lifestyle
    d. Dehydration

Discussion and Application

1. What did I know about altered elimination before today?

2. What body processes are affected by altered elimination? How does altered elimination affect those processes?

3. What are the potential etiologies for altered elimination? How does altered elimination develop?

4. Who is most at risk for developing altered elimination? How can these alterations be prevented?

5. What are the human differences that affect the etiology, risk, or course of altered elimination?

6. What clinical manifestations are expected in the course of altered elimination?

7. What special diagnostic tests are useful in determining the diagnosis and course of altered elimination?

8. What are the goals of care for individuals with altered elimination?

9. How does the concept of altered elimination build on what I have learned in the previous chapter and in the previous courses?

10. How can I use what I have learned?

RESOURCES

National Kidney and Urologic Diseases Information Clearinghouse:
http://kidney.niddk.nih.gov/index.htm

National Institute of Diabetes and Digestive and Kidney Disease, National Institutes of Health:
http://www.niddk.nih.gov

REFERENCES

1. Hartel M, Wente MN, Sido B, et al. Carcinoid of the ampulla of Vater. *J Gastroenterol Hepatol.* 2005;20(5):676–681.
2. Reed BY, Heller HJ, Gitomer WL, et al. Mapping a gene defect in absorptive hypercalciuria to chromosome 1q23.3–q24. *J Clin Endocrinol Metab.* 1999;84(11):3907–3913.
3. Zilberman DE, Yong D, Albala DM. The impact of society changes on patterns of urolithiasis. *Curr Opin Urol.* 2010;20(2):148–153.
4. Hall PM. Nephrolithiasis: treatment, causes and prevention. *Cleve Clin J Med.* 2009;76(10):583–591.
5. Srisubat A, Potisat S, Lojanapiwat B, et al. Extracorporeal shock wave lithotripsy (ESWL) versus percutaneous nephrolithotomy (PCNL) or retrograde intrarenal surgery (RIRS) for kidney stones. *Cochrane Database Syst Rev.* 2009;4:CD007044.
6. Coe FL, Evan A, Worcester E. Kidney stone disease. *J Clin Invest.* 2005;115(10):2598–2608.
7. Straub M, Hautmann RE. Developments in stone prevention. *Curr Opin Urol.* 2005;15(2):119–126.
8. Stothers L, Thom D, Calhoun E. Urinary incontinence in men. In: Litwin MS, Saigal C, eds. *Urologic Diseases in America.* US Department of Health and Human Services, Public Health Service, National Institutes of Health, National Institute of Diabetes and Digestive and Kidney Diseases. Washington, DC: US Government Publishing Office; 2004.
9. Nygaard I, Thom D, Calhoun E. Urinary incontinence in women. In: Litwin MS, Saigal C, eds. *Urologic Diseases in America.* US Department of Health and Human Services, Public Health Service, National Institutes of Health, National Institute of Diabetes and Digestive and Kidney Diseases. Washington, DC: US Government Publishing Office; 2004.
10. Vandoninck V, Bemelmans BL, Mazzetta C, et al. The prevalence of urinary incontinence in community-dwelling married women: a matter of definition. *BJU Int.* 2004;94(9):1291–1295.
11. Yoshida M, Masunaga K, Nagata T, et al. The forefront for novel therapeutic agents based on the pathophysiology of lower urinary tract dysfunction: pathophysiology and pharmacotherapy of overactive bladder. *J Pharm Sci.* 2010;112(2):128–134.
12. Patel V, Chowdhury R, Igarashi P. Advances in the pathogenesis and treatment of polycystic kidney disease. *Curr Opin Nephrol Hypertens.* 2009;18:99–106.

13. NIDDK. *Kidney and Urologic Disease Statistics for the United States.* Available at: http://kidney.niddk.nih.gov/kudiseases/pubs/kustats/index.htm#kidney. Accessed on February 6, 2010.

14. Niemczyk M, Niemczek S, Paczek L. Autosomal dominant polycystic kidney disease and transplantation. *Ann Transplant.* 2009;14(4);86–90.

15. Wilkins T, Baird C, Pearson AN, et al. Diverticular bleeding. *Am Fam Physician.* 2009;80(9):977–983.

16. Loening-Baucke V. Chronic constipation in children. *Gastroenterology.* 1993;105(5):1557–1564.

17. Rasquin-Weber A, Hyman PE, Cucchiara S, et al. Childhood functional gastrointestinal disorders. *Gut.* 1999;45(suppl 2):II60–II68.

18. Di Lorenzo C, Benninga MA. Pathophysiology of pediatric fecal incontinence. *Gastroenterology.* 2004;126(suppl 1):S33–S340.

19. Kuhn BR, Marcus BA, Pitner SL. Treatment guidelines for primary nonretentive encopresis and stool toileting refusal. *Am Fam Physician.* 1999;59(8):2171–2178, 2184–2186.

20. Drossman DA. The functional gastrointestinal disorders and the Rome II process. *Gut.* 1999;45(suppl 2):II1–II5.

Chapter 17

Degenerative Changes in Aging

LEARNING OBJECTIVES

1. Define and use the key terms listed in this chapter.
2. Describe the basis of theoretical explanations of aging.
3. Recognize the implications of degenerative changes in aging on the health of the individual.
4. Identify common manifestations of age-related degenerative changes.
5. Detail methods to maximize health status in the elderly population.
6. List the common diagnostic procedures used to identify degenerative changes in aging.
7. Describe treatment strategies appropriate for degenerative changes in aging.
8. Apply concepts of age-related alterations in cells, tissues, and organ systems to select clinical models.

INTRODUCTION

"You're only as old as you feel" is a phrase often quoted, but what is it that makes us feel old? Aging is a normal, expected process that occurs in all living individuals. Even though it is a normal, physiologic process, the effects can cause clinical manifestations that range from minimally impaired function to serious disability. Knowledge of the degenerative changes that are involved in the aging process can provide the basis of adaptations that can promote the greatest degree of function and independence.

Module 1

Theoretical Causes of Aging

Aging is commonly defined as the gradual deterioration of a mature organism resulting from time-dependent, irreversible changes in structure. Senescence is often used interchangeably with aging and refers to postmaturational processes that lead to diminished homeostasis and increased vulnerability. Aging is a time-related process that determines responses leading to illness and death. Life expectancy, the age at which 50% of a given population is expected to survive, is a term used to describe demographics associated with aging. Based on a recent analysis of population data from 2004, life expectancy for males was 75.2 years and 80.0 years for females.[1] Life expectancy for the Black population rose to 73.1 years but remained lower than the 78.3 year life expectancy for the White population, pointing to significant difference in life expectancy between races.

Aging Theories

Theories of aging have been developed to explain physiologic processes that lead to clinical manifestations. The mechanisms that program cells to age are not clearly understood, but they are known to contribute to impaired structure and function. Aging is associated with reduced functional capacity because the body fails to produce sufficient numbers of replacement cells, especially those that are not capable of mitotic division. Identifying the cellular mechanisms underlying degenerative changes of aging is necessary for effective diagnosis and treatment of related pathology.

Theories of aging are usually categorized as developmental or stochastic. **Developmental theories** point to the influence of genetics as the major determinant of aging. **Stochastic theories** support the idea that aging is the result of cumulative cellular damage. The process of aging is likely multifactorial, reflecting mechanisms of both genetics and injury. Damage to cells may be due to cumulative extrinsic events that cause injury to cells or from intrinsic events regulating cell death determined by genetic control. Cellular damage resulting from mechanical or chemical injury caused by accumulation of metabolites and ultraviolet radiation damage to DNA are among the potential causes thought to contribute to aging. Cell death that is programmed (apoptosis) or occurring because of injury (necrosis) often contributes to the clinical manifestations of aging (see Chapter 2).

DEVELOPMENTAL THEORIES

Developmental theories support the existence of a genetically programmed and controlled continuum of development and maturation. At earlier ages, biochemical pathways optimally maintain genes to assure reproductive function and survival of the species, with genes that determine survival at younger ages having greater influence than genes that are expressed at older ages.[2]

The **accumulated mutations theory** suggests that over time, the accumulation of genetic mutations during cell division may contribute to altered cellular function associated with aging. The gradual decline in cellular and metabolic function likely results from a combination of DNA mutation and telomere shortening. *Telomeres* are the capped structures on chromosomes that protect chromosome ends (Fig. 17.1). Each time a chromosome is replicated, the telomeres shorten. When chromosomes reach a critical length, **cellular senescence**, or the intrinsic loss of the capacity of the cell to proliferate, is triggered. Observations of decreased immune function with increased age have led to the development of the **immunologic theory of aging**. Reduced resistance to disease secondary to reduced T-cell function and enhanced autoimmune responses are common characteristics of increasing age. Another theory, the **antagonistic pleiotropy theory**, suggests that genes may have beneficial effects during early life but harmful effects as the individual ages. The origin for this selection may be based on the promotion of reproductive success rather than negative effects associated with aging. Mutations that occur later in life limit the influence of evolutionary selection. The **neuroendocrine theory** suggests the interrelationship between neurons and associated hormones as the stimulus for aging. As discussed in Chapter 11, the hypothalamic–pituitary axis is instrumental in contributing to the regulation of many bodily functions, including development, growth, puberty, reproduction, metabolism, and aging. Menopause is an example of the manifestation of altered neuroendocrine responsiveness characteristic of women with increasing age.

A condition that illustrates how genetic damage can lead to aging is Hutchinson–Gilford progeria. Progeria is a syndrome commonly characterized by accelerated aging. Children affected by progeria have a life expectancy of approximately 13 years. Progeria results from damage to the *LMNA* gene that produces the protein lamin A. Lamin A is important to

Figure 17.1 Telomere location on a single chromosome. Each chromatid is capped by a telomere. (Image modified from McClatchey KD. *Clinical Laboratory Medicine*. 2nd ed. Philadelphia: Lippincott Williams & Wilkins; 2002, with permission.)

Figure 17.2 Manifestations of progeria. A 10-year-old girl affected by progeria shows signs of accelerated aging.

the structure of the nucleus and other cellular components. A *point mutation* (see Chapter 2) in the *LMNA* gene results in a shortened gene caused by a mistake during *translation* of the protein. Children with progeria show signs of early aging at 18 to 24 months of age. Manifestations include growth failure, loss of hair and body fat, aged skin, joint stiffness, and atherosclerosis. Objective signs of progeria are seen in Figure 17.2.

STOCHASTIC THEORIES

Stochastic theories suggest that random accumulated cellular damage leads to aging. Targets for cellular damage include mitochondria and DNA. The **free radical theory** of aging links cellular damage with the production of reactive oxygen species (ROS). According to this theory, intracellular production of ROS contributes to the final

determination of life span.[3] Mitochondria are especially at risk for damage from ROS because of byproducts produced in the electron transport chain that produce energy in the form of ATP. Oxidative damage to mitochondrial DNA and other cellular structures is thought to be cumulative, leading to the manifestations of aging.

The **somatic mutation theory** states that the aging process is caused by impaired DNA repair, antioxidant defense, or errors in protein expression. Caloric restriction has been shown experimentally to prolong life expectancy. Although the underlying mechanism is unclear, longevity may be caused by a shift in energy from growth and reproduction toward repair and maintenance of the soma, or cell.

Module 2

General Manifestations of Aging

A pattern of gradual loss is characteristic of the changes associated with aging (Fig. 17.3). These changes are physiologic rather than pathologic. However, these same changes may result in altered

structure and function, leading to findings that are often associated with pathologic manifestations. Aging processes and disease states are not always clearly delineated.

■ **Figure 17.3**   Concept map: Manifestations of aging.

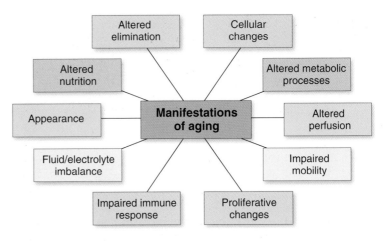

Common characteristics of aging include:

1. Increased mortality with age after maturation
2. Changes in biochemical composition in tissues
3. Progressive decrease in physiologic capacity
4. Diminished ability to respond adaptively to environmental stimuli
5. Increased vulnerability and susceptibility to disease

Cellular Changes in Aging

Cellular changes characteristic of aging include hypertrophy and the impaired ability to undergo mitosis. Cell function may be impaired by the deposition of lipids or damage from free radicals. Tissue effects of aging include the accumulation of metabolic waste products and the deposition of **lipofuscin**, a fatty brown lipid pigment, causing stiffening or rigidity. Loss of mass by atrophy is a common age-related effect that occurs in organs and bones. Although these changes are part of the normal processes of aging, the resulting changes in function may lead to the development of disease.

Aging and Appearance

Appearance is altered in aging and can potentially affect self and body image. Typical skin changes include a dry, wrinkled appearance with a varied pattern of pigmentation (Fig. 17.4). Collagen changes decrease elasticity. Decreased vascularity and increased fragility may lead to skin discoloration and thickened nail appearance. Changes in hair include loss, growth, distribution, and graying because of melanin deficiency in the hair follicle (Fig. 17.5). Sexual function in women may decrease

as an indirect result because attractiveness is influential in the development of desire in women.

● **STOP** *and* **Consider**

Why do "age spots" form as individuals age?

Fluid and Electrolyte Balance

Aging is associated with changes in body mass characterized by a decrease in muscle and an increase in fat. These changes contribute to a decrease in total body water, further enhanced by the kidney's diminished ability to regulate sodium and water balance,

■ **Figure 17.4**   Atrophic changes in the aged hand. The hand of an 84-year-old woman shows typical atrophic changes of aging.

which is important in the establishment of extracellular fluid volume and tonicity. Total body water balance is a key element in the determination of sodium concentration in the blood, which increases the risk for hyponatremia in cases of water retention and hypernatremia caused by water loss. Additional stressors in the form of disease, altered elimination, or altered nutrition may result in significant consequences related to altered fluid and electrolyte balance (see Chapter 8).

Alterations in Immune Responses

The processes of inflammation, immunity, and protection from infection are altered with aging (see Chapters 3 to 5). **Immune senescence**, progressive dysfunction of the immune system associated with aging, is characterized by both diminished and enhanced immune responses. Antigenic immune responses progressively diminish with aging because of decreased T-cell function even in the absence of any significant decrease in actual T-cell number. Thymus degeneration occurs after age 50 years, at which time it is only 15% of its peak size reached at sexual maturity. This degeneration results in decreased thymic hormone production and T-cell differentiation. Monoclonal antibody production may occur even in the absence of B-cell malignancies. Autoimmune responses may become enhanced because of the increased circulation of autoantibodies and immune complexes. IgE-mediated hypersensitivity responses are decreased and are associated with a lessening of allergy-mediated symptoms.

● **STOP** and *Consider*

How can the elderly protect themselves from infection?

Manifestations of decreased immune responsiveness include attenuated delayed hypersensitivity responses, diminished T-cell activity, and responsiveness to pathogens. Loss of previously acquired immunity may increase the reactivation of pathogens, resulting in reinfection. The incidence of

herpes zoster and tuberculosis infection is increased in the elderly. Mortality rates are increased in the elderly in response to pneumonia and influenza. Rates of nosocomial infection are also increased in this population. Impaired wound healing may result as a response to altered immune function due to aging or from decreased function induced by medications for chronic illness, such as steroids. Typical physical changes of aging, including loss of subcutaneous fat, decreased elasticity of collagen, and atrophied epidermis and supporting capillaries, also contribute to impaired healing.

Age-Related Proliferative Changes

Chronic myeloproliferative disorders, such as polycythemia vera and primary thrombocythemia, are more common in individuals greater than 60 years of age. The incidence of many of the most common cancers is also increased in many older individuals, with the greatest incidence occurring between the ages of 65 and 80 years, which is when approximately 60% of new cancer cases and deaths occur.[4] The potential causes for these findings may result from many of the characteristic changes of aging contributing to increased risk or attenuated defense to carcinogens. These potential causes include:

- Impaired immune function
- Genetic mutation accumulation
- Prolonged carcinogen exposure
- Impaired ability for DNA repair

Manifestations of alterations in proliferation are specific to the involved cells and tissues (see Chapter 7). Treatment is often based on the type of malignancy, the effects resulting from the malignancy, the person's age and quality of life, and consent.

Alteration in Neurologic Function in Aging

Age-related neurologic manifestations may include alteration in cognition, sensation, pain, and motor responses. These manifestations often result from changes in both structure and function of cells and the tissues responsible for the stimulation of physiologic responses. Neurologic function may be altered as a response to cellular processes, resulting in functional changes in both the central, somatosensory, and peripheral nervous systems (see Chapters 9 and 10). Typical structural changes include:

- Decrease in brain mass
- Enlargement of cerebral ventricles
- Decrease in number of neurons, dendritic processes, and synapses
- Decrease in myelin
- Altered production of neurotransmitters

Histologically, in the brain, evidence of lipofuscin pigment in nerve cells and amyloid in the vascular tissue are findings consistent with aging. Neurofibrillatory tangles and plaques may occur and are discussed further under the clinical model in this chapter: Alzheimer disease (AD). Evidence exists of a declining number of cells in the spinal cord, although the functional effects are not clearly linked. Most functional alterations result from the involvement of peripheral nerves and degenerative changes of the spine and muscles. Slowing of nerve conduction and less efficient axon response to injury and repair are typical with aging. Factors critical to the promotion of neurologic responses, including neurotransmitters, enzymes, and receptors, are also altered during the aging process.

Manifestations of impaired functioning often result from these structural changes. These changes include sensory deficits (taste, smell, vibration, vision, and hearing), motor dysfunction (altered gait and posture), sleep disturbances, and impaired memory and cognition. Slowing of central processing may prolong the time it takes to complete tasks. Declines in motor strength, reflex responses, and reaction time are related to sensorimotor changes. Changes associated with aging include mild forgetfulness, a decrease in vocabulary, and learning difficulties. These changes typically do not occur until the seventh decade of life.

Cognitive function can be compromised by the coexisting conditions related to decline in mental health. Often related to environment and social conditions, depression and anxiety among the elderly is more prevalent in long-term care settings compared with elderly who are community dwelling. Psychological disorders may complicate physical health, reducing motivation or ability to maintain health through everyday activities, such as properly administering medications, assuring adequate nutrition, obtaining adequate exercise, and maintaining personal hygiene.

Impaired Mobility

Physical activity is decreased among the elderly, who are often limited by musculoskeletal or neurologic alterations in aging. The occurrence of **osteopenia** (reduced calcification and/or skeletal bone mass) and **osteoporosis** (atrophy of skeletal tissue) in individuals over age 50 years is increased, placing this population at risk for injury caused by falls. Women experience a more rapid phase of bone loss after menopause, known as **menopausal bone loss**, followed by a slower loss phase that affects both men and women (**senescent bone loss**). Menopausal bone loss is cytokine-induced (IL-6), occurring in the absence of adequate levels of protective ovarian hormones. This response is associated with delayed apoptosis of osteoclasts and enhanced apoptosis of osteoblasts, resulting in an imbalance favoring bone loss. Senescent bone loss is related to diminished bone remodeling and formation. Osteoblast production is decreased, slowing the rate of bone formation and reducing bone mineral density. Osteoporosis is discussed in more detail in this chapter as a clinical model.

STOP *and Consider*

What types of physical activities are considered weight bearing? What types are not?

Loss of bone with progressive age affects the *axial (trabecular)* and *appendicular (cortical)* skeleton and is manifested by pain, stiffness, loss of height, and development of **kyphosis**, an exaggerated anterior concave curvature of the thoracic spine. Fractures of the vertebrae and hips are common. Cartilage changes may also impair mobility, decreasing function via joint limitations. Enzyme activity in chondrocytes may lead to crystal deposition, promoting the development of **chondrocalcinosis** (calcification of cartilage). Cartilage may thin in weight-bearing joints, such as the knees, causing pain and decreased mobility.

Loss of lean body mass typical in aging is primarily caused by the decreased number and size of skeletal muscle fibers. **Sarcopenia**, or loss of skeletal muscle, is a common age-related change that limits function. Causes of sarcopenia include:

- Decreased physical activity
- Changes in the nervous system (central and peripheral)
- Protein undernutrition

Faster-contracting muscle fibers (type II) are lost more quickly compared to the slower-contracting fibers (type I), leading to loss of isometric contractile force. Posture and the ability to perform rhythmic movements are affected more slowly. Decreased mobility caused by other comorbid conditions can greatly accelerate the process of muscle loss in the elderly.

Age-Related Changes in Perfusion and Ventilation

Age-related changes in the cardiovascular system may lead to altered perfusion (see Chapter 14). Variables affecting cardiac function include:

- Compliance
- Cardiac filling
- Preload
- Afterload
- Contractility
- Ejection fraction
- Stroke volume
- Heart rate
- Cardiac output

Connective tissue changes promote decreased elasticity in the smooth muscle of the vascular system. Increased afterload caused by arterial stiffening and limited distention may alter cardiac output. Left ventricular wall thickness may increase because of hypertension, a common comorbid condition in the elderly. Atherosclerosis may result from increased intimal thickness from cellular accumulation, often coupled with damage to the internal elastic layer of the vascular smooth muscle. Alterations in cardiovascular functioning may affect any organ system, promoting the development of organ-specific manifestations. Decreased cerebral blood flow may be linked to alterations in neurologic function, further determined by the specific area of the brain involved.

Pulmonary changes in aging, coupled with decreased density of pulmonary capillaries, may limit the availability of oxygen to adequately supply tissues (Chapter 13). Typical changes include:

- Decreased inspiratory reserve volume
- Increased residual volume
- Reduced ventilatory capacity
- Reduced ventilation–perfusion ratio

Decreased muscle and bone mass in the chest cavity may increase the work of breathing. In non-smokers, these typical changes affecting ventilation, gas exchange, and compliance are not associated with significant manifestations. Dyspnea may indicate airway obstruction, often seen in individuals with comorbid conditions such as emphysema. Limited immune defense along with dysphagia, loss of cough mechanisms, and decline of mucociliary transport may predispose elderly individuals to pulmonary infection and aspiration.

Age-Related Changes in Metabolic Processes

Atrophy, decreased hormonal secretion, impaired receptor/ligand binding, and alterations in intracellular signaling may influence the changes typical in the hormonal processes associated with aging. Because hormonal and metabolic effects are body-wide, the manifestations of alterations often affect many organ systems. The most commonly affected processes include:

- Mineral metabolism
  - Calcium
  - Phosphate
  - Magnesium
- Vitamin and trace mineral metabolism
- Acid–base metabolism
- Nutrient metabolism
  - Obesity
  - Undernutrition
- Endocrine metabolism
  - Thyroid
  - Parathyroid
  - Adrenal
  - Pituitary
    - Anterior
    - Posterior
  - Ovarian/testicular

Calcium levels in the elderly are regulated by parathyroid hormone (PTH), vitamin D, and calcitonin. **Calcitonin**, a hormone produced by the parathyroid, thyroid, and thymus glands, promotes the deposition of calcium and phosphate in bone. **Parathyroid hormone (PTH)** promotes removal of calcium and phosphate from bone, opposing the effects of calcitonin. The activated form of vitamin D, **1,25-dihydroxycholecalciferol**, promotes calcium absorption in the intestine. Calcium levels vary depending on the concentration of plasma proteins (i.e., albumin), the concentration bound to anions (i.e., phosphate and bicarbonate), and the blood pH altering calcium–protein binding (decreased in acidosis, increased in alkalosis). Calcium levels may be affected by age-related decreased intestinal absorption of calcium, a blunted response to vitamin D activation, and the age-related increase in PTH (Fig. 17.6). Nutritional intake of calcium and vitamin D is also important in the regulation of calcium metabolism. Proliferative disease, particularly breast cancer, lung cancer, and multiple myeloma, may result in dangerously high levels of serum calcium.

Figure 17.6 Metabolism of vitamin D and the regulation of calcium. Calcium regulation involves multiple organ systems. Reduced function in any of the involved systems may result in altered calcium homeostasis. (Image from Rubin E, Farber JL. *Pathology*. 4th ed. Philadelphia: Lippincott Williams & Wilkins; 2005, with permission.)

STOP *and Consider*

Why would metastatic disease increase calcium levels in the blood?

Phosphate levels are typically lower in the elderly. Phosphate intake is decreased in the elderly and is coupled with poor intestinal absorption. Increased activity of the parathyroid gland may result in the promotion of renal excretion of phosphate related to altered tubular absorption. Vomiting and metabolic acidosis may also further contribute to hypophosphatemia. Chronic renal failure may result in hyperphosphatemia. Hypomagnesemia is also common among the elderly and often results from decreased dietary intake, excessive renal excretion, or loss via the gastrointestinal system (i.e., vomiting, diarrhea, or impaired absorption). Maintenance of acid–base balance is impaired because of a diminished ability of the aging respiratory and renal systems to correct alterations. Impairment of these homeostatic mechanisms represents a significant risk of altered acid–base balance in the elderly.

Decreased T3 levels and elevated TSH levels characterize typical thyroid function alterations in the elderly. The incidence of hypothyroidism increases with age and may manifest subclinically or with overt symptoms. The prevalence of hyperthyroidism does not increase with age. Temperature regulation is also compromised in the elderly, more so if coupled with chronic illness. The ability to cool the body via sweating is impaired because of a decrease in the number, size, and activity of sweat glands, making the elderly particularly susceptible to heat stress. Frail elderly individuals are especially at risk for hypothermia because of diminished cold perception, altered responsiveness to catecholamine-induced vasoconstriction and shiver, and limited ability to produce heat.

Alterations in Nutrition and Elimination in Aging

Processes that regulate digestion and elimination are altered in aging because of morphologic and functional changes within the enteric nervous system,[5] a division of the autonomic nervous system (see Chapter 16). Impaired nutrition that leads to deficiencies in macronutrients and micronutrients are common among the elderly (see Chapter 15). These deficits can lead to cognitive impairment, increased risk of infection caused by impairment of immune function, anemia, and poor wound healing. Inadequate intake of protein and energy-producing foods may result in undernutrition, often associated with deficiencies in water-soluble vitamins B and C as well as fat-soluble vitamins A, D, E, and K.

The problem of undernutrition is even more prevalent among elderly in long-term care and in hospitals, which increases the risk for the development of chronic illness. Impaired nutrition may be caused by tooth loss or poorly fitting dentures, making the process of chewing food difficult. Often in aging, the physiologic response to hunger is blunted, coupled with a feeling of fullness from less food. The reasons for these responses are unclear, but they may be linked to the effects of the hormone leptin, as discussed in Chapter 15 (Fig. 17.7). Leptin levels are correlated with the amount of body fat in elderly women, although an inverse relationship is found among elderly men.[4] Levels of cytokines have also been suggested to be involved in the development of anorexia among the elderly, which leads to undernutrition.

Obesity may also lead to the development or exacerbation of chronic conditions in the elderly. An improved level of activity, determined by functional ability, is the safest way to achieve a normal body weight. Elderly individuals with a history of obesity

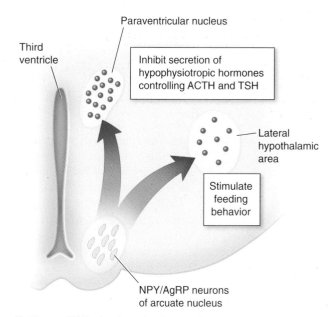

Figure 17.7 Leptin action in appetite regulation. Reduction in leptin is detected by neurons in the arcuate nucleus, inhibiting secretion of ACTH and TSH at the level of the paraventricular nucleus and stimulating the release of NPY/AgRP, prompting feeding behaviors. (Image from Bear MF, Connors BW, Parasido MA. *Neuroscience: Exploring the Brain*. 3rd ed. Philadelphia: Lippincott Williams & Wilkins; 2005, with permission.)

may have clinical manifestations of dyslipidemia and coronary artery disease.

Functional responses of the kidneys decrease with age. Renal changes characteristic in aging include:

- Reduced renal blood flow
- Decreased glomerular filtration rate
- Reduced renal mass
- Decline in proximal tubular function
- Reduced renin and aldosterone levels

Reduction in nephron number may alter the renal function of urine concentration, placing additional importance on the regulation of total water balance. Drug excretion may be impaired, increasing the risk of toxicity.

Impaired gastrointestinal elimination in elderly individuals is most frequently manifested as constipation, diarrhea, fecal incontinence, and impaction. The stress of fluid and electrolyte loss via diarrhea represents a significant threat to water balance, often resulting in severe dehydration. Increased rectal compliance and impaired rectal sensation represent age-related changes that predispose elderly individuals to constipation. Fecal incontinence is caused by decreased resting and maximal anal sphincter pressures.

Functional megarectum, delay at the rectosigmoid outlet, and pelvic floor dysfunction may all contribute to age-related constipation. Fecal impaction, overflow incontinence, and urinary retention may be consequences of constipation (see Chapter 16).

Module 3

Managing Degenerative Changes in Aging Populations

It is estimated that 20% of Americans will be aged 50 to 64 by the year 2015.[6] Primary and secondary prevention of injury and illness are the major challenges in the management of age-related degenerative changes. Management strategies must be individualized because of the wide range of manifestations exhibited among the elderly. Strategies must take into account comorbid conditions, physical health, cognitive status, functional ability, and social support. Strategies for illness prevention among the elderly population include an exercise regimen, weight control, cancer screening, avoidance of smoking and binge drinking, and influenza and pneumococcal vaccination.

Elders should visit their primary care providers to institute a management plan that encompasses primary and secondary prevention strategies. A careful evaluation of the home environment is essential for accident prevention. Family members or individuals responsible for providing elder care should be aware of changes in functional or cognitive abilities in their charges. Assurance of appropriate medication administration may prevent injury related to improper dosing.

Exercises may involve specific activities designed to promote function and strength simultaneously. Activities designed to promote conditioning are important to maintain musculoskeletal function, which affects many other body systems, including those regulating perfusion and ventilation. Decreased vascular stiffening and enhanced aerobic capacity may directly result from adequate physical conditioning. Elders with limited mobility or functional ability may benefit from physical therapy to delay deconditioning.

A well-balanced diet that includes essential protein intake, macronutrients, and micronutrients is important to maintain homeostasis. Assurance of adequate fluid intake is essential to volume regulation and may lessen the incidence of constipation.

Module 4

Clinical Models

Clinical models for this chapter were selected to demonstrate the application of previously described processes within aging populations. As you read the descriptions that follow, consider the cellular mechanisms that contribute to the alterations in tissues and body systems associated with aging.

Osteoporosis

Osteoporosis is the most common type of bone disease affecting many older Americans. According to a recent report by the U.S. Surgeon General, 10 million Americans older than 50 years of age are estimated to have osteoporosis. Annually, 1.5 million people are diagnosed with a fracture related to osteoporosis. It is estimated that one out of every two women over 50 years of age will be the victim of this type of fracture. The incidence of hip fracture is two times greater in women than men older than 50 years of age. Because of an increasing number of older individuals in the population, the number of hip fractures in the United States may double or triple by the year 2020.[7] Osteoporosis affects both genders, with a greater prevalence among women, in which it occurs eight times more frequently.

Characterized by loss of bone mass and degeneration of bone tissue, osteoporosis (porous bone) leads to increased fragility of the bone and likelihood of fracture (Fig. 17.8). The economic burden related to complications of osteoporosis takes a significant toll on individuals, families, and society. Currently, strategies exist to limit the adverse outcomes related to osteoporosis. These strategies and the challenges of implementation are reviewed in this clinical model.

PATHOPHYSIOLOGY

Osteoporosis occurs because of an imbalance in the bone remodeling process; bone resorption by osteoclasts is favored over bone formation by

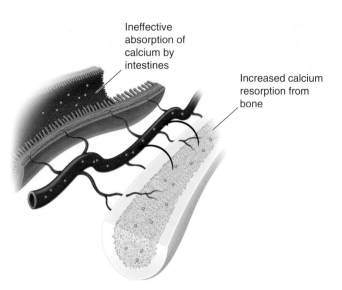

Ineffective absorption of calcium by intestines

Increased calcium resorption from bone

■ **Figure 17.8** Osteoporosis in aging. Impaired intestinal calcium absorption and increased osteoclastic activity relative to osteoblastic activity contribute to age-related osteoporosis.

inadequate levels of these minerals, which are the building blocks of bone (Fig. 17.9). Vitamin D, taken in by diet or produced in response to sunlight, promotes the intestinal absorption of calcium and phosphate. The process of bone formation is enhanced by mechanical stress and the hormone calcitonin, inhibiting the activation of osteoclasts and promoting the deposition of calcium and phosphate into bone. Although a variety of tissues produce calcitonin, the major source of calcitonin is the parafollicular cells of the thyroid gland. PTH opposes calcitonin, activating osteoclasts and promoting removal of calcium and phosphate from bone, which results in bone resorption. Tubule reabsorption in the kidneys minimizes excretion of both calcium and phosphorus in the urine.

● **STOP** *and Consider*

What influence does geographic location have on vitamin D production?

CLINICAL MANIFESTATIONS

Pathologic findings associated with osteoporosis include loss of coarse cancellous bone and thinning of the cortex. The trabeculae in the coarse cancellous bone become structurally impaired, and cortical bone becomes thin and porous, increasing the fracture risk.

Often known as the "silent disease," osteoporosis is not manifested until fracture, spinal deformity, or loss of height occurs. Because of the high quantity of cancellous bone in the vertebrae, spinal fractures

osteoblasts, resulting in loss of bone mass. *Primary osteoporosis* is more common than *secondary osteoporosis* in both genders. Characterized by an increase in osteoclast activity, primary osteoporosis is often stimulated by estrogen withdrawal in postmenopausal women, which is caused by activation of estrogen-sensitive cytokines. Secondary osteoporosis, a less common form, results from other causes, including hormonal or genetic factors (Table 17.1). Reduced osteoblast function characterizes this form of osteoporosis.

Calcium and phosphate promote bone calcification, and their metabolism is tightly regulated to maintain normal extracellular levels. Metabolic alterations can result in, or cause, excessive or

Table 17.1 Conditions Leading to Secondary Osteoporosis

Condition	Etiology	Effect
Corticosteroid administration	Impaired vitamin D–dependent intestinal calcium absorption leading to increased PTH secretion	Inhibition of osteoblastic activity
Hyperparathyroidism	Increased PTH secretion	Increased osteoclast activity
Hyperthyroidism	Increased thyroid hormone	Increased osteoclast activity
Hypogonadism		
Women	Estrogen deficiency stimulates estrogen-sensitive cytokines	Increased osteoclast activity
Men	Deficiency of anabolic androgens	Decreased osteoblast activity
Hematologic malignancies	Osteoclast activating factor secreted from plasma cells	Increased osteoclast activity
	PTH-related protein secretion from tumor	

■ **Figure 17.9** Bone remodeling in osteoporosis. Vitamin D promotes the intestinal absorption of calcium. Vitamin D is converted to its active form (1,25(OH$_2$)D by the renal enzyme 1 α-hydroxylase. Age-related decrease in kidney function limits the availability of 1 α-hydroxylase. Decreased 1 α-hydroxylase stimulation by PTH and an age-related blunted response of the renal tubules to PTH contribute to the development of an imbalance of bone remodeling, favoring resorption. TNF, tumor necrosis factor; PTH, and parathyroid hormone. (Image from Rubin E, Farber JL. *Pathology.* 4th ed. Philadelphia: Lippincott Williams & Wilkins; 2005, with permission.)

represent significant sequelae of osteoporosis. Factors contributing to osteoporosis risk include:

- Genetic predisposition
  - Family history of first-degree relative with osteoporosis
- Peak bone mass
  - Reduced maximal amount of bone in a given person
  - Body mass index less than 25%
- Loss of estrogen
- Aging
- Inadequate calcium and vitamin D intake
- Cigarette smoking
- Excessive alcohol
- Sedentary lifestyle

Although this disease is more common in women, awareness of osteoporosis in men is increasing.[8] Compared to women, men have fewer spine and hip fractures because of increased bone mass and strength. Reduced bone size and loss caused by cortical and trabecular thinning characterizes the development of bone fragility in men. Increased bone remodeling in elderly men is often caused by secondary hyperparathyroism, calcium malabsorption, and vitamin D deficiency.

DIAGNOSIS

Osteoporosis can be identified by the presence of an unexplained fracture. The goal of diagnosis is to identify early bone loss before significant risk develops. Risk for osteoporosis can be determined by tests of bone density and bone quality, recommended as part of routine screening in all women over age 65 and in men and younger women who have had a previous fragility fracture.[9] The **dual energy X-ray absorptiometry (DEXA)** is a specialized, low-level radiographic technique used to measure bone density. Density of both the trabecular and cortical bones can be determined in a single test, and changes in bone density can be determined if the DEXA is done serially, usually annually or biannually. Results of DEXA testing are reported as a T score, based on the following guidelines issued by the World Health Organization:

- Normal bone density
  - Bone mass greater than 833 mg/cm^2
  - T score more than -1.0
- Osteopenia
  - Bone mass between 833 and 648 mg/cm^2
  - T score from -1.0 to -2.5
- Osteoporosis
  - Bone mass less than 648 mg/cm^2
  - T score less than -2.5

A comparison of an individual T score to persons in the population of the same age and gender is documented using a Z score. Report of a Z score of less than -1.5 suggests a secondary, rather than primary, cause for osteoporosis.

Bone quality can be determined by the use of quantitative ultrasound. Measurement of the passage of an ultrasound beam through the trabecular bone in the heel portion of the foot determines bone structure, strength, and degree of elasticity. Although using an ultrasound measurement of bone quality has many benefits, including cost, time, and convenience, such measurements may not be as accurate as DEXA scanning. Findings of adequate bone quality in the peripheral bone of the heel may not represent similar findings in the central locations of the hip and spine, reducing the ability to generalize findings from one site to the other.

TREATMENT

Prevention of osteoporosis is the ideal treatment. Recommendations for promoting bone health include:

1. Get your daily recommended amounts of calcium and Vitamin D.
2. Engage in regular weight-bearing exercise.
3. Avoid smoking and excessive alcohol.
4. Talk to your doctor about bone health.
5. Have a bone density test and take medication when appropriate.

Calcium intake recommendations include 1,200 mg/day for postmenopausal women and elderly men in divided doses for best absorption. Vitamin D (400 to 600 IU/day) should be included to promote calcium absorption and metabolism.[11] Preventive therapy may be considered for individuals with a T score of less than -1, but treatment should begin when the T score is less than -2.5 (see Table 17.2). Weight bearing is important in the stimulation of osteoblastic activity and bone calcification. Even

immobile individuals should have a regimen designed to promote bone health or, at a minimum, decrease bone loss.

Most current pharmacologic treatments of osteoporosis are limited to the use of drugs that inhibit or reduce bone resorption, also known as **antiresorptive** medications. The effectiveness of these medications is caused by the attenuation of the resorptive process with no effect on the formation process, thereby altering the balance in favor

From the Lab

There are no consistent guidelines for laboratory testing to determine causes of secondary osteoporosis. Tests to determine underlying causes of osteoporosis may include a complete blood count, blood chemistry tests (calcium, phosphorus, total protein, liver enzymes, alkaline phosphatase, and electrolytes), urinary studies (calcium excretion), and hormonal testing (serum thyrotropin, vitamin D, parathyroid hormone, and cortisol).[10]

of bone formation. Treatments, including calcium, vitamin D, calcitonin, and bisphosphonates, have been shown to be effective in individuals with bone loss caused by corticosteroid use and in postmenopausal women. Bisphosphonates (alendronate and risedronate), calcitonin, estrogens, PTH, and raloxifene are drugs currently approved by the U.S. Food and Drug Administration (FDA) for use to prevent or treat osteoporosis. Teriparatide (Forteo), a form of PTH, is an anabolic agent representing the first treatment for osteoporosis that works by increasing the formation of bone. Teriparatide, when given in a small daily dose,

Table 17.2 Pharmacologic Prevention and Treatment of Osteoporosis

Treatment	Class	Indication	Effect	Comments
Estrogen	Hormone	Prevention	Increased bone density	Risk of endometrial hyperplasia when uterus is present and unopposed by progestin, deep vein thrombosis, and breast cancer
Alendronate (Fosamax)	Bisphosphonate	Prevention	Increased bone density	Upper GI distress, myalgias, and arthralgias
		Treatment	Reduction in vertebral and hip fracture	
Risedronate (Actonel)	Bisphosphonate	Prevention	Increased bone density	Upper GI distress, myalgias, and arthralgias
		Treatment	Reduction in hip fracture	
Raloxifene (Evista)	SERM	Prevention	Increased bone density	Hot flashes, DVT
		Treatment	Reduction in vertebral fracture	
Calcitonin (Miacalcin)	Hormone	Treatment	Reduction in vertebral fracture	Rhinorrhea
Teriparatide	Hormone	Treatment	Increased bone formation	Dizziness and leg cramps

GI, gastrointestinal; SERM, selective estrogen receptor modulator; DVT, deep vein thrombosis.

promotes stimulation of new trabecular and cortical bone.

Parkinson Disease

Parkinson disease (PD) is a chronic, progressive neurologic condition that affects the pigmented dopaminergic neurons of the substantia nigra and locus ceruleus of the basal ganglia. Degeneration of neurons is associated with impaired motor function, and onset occurs predominantly in individuals of middle to old age. First described in the early 1800s as "shaking palsy" by Dr James Parkinson, the disease did not bear his name until half a century later, when Jean-Martin Charcot honored the early pioneer.[12] Although much has been learned, the condition still has no cure.

According to the National Institute on Neurologic Disorders and Stroke, approximately 500,000 people in the United States are diagnosed with PD.[13] Annually, approximately 50,000 new cases are reported. More common in men than in women, the average age of onset is 60 years, with prevalence and incidence increasing with age.

PATHOPHYSIOLOGY

The basal ganglia are important in the control of movement through regulation of inhibitory and excitatory stimuli. The basal ganglia are comprised of the forebrain structures of the striatum (caudate nucleus and putamen) and globus pallidus interna, the subthalamic nucleus (diencephalon), and the substantia nigra (midbrain) (Fig. 17.10). The substantia nigra is named for the black appearance of cells caused by the pigment melanin. Secreted by the cells of the substantia nigra, the neurotransmitter *dopamine* is transported to the striatum via the nigrostriatal pathway. PD is characterized by degeneration of the nigrostriatal pathway, which leads to a reduction in the neurotransmitter dopamine. Dopamine modulates balance between the excitatory and inhibitory neural motor pathways.

Impaired transport of dopamine alters excitability of the striatum and the release of other neurotransmitters. Neurons in the substantia nigra lose their pigment and their characteristic black color. In addition to pigment loss in the cells of the substantia nigra, neurons are atrophied, with some

Figure 17.10 Pigmented neurons of the substantia nigra. Neurons of the substantia nigra and the locus ceruleus are heavily pigmented with neuromelanin.

containing Lewy bodies. **Lewy bodies** are protein aggregations composed of the protein α-synuclein located primarily in the cells of the substantia nigra.

No specific mechanism explaining PD has been found. Neuronal injury from oxidative damage is suspected to play a role in the pathology associated with PD, potentially causing impaired mitochondrial function and antioxidant protection of neurons. The onset of the disease may also be related to a decline in the endogenous defense mechanisms associated with aging. Depigmentation of neurons may contribute to an inflammatory response to extracellular melanin in surrounding brain tissue.

PD can be an inherited disease, or it may occur sporadically. Although the genetic predisposition to PD in families is well known, recent developments in molecular biology have led to the identification of several genetic loci responsible for familial PD.[14] Recent insights may lead to more effective treatments and markers of disease before the onset of symptoms.

CLINICAL MANIFESTATIONS

Most neural degeneration in PD occurs before the onset of the manifestations of this disease, also

Figure 17.12 Mobility deficits in Parkinson disease. Musculoskeletal manifestations of Parkinson disease include tremors, rigidity, bradykinesia, and postural instability affecting the entire body. (Image modified from Rosdahl CB, *Book of Basic Nursing.* 7th ed. Philadelphia: Lippincott-Raven; 1999, with permission.)

Figure 17.11 Pathophysiology and clinical manifestations of Parkinson disease. The nuclei in the substantia nigra project fibers to the corpus striatum, the pathway of dopamine transport. Loss of dopaminergic neurons in the substantia nigra is associated with manifestations of Parkinson disease. (Image modified from Smeltzer SC, Bare BG. *Textbook of Medical-Surgical Nursing.* 10th ed. Philadelphia: Lippincott Williams & Wilkins; 2003, with permission.)

known as the preclinical period. The four primary manifestations of overt PD include (Fig. 17.11):

1. Tremor
2. Rigidity
3. Bradykinesia
4. Postural instability

Tremors usually involve the hands, arms, legs, and face, and they occur when the body is at rest. Tremors are progressive, initially manifesting in an isolated area and often beginning in one hand.

Bradykinesia (slowed movement) is associated with initiation of movement and may progress to **akinesia**, or the inability to move (Fig. 17.12). Sudden halting of movement is also a cardinal sign of bradykinesia. Individuals with PD often walk with a shuffling gait and stooped posture. Rigidity caused by resistance to movement by both flexors and extensors manifest as jerky movements, also known as *cogwheel rigidity.* Involvement of the tongue, throat, and palate may increase the likelihood of feeding difficulties and aspiration caused by muscle rigidity. Speech may also be affected by oral manifestations, resulting in monotone, expressionless inflections in voice. Stiffness of the limbs and trunk, bradykinesia, and postural instability contribute to decreased coordination and impaired balance. A flat, or expressionless, affect may be the result of facial stiffness (Fig. 17.13).

Indirect manifestations of PD involve the influence of basal ganglia in autonomic nervous system responses. Increased sebaceous, sweat, and saliva secretions are common. Other autonomic dysfunctions, including altered blood pressure and thermal

■ Figure 17.13 Facial features of Parkinson disease. Blunted expression, decreased blinking, and stare are characteristic manifestations. (Bickley LS, Szilagyi P. *Bates' Guide to Physical Examination and History Taking.* 8th ed. Philadelphia: Lippincott Williams & Wilkins; 2003, with permission.)

regulation, constipation, incontinence, and impotence, may occur. Cognitive and personality changes may be associated with PD. Dementia is also a common manifestation of PD.[15]

● **STOP** *and Consider*

Why are individuals on antipsychotic medications at risk for the development of Parkinsonian-like symptoms?

DIAGNOSIS

No single, definitive test exists to diagnose PD. Clinical findings based on the history and manifestations of the disease are used to obtain diagnosis. The Movement Disorder Society Task Force for Rating Scales for Parkinson disease confirms the reliability of the Hoehn and Yahr (HY) scale as an indicator of stage progression and severity.[16] The HY scale includes the following criteria:[17]

- Stage one
  - Signs and symptoms on one side only
  - Symptoms mild
  - Symptoms inconvenient but not disabling
  - Usually presents with tremor of one limb
  - Friends have noticed changes in posture, locomotion, and facial expression
- Stage two
  - Symptoms are bilateral
  - Minimal disability
  - Posture and gait affected
- Stage three
  - Significant slowing of body movements
  - Early impairment of equilibrium upon walking or standing
  - Generalized dysfunction that is moderately severe

- Stage four
  - Severe symptoms
  - Can still walk to a limited extent
  - Rigidity and bradykinesia
  - No longer able to live alone
  - Tremor may be less than earlier stages
- Stage five
  - Cachectic stage
  - Complete invalidism (i.e., disability)
  - Cannot stand or walk
  - Requires constant nursing care

TREATMENT

Pharmacologic management is a first-line treatment for PD. Levodopa is a dopamine precursor used as therapy to replace dopamine. Effective at ameliorating the symptoms associated with PD, there are many side effects, including nausea and vomiting, that make the drug difficult to tolerate. After prolonged use, additional dosing is often required and may result in other side effects, including *dyskinesias* and periods of time when the medication seems ineffective. When combined with the drug carbidopa (Sinemet), lower doses of levodopa and a decline in the incidence of side effects are possible while retaining effectiveness. A combination drug that adds entacapone to carbidopa and levodopa in the same formulation (Stalevo) extends the duration of action of levodopa. Symmetrel, an indirect-acting dopamine agonist, promotes the release of stored dopamine, blocks dopamine reuptake at synapses, and inhibits the excitatory neurotransmitter glutamate by inhibiting receptor binding. Anticholinergic agents often increase the effectiveness of levodopa, although the undesirable side effects of dry mouth, blurred vision, and urinary retention may occur. Dopamine agonists activate receptors and are a useful strategy for the treatment of PD. Drugs in this class include bromocriptine (Parlodel), pramipexole (Mirapex), and ropinirole (Requip). The drug Apokyn (apomorphine) is used for the treatment of hypomobility or "off periods" when immobility prevents completion of activities of daily living.

Surgical options for the treatment of PD include pallidotomy and **deep brain stimulation (DBS)**. These strategies are reserved for more advanced disease because of the risk involved with the treatments. **Pallidotomy**, an irreversible procedure involving destruction of the globus pallidus, is designed to decrease excitatory nerve firing in the damaged tissue. DBS is a reversible procedure designed to alter abnormal function of the brain tissue through insertion of a neurostimulator designed to deliver electrical signals to a targeted area of the brain. Stimulation is intended to block abnormal nerve signals, resulting in tremor and other PD symptoms. The exact location of the brain tissue responsible for the generation of nerve signals causing PD symptoms is identified before the procedure via a magnetic resonance imaging (MRI) or computed tomography (CT) scan.

Alzheimer Disease

AD is the most common neurodegenerative disorder and most frequent cause of dementia in the elderly, affecting more than 4 million people in the United States. According to the National Institutes on Aging, the incidence of AD increases with age but is not considered a normal consequence of aging.

PATHOPHYSIOLOGY

The histopathology of AD is characterized by the presence of neurofibrillary tangles and senile plaques. **Senile plaques** are caused by accumulations of proteins surrounding deposits of **β-amyloid protein** (also known as amyloid β [Aβ]), which are surrounded by inflammation (Fig. 17.14). The *β-amyloid* gene produces a large protein, **amyloid precursor protein (APP)**, serving as the basis of the β-amyloid protein. **Neurofibrillary tangles** are made up of the protein *tau*. Tau is also contained in the degenerating

nerve terminals in plaques. Tau fibers become twisted into a helical structure, forming tangles (Fig. 17.15). Cellular changes result in atrophy caused by loss of neurons in the hippocampus, cortex, and association areas of the neocortex.

Flaws in the accumulation, production, or disposal of Aβ are associated with the pathogenesis of AD, including development of tangles, plaques, and neuronal death.[18] β-amyloid protein accumulates in plaques beginning in small clusters (*oligomers*), followed by formation into chains (*fibrils*), and then finally into fibers organized as *beta sheets*. As plaque development progresses, brain cell-to-cell communication becomes disrupted. Immune cells become activated, destroying and ingesting injured cells.

The specific mechanism of disease has not been fully explained. The influence of other factors, such as neurotransmitters and inflammation, are under investigation. Familial predisposition for early-onset AD prompted the identification of three genes linked to this condition. Autosomal-dominant inheritance of the early-onset forms of AD are associated with mutations in the genes for *APP* (chromosome 21),

From the Lab

Development of an early marker of disease before the onset of symptoms has been a focus of investigation in PD. No tests have demonstrated adequate sensitivity or specificity of practical use for the early diagnosis of PD.

presenilin 1, and *presenilin 2* (chromosome 14 and 1), accounting for approximately half of the early-onset forms of AD.[19] Other genes may also be

β-amyloid plaques outside neurons

Alzheimer's   Normal

β-amyloid in blood vessel

β-amyloid protein core

Neurites

White matter   Cerebral cortex (gray matter)   Neuron cell body   Axon

■ **Figure 17.14**   β-Amyloid plaques in Alzheimer disease. (Asset provided by Anatomical Chart Company)

■ **Figure 17.15** Neurofibrillary tangles in Alzheimer disease. (Asset provided by Anatomical Chart Company)

implicated in the transmission of familial forms of AD. Late-onset AD, accounting for approximately 90% of AD cases, results from a combination of environmental influences and late-onset acting genes. The protein apolipoprotein E (ApoE), encoded by a gene located on chromosome 19, is linked to the increased incidence of late-onset AD. The altered protein resulting from a mutation of this gene may be related to AD pathology caused by the acceleration of plaque formation. Aβ protein may also be involved in the stimulation of oxidative stress and the induction of inflammatory responses, increasing the risk of neuronal injury.

CLINICAL MANIFESTATIONS

AD is characterized by a global cognitive decline. Memory, reasoning, judgment, and orientation (e.g., person, place, and time) are altered. Initial symptoms mimic processes of natural aging and include:

- Memory loss
- Language loss
- Confusion
- Restlessness
- Mood swings
- Difficulty in interpreting visual information

Eventual loss of personality and function are late signs of AD. Psychotic symptoms are common among individuals with AD. Guidelines for staging of AD include:[20]

- Stage 1
  - No cognitive impairment
- Stage 2
  - Mild cognitive decline
  - Evident only to self
    - Memory lapse
    - Forgetfulness of familiar words
    - Altered memory of location of everyday objects
- Stage 3
  - Mild cognitive decline
  - Early-stage AD
  - Evident among friends, family, or coworkers
  - Difficulty with word or name finding
  - Decreased performance at work or home
  - Difficulty with reading retention
  - Misplacing valuable objects
  - Impaired organization or planning
- Stage 4
  - Moderate cognitive decline
  - Mild/early-stage AD
  - Evident by examiner
    - Decline in knowledge of current events or occasions
    - Impaired mathematical ability
    - Impaired performance of complex tasks (e.g., bill paying, planning meals)
    - Difficulty remembering personal history
    - Change in personality (subdued or withdrawn)
- Stage 5
  - Moderately severe cognitive decline
  - Moderate/mid-stage AD
    - Exhibits major memory and cognitive deficits
    - Requires assistance in day-to-day activities
- Stage 6
  - Severe cognitive decline
  - Moderately severe/mid-stage AD
    - Significant personality changes
    - Increased need for help in activities of daily living
    - Worsening memory
      - Loss of awareness of surroundings and recent experiences
      - Occasional loss of memory of spouse's/primary caregiver's name
      - Disrupted sleep/wake cycle
      - Assistance needed with toileting details
      - Increasing episodes of incontinence
      - Sense of paranoia, delusions, and hallucinations
      - May wander or become lost
- Stage 7
  - Very severe cognitive decline
  - Severe/late-stage AD
    - Loss of ability to respond to the environment, including speech and movement
    - Loss of communication ability

Table 17.3 Drugs Used in the Treatment of Alzheimer Disease

Drug	Classification	Action in Alzheimer Disease
Donepezil (Aricept)	Cholinesterase inhibitor	Improvement in cognitive, global functioning and activities of daily living
Rivastigmine tartrate (Exelon)	Cholinesterase inhibitor	Improvement in cognition, participation in activities of daily living, and global functioning in mild to moderately severe disease
Galantamine (Razadyne)	Cholinesterase inhibitor	Improvement in cognitive function in mild to moderate disease
Tacrine (Cognex)	Cholinesterase inhibitor	Improvement of cognition in mild to moderate disease
Memantine (Namenda)	NMDA receptor antagonist	Improvement in cognitive, social, and motor impairment in moderate to severe disease

NMDA, N-methyl-D-aspartate.

- Requires increasing assistance with eating and toileting
- Impaired swallowing, positioning, and reflex response

DIAGNOSIS

A definitive diagnosis of AD can be made only at the time of autopsy when typical characteristics of plaques and tangles can be seen. Other testing can be done that, when combined with clinical presentation and history, may support a diagnosis of AD. The symptoms of AD can mimic other diseases; therefore, AD often becomes the diagnosis when other conditions are excluded. A thorough neurologic evaluation should be completed, which includes a mental status examination to determine sense of time and place, communication ability, memory, comprehension, and ability to complete simple math problems. Evaluation of reasoning ability, balance, and visual/motor coordination should also be completed. A brain scan, MRI, or CT scan may be done to rule out other pathology.

TREATMENT

AD is approaching epidemic proportions, yet there is no cure or preventive treatment available. Treatment of AD includes supportive care for the individuals and their families. Focus on maximizing quality of life and general health is the cornerstone of care. Medications approved by the FDA for use in the treatment of AD are designed to temporarily delay memory decline (Table 17.3). Many medications under investigation are targeting the formation of amyloid β in an effort to reduce aggregation, production, and disposal. No medication is currently available that works by halting the progress of neurodegeneration.

Summary

- Aging is a normal condition that can be complicated by degenerative changes affecting health status.
- The cellular basis of aging reflects the influences of genetics and cumulative effects of damage over time. This multifactorial process contributes to the typical manifestations of aging.
- Manifestations of aging reflect physiologic changes characteristic of human patterns of development. Changes in the soft tissues of the skin and hair contribute to the typical outward appearance of aging.
- Altered structure and function resulting from degenerative aging changes may lead to functional impairment or may be exacerbated by chronic pathologic conditions.
- Alterations in fluid and electrolyte balance, immune responses, cellular proliferation, neurologic function, mobility, perfusion, nutrition, elimination, and metabolic processes represent areas of potential pathologic sequelae related to body system changes in aging.
- Although there is no way to halt the aging process, health promotion across the life span may improve quality of life and attenuate many age-associated degenerative changes.

Case Study 17.1

A.Z., a 65-year-old woman, was having a follow-up visit with her physician. She was concerned about a change in her sleeping habits, including taking at least 30 minutes to fall asleep. She woke up after only about 5 to 6 hours of sleep and found herself unable to fall asleep again. She consequently got sleepy in the afternoon and took frequent naps.

1. What are some causes of age-associated sleep disorders?

2. What are the typical changes in sleep patterns that occur in response to age?
3. What causes age-related changes in sleep patterns?
4. What are the risks related to the use of pharmacologic sleeping aids in the elderly?
5. What nonpharmacologic strategies can be used to help promote sleep?

Log onto the Internet. Search for a relevant journal article or Web site that details sleep disorders in the elderly to confirm your predictions.

Practice Exam Questions

1. Genetic influences as the major determinants of aging are the focus of which of the following theories?
   a. Developmental theory
   b. Stochastic theory
   c. Free radical theory
   d. Error theory

2. Typical changes in total body water in the elderly include:
   a. Increased total body water caused by increase in muscle mass
   b. Increased total body water caused by increased fat mass
   c. Decreased total body water caused by decrease in muscle mass
   d. Decreased total body water caused by decreased fat mass

3. Immune senescence is characterized by:
   a. Increased antigenic immune response
   b. Enhanced T-cell function
   c. Enhanced IgE-mediated hypersensitivity
   d. Enhanced autoimmune response

4. Age-related changes affecting neurologic function include:
   a. Increased myelin
   b. Decreased number of neurons
   c. Enhanced nerve conduction
   d. Improved axonal repair mechanisms

5. An imbalance in bone remodeling characteristic of osteoporosis is caused by:
   a. Enhanced bone formation caused by increased activity of osteoclasts
   b. Enhanced bone formation caused by increased activity of osteoblasts

   c. Increased bone resorption caused by increased activity of osteoclasts
   d. Increased bone resorption caused by increased activity of osteoblasts

6. Age-related changes contributing to impaired healing include:
   a. Increased skin elasticity
   b. Enhanced subcutaneous fat
   c. Decreased superficial capillary perfusion
   d. Atrophied capillary support to dermis

7. Osteoporosis is the result of an imbalance favoring increased:
   a. Osteoblastic activity
   b. Osteclastic activity
   c. Vitamin D absorption
   d. Calcium absorption

8. Parkinson disease is characterized by:
   a. Neurofibrillary tangles
   b. Amyloid plaque
   c. Lewy bodies
   d. Tau

9. Which one of the following neurotransmitters is deficient in Parkinson disease?
   a. Dopamine
   b. Serotonin
   c. Norepinephrine
   d. Acetylcholine

10. Memory loss in Alzheimer disease results from impaired neural conduction in the:
    a. Frontal lobe
    b. Basal ganglia
    c. Limbic system
    d. Hippocampus

Discussion and Application

1. What did I know about degenerative changes in aging before today?

2. What body processes are affected by degenerative changes in aging? How do degenerative changes in aging affect those processes?

3. What are the potential etiologies for degenerative changes in aging? How do degenerative changes in aging develop?

4. Who is most at risk for developing complications related to degenerative changes in aging? How can these alterations be prevented?

5. What are the human differences that affect the etiology, risk, or course of degenerative changes in aging?

6. What clinical manifestations are expected in the course of degenerative changes in aging?

7. What special diagnostic tests are useful in determining the diagnosis and course of degenerative changes in aging?

8. What are the goals of care for individuals with degenerative changes in aging?

9. How does the concept of degenerative changes in aging build on what I have learned in the previous chapter and in the previous courses?

10. How can I use what I have learned?

RESOURCES

Alzheimer's Association:
http://www.alz.org

National Center for Chronic Disease Prevention and Health Promotion: Healthy Aging:
http://www.cdc.gov/aging/index.htm

National Institute of Neurological Disorders and Stroke:
http://www.ninds.nih.gov

National Institute on Aging:
http://www.grc.nia.nih.gov

National Osteoporosis Foundation:
http://nof.org

National Parkinson Foundation:
http://www.parkinson.org/

REFERENCES

1. Arias E. United States life tables, 2004. *Natl Vital Stat Rep.* 2007;56(9):1–40.
2. Hughes K, Reynolds R. Evolutionary and mechanistic theories of aging. *Annu Rev Entomol.* 2005;50:421–445.
3. Balaban RS, Nemoto S, Finkel T. Mitochondria, oxidants, and aging. *Cell.* 2005;120(4):483–495.
4. Beers M, Berkow R, eds. *Merck Manual of Geriatrics.* Whitehouse Station, NJ: Merck and Co.; 2005.
5. Wade PR. Aging and neural control of the GI tract. I. Age-related changes in the enteric nervous system. *Am J Physiol Gastrointest Liver Physiol.* 2002;283(3):G489–G495.
6. Centers for Disease Control and Prevention, AARP, American Medical Association. Promoting preventive services for adults 50-64: community and clinical partnerships. Atlanta: National Association of Chronic Disease Directors; 2009. Available at http://www.cdc.gov/aging/pdf/promoting-preventive-services.pdf. Accessed on February 20, 2010.
7. US Department of Health and Human Services. *Bone Health and Osteoporosis: A Report of the Surgeon General.* Rockville: US Department of Health and Human Services, Office of the Surgeon General; 2004.
8. Stokstad E. Bone quality fills holes in fracture risk. *Science.* 2005;308(5728):1580.
9. Raisz LG. Clinical practice. Screening for osteoporosis. *N Engl J Med.* 2005;353(2):164–171.
10. Crandall C. Laboratory workup for osteoporosis. Which tests are most cost-effective? *Postgrad Med.* 2003;114(3):35–38, 41–44.
11. Institute of Medicine. *Dietary Reference Intakes for Calcium, Phosphorus, Magnesium, Vitamin D, and Fluoride.* Washington, DC: Institute of Medicine; 1997.
12. Burch D, Sheerin F. Parkinson's disease. *Lancet.* 2005;365(9459):622–627.
13. National Institute of Neurologic Diseases and Stroke. *Parkinson's Disease Backgrounder.* Washington, DC: National Institutes of Health.
14. Hatano T, Kubo S, Sato S, et al (). Pathogenesis of familial Parkinson's disease: new insights based on monogenic forms of Parkinson's disease. *J Neurochem.* 2009;111(5):1075–1093.
15. Aarsland D, Andersen K, Larsen JP, et al. Prevalence and characteristics of dementia in Parkinson disease: an 8-year prospective study. *Arch Neurol.* 2003;60(3):387–392.
16. Goetz CG, Poewe W, Rascol O, et al. Movement disorder society task force report on the Hoehn and Yahr staging scale: status and recommendations. *Mov Disord.* 2004;19(9):1020–1028.
17. Hoehn MM, Yahr MD. Parkinsonism: onset, progression and mortality. *Neurology.* 1967;17:427–442.
18. Tanzi RE, Bertram L. Twenty years of the Alzheimer's disease amyloid hypothesis: a genetic perspective. *Cell.* 2005;120(4):545–555.
19. Miyoshi K. What is 'early onset dimentia'? *Psychogeriatrics.* 2009;9(2):67–72.
20. Cummings JL, Frank JC, Cherry D, et al. Guidelines for managing Alzheimer's disease: Part 1. Assessment. *Am Fam Physician.* 2002;65(11):2525–2534.

Chapter 18

Combining Complex Pathophysiologic Concepts: Diabetes Mellitus

LEARNING OBJECTIVES

1. Define and use the key terms listed in this chapter.
2. Recognize the effects of combining pathophysiologic concepts on the health of the individual.
3. Identify how previous concepts within this text relate to diabetes mellitus.
4. Differentiate type 1, type 2, and gestational diabetes.
5. Identify common clinical manifestations of diabetes.
6. Recognize short-term and long-term complications of diabetes.
7. Describe diagnostic tests and treatment strategies appropriate for diabetes.

INTRODUCTION

The human body is highly complex. We have attempted to distinguish functional alterations in human health by introducing you to concepts of pathophysiology. What you have probably figured out by now is that very few health conditions fit purely into one or two conceptual categories. For example, myocardial infarction (MI) is a problem of *perfusion*. MI also has roots in altered *nutrition, genetics,* and the *environment*. MI results in myocardial *inflammation* and induces a *stress response*. *Hormones,* such as cortisol, are released during stressful situations to aid in reestablishing homeostasis. The ineffective myocardium is less able to move fluids through the circulation, resulting in altered *fluid balance*. Pulmonary congestion may result, leading to altered *ventilation and diffusion*. The goal of this chapter is to illustrate the impact of combining complex pathophysiologic concepts using diabetes mellitus as the select clinical model.

Glucose, Insulin, Energy, and the Pancreas

Energy, in the form of glucose, is essential for optimal human functioning. Glucose is a monosaccharide, which is derived from dietary carbohydrates. Excess glucose is stored as glycogen in the liver. Glucose in the blood triggers the release of insulin. **Insulin** is an anabolic hormone required for the uptake of glucose by many cells, particularly those of the liver, muscle, and adipose cells. Insulin is *not* required for glucose uptake in the brain, red blood cells, kidney, and lens of the eye.

STOP *and Consider*

In the absence of insulin, glucose is still able to move into cells of the brain, blood, kidney, and lens. This seems a beneficial property. What do you think is the drawback of inadequate insulin resulting in excessive circulating glucose to these cells?

Anabolic hormones, including insulin, are responsible for building complex compounds in the body, such as building proteins from amino acids. Insulin has several key functions:

- Promoting glucose usage, thereby decreasing blood glucose levels
- Promoting protein synthesis
- Promoting the formation and storage of lipids
- Facilitating transport of potassium, phosphate, and magnesium into the cells

Insulin production and availability is closely connected to the pancreas. The pancreas is located behind the lower portion of the stomach and is innervated by the autonomic nervous system. The pancreas has both endocrine and exocrine functions. The **endocrine pancreas** secretes hormones, such as insulin and glucagon. The acini cells of the **exocrine pancreas** secrete digestive enzymes and alkaline fluids through the pancreatic duct into the duodenum. Chapter 15 is concerned with the role of the pancreas as a digestive accessory organ. This chapter is concerned with the endocrine, or hormone-secreting, function of the pancreas.

Throughout the pancreas are clusters of cells called the **islets of Langerhans** (Fig. 18.1). The islets of Langerhans contain three major types of hormone-secreting cells:

- *Alpha* cells secrete glucagon, which mobilizes glycogen from the liver and suppresses insulin secretion; glucagon is critical in maintaining blood glucose levels between meals
- *Beta* cells secrete insulin, which promotes glucose utilization

Figure 18.1   Islets of Langerhans in the pancreas.

- *Delta* cells secrete somatostatin and gastrin, which regulates alpha and beta cell function by suppressing the release of insulin, glucagon, and pancreatic polypeptides

The pancreas also contains F cells, which are located primarily at the periphery of the islets, although a few F cells are scattered throughout the ducts and acini. F cells secrete pancreatic polypeptides, which suppress digestive enzyme release from the exocrine pancreas.

STOP *and Consider*

If you skipped breakfast and had a really low blood glucose level, which cells of the islets of Langerhans would you expect to be stimulated?

The hormones secreted from the islets of Langerhans are important controlling devices of carbohydrate, protein, and fat metabolism. As with other hormones, feedback systems are critical to maintaining homeostasis. With insulin, secretion is *increased* when there are elevations in (1) blood glucose; (2) amino acids; (3) potassium, phosphate, and magnesium; and (4) glucagon and gastrin. Insulin is needed to promote glucose uptake and metabolism of nutrients. Certain situations also promote a *decrease* in insulin secretion, such as low blood glucose, high levels of insulin (through negative feedback mechanisms), and the stimulation of alpha cells. In these cases, insulin is not needed because it would exacerbate the state of hypoglycemia.

● **STOP** *and* **Consider**

How does eating a large meal or skipping a meal affect insulin levels in the body?

◢ Diabetes Mellitus

Diabetes mellitus is a group of disorders, characterized by the inability to regulate the amount of glucose in the body, leading to inadequate metabolism of protein, fats, and carbohydrates. The different types of diabetes are summarized in Table 18.1 and explained in detail in this chapter. Diabetes insipidus, a condition of inadequate antidiuretic hormone, was discussed in Chapter 11. Many other secondary conditions can lead to diabetes; these are summarized in Box 18.1.

One or a combination of the following characterizes the basic pathophysiology in various types of diabetes:

1. A complete destruction of pancreatic beta cells leading to a lack of insulin secretion
2. Reduced insulin secretion from impaired beta cell function in response to glucose stimulation
3. A peripheral resistance to insulin

The absence, deficit, or resistance to insulin leads to a state of **hyperglycemia**, which is a significant elevation in blood glucose level, coupled with the inability to transport glucose and amino acids into those cells that require insulin for transport. Liver, muscle, and adipose cells become deprived of glucose as an energy source and must turn to other less efficient sources, such as body fats or even proteins, for energy.

Box 18.1 Secondary Conditions That Can Lead to Insulin Deficit or Resistance

- Diseases of the pancreas that destroy pancreatic beta cells
  - Pancreatitis
  - Cystic fibrosis
  - Pancreatic cancer
- Hormonal syndromes that interfere with insulin secretion or cause peripheral insulin resistance
  - Pheochromocytoma
  - Acromegaly
  - Cushing syndrome
- Stress, such as that occurs with severe medical illness or surgery, because increases in glucagon, catecholamines, cortisol, and growth hormone levels antagonize the secretion or effects of insulin
- Certain medications
  - Phenytoin
  - Glucocorticoids
  - Estrogens

INSULIN DEFICIT: TYPE 1 DIABETES MELLITUS

Type 1 diabetes is a chronic problem of carbohydrate, fat, and protein metabolism. The body is unable to metabolize nutrients because of an absolute or significant deficiency of insulin. Approximately 10% of individuals with diabetes are categorized as type 1. This type of diabetes was previously known as insulin-dependent diabetes mellitus (IDDM) or juvenile-onset diabetes to reflect the most common treatment modality (insulin replacement) and age at diagnosis

Table 18.1 Comparison of Types of Diabetes Mellitus

	Onset	Cause	Treatment
Type 1	Puberty or childhood (peak at 10–14 years)	Insulin deficit	Insulin replacement balanced with exercise and diet
Type 2	Adult years (peak at age 45 years); prevalence increases in those under age 45 years	Insulin resistance or impaired ability of the tissues to use insulin; insufficient insulin in relation to the needs of the body	Diet, exercise, oral glycemic agents, and possibly insulin
Gestational	Pregnancy (peak at fifth or sixth month gestation)	Insulin resistance during pregnancy as a result of too much hormone production in the body (for the placenta); inability to make the additional insulin that is needed during pregnancy	Diet, exercise, sometimes insulin, delivery of baby

(approximately 10 to 14 years of age). These labels have been replaced with type 1 to reflect the possibility that those individuals with type 2 diabetes can also be children and may be treated with insulin. The current labels (type 1 or type 2) more clearly distinguish the reason for hyperglycemia.

Pathophysiology

The etiology of type 1 diabetes is multifactorial and includes both genetic and environmental influences leading to autoimmune destruction of beta cells. The importance of genetic susceptibility has been demonstrated in studies of identical twins (25% to 50% greater risk in second twin if one twin is diagnosed) and the presence of certain antigens expressed on the major histocompatibility complex (MHC; see Chapter 4) in those with type 1 diabetes. Exposure to a trigger in the environment, such as a virus or toxin, then stimulates cell-mediated destruction and a process of autoimmunity that promotes destruction of the beta cells. Most beta islet-cell antibodies are directed against glutamic acid decarboxylase (GAD), a chemical within the beta cells. Examples of triggering environmental agents include infection with mumps, group-B coxsackie viruses, or intra-uterine rubella exposure.

Cell-mediated immune mechanisms (more specifically, the presence of cytotoxic T lymphocytes) destroy beta cells. Autoimmune destruction triggers a chronic inflammatory response. Inflammation contributes to further destruction of beta cells and impaired insulin secretion. In the early stages of this cell-mediated immune destruction, antibodies against beta cells are circulating, but hyperglycemia is not yet present. This is considered a state of "prediabetes" and can last for several years. Clinical manifestations and detection of diabetes usually occur when autoimmune processes destroy 80% to 90% or more of the beta cells of the pancreas. Over time, the exocrine pancreas becomes fibrotic with the subsequent atrophy of acinar cells.

Type 1 diabetes also affects alpha cell function, resulting in increased levels of glucagon. Recall that the glucagon suppresses insulin production. This, coupled with beta cell destruction, leads to a state of hyperglycemia and hyperketonemia. Hyperglycemia is a result of accumulations of circulating blood glucose unmatched by insulin for use in the cell. The body is starving for energy and turns to fat stores and protein for energy. Insulin inhibits lipolysis (fat breakdown). Therefore, the reduction or absence of insulin allows the unregulated mobilization of fats for energy. As a result, fat oxidation produces **hyperketone-mia** (excess circulating ketone bodies), composed of acetoacetic acid, acetone, and β-hydroxybutyric acid, leading to a state of metabolic **ketoacidosis** (see Chapter 8).

Hyperglycemia, even when not associated with ketoacidosis, is problematic and can lead to osmotic diuresis. Osmotic diuresis is a condition in which excess glucose promotes the attraction of water into the kidneys, thereby eliminating glucose, electrolytes, and water through the urine. This can lead to severe dehydration. Hyperglycemia also undermines white blood cell function, promotes infection, and impairs wound healing.

STOP *and Consider*

How does an insulin deficit compare to marasmus as described in Chapter 15?

Clinical Manifestations

The clinical manifestations of type 1 diabetes mellitus are related to severe hyperglycemia and hyperketonemia, as well as to inadequate energy and nutrient metabolism (Fig. 18.2). These manifestations often appear abruptly despite months or even years of beta cell destruction. The clinical manifestations most commonly associated with type 1 diabetes include:

- **Polydipsia**—excessive thirst
- **Polyuria**—excessive urination
- **Polyphagia**—excessive hunger

Other symptoms include **nocturia** (urination at night), fatigue, lethargy, weight loss, and blurred vision. The clinical manifestations, along with the pathophysiologic origins, are outlined in Table 18.2.

Research Notes

Those who perform blood glucose testing three to four times per day were found in one study to have clinically and statistically better HbA$_{1c}$ levels. However, only 54% of those with diabetes reported testing this frequently.[1]

Diagnostic Criteria

The diagnosis of type 1 diabetes mellitus is based on a thorough patient history and physical examination, including specific laboratory and diagnostic tests. The presence of polyuria, polydipsia, polyphagia, weight loss, and fatigue, along with an elevation in the fasting blood glucose above 126 mg/dL or the random blood glucose level above 200 mg/dL, is usually sufficient for diagnosis.

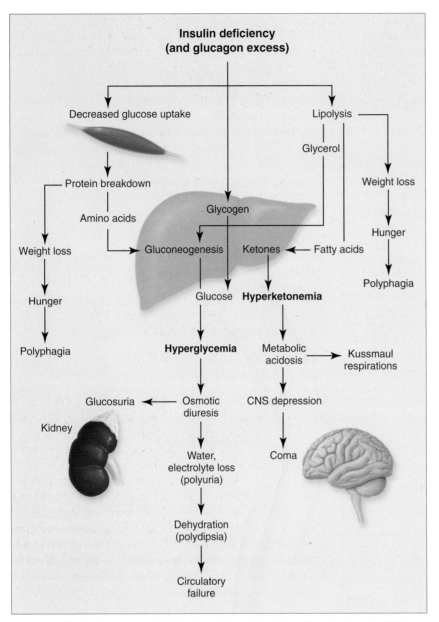

**Insulin deficiency
(and glucagon excess)**

Decreased glucose uptake

Lipolysis

Glycerol

Protein breakdown

Weight loss

Amino acids

Glycogen

Weight loss

Hunger

Gluconeogenesis   Ketones ← Fatty acids

Hunger

Polyphagia

Glucose   **Hyperketonemia**

Polyphagia

Hyperglycemia   Metabolic
acidosis → Kussmaul
respirations

Glucosuria ← Osmotic
diuresis   CNS depression

Kidney

Water,
electrolyte loss
(polyuria)   Coma

Dehydration
(polydipsia)

Circulatory
failure

■ **Figure 18.2**   Concept map. Mechanisms of hyperglycemia and hyperketonemia. CNS, central nervous system. (Image modified from Porth CM. *Essentials of Pathophysiology: Concepts of Altered Health States*. Philadelphia: Lippincott Williams & Wilkins; 2003, with permission.)

🔬 *From the Lab*

Glycosylated hemoglobin (HbA$_{1c}$) is a blood test that depicts hemoglobin and red blood cell exposure to glucose over the previous 3 to 4 months. In prolonged hyperglycemia, found in both type 1 and type 2 diabetes, the hemoglobin that travels on the red blood cell becomes irreversibly combined with glucose, a situation termed glycosylation, for the life of that red blood cell (120 days). HbA$_{1c}$ is therefore a useful determinant of "average" exposure of red blood cells to glucose over that period. The higher the HbA$_{1c}$, the more hyperglycemic, or uncontrolled, the diabetes has been. The goal for those with diabetes should be 7% or below. Persons with elevations in HbA$_{1c}$ are at greater risk for long-term complications, including cardiovascular disease and death.[2]

Checking urine for ketones can also provide information on the presence of hyperketonemia; urine ketone levels are proportional to blood ketone levels. Islet-cell autoantibodies can be detected in the early stages of type 1 diabetes as well as autoantibodies against GAD, an enzyme produced by pancreatic islet cells, which persist over time. Table 18.3 provides a guide to laboratory tests useful in the diagnosis of type 1 diabetes.

Treatment

Treatment of diabetes mellitus requires a balance of the following:

1. Carbohydrate (food) intake
2. Exercise
3. Insulin replacement therapy

The goal of treatment is to stabilize blood glucose levels within the expected range (70 to 120 mg/dL). Blood glucose levels are measured frequently using self-blood glucose monitoring systems (Fig. 18.3). Food intake increases blood glucose levels. Therefore, food intake must equal the available insulin and metabolic needs of the body. The diet should include complex carbohydrates, protein, and unsaturated fat sources while limiting simple sugars, cholesterol, and saturated fats. Typically, the carbohydrate to insulin ratio needed is around 10 to 15 g of carbohydrate to 1 unit of rapid-acting insulin. Exercise decreases blood glucose levels through increased glucose usage by muscle tissue. Increases in exercise must be matched with reductions in insulin or increases in food intake.

Insulin replacement therapy is integral to the treatment plan for type 1 diabetes. Insulin is destroyed in the gastrointestinal tract if taken orally, so it must be injected subcutaneously via intermittent injections or with an insulin infusion pump. The onset,

Table 18.2 Clinical Manifestations and Corresponding Pathophysiologic Process in Type 1 Diabetes Mellitus

Clinical Manifestation	Pathophysiologic Process	Potential Complications
Polyuria, nocturia, and glucosuria (excess glucose in the urine)	Hyperglycemia osmotically draws fluids into the intravascular space; glucose also acts as a diuretic; this leads to large volumes of urine being filtered by the kidneys and excreted; also, the renal threshold for glucose is exceeded; the kidneys allow this excess glucose to spill out into the urine	Dehydration
Polydipsia and dry mouth	Hyperglycemia osmotically draws fluids from the cells into the intravascular space; this leads to cellular dehydration and the stimulation of thirst by the hypothalamus	Dehydration
Polyphagia, weight loss, and fatigue	Insulin deficit disallows use of glucose for energy; storage of fats, proteins, and carbohydrates begin to deplete; cells are in a state of starvation because of lack of nutrients, thereby inducing hunger	Starvation, coma, and death
Blurred vision	Lens and retina are exposed to hyperosmolar fluids	Vision impairment and blindness

peak, and duration of action can vary among different types of insulin and include:

1. Rapid onset, short-acting (also called regular)
2. Intermediate-acting
3. Slow onset, long-acting

Table 18.4 distinguishes the different forms of insulin based on onset, peak, and duration of action. The goal is to coordinate food intake with insulin availability in the body. Injecting insulin without adequate dietary intake induces **hypoglycemia**, or low blood glucose levels.

Insulin infusion pumps are an alternative to daily injections. An insulin pump looks like a pager and can be worn inconspicuously on a belt, in a pocket, or on an elastic band wrapped around an arm or leg. The insulin is delivered through a plastic catheter into subcutaneous tissue of the abdomen. An insulin pump is able to simulate the pancreas' delivery of insulin more closely than insulin injections. Most people on the pump find that they are able to achieve better control of their blood glucose levels because the insulin is delivered continuously (at a basal rate) and in a bolus for mealtimes or times of physical activity. When an insulin pump is used, blood glucose levels must be checked more frequently.

Table 18.3 Comparison of Laboratory Tests for Type 1 Diabetes Mellitus

Diagnostic Test	Expected Values	Significant Findings (Values Are Approximate and May Vary by Source)
Random blood glucose	70–120 mg/dL	>200 mg/dL along with clinical manifestations
Fasting blood glucose	70–120 mg/dL	>126 mg/dL on two occasions after fasting
Glucose tolerance test: individual is given 50–100 g of glucose dissolved in water; blood glucose is measured at 1, 2, and 3 hours	120–160 mg/dL at 1 hour 70–120 mg/dL at 2 hours	>190 mg/dL after 1 hour >165 mg/dL after 2 hours
Glycosylated hemoglobin (HbA$_{1C}$)	2%–6%	8% and greater signifies prolonged hyperglycemia
Urinalysis	Negative for glucose	Glucose >15 mg/dL
	Negative for ketones	Ketones present

■ **Figure 18.3** Self-monitoring of blood glucose levels.

INSULIN RESISTANCE AND REDUCTION: TYPE 2 DIABETES

Type 2 diabetes mellitus is a problem of insulin resistance (reduced tissue sensitivity to insulin) *and* a reduction in adequate insulin secretion. Most (90%) individuals with diabetes are estimated to have type 2. This form was previously referred to as non–insulin-dependent diabetes or adult-onset diabetes, although some individuals with type 2 may require insulin replacement, and the incidence is increasing in children. Maturity-onset diabetes of the young (MODY) is a rare form of type 2 diabetes that has a strong genetic component (autosomal dominant inheritance) and is found to affect individuals younger than 25 years of age. The metabolic syndrome (syndrome X) is a condition that includes insulin resistance and a constellation of other metabolic problems, including obesity, high triglyceride levels, low high-density lipoprotein levels, hypertension, and coronary heart disease. Individuals diagnosed with type 2 diabetes must also be evaluated for metabolic syndrome to determine the full range of metabolic alterations. Gestational diabetes (discussed later) is also considered a form of type 2 diabetes that presents during pregnancy.

Pathophysiology

Similar to type 1 diabetes, the exact cause of type 2 is unknown; however, genetic and environmental factors appear to contribute for its development. The most significant risk factor is obesity, which results from both genetic and environmental influences. Approximately 90% of those who develop type 2 diabetes are obese. All overweight individuals have insulin resistance, but only those who are unable to compensate by increasing beta cell production of insulin go on to develop type 2 diabetes. Other risk factors include age over 30 years, a family history of type 2 diabetes, and Native American, Hispanic, or Black race.

Unlike type 1 diabetes, there is no autoimmune destruction of the pancreas. Rather, insulin *resistance,* or a decreased sensitivity to insulin in metabolic tissues, such as the liver, skeletal muscle, and adipose tissue, results in insufficient insulin usage (Fig. 18.4). Obesity promotes peripheral insulin resistance by releasing free fatty acids and cytokines from adipose cells. These chemicals interfere with insulin signals, disrupt insulin receptors on the target cell plasma membranes, and prohibit insulin from facilitating the entry of glucose into liver, muscle, and adipose tissues. Individuals with type 2 diabetes also exhibit reduced insulin secretion in response to glucose exposure. In type 2 diabetes, subadequate levels of insulin and peripheral resistance to insulin uptake leads to the following:

1. Beta cells do not adequately respond to circulating blood glucose levels.
2. The release of glycogen from the liver coupled with the suppression of insulin by glucagon promotes excessive circulating glucose.

Table 18.4 Comparison of Types of Insulin

Insulin	Rapid-acting (i.e., Lispro)	Short-acting (i.e., Regular, Humulin R)	Intermediate-acting (i.e., NPH)	Long-acting (i.e., Ultralente)	Other (i.e., Glargine)
Onset of action	15 minutes	30 minutes	2–4 hours	6–10 hours	2–4 hours
Peak (in hours)	1	2–3	4–12	8–12	Peakless
Duration (in hours)	2–4	3–6	12–18	18–26	Up to 24
When to administer	Immediately before a meal	Throughout the day	Throughout the day	Nighttime	Nighttime

NPH, Neutral Protamine Hagedorn (Hagedorn discovered in 1936 that when protamine was added to insulin, it prolonged the effects).

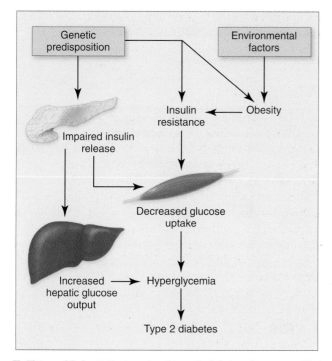

Figure 18.4 Pathogenesis of type 2 diabetes. (Image modified from Porth CM. *Essentials of Pathophysiology: Concepts of Altered Health States*. Philadelphia: Lippincott Williams and Wilkins; 2003, with permission.)

cular disease, recurrent infections, or neuropathy. The presence of obesity and hyperlipidemia should heighten suspicion that type 2 diabetes is present.

Diagnostic Criteria

Those identified within the risk categories for type 2 diabetes should be evaluated by random or fasting blood glucose measurements. Many individuals with type 2 diabetes are asymptomatic and the disease goes undiagnosed for many years. As with individuals who have type 1 diabetes, those individuals with clinical manifestations (i.e., polyuria, polydipsia, polyphagia, nocturia, and weight loss) and random plasma glucose levels above 200 mg/dL are easily diagnosed as having diabetes. A major diagnostic challenge is differentiating type 1 from type 2 diabetes. More often, individuals with type 2 diabetes are overweight adults, but this is not always the case. Upon diagnosis, it is not unusual for blood glucose levels to be less than that found with type 1 diabetes because insulin is still available. If diabetes is suspected, two separate fasting blood glucose measurements are warranted. If both are above 126 mg/dL, type 2 diabetes may be suggested. A fasting plasma glucose between 110 and

3. The insulin receptors in the liver, skeletal muscle, and adipose tissue are unresponsive, thereby making the tissues unable, or resistant, to using the insulin.

Glucagon secretion is significantly increased. Recall that glucagon mobilizes glycogen from the liver and suppresses insulin secretion. Although there is no reduction in beta cells, high serum lipid levels, as may occur with obesity, allows fat to deposit in the pancreas, which may lead to sclerosis and further impair pancreatic function. Ultimately, this results in the impaired metabolism of carbohydrates, fats, and proteins.

Clinical Manifestations

The clinical manifestations for type 2 diabetes are often insidious and nonspecific. In some cases the classic symptoms for type 1 (polyuria, polyphagia, and polydipsia) may be present. Most of the time, however, clinical manifestations that appear are related to long-term complications that may arise with diabetes, such as visual changes, changes in kidney function, coronary artery disease, peripheral vas-

Research Notes

In a study of over 25,000 volunteers over a 12-year period, the European Prospective Investigation of Cancer-Norfolk Cohort Study determined that a diet of energy-dense foods predisposes to obesity and is linked to the development of type 2 diabetes. The researchers determined that the baseline energy density for foods consumed was higher in those who developed type 2 diabetes compared to those who never developed diabetes when adjusted for lifestyle factors, social factors, and dietary factors. This study concluded that dietary intake as an isolated variable has a significant impact on diabetes and a low-energy dense diet must be considered in the prevention of diabetes.[3]

125 mg/dL indicates "impaired fasting glucose" and requires close monitoring because there is a high risk of developing diabetes over time. The presence of antibodies against the islet cells or GAD would indicate that this person does *not* have type 2 diabetes, but rather has type 1. Also, at diagnosis, approximately 25% of individuals with type 2 diabetes have retinopathy, 9% have neuropathy, and 8% have nephropathy.[4]

Treatment

Treatment of type 2 diabetes begins with weight control through an individualized nutrition and exercise plan and can include oral glycemic agents or insulin replacement therapy. The goal of treatment for type

Table 18.5 Oral Glycemic Agents Used to Treat Type 2 Diabetes Mellitus

Oral Glycemic Agent (Examples of Generic Names)	Primary Site of Action	Method of Action
Alpha-glucosidase inhibitors (acarbose, miglitol)	Intestines	Slows carbohydrate digestion
Biguanides (metformin)	Liver	Prevents excessive glucose release from the liver; makes peripheral tissues more sensitive to insulin
Meglitinides (repaglinide)	Pancreas	Stimulates more secretion of insulin from the pancreas; short-acting
Sulfonylureas (tolbutamide, glipizide, glyburide, glimepiride)	Pancreas	Stimulates more secretion of insulin from the pancreas
Thiazolidinediones (rosiglitazone, pioglitazone)	Muscle cells	Increases sensitivity of tissues (fat, muscle, liver) to insulin

2 diabetes is the same as that of type 1: to maintain optimal blood glucose levels. Physical activity is advantageous because it increases the uptake of glucose by the muscles without increasing insulin needs. Exercise also improves insulin sensitivity. The other positive outcomes of physical activity, such as decreased body fat, increase in endorphins, improved cardiovascular health, and weight control, also lower the risk for some of the long-term complications of diabetes.

If diet and exercise are inadequate to produce adequate glycemic control, individuals with type 2 diabetes may also require oral medications along with continued dietary modifications and exercise. Glycemic agents act to increase insulin release by the beta cells, increase glucose production by the liver, or increase the uptake of insulin. Table 18.5 describes common oral glycemic agents and their

From the Lab

Annual screening for albumin (protein) in the urine is recommended in all patients with diabetes, especially those with type 2 diabetes to detect early renal damage and is a risk factor for heart disease. Performing an albumin-to-creatinine ratio is the best way to start. If abnormal (i.e., >30 mg/g), a 24-hour urine specimen should be performed to determine albumin excretion. Normal urine albumin excretion is defined as less than 30 mg/day. Microalbuminuria is defined as 30 to 300 mg/day (20 to 200 µg/min). At least two of the three samples over 3 to 6 months are needed to confirm the presence of albumin in the urine.[4]

mechanism for action in treating type 2 diabetes. Insulin therapy may also be initiated if insulin replacement is warranted. The forms of insulin are illustrated in Table 18.4.

STOP *and* **Consider**

Why is it not recommended to use oral glycemic agents to treat those with type 1 diabetes?

GESTATIONAL DIABETES

Gestational diabetes is defined as any degree of glucose intolerance that occurs during pregnancy. This form of diabetes is usually temporary, but in some cases, the woman may go on to develop type 2 diabetes. Gestational diabetes occurs because of insulin resistance that occurs during pregnancy *and* because of an inability of the pancreas to make the additional insulin that is needed during the pregnancy to support the placenta. Risk factors for this type of diabetes include family history of diabetes, five or more previous pregnancies, and a previous large-for-date baby. This condition occurs in 4% to 14% of pregnancies and is usually diagnosed in the fifth or sixth month. Treatments for gestational diabetes include diet modification, exercise, and possibly insulin. Tight control of blood glucose is needed to prevent overstimulation of the fetal pancreas during pregnancy. Oral glycemic agents are not recommended because of their potentially teratogenic effects. If untreated, gestational diabetes, or even poorly controlled type 1 or type 2 diabetes in a pregnant woman, can lead to:

- Fetal macrosomia (abnormally large body size)
- Hypoglycemia from pancreatic hyperplasia and excess insulin secretion in the newborn
- Hypocalcemia
- Hyperbilirubinemia
- A 5% to 10% incidence of major developmental anomalies, such as spina bifida or heart defects.

Additional complications for the mother include a greater risk for chronic hypertension and cesarean delivery. Gestational diabetes does increase a woman's risk for developing type 2 diabetes even after the pregnancy and delivery is complete.

Acute Complications of Diabetes Mellitus

Acute complications of diabetes mellitus are related to either hypoglycemia or a state of excessive hyperglycemia. Acute complications have a rapid onset and often have significant manifestations of altered neuronal function. Particularly in those with type 1 diabetes, the regulation of glycemic control can be challenging. The Somogyi effect and dawn phenomenon illustrate acute complications of diabetes related to the attempted regulation of glycemic control.

HYPOGLYCEMIA

Hypoglycemia is a state of significantly low blood glucose that results in demonstrable clinical manifestations, such as weakness, pallor, or cool/clammy skin. Although individual variations exist, manifestations typically present when the serum glucose becomes less than 50 mg/dL. This can occur in situations such as:

- Hyperinsulinemia (high circulating insulin levels) as can occur with the administration of exogenous insulin to treat diabetes
- Inadequate food intake or vomiting, in which the presence of glucose in the body is reduced
- Frequent simple carbohydrate intake
- Strenuous exercise or infection, during which the use of glucose is excessive

Hypoglycemia is most commonly found in individuals with type 1 diabetes who are undergoing insulin replacement therapy. Insulin replacement therapy requires the careful intake of adequate nutrients to match the injected insulin. This step is particularly critical with the insulin pump because the pump admini sters a basal dose of insulin throughout the day. Therefore, the presence of insulin, coupled with skipping a meal and exercising, can lead to blood glucose levels as low as 40 to 50 mg/dL. Hypoglycemia is particularly problematic for the brain, which has an energy demand twice that of other cells in the body. Neurons are in a constant state of metabolic activity, even during sleep. Mental concentration and other forms of bioelectrical communication throughout the nervous system require high concentrations of glucose. A lack of glucose has been found to impede the synthesis of acetylcholine, a major brain neurotransmitter.

Interestingly, the ingestion of simple carbohydrates, as opposed to complex carbohydrates, can also promote a state of neuronal hypoglycemia. Complex carbohydrates are gradually broken down, stored in the liver, and released gradually into the blood in the form of glucose. Therefore, the process of intake, storage, and release of glucose from complex carbohydrates is ideal for brain function. Simple carbohydrates, such as that found in sugary foods like syrup, fruit juice, or honey, enter the blood and rapidly raise the blood sugar. This stimulates the rapid release of insulin. The insulin pulls this excess glucose into cells of the body and actually deprives the brain of glucose. Recall that neurons do not require insulin for glucose uptake and are unable to store glucose. Even though other cells in the body have stored glucose, the brain becomes hypoglycemic.

Clinical manifestations of hypoglycemia can vary among individuals but are most notably related to neuronal deprivation of glucose. Potential signs and symptoms include poor concentration, extreme hunger, clammy/cool skin, blurred vision, dizziness and confusion, difficulty with speech, lack of coordination, staggering gait, and headache. The hypoglycemic state activates the sympathetic nervous system, which causes an increase in the pulse, along with palpitations, sweating, anxiety, and tremors. Loss of consciousness, seizures, coma, and death can occur if hypoglycemia is not treated.

Prevention of hypoglycemia involves calculating and administering insulin dosages with regard to nutritional intake and physical activity. The treatment of hypoglycemia requires administration of 15 to 20 g of glucose. The method of administration depends on the level of consciousness of the person. If the person is fairly conscious and able to swallow, a concentrated carbohydrate, such as sweetened fruit juice, honey, or candy, is sufficient. If the symptoms do not improve within a few minutes, the dose can be repeated. If the person is unconscious and cannot swallow, glucagon must be administered parenterally, intramuscularly, or subcutaneously.

DIABETIC KETOACIDOSIS

Diabetic ketoacidosis (DKA) is a problem of deficient insulin and severe hyperglycemia leading to a state of metabolic acidosis and severe osmotic diuresis. It occurs most commonly in those with type 1 diabetes. DKA typically develops over a few days and is triggered by an increased demand for insulin, such as that occurs with severe stress, infection, overconsumption of food, pregnancy, or inadequate insulin administration. The onset of DKA may be the event that makes the individual aware that he or she has type 1 diabetes. Blood glucose levels can reach as high as 1000 mg/dL.

The lack of insulin causes mobilization of fatty acids for energy, leading to an increased production of ketones. The kidneys are unable to excrete the ketones and the cells are unable to use these byproducts, allowing ketones to accumulate in the blood. Recall that optimal cell function occurs within a narrow pH range (see Chapter 8). Acidosis (pH less than 7.3) leads to widespread cellular injury. Hyperglycemia promotes osmotic diuresis, loss of electrolytes, and dehydration.

The signs and symptoms of DKA are consistent with severe hyperglycemia, metabolic acidosis, and dehydration. Manifestations preceding DKA include those of type 1 diabetes: polyuria, polydipsia, polyphagia, nocturia, weight loss, and fatigue. Abdominal pain and vomiting are common. With the onset of acidosis, buffer systems are taxed and compensatory changes occur in an effort to improve the acid–base balance in the body. **Kussmaul respirations** are deep, rapid respirations that release excess acids through the lungs and into the atmosphere. The breath also has a sweet, fruity odor caused by the release of acetone, a volatile form of ketones. The decreased circulating blood volume promotes tachycardia and hypotension. Acidosis triggers a decreased level of consciousness, which can progress to coma and even death.

Treatment of DKA focuses on stabilizing blood glucose levels, correcting acidosis, replacing fluids and electrolytes, and improving tissue perfusion. These goals are accomplished through intravenous administration of insulin, fluid, and electrolyte solutions. Any triggering causes, such as infection, must also be addressed. After the individual's blood glucose and fluid balance are stabilized, treatment involves initiating or resuming strategies to manage the diabetes effectively and to prevent further occurrences of DKA over time.

STOP *and Consider*

You arrive on a scene and see that someone with diabetes is unconscious. How do you know if the person is experiencing hypoglycemia or hyperglycemia?

HYPERGLYCEMIC HYPEROSMOLAR NONKETOTIC SYNDROME

Hyperglycemic hyperosmolar nonketotic syndrome (HHNK) is primarily a problem of type 2 diabetes in older adults that is characterized by:

- Hyperglycemia, often above 600 mg/dL
- High plasma osmolarity
- Dehydration
- Lack of (or mild) ketosis
- Changes in the level of consciousness

In HHNK, severe hyperglycemia results from increased insulin resistance and excessive carbohydrate intake. Hyperosmolarity from excessive glucose and inadequate fluid intake results in water shifting from intracellular to extracellular spaces, leading to cellular dehydration and cell death. The presence of glucose in the urine impairs the ability of the kidney to concentrate urine and promotes osmotic diuresis. This exacerbates water losses.

The onset is often gradual and presents over a period of days to weeks. Hyperglycemia and solute diuresis leads to polyuria, polydipsia, polyphagia, weight loss, weakness, and signs of dehydration, such as leg cramps, poor tissue turgor, cool extremities, and tachycardia. The individual may also present with renal impairment and neurologic changes, such as seizures, hallucinations, weakness, paralysis, muscle tremors, and visual changes. Approximately one out of four of the individuals in HHNK present in a state of coma. In some cases, the individual is not known to have diabetes before the onset of HHNK. Glucose is present in the urine and ketones are typically absent or minimal. Treatment involves careful fluid replacement with a tonicity matched to the level of hyperosmolarity, along with potassium, magnesium, and phosphate replacement, and stabilization of blood glucose levels. After the individual is stabilized, ongoing care is required to prevent further occurrences of HHNK through the ongoing management of type 2 diabetes.

THE SOMOGYI EFFECT AND DAWN PHENOMENON

The **Somogyi effect** is the presence of rebound hyperglycemia as a reaction to insulin-induced hypoglycemia. Insulin-induced hypoglycemia triggers compensatory increases in catecholamines, glucagon, cortisol, and growth hormone in an effort to promote insulin resistance and increase circulating blood glucose levels. Hypoglycemia, which often occurs during the night, is met with morning or daytime hyperglycemia. This prompts the increased exogenous administration of insulin, which further perpetuates the Somogyi effect and poses a major challenge to tight control of glucose levels. Individuals with morning hyperglycemia need to test their blood glucose levels in the middle of the night to determine the presence of the Somogyi effect. If the individual is hypoglycemic, adjustments in the evening snack or insulin type or dose may be required.

The **dawn phenomenon** is a situation in which an individual's blood glucose level upon waking is higher than the level before going to bed in the evening. Because there is no food intake during the night, this finding suggests that blood glucose should decrease during the night. The dawn phenomenon, similar to the Somogyi effect, is related to the release of hormones (growth hormone, cortisol, glucagon, and catecholamines), usually between 4 and 9 a.m., which triggers insulin resistance and the release of glucose from the liver. The dawn phenomenon differs from the Somogyi effect in that hyperglycemia is not triggered by overnight hypoglycemia. Blood glucose levels steadily rise through the night. Management of the dawn phenomenon requires limiting or regulating evening snacks or possibly increasing oral glycemic agents (in type 2 diabetes) or basal insulin doses (in type 1 diabetes).

Chronic Complications of Diabetes Mellitus

The presence of diabetes immediately increases the risk of developing irreversible clinical complications because of degenerative changes throughout the body. Chronic complications of diabetes develop primarily in tissues that are affected by the high levels of glucose circulating in the blood. In those tissues that require insulin for transport of glucose, hyperglycemia causes degenerative changes by thickening the basement membrane, promoting coagulation, obstructing perfusion, inducing hypoxia, and producing tissue necrosis. In those tissues that do not require insulin for glucose transport (e.g., red blood cells, lens, kidney, and nerves), the excess glucose causes fluid to osmotically shift into these cells and causes the cells to rupture. Complications, illustrated in Figure 18.5, are frequently classified as:

1. Microvascular (relating to small vessels)
2. Macrovascular (relating to large vessels)
3. Neuropathies

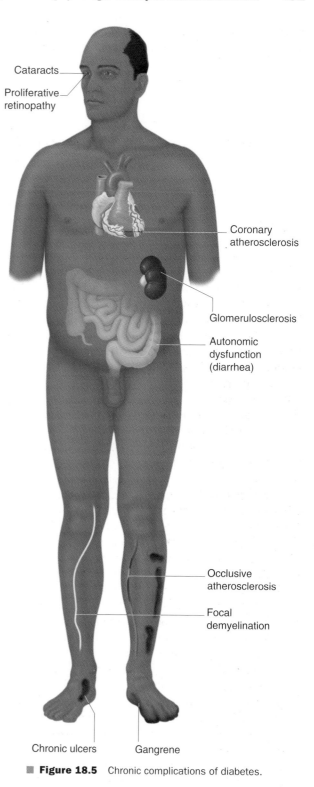

Figure 18.5 Chronic complications of diabetes.

An individual is less likely to develop chronic complications of diabetes if blood glucose levels are kept in tight control (70 to 120 mg/dL).

MICROVASCULAR COMPLICATIONS

Degenerative changes in small vessels occur most notably in the retinas, a condition called **retinopathy**, and in the kidneys, referred to as **nephropathy**. One mechanism for the development of complications is the presence of excess glucose, which binds to collagen and proteins in the blood vessel walls. This process is referred to as glycosylation. The rate of glycosylation is proportionate to the level of hyperglycemia. Glycosylation permanently alters the structure of collagen and proteins in the blood vessel walls. This alteration leads to the hardening and thickening of the capillary basement membrane, resulting in obstruction or rupture of the capillaries. Ultimately, this development leads to necrosis and loss of function in those tissues being supplied by the small vessels. In retinopathy, retinal ischemia related to obstruction and rupture of capillaries can lead to blindness. The development of complications may also be related to an accumulation of sorbitol, a sugar alcohol, derived from the metabolism of excessive glucose by aldose reductase (an enzyme) in tissues that do not require insulin. Sorbitol is theorized to promote the osmosis of fluid into the lens of the eye and may also be directly toxic to cells. Reactive oxygen species (free radicals) may also be involved in the development of diabetes complications due to release of free radicals as a result of tissue injury from excessive glucose exposure.

Based on these potential mechanisms, the development of nephropathy is a consequence of:

1. Protein breakdown caused by high glucose levels and inadequate insulin
2. Excessive osmotic diuresis and glucosuria that occurs with hyperglycemia
3. Intraglomerular hypertension, which is worsened in the presence of systemic hypertension

With nephropathy, changes in the glomerular capillaries increase the intraglomerular pressure, causing hypertension within the kidney. Chronic renal hypertension contributes to glomerular sclerosis, hypoxia, and, ultimately, chronic renal failure. Nephropathy in individuals with diabetes is the leading cause of end-stage renal disease, accounting for almost half of new cases of renal failure. The presence of continuous proteinuria is a key manifestation of diabetic nephropathy and progressive renal disease. Protein restriction, dialysis, or renal transplant may be indicated for those who develop chronic renal failure secondary to diabetic nephropathy. Essential to the avoidance of microvascular complications are strict blood glucose control, maintenance of HbA$_{1c}$ levels below 7%, treatment of hypertension, and avoidance of smoking.[5]

MACROVASCULAR COMPLICATIONS

Macrovascular diseases involve large vessels and include coronary artery disease, cerebrovascular disease (stroke), and peripheral vascular disease (see Chapter 14). The major mechanisms for the development of macrovascular complications are related to the role of diabetes in the development of atherosclerosis. Hyperglycemia, hyperlipidemia, and hypertension contribute to the development of atherosclerotic plaques by injuring the intima. Lipids are deposited in the walls of large vessels. Low-density lipoproteins are typically found in high concentrations in those with diabetes, particularly type 2. High-density lipoproteins, considered a protective form of cholesterol, are found in low concentrations. Platelets adhere to the damaged endothelial cells in the intima. Large vessels become sclerotic and obstructed. These complications lead to hypoxia and eventually anoxia, which lead to necrosis of peripheral tissues (Fig. 18.6). Depending on the location, plaque formation can result in the coronary arteries, leading to MI; in the cerebral arteries, leading to stroke; or in the peripheral arteries, leading to peripheral vascular disease, gangrene, and may require amputation.

The presence of macrovascular complications in individuals with diabetes is staggering. More than half of people with diabetes will die of heart disease or stroke; those with diabetes are two to four times more likely to have heart disease or suffer from a stroke than those without diabetes.[4] One of every three patients with diabetes who are older than 50 years is estimated to have peripheral vascular disease and **intermittent claudication**, a condition of fatigue or aching in the leg muscles even when walking short distances. The risk of a leg amputation is 15 to 40 times greater for a person with diabetes.[4] Amputation is one of the most important predictors for mortality in patients with type 1

■ **Figure 18.6** Peripheral ulcerations related to vascular and neurologic impairment. (Image from Marks R. *Skin Disease in Old Age.* Philadelphia: JB Lippincott; 1987, with permission.)

diabetes, and the mortality rate after amputation has been reported to be two to eight times higher than those without amputations.[6] At diagnosis, an estimated 50% of those with type 2 diabetes present with macrovascular or microvascular complications.

NEUROPATHIES

Neuropathy is nerve degeneration that results in delayed nerve conduction and impaired sensory function. Neuropathies can occur in somatic, peripheral, and autonomic nerve cells. Neuropathies are a result of (1) thickening, sclerosis, obstruction, and ischemia of the vessels that supply nerve fibers, and (2) demyelinization caused by impaired metabolism. These degenerations are often distinguished as somatic versus autonomic. Somatic nerve degeneration and delayed conduction lead to decreased sensation, numbness, tingling, weakness, muscle wasting, and pain. Autonomic neuropathies lead to bladder incontinence, impotence, diarrhea, erectile dysfunction, and postural hypotension. The prevalence of autonomic neuropathy increases with age, duration of diabetes, and increased hemoglobin A_{1c}.

INFECTION

Individuals with diabetes are also at increased risk for the development of infection. This is related to several aspects of hyperglycemia related to microvascular, macrovascular, and neuropathic complications:

- Excess glucose in blood provides an optimal environment for some pathogens, allowing rapid proliferation.
- Tissue ischemia from microvascular and macrovascular degeneration damages tissue integrity and allows ready access to pathogens.
- Red blood cell destruction and high levels of glycosylated hemoglobin prevent release of oxygen to the tissues.
- White blood cells are impaired without adequate glucose transport and are unable to engulf and remove pathogens.
- Neuropathies prevent the individual from being able to sense breaks in the skin integrity, allowing pathogens easy access.
- Retinopathy may prevent the individual from being able to adequately inspect for manifestations of infection and will delay treatment.

As with all complications of diabetes, tight glycemic control is key in prevention. Other prevention strategies include smoking cessation, management of hypertension, weight loss, and lowering of lipids. Education on preventing complications can follow the alphabet:[7]

- A = advice to follow diet, weight loss, exercise program, and lifestyle modifications
- B = blood pressure reduction
- C = cholesterol reduction
- D = diabetes hyperglycemia control
- E = eye screening
- F = foot care

Summary

- This chapter illustrates the integration of concepts from all previous chapters to appreciate the complexities of human disease. Diabetes is presented as the primary clinical model.
- Insulin is needed to promote glucose uptake and metabolism of nutrients.
- Diabetes results from either (1) a lack of insulin secretion by the beta cells of the pancreas or (2) a resistance to insulin. This leads to a state of hyperglycemia.
- Insulin absence or resistance prohibits using insulin to transport glucose and amino acids into those cells that require insulin for transport.
- The three main types of diabetes (type 1, type 2, and gestational) differ in the way that the body produces or responds to insulin.
- Type 1 diabetes exhibits an absolute or significant deficit of insulin; the cause is multifactorial and includes both genetic and environmental influences that lead to autoimmune destruction of beta cells. Common clinical manifestations include polyuria, polydipsia, and polyphagia. Treatment of type 1 diabetes mellitus requires a balance of carbohydrate/dietary intake, exercise, and insulin replacement therapy.
- Type 2 diabetes is a problem of insulin resistance or suboptimal insulin presence in the body. The exact cause is unknown; however, genetic and environmental factors, particularly obesity, appear to contribute to its development. The clinical manifestations for type 2 diabetes are often insidious and nonspecific. Treatment involves weight management, nutrition monitoring, and (possibly) oral glycemic agents or, in some cases, insulin replacement.
- Gestational diabetes is defined as any degree of glucose intolerance that occurs during pregnancy. This form of diabetes is usually temporary, but in some cases, women may go on to develop type 2 diabetes. Gestational diabetes occurs because of insulin resistance that occurs during pregnancy *and* because the pancreas is unable to make the additional insulin needed during the pregnancy to support the placenta.
- Acute complications can occur in all types of diabetes and include DKA and hypoglycemia. The

Somogyi effect and dawn phenomenon are acute complications related to the treatment and management of diabetes, particularly in those individuals who require insulin replacement.

- Hyperglycemia hyperosmolar nonketotic syndrome is an acute complication of type 2 diabetes. It primarily occurs in older adults and is marked by hyperglycemia, hyperosmolarity, glucosuria, and dehydration without the presence of ketosis.
- Chronic complications involve microvascular, macrovascular, and neuropathic degeneration. The complications of diabetes can be minimized with control of blood glucose levels.

Case Study 18.1

P.K. is a 73-year-old man with long-standing diabetes. Today, he presents to the emergency department in a coma. You review his past history and note that he was diagnosed with type 2 diabetes about 12 years ago. He experienced a stroke about a year ago and has been living in a long-term care facility since then. His care providers indicate that his blood glucose levels are monitored daily. The levels are typically around 160 to 200 mg/dL, but these have been steadily climbing over the past 2 weeks. He is on an oral glycemic agent. He does not exercise due to residual weakness from the stroke, and he does have frequent visitors who like to bring him hard candies. He had an appointment scheduled this week to meet with his primary care physician to evaluate a leg ulcer that is possibly infected. The care providers indicate that his urine output has increased over the past 2 weeks. They are not sure if his fluid intake has increased. When they went into

his room this morning, he was unresponsive. His current blood glucose level is 721 mg/dL. His urine is positive for glucose and negative for ketones. Based on the information provided:

1. *What is the most likely cause for the altered level of consciousness?*
2. *What risk factors are present in this patient that lead to your conclusion in Question 1?*
3. *What is happening in this patient's body?*
4. *What are the potential causes for the onset of this condition?*
5. *What treatment strategies would you anticipate?*

Case Study 18.2

G.H., a 12-year-old female with type 1 diabetes, is at a birthday party after school. At around 4 p.m., pizza, ice cream, and cake are served. G.H. has one slice of pizza because she knows she cannot have too much sugar. At around 4:30 p.m., G.H.'s friends decide to play a game of soccer. G.H. plays for about 30 minutes and then needs to leave for gymnastics practice from 5:15 to 6:30 p.m. On the way home from practice, G.H.'s mom asks how her day was, and G.H. cannot remember where she was earlier that day. She begins to combine words together and slur her speech. G.H. also complains of a headache.

1. *What is happening to G.H.?*
2. *What were the actual or potential contributing factors?*
3. *What should G.H.'s mom do?*
4. *What could happen if no action is taken?*

Practice Exam Questions

1. Which of the following is caused by the release of insulin?
   a. Decreased blood glucose level
   b. Increased blood glucose level
   c. Increased lipid breakdown
   d. Increased protein breakdown

2. Which of the following is not true of type 1 diabetes?
   a. Can be treated with oral glycemic agents
   b. Pancreas is completely unable to produce insulin

   c. Acute onset
   d. Definite genetic link

3. Which of the following is not true about type 2 diabetes?
   a. Accounts for up to 95% of diabetics
   b. Gradual onset
   c. Significant weight loss occurs as a symptom
   d. Risk factors are hypertension, family history, and obesity

4. Which of the following is not a sign of DKA?
   a. Kussmaul respirations
   b. Dehydration
   c. Ketonuria
   d. Low blood glucose level

5. Which laboratory test is the best predictor of blood glucose control over the previous few months?
   a. HbA_{1c}
   b. Fasting blood glucose
   c. Urinalysis
   d. Feasting (postprandial) blood glucose

6. Neuropathies are a potential complication of diabetes. Why do these occur?
   a. Infection in the nerves
   b. Thickening and ischemia of the vessels that supply the nerve fibers
   c. Inability to provide continuous glucose to the brain and spinal cord
   d. Excessive glucose exposure to the brain and spinal cord

7. What is the major difference between the Somoygi effect and the dawn phenomenon?
   a. One is caused by the release of certain hormones
   b. One occurs between 4 and 9 a.m.
   c. One triggers insulin resistance and the release of glucose from the liver
   d. One is characterized by hyperglycemia that is not triggered by overnight hypoglycemia

8. What would happen if your patient did not have alpha cells of the pancreas?
   a. They would not be able to secrete insulin
   b. They would not be able to secrete somatostatin and gastrin
   c. They would not be able to secrete glucagon
   d. They would not be able to secrete pancreatic polypeptides

9. What would be an unusual sign in a child that may alert the parent to the presence of diabetes?
   a. Bedwetting in a child that was previously dry through the night
   b. Irritability
   c. Asking for water to drink in the middle of the night
   d. All of these

10. What is your explanation to the parents who do not want to give their child insulin injections to treat type 1 diabetes because they have heard that pills can be used to treat this condition?
    a. Insulin is destroyed in the gastrointestinal tract if taken orally, so it must be injected subcutaneously
    b. The child can go ahead and take the oral medication because he does have type 1 diabetes
    c. The child cannot take the pills because we can't be sure that he would take the entire dose
    d. The pills are reserved for those over the age of 12

Discussion and Application

1. What did I know about diabetes prior to today?

2. What body processes are affected by diabetes? What are the expected functions of those processes? How does diabetes affect those processes?

3. What are the potential etiologies for diabetes? How does diabetes develop?

4. Who is most at risk for developing diabetes? How does this differ with the three types of diabetes (type 1, type 2, and gestational)?

5. What are the human differences that affect the etiology, risk, or course of diabetes?

6. What clinical manifestations are expected in the course of diabetes?

7. What special diagnostic tests are useful in determining the diagnosis of diabetes?

8. What are the goals of care for individuals with diabetes?

9. How does the concept of diabetes bring together what I have learned in the previous chapters and in previous courses?

10. How can I use what I have learned?

RESOURCES

Updated news and current research on diabetes as well as general information:

http://www.diabetes.org

A complete summary of diabetes and information for diabetes management:

http://diabetes.niddk.nih.gov/dm/pubs/type1and2/what.htm

Updated research in the world of diabetes:

http://www.nlm.nih.gov/medlineplus/diabetes.html

REFERENCES

1. Tanenberg R, Bode B, Lane W, et al. Use of the continuous glucose monitoring system to guide therapy in patients with insulin-treated diabetes: a randomized controlled trial. *Mayo Clin Proc.* 2004;79:1521–1526.

2. Selin E, Marinopoulos S, Berkenblit G, et al. Meta-analysis: glycosylated hemoglobin and cardiovascular disease in diabetes mellitus. *Ann Intern Med.* 2004;141:421–431.

3. Wang J, Luben R, Khaw K, et al. Dietary energy density predicts the risk of incident type 2 diabetes. *Diabetes Care.* 2008;31:2120–2125.

4. Ligaray K, Isley W. Diabetes mellitus, type 2. Available at: http://emedicine.medscape.com/article/117853-overview. Accessed March 15, 2010.

5. Gross J, de Azevedo M, Silveiro S, et al. Diabetic nephropathy: diagnosis, prevention, and treatment. *Diabetes Care.* 2005;28:164–177.

6. Cusick M, Melleth A, Agron E, et al. Associations of mortality and diabetes complications in patients with type 1 and type 2 diabetes: early treatment diabetic retinopathy study report no. 27. *Diabetes Care.* 2005;28:617–626.

7. Metoo D. Clinical skills: empowering people with diabetes to minimize complications. *Br J Nurs.* 2004;13:644–650.

Glossary

1,25-dihydroxycholecalciferol: activated form of vitamin D; promotes calcium absorption in the intestine

abscess: a pocket of purulent exudate

absorption: a complex process of taking in nutrients and moving these to the circulation to be used by cells

accommodate: ability of the lens to change its shape

accumulated mutations theory: developmental theory of aging suggesting that genes that determine survival at younger ages have greater influence than genes expressed at older ages

acid: substance that donates hydrogen ions

acoustic reflex measurement: test to determine movement of the tympanic membrane in response to sound

acromegaly: condition of hyperplasia prompted by hormone stimulation of excessive growth after closure of the epiphyseal growth plates of the long bones

action potential: electrical events that travel along an entire neuron by allowing charged ions to flood through channels in the semipermeable membrane around the nerve cell

active transport: energy-dependent transport of particles across the cell membrane against a gradient

activities of daily living (ADLs): performance of usual functions of everyday life (e.g., eating, dressing)

acuity: clarity; ability to locate the site of the initiation of a stimulus

acute: describes manifestations or illnesses that are usually abrupt in onset and last a few days to a few months

acute respiratory distress syndrome (ARDS): a condition of severe acute inflammation and pulmonary edema without evidence of fluid overload or impaired cardiac function

acute tubular necrosis: condition of the kidney characterized by sloughing of tubular cells

adaptation: alteration in function that allows cells, tissues, and organs to adjust to new conditions; survival due to the capacity to adjust to an adverse environment

adaptive immunity: cell-mediated and humoral immunity; specific immune response occurring during a lifetime

Addison disease: a condition of adrenal cortical insufficiency most commonly caused by the autoimmune destruction of the adrenal cortex

adenocarcinoma: a malignant tumor of epithelial cells

adenoid hypertrophy: enlargement of lymphoepithelial adenoid tissue in the back of the nasal area

adenoma: benign tumor of glandular epithelial origin

adenosine triphosphate (ATP): principal source of cellular energy; product of a chemical reaction between oxygen and nutrient products such as glucose, fatty acids, amino acids, and enzymes

adherence: the attraction and binding of cells to a specific location to promote healing

adhesions: fibrous connections between serous cavities and nearby tissues that do not allow the surrounding tissues to move freely

adjuvant: substance that increase immune response to antigens

adventitious: refers to an alteration in lung sounds, as with wheezing or crackles

aerobic bacteria: microorganisms that require oxygen for growth

affective disorder: condition involving mood, emotional feeling, and tone related to thought; includes external manifestations

afferent neurons: neurons that carry impulses from receptors to the distant targets of the brain and spinal cord; also known as sensory neurons

afterload: the amount of pressure in the ventricle toward the end of the cardiac contraction

air trapping: decreased effective O_2 intake and especially CO_2 release by retaining air within the alveoli because of loss of elasticity

akinesia: inability to move

allele: a series of two or more different genes occupying the same location on a specific chromosome

allergen: protein promoting altered reactivity responses by the immune system

alloantibodies: antibodies produced against alloantigens

alloantigens: proteins that vary between individuals

allograft: graft between unrelated individuals

alternative splicing: different ways of assembling exons to produce a variety of mature mRNAs

amblyopia: a condition resulting from a muscle imbalance; commonly known as "lazy eye"

amenorrhea: the absence of menstruation

amniocentesis: insertion of a needle into the uterine cavity to obtain a sample of amniotic fluid

amphoteric: able to function as either acid or base

amyloid hypothesis: theory suggesting that flaws in the accumulation, production, or disposal of Aβ are responsible for the pathogenesis of Alzheimer disease, including development of tangles, plaques, and neuronal death

amyloid precursor protein (APP): large protein produced by the β-amyloid gene

anaerobic bacteria: bacteria that do not require oxygen for growth

anaphylactic shock: a condition of impaired tissue perfusion from shock because of a massive immune (type 1 or IgE-mediated) hypersensitivity response

anaphylaxis: extreme manifestation to foreign protein or other substance

anaplasia: a neoplasm's loss of differentiation

anemia: the reduction in the mass of circulating blood cells and subsequently reduced hemoglobin levels

aneuploidy: abnormal chromosome number

aneurysm: local outpouching caused by weakness in the vessel wall

angina pectoris: chest pain or pressure that is intermittent and associated with myocardial ischemia, a reduction in blood flow to the coronary arteries caused by atherosclerosis often accompanied by vasospasm

angioedema: sudden subcutaneous edema

angiogenesis: the generation of new blood vessels

anion exchange: transport of one negatively charged ion for another in opposite directions across the cell membrane

anion gap: calculation of the major measured cations and anions in the plasma; provides an indication of electrolyte and acid–base balance

anions: ions with a negative charge

ankylosis: a debilitating fixation of a joint from extensive fibrosis

anorexia: loss of appetite

anorexia nervosa (AN): an eating disorder characterized by a refusal to maintain a minimally healthy body weight, an intense fear of gaining weight, body image distortion, and amenorrhea

anovulation: the absence of ovulation

anoxia: the absolute deprivation of oxygen

antagonistic pleiotropy theory: developmental theory of aging suggesting that genes may have beneficial effects during early life, but harmful effects as the individual ages

anterolateral pathway: neurologic pathway involving both the anterior and lateral spinothalamic pathways; characterized by multiple synapses and slow conduction; transmits the sensations of pain, temperature, crude touch, and pressure not requiring the specific location of the origin of the stimulus

Arthus reaction: complex-mediated immune response in the skin resulting in an area of localized tissue necrosis

antibodies: immunoglobulins that react with an antigen in a specific way; produced by activated plasma cells

antigen: a substance that induces a state of sensitivity or an immune response

antigen-presenting cells: cells that process and present antigen for recognition by immune cells

antigen variation: alteration of pathogen protein particles to evade recognition and stimulation of memory in the immune system

antigenic variability: a process of eluding the human host defenses; often a result of altering the antigens present within or on the surface of the microorganism

antigenicity: the level to which a pathogen is viewed by the host immune system as foreign

antiport: system of substances transported in the opposite direction

antiresorptive: tendency to slow or block absorption

antiresorptive medication: drugs that inhibit or reduce bone resorption; used to treat osteoporosis

anuria: absent urine output

apoptosis: programmed cell death that is prompted by a genetic signal and designed to replace old cells with new; also known as "cellular suicide"

aquaporins: channels in the cell membrane; allow water movement between compartments

aqueous humor: nutritive, watery fluid produced by the ciliary body

arachidonic acid: a plasma membrane–derived substance that generates various chemical mediators through a complex chemical conversion

arteriovenous (AV) fistula: surgical attachment of an artery to a vein; used to obtain access to circulation for hemodialysis

arteriovenous shunt: surgical procedure connecting the artery to the vein using a synthetic tube

arthritis: a generic term for degeneration or inflammation of the joints

ascending: the upward movement of an infection

ascites: accumulation of fluid in the peritoneal cavity

aspiration: a problem of inhaling a foreign substance into the lungs

asthma: a chronic inflammatory disorder of the airways resulting in intermittent or persistent airway obstruction caused by bronchial hyperresponsiveness, inflammation, bronchoconstriction, and excess mucous production

astigmatism: irregular curvature of the cornea or lens preventing the focusing of images; blurring vision

astrogliosis: formation of a glial scar caused by proliferation of astrocytes in response to local tissue injury

asymptomatic: the absence of any noticeable symptoms, even though laboratory or other diagnostic tests may indicate that a disease is present

ataxic: inability to control balance

atelectasis: a condition of collapse and nonaeration of the alveoli

atherosclerosis: a condition of irregularly distributed lipid deposits in the inner lining, or intima, of large or medium arteries

athetoid: inability to control muscle movement

atopic: describes individuals having a genetic predisposition to developing hypersensitivities

atopy: the process by which IgE responses are stimulated from exposure to typically benign substances

atretic: is a decrease in cell size (atrophic)

atrioventricular (AV) node: connects the conduction of impulses between the atria and ventricles

atrophic macular degeneration: retinal deterioration resulting from deposition of drusen, under the macula next to the basement membrane of the retinal pigment epithelium; also known as dry macular degeneration

atrophy: decrease in the size of the cell

attenuated: weakened; reduced ability to cause disease

Auerbach plexus: part of the enteric nervous system; found between the longitudinal and circular muscle layers of the large intestine; also known as the myenteric plexus

auscultation: to listen with a stethoscope

autoclave: a device that uses steam heat at high pressures to sterilize objects

autograft: grafts from different sites on the same person

autoimmune: immune responses directed at an individual's own tissues

autonomic nervous system (ANS): component of the peripheral nervous system; includes the sympathetic nervous system (SNS) and the parasympathetic nervous system (PNS); controls involuntary function of organs

autonomy: the unregulated cell growth of neoplasms

autoreceptors: receptors involved in detection of chemicals to regulate the cell's own function

autosomes: chromosomes other than a sex chromosome; totals 44 chromosomes in each body cell

axon: neuronal structure that carries impulses away from the cell body

axon hillock: point at which the axon joins the cell body

B lymphocytes: lymphocytes that differentiate into plasma cells in the bone marrow; produce and secrete antibodies after contact with an antigen

B-cell receptor: receptor bound to the cell membrane of the B cell; association with antigen activates plasma cells to produce and secrete antibodies

bacteremia: a state in which bacteria gain access to the blood

bacteria: single-celled microorganisms that can reproduce outside of host cells

baroreceptors: located throughout the blood vessels and the heart; sense pressure changes in the arteries and alert the cardiac control center in the brainstem

barotrauma: injury resulting from the inability of the ear to equalize pressure

basal ganglia: structure of the brain (ADD) with a major role in coordinated muscle movements

base: substance that accepts hydrogen ions

base deficit: amount of base needed to achieve a pH of 7.4 in the blood sample

base excess: amount of fixed acid needed to achieve a pH of 7.4 in the blood sample

base pairs: nitrogen base combinations; DNA base pairs include cytosine and guanine, and adenine and thymine

basement membrane: the outer membrane of the vessels that separates the vessel from the tissues of the body

basophil: granulocyte that complements the actions of mast cells; important in establishing allergic reactions

benign: describes a tumor that remains localized and closely resembles the tissue of origin

β-amyloid protein: accumulations leading to the production of senile plaques, characteristic of Alzheimer disease; also known as amyloid β or Aβ

bifurcations: regions wherein a vessel branches

bilayer: two interconnected layers of the plasma membrane; the lipid (fat-soluble) layer contains phospholipid and glycolipid

bilirubin: yellow, lipid-soluble byproduct of hemoglobin; elevated levels result in jaundice

bioavailability: refers to a mineral that is unbound and must remain unbound (also called an ionic state) to be absorbed

biomedicine: a systematic scientific study of biologic processes within the framework of Western medicine

binding affinity: tightness or strength of ligand/receptor interaction

bladder: muscular organ serving as a reservoir for urine; lined with transitional epithelium and innervated by the pelvic nerves

bladder training: process of learning to hold urine for increasing intervals as a management strategy for incontinence

blast cell: any immature cell

blastomere: early embryo

blood–brain barrier (BBB): reduced permeability of capillaries in the brain to protect against exposure to potentially hazardous substances

blood pressure: the pressure or tension of the blood within the systemic arteries

blood transfusion: the most common form of tissue transplant; infusion of donor blood into recipient

blood typing: the process by which the recipient's blood type is determined

blunt force injury: injury that occurs when the head strikes a hard surface or is struck by a rapidly moving object

body mass index (BMI): a measure of body fat calculated by measuring weight in kilograms and dividing this by height in meters squared ($BMI = kg/m^2$)

body-self neuromatrix: neural network in the brain containing somatosensory, limbic, and thalamocortical components; integrates multiple sources of input resulting in the cognitive, affective, and sensory perceptions of pain

bowel resection: surgical procedure involving the removal of intestine

brachial plexus palsy: trauma to the brachial nerve plexus resulting in flaccid paralysis of the affected arm

bradykinesia: decreased spontaneity of movement; slowed movement associated with initiation of movement or sudden halting of movement

bronchiectasis: the irreversible dilation and destruction of the bronchial tree most often caused by chronic obstruction or infection

bronchopulmonary dysplasia (BPD): condition in which cellular alterations lead to chronic, irreversible tissue changes in the respiratory tree of the lungs

bronchospasm: contraction of the smooth muscle in the bronchi and bronchioles of the lungs, decreasing airway size

Brudzinski sign: a test of meningeal irritation where the patient is supine and the neck is quickly flexed; this activity elicits pain along with involuntary flexion of the hips and knees

buffer system: mixing of acid and base to resist pH change; system for trading stronger acids and bases for weaker varieties to achieve acid–base balance

cachexia: a syndrome of unexplained weight loss and tissue wasting related to the stimulation of inflammatory mediators, along with excess energy use, by the proliferating neoplastic cells

calcitonin: hormone promoting the deposition of calcium and phosphate in bone; produced primarily by the parafollicular cells of the thyroid gland, with other sources including the parathyroid and thymus glands

caloric test: test that uses warm and cool water or air irrigation to induce nystagmus; diagnostic of Ménière disease

calpain: type of proteolytic enzyme

cancer: a term used to describe highly invasive and destructive neoplasms

capacitor: structure that stores current

carcinogen: a known cancer-causing agent

carcinogenesis: a term used to describe the origin, promotion, or development of cancerous neoplasms

carcinoma in situ: a unique term used to describe carcinomas that are confined to the epithelium and have not yet penetrated the basement membrane

cardiac contractility: the ability of the heart to increase the force of contraction without changing the diastolic (resting) pressure

cardiac cycle: refers to one contraction and one relaxation phase of the heart

cardiac dysrhythmias: a category of problems with maintaining an efficient heart rhythm, such as impairments of the sinoatrial (SA) node, atrioventricular (AV) node, cardiac cells that join the SA and AV nodes, or conduction systems in the atria or ventricles

cardiac hypertrophy: a disease of cardiac muscle that results from excessive workload and functional demand

cardiac output (CO): the volume of blood pumped from the ventricles in 1 minute

cardinal signs: the local manifestations of acute inflammation; include redness, heat, swelling, pain, and loss of function

cardiogenic shock: the result of inadequate or ineffective cardiac pumping

carriers: heterozygous for a recessive genetic mutation; able to transmit the genetic mutation to subsequent generations in the absence of a disease phenotype

caseous necrosis: a distinctive, yellow, pasty, cheese-like necrosis of tuberculosis

casts: structures found in urine consisting of a protein meshwork of entrapped cells formed in the distal collecting tubules and collecting ducts

cataracts: clouding of the lens in the eye; causes blurred vision by scattering incoming light

cations: ions with a positive charge

cation exchange: transport of one positively charged ion for another in opposite directions across the cell membrane

cauda equina: extension of nerves in the spinal cord extending below the sacral level through the exit of the vertebral column

cavitation: area of necrosis that erode surrounding structures of the lungs, including the bronchioles, bronchi, and surrounding blood vessels

CD4 T lymphocytes: subtype of helper T lymphocyte that expresses the molecule CD4 on its cell surface

CD8 T lymphocytes: subtype of cytotoxic T lymphocyte that expresses the molecule CD8 on its cell surface

celiac disease: also called gluten-sensitive enteropathy; a disorder of gluten malabsorption caused by a T cell–mediated hypersensitivity to gluten in persons who are genetically predisposed to developing this condition

cell: smallest component of the living individual

cell body: cell structure containing cytoplasm and organelles responsible for the specialized function of the cell; also known as a soma

cell-mediated immunity: a component of adaptive immunity; cytotoxic T cell–mediated destruction of pathogen and infected host cell

cellular casts: compacted collection of protein, cells, and debris that are formed in kidney tubules

cellular response: the role of inflammation in alerting the products of healing to attend to the site of injury

cellular senescence: developmental theory suggesting that aging is caused by an intrinsic loss of the capacity of the cell to proliferate, triggered by a critical loss of telomere

central auditory processing disorder: disorder involving an alteration in auditory signal processing in the brain

central nervous system (CNS): component of the nervous system comprising the brain and spinal cord

centromere: structure linking the chromosome pairs of the somatic cells of the body; divides the chromosome into two arms; constant position for each chromosome

cerebral aqueduct: connecting point of the third and fourth ventricles; also known as the aqueduct of Sylvius

cerebral atrophy: decrease in neuronal cell size and number leading to impaired neuronal communication and reduced brain tissue mass

cerebrospinal fluid (CSF): fluid bathing the surface of the central nervous system structures of the brain and spinal cord; flows through four fluid-filled interconnecting ventricles in the brain

cerumen: secretion by glands in the ear

cheilitis: a problem with fissure development in the corners of the mouth often associated with riboflavin deficiency

chemical injury: injury to cells caused by damage from toxins

chemical mediators: potent substances that facilitate the process of widening and loosening the blood vessels at the site of injury; are active in all phases of the inflammatory response

chemical synapse: transmit impulses across a small gap between cells via stimulation of neurotransmitters

chemotactic factors: substances that attract specific types of cells

chemotaxis: the calling forth of inflammatory cells to the injured site

chondrocalcinosis: calcification of cartilage

chondroma: benign tumor that stems from chondrocytes

chondrosarcoma: a malignant tumor of chondrocytes

chorea: irregular, involuntary movements of extremities or facial muscles

choroid plexus: structure located in the two lateral and single third and fourth ventricles of the brain; responsible for production of cerebrospinal fluid

choroidal neovascularization: formation of new blood vessels under the retina and macula; associated with wet (exudative) macular degeneration

chromatin: nuclear genetic material made of DNA; condenses into chromosomes during mitosis

chromatolysis: swelling of a neuron because of injury

chromosomes: double-stranded DNA containing threadlike sections of genes that form an individual's genetic code; most commonly found in the cell nucleus; responsible for reproduction of physical and chemical structures; human somatic cells contain 46 chromosomes: 22 paired autosomes and 1 pair of sex chromosomes

chronic: describes manifestations or illnesses that are often more insidious and generally last 6 months or longer

chronic bronchitis: the presence of a persistent, productive cough that lasts for 3 months or longer for 2 or more consecutive years

chronic obstructive pulmonary disease (COPD): a generic term that describes all chronic obstructive lung problems including asthma, emphysema, and chronic bronchitis, separately or in combination

ciliary body: ocular structure producing the aqueous humor

ciliary muscle: regulates lens shape to focus an object at close range

cirrhosis: an end-stage liver disease marked by interference of blood flow to the liver and widespread hepatocyte damage

climacteric: gradual transition between normal reproductive cycles and menopause; also known as perimenopause

clinical manifestations: the presenting signs and symptoms of an illness

clonal expansion: the proliferation of B and T lymphocytes activated by clonal selection to produce a clone of identical cells; enables the body to have sufficient numbers of antigen-specific lymphocytes to mount an effective immune response

clonal selection: the selection and activation of specific B lymphocytes and T lymphocytes by the binding of epitopes to B-or T-cell receptors with a corresponding fit

clonic: rapid successions of alternating muscle contraction and relaxation

closed head injury: injury to the head that causes tissue damage without exposing tissue to the external environment

clotting system: promotes coagulation through the activation of clotting factors in a cascade sequence and suppresses coagulation through the release of anticoagulation factors

clubbing: a painless enlargement and flattening of the tips of fingers or toes due to chronic hypoxia

clusters of differentiation: determine specific functions and responses of T-cell subtypes

cochlea: bony structure located in the inner ear; important for hearing

cochlear implant: artificial devices surgically placed behind the ear to enhance hearing

codon: sequence of three forms of nitrogen bases forms; nucleotide triplet; fundamental triplet code necessary for protein synthesis; basic compounds produced are amino acids

cogwheel: muscle rigidity (jerking) in response to limb flexion attempt

coinfection: a phenomenon of hosting two or more pathogens simultaneously

collagen: also known as scar tissue; a substance manufactured by fibroblasts that fills in the gaps left after the removal of extensively damaged tissues or those tissues made up of cells that are unable to regenerate

colonoscopy: a procedure using an endoscope to perform direct visualization of the colon

colostomy: establishment of an artificial opening of the large intestine externally on the abdomen

columnar epithelium: single layer of epithelial cells taller than they are wide

communicable diseases: diseases that are spread from person to person, often through contact with infected blood and body fluids

communicating hydrocephalus: increased ventricular accumulation of cerebrospinal fluid due to impaired cerebrospinal fluid absorption

complement system: a key source of chemical mediators within the plasma; has many roles, particularly as it relates to inflammation, immunity, and the resolution of infection

compliance: the expected distensibility, or expandability, of the lung tissue and chest wall

complications: negative sequelae from a disease

concentration gradient: mechanism of passive transport that promotes the movement of particles from an area of high to lower concentration

concept: an abstract idea generalized from particular instances

conductive hearing loss: hearing loss localized to the outer or middle ear; may be temporary or permanent

cone: photoreceptor located in the retina; essential for sharp and color vision

congenital defects: damage to a developing fetus

congestive heart failure: occurs when the left ventricle of the heart is ineffective and blood backs up into the pulmonary vein and subsequently into the lung tissues; results in pulmonary edema; also called left heart failure

conjugated vaccine: antigens that promote activation of more than one cell type

conjunctivitis: inflammation of the mucous membrane lining the eye

consolidation: a solid mass in the lung tissue

constant region: structure forming the base of the Y-shaped antibody; the most stable component

constipation: absent or incomplete bowel movement; may represent a consequence of impaired gastrointestinal mobility or obstruction

contractures: areas of thick, shortened, and rigid tissue from a loss of elasticity

contralateral: referring to the opposite side of the body

cor pulmonale: an alteration in the structure and function of the right ventricle caused by a primary disorder of the respiratory system

cornea: clear, transparent structure covering the exterior wall of the eye

corpus callosum: nerve fiber bundles promoting communication between the right and left hemispheres of the brain

cortisol: is a major glucocorticoid secreted from the adrenal cortex that regulates metabolism, inflammatory/immune processes, and the stress response

costovertebral angle (CVA): anatomic area including the lower abdomen anteriorly and posteriorly; site of associated dermatomes of the kidney

cotransport: substances transported together in the same direction

countercurrent exchanger: flow of blood in the vasa recta capillaries aligned with filtrate flow in the loop of Henle; slow descending blood flow allows water transport from the medullary interstitium into the capillary blood, and slow ascending blood flow allows solute transport from the vasa recta into the interstitium, preserving medullary gradient and preventing washout of interstitial solutes

countercurrent mechanism: process of filtrate concentration in the loop of Henle in the medulla of the kidney; includes the countercurrent multiplier and the countercurrent exchanger

countercurrent multiplier: process of water and solute transport in the loop of Henle maintaining the vertical medullary gradient

countertransport: substances transported in the opposite direction

cretinism: a condition of mental retardation and impaired growth from a congenital lack of thyroid hormone production and secretion.

cross matching: the process by which antibody compatibility between donor and recipient blood is determined

cryptorchidism: a congenital condition of one or two undescended testes

crypts: mucosal epithelial depressions of the colon

Cushing disease: a condition of hypercortisolism specifically related to pituitary corticotrope tumors

Cushing syndrome: a condition of excess glucocorticoid secretion from the adrenal cortex

cyanosis: a result of a greater proportion of desaturated hemoglobin in the blood, which gives the blood a bluish hue

cytochrome oxidase (COX): enzyme important in catalyzing oxidation–reduction mitochondrial reactions in cellular respiration

cytokine: a hormonelike cell protein that regulates the activity of many other chemical mediators in an effort to trigger, enhance, and then discontinue the inflammatory response

cytoplasm: colloid substance surrounding the cell nucleus composed of water, proteins, fats, electrolytes, glycogen, and pigments

cytoskeleton: tubule and filament structures, contributing to cell shape, movement, and intracellular transport; composed of microtubules and thin, intermediate, and thick microfilaments

cytosol: the cytoplasm of bacteria that contains extensive ribosomes, proteins, and carbohydrates, but does not contain mitochondria, endoplasmic reticulum, or other membranous components

cytotoxic T lymphocyte: subset of T lymphocyte that directs destruction of the antigen or cells carrying the antigen

dawn phenomenon: a situation in which an individual's blood glucose level upon waking is higher than that before going to bed in the evening

dead space: an area where gas exchange cannot take place

death: cessation of life; cessation of the integration of cellular, tissue, and organ functions

decerebrate posturing: increased extensor muscle excitability caused by neurologic injury

decibels (dB): the unit of measurement of intensity or loudness of the sound

decorticate posturing: increased flexor muscle excitability caused by neurologic injury

debridement: a process of mechanically removing debris, including necrotic tissue, from a wound

deep brain stimulation (DBS): reversible procedure designed to alter abnormal function of the brain tissue; neurostimulator delivers electrical signals to a targeted area of the brain, blocking abnormal nerve signals and resulting in tremor and other Parkinson disease symptoms

deep partial-thickness burns: formerly known as second-degree burns; burns that damage epidermal skin layers and penetrate some dermal skin layers

defecation: the process of stool elimination

deficit injury: damage caused by deprivation of oxygenation, hydration, and nutrition

degranulation: the release of chemical mediators in the form of extracellular granules

dehiscence: a problem of deficient scar formation in which the wound splits or bursts open, often at a suture line

delayed hypersensitivity reaction: reaction after allergen contact that is slow in onset and peaks after 36 to 48 hours; associated with a type IV cell–mediated hypersensitivity reaction

demyelination: degradation of myelin

dendrites: branching protoplasmic processes of the nerve cell

dendritic cells: process and display of antigens to T lymphocytes; take up antigens when they are encountered in the circulation

deoxyribonucleic acid (DNA): type of nucleic acid containing a sugar (deoxyribose); usually found in the cell nucleus and mitochondria; responsible for the storage of genetic information; made up of four nitrogenous bases, including adenine (A) and guanine (G), cytosine (C) and thymine (T)

depolarization: result of rapid movement of sodium into the cell through sodium channels in the cell membrane

dermatomes: body regions to which spinal nerves transmit impulses

dermatophyte infections: fungal infections of the skin, hair, and nails

detrusor muscle: tissue comprising the body of the bladder; contraction assists with bladder emptying and elimination of urine

developmental theory: theory implicating the influence of genetics as the major determinant of aging

diabetes insipidus (DI): a condition of insufficient antidiuretic hormone resulting in the inability of the body to concentrate or retain water

diabetes mellitus: a disorder of the body's metabolism of protein, fats, and carbohydrates because of an absolute lack of insulin or insulin resistance

diagnosis: a label for the altered health condition

diapedesis: a process that allows leukocytes to move between and through endothelial cells in order to engulf and destroy the offending agent and remove dead tissue

diarrhea: loose, watery stools

diastole: the relaxation of the heart that allows blood to fill the ventricles

diastolic blood pressure: the amount of pressure that remains in the aorta during the resting phase of the cardiac cycle

diastolic failure: failure that occurs with stiffness of the ventricle and loss of relaxation ability, which impairs the heart's ability to optimally fill with blood between cardiac contractions

differentiation: a process of changing the physical and functional properties of a cell to allow greater specificity and functionality to that cell

diffusing capacity: a measurement of carbon monoxide (CO), oxygen, or nitric oxide transfer from inspired gas to pulmonary capillary blood; is reflective of the volume of a gas that diffuses through the alveolar capillary membrane each minute

diffusion: movement of particles from an area of high to lower concentration

digestion: the process by which food is broken down mechanically and chemically in the gastrointestinal tract and converted into absorbable components

diplegia: involving both legs

diploid: the number of chromosomes a human body cell contains; 23 pairs of chromosomes, or a total of 46

diplopia: resulting from a lack of coordination of the extraocular muscles; may result in double vision

direct extension: a process of tumor cells moving into adjacent tissues and organs

discoid: red, raised, round rash

discriminative pathway: neurologic pathway communicating sensory information, including discriminative touch and spatial orientation

disease: an impairment of cell, tissue, organ, or system functioning

disseminated intravascular coagulation (DIC): a condition of uncontrolled activation of clotting factors resulting in widespread thrombi formation followed by depletion of coagulation factors and platelets; leads to massive hemorrhage

distal axonopathy: axonal injury of neurons in distal areas of the body, such as hands and feet

diuretics: drugs that increase urine production

diverticula: more than one diverticulum

diverticulitis: infection of the diverticula

diverticulosis: condition characterized by the presence of diverticula

diverticulum: small sac or outpouching along the wall of the colon; plural diverticula

dominant: an allele possessed by one of the parents of a hybrid that is expressed in the latter to the exclusion of a contrasting allele (the recessive) from the other parent

dorsal horns: posterior extensions of the spinal cord containing sensory neurons; receive afferent impulses via the dorsal roots and other neurons

drusen: small, yellow deposits; deposition under the macula is characteristic of dry (atrophic) macular degeneration

dry (atrophic) MD: retinal deterioration resulting from deposition of drusen, under the macula next to the basement membrane of the retinal pigment epithelium; also known as atrophic macular degeneration

dual energy X-ray absorptiometry (DEXA): specialized, low-level radiographic technique used to measure bone density

dyskinesia: difficulty in performing voluntary movements

dyskinetic: inability to control muscle movement

dysmenorrhea: pain with menstrual periods

dyspareunia: painful intercourse

dyspepsia: a vague epigastric discomfort associated with nausea and heartburn

dysplasia: actual change in cell size, shape, uniformity, arrangement, and structure

dyspnea: the subjective feeling of shortness of breath or the inability to get enough air

dystonia: abnormal tone

dysuria: pain with urination

ecchymoses: bruises from superficial bleeding into the skin

ectocervix: outside of the cervix lined with squamous epithelium

ectopic: refers to hormone secretion from a site outside of an endocrine gland

edema: the presence of excessive watery fluid that accumulates in the tissues

efferent neurons: neurons that carry impulses from central nervous system to the periphery

elastin: a substance that allows stretching and recoil of tissue

electrical synapses: transmit impulses via passage of current-carrying ions through small openings or gaps

electrolytes: ionizable substances in solution; conduct electricity in solution

electronystagmography (ENG): group of tests that determine vestibular function based on eye movement

elemental body: the metabolically inactive stage in the life cycle of chlamydiae in which the microorganism attaches to and internalizes the host cell

elicitation phase: second phase of delayed hypersensitivity reaction; memory cells in the dermis are stimulated after presentation with antigen by Langerhans cells, prompting activation of memory T cells and stimulation of cell-mediated responses

embolus: any plug of material, such as thrombi, air, neoplasms, microorganisms, or amniotic fluid, that travels in the circulation and can obstruct the lumen of a vessel

embryonic carcinomas: resemble primitive undifferentiated embryonic tissue

emphysema: an irreversible enlargement of the air spaces beyond the terminal bronchioles, most notably in the alveoli, resulting in destruction of the alveolar walls and obstruction of airflow

encephalopathy: brain disorder

encopresis: a condition of fecal incontinence characterized by inappropriate fecal soiling; frequently seen in the pediatric population; also known as functional nonretentive soiling

endemic: a condition in which the incidence and prevalence are stable and predictable

endocardium: the inner lining of the heart that forms a continuous layer of endothelium that joins the arteries and veins to the heart, forming a closed circulatory system

endocervical canal: area between the external and internal cervical os; lined with columnar epithelium

endocrine: hormone secretion with systemic effects

endocrine pancreas: an organ that secretes hormones, such as insulin and glucagon

endocrine system: a collective group of tissues that are capable of secreting hormones

endocytosis: transport mechanism involving vesicular enclosure of particles from the extracellular environment into the cytoplasm for use by the cell

endogenous: from within the body system

endolymph: fluid filling the cochlea

endometriosis: a condition involving endometrial tissue that is located outside of the uterus

endoplasmic reticulum: cellular organelle composed of a complex network of tubules; important in the production of proteins and fats and ion regulation; subtypes include rough and smooth

endothelial cells: cells that form a tight junction within the inner lining of the blood and lymphatic vessels and the heart

endotoxin: a complex of phospholipid–polysaccharide molecules that form the structural component of the gram-negative cell wall and causes inflammatory mediators to be released, leading to a massive inflammatory response

energy: the capacity to do work

enteric nervous system: subdivision of the peripheral nervous system; provides innervation to the muscle of fibers of the intestine via the myenteric (Auerbach) and Meissner plexus, controlling gastrointestinal movement and sensation

enuresis: urinary incontinence; inability to voluntarily prevent the discharge of urine

eosinophils: granulocyte with greatest protection against parasites

epidemic: a dramatic increase in the incidence of a health condition in a population

epidemiology: the study of disease in populations

epigenetic: regulation of the expression of gene activity without alteration of genetic structure

epiphyseal: long bone ossification site

epistaxis: episodes of nose bleeds

epithelioid cells: phagocytes that gather and contain smaller substances by forming a wall, or fibrotic granuloma, around the affected area

epithelioma: a benign tumor of the squamous epithelium

erectile dysfunction (ED): the inability to achieve or maintain an erection sufficient for satisfactory sexual performance

erythema: redness caused by increased blood flow to the tissues

erythrocyte sedimentation rate: also referred to as a sed rate, or ESR; a nonspecific method of testing for inflammation

erythrocytes: red blood cells (RBCs); comprise a large proportion of the blood and are needed to provide tissue oxygenation

erythropoiesis: the formation of new red blood cells

erythropoietin: a protein that stimulates the formation of red blood cells for growth

eschar: a thick, coagulated crust that develops after a thermal or chemical burn that cauterizes the skin

esotropia: suppression of one visual images by the brain, preserving normal vision

essential fat: a lipid required for physiologic functioning

essential nutrients: those that must be consumed regularly in the diet, because the body is unable to synthesize the nutrient in quantities sufficient to meet its needs

etiology: the cause of the disease

evolution theory: developmental theory suggesting that aging is the result of the forces of natural selection

exacerbation: a period in which symptoms flare and can be severe

exocrine pancreas: an organ that contains acini cells, which secrete digestive enzymes and alkaline fluids through the pancreatic duct into the duodenum

exocytosis: the process of movement of granules or particles out of the cell; fusion of the membrane surrounding the granule with the cell membrane, followed by rupture and release of contents

exogenous: from the external environment

exon: segment of DNA coded for protein production

exophthalmos: a protrusion of the eyeballs that sometimes occurs with hyperthyroidism

exotoxins: potent substances produced by many bacteria, which result in host cell dysfunction or lysis

expectorate: to spit out the mucus that is ejected during a cough

expiration: the process of removing carbon dioxide out of the body through the lungs

expressivity: the evidence of the gene in the phenotype

external anal sphincter: skeletal muscle surrounding the internal rectal sphincter; innervated by the pudendal nerve of the somatic nervous system; providing voluntary control of defecation

external auditory meatus: opening of the ear canal

external urethral sphincter: skeletal muscle of the bladder neck; allows for voluntary release of urine; innervated by the pudendal nerve

extracellular compartment: body fluid in the interstitial tissue and plasma outside the cells; contains two thirds of the body water; accounts for 40% of body weight

extracellular matrix: (ECM) the layers of architectural structures that support the cells

extracorporeal shockwave lithotripsy (ESWL): procedure of renal calculi removal involving acoustic shock waves to break up the stone; the most common procedure for kidney stone removal

extrapyramidal disorders: movement disorders affecting the structures of the basal ganglia, substantia nigra, and subthalamic nucleus

extrapyramidal system: nervous system outside of the pyramidal nervous system; attenuated erratic motions; maintains muscle tone and trunk stability; composed of the subcortical nuclei of the basal ganglia

exudate: the watery fluid with a high protein and leukocyte concentration that accumulates at the site of injury

exudative macular degeneration: macular degeneration characterized by the formation of new blood vessels under the retina and macula, known as choroidal neovascularization; macular damage caused by leakage of fluid and bleeding from new vessels, altering the shape of the macula and distorting central vision; also known as wet macular degeneration

facilitated diffusion: assisted movement of substances across the cell membrane; not energy dependent

facultative parasites: microorganisms that may live on the host but can also survive independently

familial tendency: propagation of a condition among family members

feedback mechanism: regulatory mechanism; response of input to a system by generation of output in a given system

fetal alcohol syndrome (FAS): condition resulting from exposure of a fetus to alcohol; characterized by mental handicap, growth deficit, and physical disability

fibrillation: a problem of the heart chamber vibrating instead of effectively pumping

fibrinolysis: the dissolution of blood clots

fibroblasts: cells that produce and replace the connective tissue layer to support the constructive phase of wound healing

filtration pressure: the force that promotes movement of fluid across a pressure gradient

fistula: an abnormal track or passage that forms between two segments of bowel or other epithelial tissue

flaccid: relaxed, without tone

forced expiratory volume in 1 second (FEV$_1$): the maximal amount of air expired from the lungs in 1 second

forced vital capacity (FVC): the maximal amount of air that is exhaled from the lungs during a forced exhalation

fovea: area in the center of the macula with the highest density of cones

frank: visible blood in the stool

free radical injury: damage to cells resulting from reactive oxygen species

free radical theory: stochastic theory of aging suggesting that intracellular production of reactive oxygen species (ROS) contributes to the final determination of life span

friability: a state where tissue readily bleeds

full-thickness burns: formerly known as third-degree burns; burns that damage the epidermis, dermis, and can penetrate subcutaneous layers as well

fully saturated: a state in which all of the available seats for hemoglobin molecules are occupied on the red blood cell

fulminant hepatitis: liver failure from severe acute hepatitis

function: the action or workings of the various properties of the body

functional electrical stimulation (FES): technique used to generate artificial autonomic reflexes to promote mechanisms regulating bowel and bladder function

functional incontinence: unintentional loss of urine; characterized by normal bladder control coupled with an impaired ability to transport to toilet facilities

functional nonretentive soiling: voluntary or involuntary evacuation of stool; occurs in the absence of an appropriate toileting situation; often results from resistant behaviors in the child or ineffective toilet-training management strategies

gamete: ova and sperm; contains only one of the chromosome pairs, known as the haploid number

ganglion: collection of nerve cell bodies in the peripheral nervous system

gap junction: intercellular junctions with 2 nm gaps characterized by enhanced cell to cell communication

gastritis: an inflammatory condition of the gastric mucosa of the stomach

gate control theory: modification of the specificity theory; stimulation of the large type A beta and alpha inhibitory fibers "close the gate," preventing crossover and inhibiting pain impulse conduction along type A delta and type C fibers, diminishing pain perception

gene amplification: a process of altering chromosomes by accelerating the replication and number of copies of a gene

general adaptation syndrome: a term used to describe the neuroendocrine response to a stressor and the corresponding physiologic changes

genes: individual units of inheritance located on the chromosomes; determine cell protein characteristics

genetic code: hereditary units containing information for the production of proteins

genomic imprinting: an epigenetic phenomenon; mechanism that controls expression of genes based on parental origin

genomics: study of the human genome; includes the functions and interactions of all genes comprising an individual

genotype: genetic makeup of an individual

Ghon complex: a combination of the Ghon focus and additional granulomas that develop through the lymph channels in the lungs

Ghon focus: the formation of a granuloma, or walled-off area of bacteria, which is considered the primary lung lesion in tuberculosis

giant cells: phagocytes that can engulf particles much larger than the typical macrophage

gigantism: condition of hyperplasia characterized by excessive growth; growth hormone excess before the closure of the epiphyseal growth plates of the long bones

glia: neural support cells in the brain; provide support and nutrition, maintain homeostasis, and form myelin

global ischemia: consequences of inadequate blood supply to meet the needs of the brain tissue; results in hypoxia

glomerulus: capillary network of the nephron; located in the renal cortex; produces early urinary filtrate

glutamate: excitatory neurotransmitter

glutens: specific proteins found in wheat, rye, and barley

glycolipid: sugar bound to lipid heads of the plasma membrane

glycoproteins: regulate cell movement across the matrix, provide a place for attachment of the cells to the matrix, and prompt the cells to function

glycosylated hemoglobin (HbA$_{1c}$): a blood test that depicts hemoglobin and red blood cell exposure to glucose over the previous 3 to 4 months

goiter: an enlargement of the thyroid gland caused by follicular epithelial hyperplasia from excessive thyroid hormone exposure

Golgi apparatus: cellular organelle with a membranous structure; prepares substances by the endoplasmic reticulum for secretion out of the cell

grading: a process of differentiating the level of anaplasia depicted by the tumor

graft versus host disease (GVHD): a condition in which transplanted donor T lymphocytes mount an immune response against the host

gram-negative: bacteria with cell walls that do not retain a dark blue color when Gram stain is applied and instead turn red when counterstained in the laboratory

gram-positive: bacteria with cell walls that preserve the Gram stain and turn dark blue in the laboratory

granulation tissue: connective tissue characterized by extensive macrophages and fibroblasts and the promotion of angiogenesis

granulocytes: phagocytic cells named for the cytoplasmic granules common to all types; polymorphonuclear leukocytes, including neutrophils, eosinophils, and basophils

granulomas: nodular inflammatory lesions that encase harmful substances

Graves disease: an autoimmune condition that causes excessive stimulation of the thyroid gland

gray matter: tissue of the central nervous system composed primarily of cell bodies; contains synapses between sensory neurons, motor neurons, and interneurons

gustation: the sensation of taste

glycerol test: diagnostic test used to identify inner ear volume excess typically seen in Ménière disease

gyri: irregular convolutions on the brain surface

haploid: cells containing single chromosomes, rather than pairs; chromosome number totals 23 (22 autosomes, 1 sex chromosome); characteristic of gametes

haustra: pouches between taenia coli in the large intestine

health: the condition of being sound in body, mind, and spirit

heart block: the obstruction of cardiac conduction, often at the atrioventricular node, leading to heart dysrhythmias

heart failure: reflects an inadequacy of heart pumping so that the heart fails to maintain the circulation of blood

heart rate: the number of heartbeats that occur in 1 minute

helper T lymphocyte: subset of T lymphocyte that enhance humoral and cell-mediated responses of the immune system

hematoma: larger accumulations of blood in the tissue

hematuria: blood in the urine

hemiplegia: involving one arm and one leg on the same side of the body

hemodialysis: treatment using special filters to remove wastes that the kidneys no longer can do on their own through the mechanisms of diffusion, osmosis, and ultrafiltration

hemoglobin A (HbA): adult form of hemoglobin

hemoglobin F (HbF): fetal form of hemoglobin

hemoglobin S (HbS): sickled form of hemoglobin

hemolysis: breakdown of red blood cells

hemolytic: destruction of blood cells

hemoptysis: coughing up blood from the respiratory tract; defined by the presence of red blood cells in the sputum

hemorrhage: the loss of blood through the vessel wall

hepatic steatosis: fatty liver

hepatomegaly: enlarged liver

hepatorenal syndrome: renal failure caused by severe renal vasoconstriction in patients with liver disease

heredity: passage of characteristics from parent to offspring

Hertz (Hz): unit measurement of frequency; equivalent to one cycle per second

heterozygous: different alleles on each chromosome

heteroplasmy: random distribution of genes leading to a variable distribution in tissues

hirsutism: a condition of excessive body and facial hair

histology: a branch of anatomy that deals with the minute structure of cells and tissues, which are discernible with a microscope

Hodgkin lymphoma: a malignant disorder of the lymphoid tissue often characterized by the painless, progressive enlargement of cervical (neck) lymph nodes

Homans sign: a test of foot dorsiflexion, which, in the presence of deep vein thrombosis, causes pain in the back of the lower leg

homeostasis: a dynamic steady state marked by appropriate regulatory responses in the body

homozygous: identical alleles on each chromosome

hormones: chemical substances, formed in a tissue or organ and carried in the blood, that stimulate or inhibit the growth or function of other tissues or organs

host: the individual who is exposed to and contracts an infection

human immunodeficiency virus (HIV): enveloped retrovirus that infects CD4 T cells, dendritic cells, and macrophages; virus associated with the secondary immunodeficiency, acquired immunodeficiency syndrome (AIDS)

human leukocyte antigens (HLAs): the major histocompatibility complex proteins in humans; HLA genes encode antigen specificity; important in transplant rejection

human papilloma virus (HPV): DNA virus; specific viral strains cause cutaneous and genital warts and severe cervical intraepithelial lesions

humoral immunity: adaptive immunity involving antibodies

Hutchinson–Gilford progeria: syndrome commonly characterized by accelerated aging; results from damage to the LMNA gene that codes for the protein lamin A

hydrophilic: possessing affinity to water

hydrophobic: lacking affinity to water

hydrostatic forces: force promoting fluid movement between extracellular compartments; promotes movement of fluid based on the pressure gradient; also known as filtration pressure

hydroureter: accumulation of fluid in the urinary ureter; represents a consequence of complete ureteral obstruction

hygroma: cystic structure containing serous fluid

hyperacute graft rejection: rapid rejection of grafts

hypercalcemia: blood calcium levels greater than 10.5 mg/dL

hypercapnia: a state of increased carbon dioxide in the blood

hyperchloremia: blood chloride levels greater than 108 mEq/L

hyperglycemia: an elevation in the blood glucose level

hyperkalemia: potassium blood levels greater than 5 mEq/L

hyperketonemia: a condition of elevated circulating ketones that results from a loss of insulin, which is an inhibitor of lipolysis

hyperlactatemia: elevation of lactic acid in the blood

hypermagnesemia: magnesium levels greater than 2.5 mEq/L

hypernatremia: greater than 145 mEq/L of sodium in the blood

hyperopia: error in refraction commonly referred to as farsightedness

hyperphosphatemia: blood phosphate levels greater than 4.5 mg/dL

hyperpituitarism: a generic term indicating the increased secretion of one or more pituitary hormones

hyperplasia: increase in the number of cells

hyperpolarization: when the resting membrane potential is less negative than normal

hypertension: an elevation in blood pressure commonly defined by a systolic pressure above 140 mm Hg or a diastolic pressure above 90 mm Hg

hyperthyroidism: a state of excessive thyroid hormone as a result of excessive stimulation of the thyroid gland, diseases of the thyroid gland, or excess production of thyroid-stimulating hormone by a pituitary adenoma

hypertonic: solutions having a greater osmolality than the intracellular fluid

hypertrophy: increase in cell size

hypervolemia: excessive increase of fluid in the extracellular compartment

hyphae: tubular branches formed by mold colonies

hypocalcemia: calcium blood levels of less than 8.5 mg/dL

hypochloremia: blood chloride levels of less than 98 mEq/L

hypochromic: indicates pale red blood cells on microscopic examination

hypoglycemia: low blood glucose levels

hypokalemia: potassium blood levels of less than 3.5 mEq/L

hypomagnesemia: magnesium blood levels of less than 1.5 mEq/L

hyponatremia: less than 135 mEq/L of sodium in the blood

hypophosphatemia: blood phosphate levels less than 2.5 mg/dL

hypopituitarism: a generic term indicating the decreased secretion of one or more pituitary hormones

hypopolarization: when the resting membrane potential is more negative than normal

hypotension: a condition of reduced blood pressure

hypothalamic–pituitary axis: the neuronal system that regulates hormone secretion and inhibition

hypothyroidism: a state of deficient thyroid hormone

hypotonic: solutions having a lower osmolality than the intercellular fluid

hypovolemia: decreased vascular volume

hypovolemic shock: the result of inadequate blood/plasma volume

hypoxemia: decreased oxygen in the arterial blood leading to a decrease in the partial pressure of oxygen (PaO_2)

hypoxia: cellular deprivation of oxygen

iatrogenic: the term used to describe illnesses that are the inadvertent result of medical treatment

icteric phase: a stage of liver disease marked by jaundice

idiopathic: describes a condition that does not have a clear etiology

illness: a state that results in suffering or distress

immune response: the third line of defense, which wages a specific defense mechanism targeted at certain harmful invaders in the body

immune senescence: progressive dysfunction of the immune system associated with aging; characterized by both diminished and enhanced immune responses

immunity: process conferring protection against disease; includes active and passive

immunodeficiency: condition resulting from an inadequate immune defense; may be primary (directly caused by an alteration in immunity) or secondary (a consequence of another disease process)

immunoglobulins (Ig): a group of structurally related proteins important in immune function; composed of a variable region promoting antigen specificity and a constant region; classifications include IgG, IgA, IgM, IgD, and IgE

immunologic memory: process by which memory cells respond much more rapidly when reexposed to the same antigen; dramatically shortens and intensifies the immunologic response

immunologic theory of aging: developmental theory of aging associated with reduced resistance to disease secondary to reduced T-cell function and enhanced autoimmune responses

immunology: study of the structure and function of the immune system as well as the phenomena of immunity-induced sensitivity and allergy

immunotherapy: use of vaccines to stimulate the immune system to attack antigens associated with disease

incidence: the rate of occurrence of a health condition at any given time

incus: one of the three bones comprising the ossicle of the ear; also known as the anvil

infarct: an area of necrosis resulting from a sudden insufficiency of arterial or venous blood supply

infarction: the process of obstructing a blood vessel

infectious disease: also called infection; a state of tissue destruction resulting from invasion by microorganisms

infectivity: the proportion of exposures needed to cause infection in an individual based on the pathogens' ability to enter, survive in, and multiply in the host

infertility: the inability to achieve pregnancy after 1 year of unprotected intercourse

inflammatory response: the second line of defense, which is a nonspecific defense mechanism to protect from harmful invaders and to prepare an injury site for healing

ingest: particle entry into the cytoplasm through incorporation into a vesicle via a portion of the cell membrane

inhibin: a hormone that alerts the pituitary gland to suppress the secretion of gonadotropins

initiating event: a situation that causes a mutation in a cell

injury: any form of damage, harm, or loss to the cell, tissue, organ, or organ system

innate immunity: responsible for early, rapid response to pathogens without prior exposure

insidious: gradual in onset

inspiration: the process of breathing in to acquire oxygen

insulin: an anabolic hormone required for the uptake of glucose by the many cells, particularly those of the liver, muscle, and adipose cells

insulin-like growth factor 1 (IGF-1): hormone secreted by the liver; promotes growth in bones, cartilage, soft tissues, and organs

integral protein: form of transmembrane protein; forms a channel in the plasma membrane for transport of ions

intermittent claudication: a condition of fatigue or aching in the leg muscles even when walking short distances

internal rectal sphincter: thick layer of smooth muscle at the distal end of the rectum; provides tonic constriction under sympathetic control

internal urethral sphincter: ring of circular smooth muscle comprising the bladder neck; relaxation promotes release of urine from the bladder

interneuron: neurons connecting motor and sensory neurons; transmit signals between afferent and efferent neurons; most abundant neuron type

interventricular foramen: area of passage of the cerebrospinal fluid between the lateral to the third ventricle; also known as the foramen of Monro

intracellular compartment: fluid inside the cells; contains two thirds of the body water, accounting for 40% of body weight

intraneuronal inclusions: distinctive structures formed in the nucleus or cytoplasm

intrinsic enteric nervous system: source of innervation to the gastrointestinal nervous system

intron: segment of DNA not involved in protein expression

involution: decrease in the size of tissues and organs

ions: electrically charged particles resulting from gain or loss of one or more electrons; negatively charged particles known as anions; positively charged particles known as cations

iris: colored part of the eye

iron-deficiency anemia: a problem of hemoglobin and red blood cell development caused by inadequate iron stores

irrigation: process of rinsing an area with fluid or air

ischemia: local response to decrease in blood supply

islets of Langerhans: clusters of cells, located throughout the pancreas, that are responsible for the secretion of hormones

isoflavone: nonsteroidal estrogen found in high concentrations in soy products; also known as phytoestrogens

isolated systolic hypertension: an elevation in systolic blood pressure without an elevation in the diastolic blood pressure

isotonic: solutions with same osmolality as the intracellular fluid

jaundice: the yellow-tinged color of the skin and sclera of the eyes in those with liver disease

karyotype: picture of arranged, paired, like chromosomes in order from largest to smallest

keloids: hypertrophic scars that result from excessive collagen production at the site of injury

Kernig sign: a test used to elicit meningeal pain; the patient is placed supine with the knees bent and hips flexed, one knee is lifted upward, thereby eliciting pain

ketoacidosis: a state of metabolic acidosis, which signifies that the body is accessing fat and protein sources for energy and is releasing ketones, which are highly acidic, in the process

kinin system: a series of potent vasoactive chemical mediators, such as bradykinin, that play a role in vasodilation, vasoconstriction, cell migration, the pain response, and the activation of other cells active in the inflammatory response

Kupffer cells: phagocytes housed in the liver

Kussmaul respirations: deep, rapid respirations that present as a compensatory measure to release excess acids through the lungs and into the atmosphere

kwashiorkor: protein deprivation in persons consuming adequate carbohydrates

kyphosis: exaggerated anterior concave curvature of the thoracic spine associated with osteoporosis

labile cells: those that constantly regenerate through mitosis, particularly epithelial cells of the skin, gastrointestinal tract, and urinary tract, and blood cells in the bone marrow

labyrinthitis: inflammation of the labyrinth of the inner ear; precipitation of severe vertigo and sensorineural hearing loss

lacrimal glands: primary producers of tears

lacteal: lymphatic channel within each small intestinal villus critical for the absorption of fats

lactic acidemia: elevation of lactic acid in the blood

lactic acidosis: pH less than 7.35 because of elevation in lactic acid in the blood

Langerhans cells: immature dendritic cells in the skin; carry surface receptors for immunoglobulin and complement, important in the immune response

lanugo: a fine downy hair that covers the body in some patients with anorexia nervosa

large intestine/colon: organ of the gastrointestinal system; composed of the cecum, appendix, colon, rectum, and anal canal; further divided into the ascending, transverse, descending, and sigmoid portions

laser-assisted in situ keratomileusis (LASIK): surgical procedure used to treat myopia, hyperopia, and astigmatism

latency: a period of dormancy

leiomyomas: fibrous tumors of the uterus

lens: eye structure responsible for fine-tuning of focus

leukocytes: white blood cells; a group of cells active in defending the body against microorganisms and in promoting an immune response

leukocytosis: an elevation in the white blood cell, or leukocyte, with a count usually above $10,000/mm^3$

Lewy body: protein aggregations composed of the protein α-synuclein located primarily in the cells of the substantia nigra; associated with neurodegenerative disease, particularly Parkinson disease

life expectancy: the age at which 50% of a given population is expected to survive

ligands: molecules that bind to specific receptors; involved in signal transduction

lipids: a group of substances that are rich in energy and insoluble in water

lipid bilayer: an organized structure of two interconnected layers composed of nonpolar hydrophobic lipid tails connected to polar hydrophilic heads

lipofuscin: fatty brown lipid pigment; intracellular deposition causes stiffening or rigidity of cellular structure

local: refers to those manifestations that are directly at the site of illness, injury, or infection and are confined to a specific area

local mediators: substances involved in cellular responses in the immediate area

local spread: the proliferation of the neoplasm within the tissue of origin

loop diuretics: drugs that increase urine production through reduced reabsorption of sodium in the thick ascending loop of Henle, causing a decreased osmolality in the interstitial fluid of the collecting ducts and impairing the ability to concentrate urine at the loop

lymph fluid: filtration product of extracellular fluid from tissues

lymph node: joined segment of lymphatic vessels

lymphadenitis: the enlargement and inflammation of the nearby lymph nodes, which can occur as a function of filtering or draining harmful substances at the injury site

lymphadenopathy: swelling or enlargement of the lymph nodes

lymphatic system: circulates lymphocytes in lymph fluid; work in concert with the blood vessels to promote an effective immune response

lymphedema: obstructed lymph flow with movement of fluid into the interstitium

lymphocyte ignorance: the process of converting lymphocytes from nonresponsive to self-reactive

lymphoid progenitor: cellular origin of natural killer cells, T and B lymphocytes

lysis: the breakdown and removal of cells

lysosomes: cellular organelle composed of small sacs surrounded by membrane; responsible for hydrolytic digestion of cellular debris

maceration: the softening and breaking down of tissue

macronutrients: proteins, carbohydrates, and fats

macrophage: large, long-lived phagocytic leukocyte found within body tissues associated with a prolonged inflammatory response

macroscopic analysis: visual determination of color and clarity

macula: area of the retina responsible for central vision, color vision, and fine detail

mainstream smoke: active exposure to smoke

major histocompatibility complex (MHC): molecules promoting recognition of the body's "self" antigens from foreign "nonself" antigens; trap an antigen within the cell and then transport it to the cell surface where it can be displayed to T cells; subsets include MHC class I and class II molecules

major histocompatibility complex class I (MHC I): subset of MHC molecules recognized by CD8 cytotoxic T cells

major histocompatibility complex class II (MHC II): subset of MHC molecules recognized by CD4 helper (T_H1 and T_H2) T cells

malabsorption: indicates a lack of movement of specific nutrients across the gastrointestinal mucosa

malabsorption syndrome: a condition in which several nutrients are not adequately absorbed

malar: rash over cheeks; characteristic manifestation of systemic lupus erythematosus (SLE)

malignancy: invasive and destructive cellular growth, as in cancer

malignant: describes tumors that are invasive, destructive, spread to other sites, and do not resemble the tissue of origin

malleus: one of the three bones comprising the ossicle of the ear; also known as the hammer

malnutrition: a state of inadequate or excessive exposure to nutrients

marasmus: a condition of starvation related to deprivation of all food

mass movements: strong peristaltic movements, occurring three to four times a day; promotes the propulsion of stool

mast cells: leukocytes that are housed throughout the body within connective tissue and near all blood vessels; they are responsible for production and immediate release of chemical mediators

mastoiditis: bacterial infection and inflammation of the air cells of the mastoid bone

matrilineal: transmitted through female or maternal lines

mean arterial pressure: an adequate measure of *systemic:* tissue perfusion; is calculated as one third the pulse pressure plus diastolic pressure

mechanical injury: damage caused by impact of a body part

Meckel diverticulum: rare congenital condition characterized by the presence of a blind pouch in the colon

meconium: infant's first stool; represents the digestion of amniotic fluid and is sterile, black, sticky, and odorless

meiosis: process of sex cell (gamete) division; cell division resulting in gametocytes containing half (haploid) the number of chromosomes found in a somatic cell

Meissner's plexus: part of the enteric nervous system, located in the submucosa of the large intestine; transmits sensory impulses through stretch receptors

melena: black stool indicative of upper gastrointestinal bleeding

membrane attack complex (MAC): a cascade of events in the inflammatory process that leads to cell lysis

membrane pore: membrane passage between the extracellular and intracellular environment

membrane potential: difference in electrical charge between the inside and outside of the cell

memory cells: differentiated B cells capable of responding much more rapidly when re-exposed to the same antigen; dramatically shortening and intensifying the immunologic response

menarche: the time of the first menstrual period

Mendelian pattern of inheritance: predictable trait transmission based on autosomal dominant or recessive genotypes

Ménière disease: condition associated with severe vertigo, sensorineural hearing loss, and tinnitus; related to overproduction or decreased absorption of endolymph

meninges: membranes surrounding the brain and spinal cord of the central nervous system; contains cerebrospinal fluid; includes the pia, arachnoid, and dura mater

menometrorrhagia: shortened menstrual interval, heavy bleeding

menopausal bone loss: rapid phase of bone loss in women after menopause

menopause: permanent cessation of menses for a 12-month period

menorrhagia: excessive flow or prolonged duration of menses with regular menstrual interval

messenger RNA (mRNA): template for protein synthesis; depends on a codon sequence based on that of the complementary strand of DNA (cDNA); cytoplasmic area where protein is made in amino acid sequences

metabolic acidosis: alteration in acid–base balance characterized by reduction of HCO_3^-, prompting an increase in pH

metabolic alkalosis: alteration in acid–base balance characterized by increased levels of HCO_3^- resulting in a decrease of pH

metaplasia: changing of one cell type to another

metastases: process that occurs when neoplasms are spread to distant sites often by way of the lymphatics or blood vessels

metrorrhagia: irregular menstrual intervals

microbiology: a section of biology dealing specifically with the study of microscopic forms of life

microcytic: cells are small; the term microcytic is often used to describe small red blood cells in certain types of anemia

microglial nodules: structure formed by the union of microglia and astrocytes

micronutrients: vitamins and minerals

microscopic analysis: analysis of urine components under magnification; low-power magnification may detect crystals, casts, squamous cells, and other large components; white and red blood cells and bacterial forms may be detected with high-power magnification

microstimulation: electrical stimulation to preganglionic neurons and interneurons controlling bladder function

micturition: process of urine elimination

minerals: inorganic substances critical to the regulation of hundreds of cellular processes; minerals constitute bone, hemoglobin, enzymes, hormones, and chemical mediators; charged (ionic) minerals mediate impulse conduction within the nervous system; minerals maintain water balance, acid–base balance, and osmotic pressure and are critical for muscle contraction and form the structural components of bones and teeth

mitochondria: cellular organelle containing enzymes involved in citric acid cycle, fatty acid oxidation, and oxidative phosphorylation; principal producer of the cellular energy source adenosine triphosphate

mitosis: process of reproduction of nuclear chromosomes in somatic cells; reproductive phases include prophase, prometaphase, metaphase, anaphase, and telophase; results in the creation of daughter cells with the same chromosome number and genetic makeup as the cell of origin

mixed hearing loss: combination of both sensorineural and conductive hearing loss

molecular mimicry: close resemblance between foreign antigen and self-antigen

mold: a multicellular form of fungus

monoamines: class of neurotransmitters, including norepinephrine, dopamine, and serotonin

monoclonal origin: the process of starting with a single mutated cell and developing into cancer

monocyte: large, mononuclear leukocytes representing 3% to 7% of the total number of circulating leukocytes associated with a prolonged inflammatory response

mononeuropathy: nerve damage limited to a single area

monosomy: one copy of a chromosome, in place of the normal pair; the result of nondisjuncture

morbidity: a poor quality of life resulting from a disease

morphology: a branch of biology that deals with the form and structure of animals and plants; looks more specifically at how cells and tissues change in form after encountering disease

mortality: the death rate resulting from a disease

mosaicism: combination of cell lines with regular and altered numbers of chromosomes

motor neurons: carry impulses from the central nervous system to an effector muscle

multifactorial: having a number of events that led to the development of the condition

mutation: change in genes or sequence of base pairs that make up the chromosomes; genetic alteration perpetuated in subsequent cellular divisions

mutator genes: genes that repair mutated DNA and protect the genome

mycelium: a cluster of hyphae formed from mold colonies

mycoses: infections with fungi as the pathogen

myeloid progenitor: origin of immune system cells, including monocytes, dendritic cells, granulocytes, and mast cells

myenteric (Auerbach) plexus: part of the enteric nervous system; found between the longitudinal and circular muscle layers of the large intestine; provides increased tonic and rhythmic contractions

myocardial infarction: the total occlusion of one or more coronary arteries resulting in ischemia and death of myocardial tissues

myocardium: the thick muscular layer of the heart

myofascia: outer membrane of muscle tissue

myopia: error in refraction; commonly known as nearsightedness

myringotomy: incision of the tympanic membrane to drain fluid

myxedema: a condition of hypothyroidism marked by the accumulation of boggy, nonpitting edematous tissue, especially of the face, mucous membranes, hands, and feet, from protein–carbohydrate complexes that accumulate in the extracellular matrix and attract fluid into the tissues

naive lymphocytes: lymphocytes that have not yet encountered an antigen

natural killer cells: large, granular lymphocytes; nonspecific cytotoxic cells

necrosis: disorderly process of cell death associated with inflammation

negative feedback loop: a system of hormone regulation in which low levels of hormone stimulate additional release and high levels of hormone inhibit further release

neoplasia: the irreversible deviant development of cells resulting in the formation of neoplasms

nephron: functional unit of the kidney; composed of the glomerulus, proximal tubule, loop of Henle, distal tubule, and collecting duct; responsible for filtering water-soluble substances from the blood, reabsorption of filtered nutrients, water, and electrolytes, and secretion of waste

nephropathy: a problem of degenerative changes in small vessels in the kidneys

neurofibrillary tangles: twisted, helical structure of accumulated proteins, primarily including tau; commonly associated with Alzheimer disease

neuroendocrine theory: developmental theory of aging suggesting that the interrelationship between neurons and associated hormones serves as the stimulus for aging

neurogenic: pain originating within the nervous system

neurogenic shock: a result of brain or spinal cord injury in which altered neuronal transmission leads to a loss of tension in the blood vessels, allowing unregulated vasodilation, decreased peripheral vascular resistance, and reduced blood pressure; oxygenated blood is *not* shunted to vital organs, and perfusion to vital organs is reduced

neuromatrix theory: modification of the pattern theory; a widely distributed neural network in the brain (body-self neuromatrix) containing somatosensory, limbic, and thalamocortical components integrates multiple sources of input resulting in the cognitive, affective, and sensory perceptions of pain

neuromodulator: chemical released from axon terminals, which inhibits, potentiates, or prolongs effects of neurotransmitter

neuron: nerve cell; fundamental unit of the nervous system; composed of a cell body, one axon, and a variable number of dendrites

neuropathy: a problem of nerve degeneration to damage to cell body resulting in delayed nerve conduction and impaired sensory function

neuropathic: pain originating within the nervous system

neurophagia: phagocytosis and inflammatory responses caused by a dead neuron damaging

neurostimulation: electrical stimulation of efferent nerves

neurotransmitter: chemical agent affecting the function of another nearby cell or cells

neutralization: making ineffective any action, process, or potential

neutrophil: granulocyte present in the greatest number; most important in the rapid response to bacterial infection; phagocytic; the first responders in the inflammatory response

N:-methyl-D-aspartate (NMDA) receptor: receptor with affinity for glutamate

nociceptive: origination of pain outside of the nervous system

nociceptor: receptor generating a pain impulse

nocturia: frequent urination at night

nodes of Ranvier: interruptions in the myelin sheaths surrounding axons in the peripheral nervous system; rich in sodium channels to promote movement of nerve impulses over long distances

nondisjunction: failure of chromosome separation during meiosis or mitosis; results in an unequal number of chromosomes

noncommunicating hydrocephalus: increased ventricular accumulation of cerebrospinal fluid caused by obstructed cerebrospinal fluid flow

non-Hodgkin lymphoma (NHL): a generic classification made up of a broad range of B-cell and T-cell malignancies within the immune system

nonpolar: compound lacking positive or negative charge

nonself: particles that are not part of the individual

nonvolatile acid: circulating fixed acid that is unable to be excreted by the lungs; require buffering and excretion by the kidneys

nosocomial: describes illnesses that are caused by exposure to the health care environment

nuchal rigidity: a hyperextended stiff neck related to meningeal irritation

nuchal translucency: ultrasound determination of thickness of the nape of the neck

nucleus: rounded mass of protoplasm within the cytoplasm of a cell; surrounded by a nuclear envelope enclosing structures responsible for mitosis during cell division

nursing diagnoses: labels distinguished by a focus on the human response to the condition

nutrient: a food or liquid that supplies the body with the chemicals needed for metabolism

nutrition: the process of ingestion and use of nutrients for energy

nystagmus: involuntary, irregular oscillations of the eye

obesity: a state of excessive body fat in which the body mass index is greater than 30 kg/m^2

obligate parasites: parasites that require the host for metabolism and reproduction

occlusion: blockage

occult: hidden blood in the stool that is not visible

olfaction: sense of smell

oligodendrocytes: neural support cells responsible for the production of myelin around the axons of the central nervous system

oligomenorrhea: decreased frequency of menstruation

oliguria: reduced urine output

oncogenes: genes that code for proteins involved in cell growth or regulation

oncogenic: cancer causing

open traumatic injury: exposure of brain structures to the environment because of injury

opportunistic pathogens: those that cause disease only in a host with a compromised immune system

opsonization: a process of rendering bacteria vulnerable to phagocytosis

organ: fully differentiated body part with specialized functions

organ of Corti: sensory receptor in the cochlea containing hair cells

organelles: structures within a cell that perform a distinct function

organogenesis: embryologic period of organ development

orthopnea: the physical need to sit in an upright or standing position to reduce respiratory effort

osmole: unit of measure reflecting the osmotic activity that nondiffusible particles exert in pulling water from one side of the semipermeable membrane to the other

osmolality: osmolar concentration in 1 kg of water (mOsm/kg of H$_2$O); used to describe fluids within the body

osmolarity: osmolar concentration in 1 L of solution (mOsm/L); used when referring to fluids outside the body

osmoreceptors: sensory neurons in the hypothalamus that promote thirst

osmosis: movement of water across a concentration gradient; water movement to an area of higher concentration of particles (less water content) from an area of lower concentration of particles (more water content); regulated by the concentration of particles that do not diffuse across the semipermeable membrane

osmotic pressure: force generated as water moves through the membrane by osmosis

ossicles: bones of the middle ear; include the malleus, incus, and stapes

osteoma: tumor that arises from bone cells

osteopenia: reduced calcification or skeletal bone mass; precursor to osteoporosis

osteoporosis: condition characterized by decreased bone mass and deterioration of bone tissue; associated with increased bone fragility and susceptibility to fracture

otitis externa: inflammation of the skin of the external ear; commonly known as "swimmer's ear"

otitis media: infection of the middle ear

otoacoustic emission (OAE): tests used to evaluate outer hair cell function

otosclerosis: an autosomal dominant condition causing the most common cause of chronic, progressive, conductive hearing loss; characterized by impairing the conduction of vibration

oval window: marks the boundary between the middle ear and the beginning point of the inner ear

overactive bladder: involuntary leakage of urine that is accompanied or immediately preceded by a strong urge to void; also known as urge incontinent

overflow incontinence: incontinence resulting from urine volumes exceeding bladder capacity

overnutrition: a state of excessive exposure to nutrients

overweight: defined as a body mass index between 25 and 30 kg/m^2

oxidative stress: potential source of cellular damage by exposure to reactive oxygen species

oxygen free radicals: an oxygen atom carrying an unpaired electron and no charge

oxygen saturation (SaO$_2$): the amount of oxyhemoglobin; that is, the amount of hemoglobin that is combined, or saturated, with oxygen

oxyhemoglobin (HbO$_2$): the oxygen–hemoglobin combination within red blood cells

PaCO$_2$: the symbol for the partial pressure of carbon dioxide

PaO$_2$: the symbol for the partial pressure of oxygen

palliative care: used to describe treating symptoms, such as pain, without curing the cancer

pallidotomy: irreversible procedure involving destruction of the globus pallidus; designed to decrease excitatory nerve firing in the damaged tissue; employed in the management of Parkinson disease

pandemic: when an epidemic spreads across continents

panhypopituitarism: a deficiency of all anterior pituitary hormones

pannus: granulation tissue that forms over the inflamed synovium and cartilage

papilledema: edema of the optic disc

papilloma: an epithelioma that presents as fingerlike projections

paracentesis: insertion of a cannula into the peritoneal cavity for removal of ascitic fluid

paracrine: hormone effects restricted to the local environment

paraneoplastic syndrome: hormonal, neurologic, hematologic, and chemical disturbances in the body not directly related to invasion by the primary tumor or metastasis

paralytic ileus: inactive intestinal muscles producing blockage or obstruction of the intestine

parasympathetic nervous system (PNS): component of the autonomic nervous system

parathyroid hormone (PTH): promotes removal of calcium and phosphate from bone; opposes the effects of calcitonin

parenchymal: tissues with a specific function, such as tissues formed of neurons, myocardial cells, and epithelial cells

paresthesia: abnormal sensation, such as burning, pricking, tickling, or tingling

partial pressure: the force exerted by gas molecules within a certain volume

passive diffusion: a process of absorption in which nutrients randomly migrate across the mucosa from areas of higher to lower concentration or pressure

passive smoke: environmental byproduct from tobacco products used by others; also known as secondhand smoke

pathogen: a disease-causing organism, such as a virus

pathogenesis: the origination and development of disease or illness

pathogenic defense mechanisms: the ways in which many pathogens have developed ways to avoid destruction by the host, such as through thick protective capsules, which prevent phagocytosis

pathogenicity: ability of a pathogen to produce an infectious disease; involve multiple factors, including the pathogen's potency, invasiveness, ability to evade the immune system, speed of replication, production of toxins, adherence to the human host cell, and degree of tissue damage that is elicited

pathology: the study of the structural and functional changes in cells and tissues as a result of injury

pathophysiology: the physiology of altered health states; specifically, the functional changes that accompany a particular injury, syndrome, or disease

pattern theory: a group of theories that suggest that nonspecific receptors transmit specific patterns influenced by duration of pain sensation, quantity of tissue involved, and summation of impulses

penetrance: ability of a gene to express a mutation; influences the effects of mutations

percutaneous nephrolithotomy: surgical procedure used for removal of large renal calculi; involves location and removal of stone with a nephroscope

perfusion: the process of forcing blood or other fluid to flow through a vessel and into the vascular bed of a tissue for the purposes of providing oxygen and other nutrients

pericarditis: inflammation of the lining of the heart

pericardium: the outer covering of the heart, which holds the heart in place in the chest cavity, contains receptors that assist with the regulation of blood pressure and heart rate, and forms a first line of defense against infection and inflammation

perilymph: fluid filling the cochlea

perimenopause: gradual transition between normal reproductive cycles and menopause; also known as climacteric

peripheral neuropathy: disease involving the nerves of the peripheral nervous system

peripheral nervous system: component of the nervous system comprising the somatic and autonomic nervous system

peripheral organs: sites for maintenance of the lymphocytes; are the organs in which immune responses are often initiated; organs include the spleen, lymph nodes, and other lymphoid mucosal tissue, such as tonsils and the appendix

peripheral proteins: plasma membrane proteins extending into the intracellular or the extracellular environment

peristalsis: rhythmic contractions of circular muscle fibers in hollow organs; promotes forward movement of contents

peritoneal dialysis: process of waste and excess water removal using the peritoneal membrane as the semipermeable "filter"; waste moves across the peritoneum using the transport mechanisms of diffusion, osmosis, and ultrafiltration

peritonitis: inflammation of the peritoneal membrane

permanent cells: cells such as neurons, cardiac myocytes, and the lens of the eye that do not undergo mitosis and are unable to regenerate

permeable: a state where junctions are opened between the endothelial cells, allowing fluid to move into the injured tissue

peroxisomes: cellular organelle made up of small membrane-enclosed sacs; promote cell survival by oxidation of oxygen free radicals

petechiae: pinpoint hemorrhages of the skin or mucous membranes

pH: clinical measurement of acid–base balance

phagocytosis: ingesting large particles such as cells, bacteria, and damaged cellular components

phenotype: genetic traits that are apparent or observable

Philadelphia chromosome: found in approximately 95% of those with chronic myelogenous leukemia (CML) and represents a chromosome 9 and 22 translocation, which activates oncogenes

phlegm: large amounts of sputum expectorated from the oropharynx

phospholipid: phosphate [PO_4^-] bound to lipid heads of the plasma membrane

photophobia: a condition in which the eyes are extremely sensitive to light

photoreceptor: receptor sensitive to light found in the eye; rods and cones

photosensitivity: skin sensitivity to the sun resulting in rash

physical injury: cellular damage from mechanical, thermal, or chemical sources

phytoestrogen: nonsteroidal estrogens found in high concentrations in soy products; also known as isoflavones

pica: (pagophagia) the compulsion to eat ice or nonfood substances, such as dirt or clay; another manifestation of iron-deficient anemia that is not clearly understood

pinna: tissue of the outer ear

pinocytosis: adenosine triphosphate (ATP)-requiring process of ingesting very small vesicles

pitting edema: edema that leaves an impression when pressure is placed

placenta: specialized organ developed during pregnancy; sustains the fetus by providing respiration, nutrition, and excretion functions

plasma membrane: an organized structure composed of lipids, carbohydrates, and proteins arranged in a bilayer; protects the cell by creating a barrier against the potentially hostile environment surrounding it

platelets: irregularly shaped cytoplasmic fragments that release chemical mediators and are essential for clotting, or coagulation

plethora: a condition of hypervolemia in which the blood becomes increasingly viscous, leading to pruritus (itching), hypertension, and interruptions of circulation

pleuritis: inflammation of the lining of the lungs or pleural cavity

plexus: formation of an interconnection of spinal fibers

pneumonia: inflammation of the lungs occurring commonly in the bronchioles, interstitial lung tissue, or the alveoli

pneumothorax: the presence of air in the pleural space that causes the lung to collapse

poikilocytosis: the irregular shape of red blood cells that are iron deficient

polar: carrying a distribution of electrons that repels water

polarize: a condition in the excitable cell when the intracellular compartment is more negative than the extracellular space

polycystic kidney disease (PKD): a condition characterized by growth of fluid-filled cysts in kidney tissue bilaterally; often leads to chronic renal failure

polycystic ovary syndrome (PCOS): a condition of excess androgen production from the ovaries

polydipsia: a state of excessive thirst

polygenic: containing several major histocompatibility complex (MHC) class I and II genes; interaction of several genes influenced by environmental factors

polymenorrhea: shortened menstrual interval

polymorphic: describes something that occurs in more than one form

polymorphism: occurring in more than one form

polymorphonuclear leukocytes: granulocytes, including neutrophils, eosinophils, and basophils

polyneuropathy: peripheral nerve damage involving multiple axons

polyphagia: a state of excessive hunger

polyuria: frequent, large volume urination

portal circulation: a blood bypass through which deoxygenated blood from the gastrointestinal (GI) tract, spleen, and pancreas travel to the liver by way of the portal vein before moving on to the vena cava and heart

portal hypertension: elevation in the hepatic pressure of the liver

positive feedback loop: a system in which the presence of hormone stimulates an increased production of hormone until there is an interruption in the cycle

postganglionic neurons: axon fibers projecting from an autonomic group of nerve cell bodies to a target organ

postictal: physical state after recovery from seizure; manifested by extreme fatigue, headache, muscle pain, and weakness

precipitating factors: triggers that lead to the onset of disease

preganglionic neurons: axon fibers extending from cell bodies in the brain or spinal cord to a group of nerve cell bodies

preimplantation genetic diagnosis: identification of genetic abnormalities before implantation of the blastocyst in the maternal uterine lining, the decidua

preload: the work imposed on the heart just prior to contraction

presbyopia: condition of farsightedness associated with aging; results from the inability of the ciliary muscle and lens to accommodate for near vision

presbycusis: sensorineural hearing loss consistent with aging; associated with tinnitus

prevalence: the percentage of a population that is affected by a particular disease at a given time

primary active transport: active transport process requiring the direct use of energy in the form of adenosine triphosphate

primary intention: a form of healing in which the wound is approximated with all areas of the wound, connecting and healing simultaneously

primary prevention: actions or activities that prohibit a disease condition from occurring

prions: protein particles that lack DNA or RNA, which have been found to cause infectious disease in humans

prognosis: the forecast or prediction of how an individual will proceed through the health condition

programmed senescence theory: developmental theory that links the aging process with alterations in the telomere portion of chromosomes

progression: an extension of the promotion phase with one exception: now the cancerous growth no longer depends on continued exposure to the promoter

proliferation: the rapid generation of new daughter cells divided from progenitor (parent) cells

promoting event: an expansion of a mutated cell's growth and reproduction; the continued growth of the cell depends on continued exposure to the promoter

protease: any of numerous enzymes that cut or splice proteins into their smaller peptide units; also known as proteolytic enzymes

proteinases: enzymes that destroy elastin and other tissue components

proteinuria: protein in the urine

proteolysis: the process of cutting or splicing proteins into their smaller peptide units

proteosome: large cellular organelle that recognizes abnormally folded or formed proteins; involved in proteolysis

protooncogenes: "normal" genes in the body with a vital role in regulating cell function; precursors to the development of oncogenes

provisional matrix: a temporary support structure that promotes healing by decreasing blood and fluid loss at the site, and attracting and supporting fibroblasts, endothelial cells, and epidermal (skin) cells

pseudobulbar affect: uncontrollable laughing or crying because of altered control of emotional responsiveness

pseudohyphae: elongated chains formed by yeast through budding

pulse oximetry: a noninvasive method of determining hypoxemia even before clinical signs and symptoms are noted

pulse pressure: the difference between the systolic and diastolic blood pressure

pupil: opening in the iris; controls the amount of light that enters the eye

pure tone bone conduction: used to evaluate the inner ear function, independent of middle and outer ear function

purine: parent compound of the nitrogenous bases adenine (A) and guanine (G)

purpura: the presence of diffuse hemorrhages of the skin or mucous membranes

pursed lip breathing: a process of holding the lips puckered tightly together while slowly exhaling to maintain positive airway pressure in the alveoli; this minimizes air trapping and promotes expiration of carbon dioxide

purulent: exudate that contains pus

pyelonephritis: infection and subsequent inflammation of the kidneys

pyogenic: pathogens that induce fever

pyramidal motor system: composed of the corticospinal and corticobulbar tracts, providing control of voluntary movement

pyrexia: also called fever, an elevated core body temperature is a result of chemical mediators acting directly on the hypothalamus

pyrimidine: parent compound of the nitrogenous bases cytosine (C) and thymine (T)

pyuria: purulent exudate (pus) in the urine

quadriplegia: paralysis of all four extremities

quadruple test: prenatal screening test; measurement of maternal serum alpha-fetoprotein, unconjugated estradiol, human chorionic gonadotropin hormone, and inhibin A

quiescence: dormancy; temporary resting

reactive oxygen species (ROS): toxic oxygen molecules or radicals that are formed by the reaction between oxygen (O_2) and water (H_2O) during mitochondrial respiration

reassortment: a process of changing genetic composition during replication in the human host cell leading to viral offspring with altered antigenic properties

receptor: a cytoplasmic or cell surface protein molecule structured to bind specific factors

recessive: trait caused by a particular allele that does not manifest itself in the presence of other alleles that generate traits dominant to it

recombinant vaccine: subunit vaccines with highly antigenic components of a pathogen

recombinant virus: virus created to include genetic material that express a desired antigen

rectal reflex: neuromuscular stimulation for defecation; defecation stimulated by movement of stool into the rectum, also known as the defecation reflex

Reed–Sternberg cell: originates in the cell components of lymph nodes following a B lymphocyte lineage; is the neoplastic cell that is diagnostic for Hodgkin lymphoma

re-epithelialization: the movement of epithelial cells to form a covering over a wound

reflex arc: basic functional pathway of the nervous system; a process by which stimuli are received and interpreted, and then stimulate a response

regeneration: a process of reformation of parenchymal tissues, which can only occur in those cells that undergo mitotic division

regulatory T cells: suppress autoreactive lymphocytes and regulate the immune response; also known as suppressor T cells

regurgitation: a problem of incompetence of the valve; the valve is unable to properly close, allowing reflux of blood

remission: a symptom-free period

repolarization: result of movement of potassium ions out of the cell

reproduction: process by which cells replicate

resident flora: microorganisms that live on or within the body in nonsterile areas without causing harm

residual volume (RV): the volume of air that remains in the lungs after maximal expiration

resolution: healing in response to mild injury with minimal disruption to cells, such as with a small superficial scratch or mild sunburn

respiration: the process of oxygen use as a source of energy for production of adenosine triphosphate (ATP) and release of metabolic products from cells

respiratory failure: a life-threatening condition that can result from any problem that severely affects ventilation, ventilation–perfusion matching, or diffusion

resting membrane potential (RMP): membrane potential of a cell at rest

retentive incontinence: withholding of feces from fear of pain on defecation; results in constipation and overflow soiling

reticulate body: the metabolically active stage of the life cycle of chlamydiae, where the microorganism takes over the host cell

retina: ocular structure located over the posterior two thirds of the eye; contains photoreceptor cells

retinopathy: a problem of degenerative changes in small vessels of the retinas (eyes)

retractions: the pulling in of accessory muscles usually in the intercostal, substernal, and supraclavicular spaces to promote more effective inspiration

rheumatoid factor (RF): a substance that can be found in the blood and synovial fluid; signifies that antibodies (IgM, IgG, or IgA) are acting against other antibodies (mainly IgG)

rhodopsin: photopigment produced by the rods of the retina

ribonucleic acid (RNA): nucleic acid that contains a sugar (ribose); responsible for the control of protein synthesis; made up of the four nitrogenous bases, including adenine (A) and guanine (G), cytosine (C) and uracil (U)

ribosomal RNA (rRNA): form of RNA of ribosomes; associated with mRNA in the translation of the genetic code

Ringer's lactate: crystalloid intravenous fluid containing sodium, chloride, potassium, calcium, and lactate

risk factors: vulnerabilities that, when present, increase the chances that a disease may occur

rods: photoreceptor cells of the retina; produce the photopigment rhodopsin, allowing vision in dim light

saltatory conduction: pattern of nerve impulse over long distances where the impulse moves down the axon from node to node in a stepwise fashion

saccule: structural component of the semicircular canal

sarcopenia: loss of skeletal muscle associated with aging

satiety: a feeling of gastric fullness, usually associated with eating

saturated fatty acids: fatty acids that have no double bonds and elevate blood cholesterol levels, are found in animal sources, and are solid at room temperature

Schwann cells: neural support cells responsible for the production of myelin on long, single axons of the peripheral nervous system

secondary active transport: active transport mechanism involving movement of a second substance; dependent on energy derived from the active transport of the primary substance

secondary intention: a form of healing characteristic of large, open, craterlike wounds in which the wounds heal from the bottom up, posing a greater risk for infection and scarring

secondary prevention: early detection and treatment of disease through screening

secrete: the process of the release of metabolic products from cells

seeding: a form of direct extension where neoplastic proliferation occurs within peritoneal and pleural cavities surrounding the affected tissue or organ

segmental movement: circular fiber contraction and relaxation occurring at different locations, producing the characteristic contractions associated with peristalsis

self-limiting: describes an infection that ceases after a definite period of time without any specific treatment

semicircular canal: inner ear structures regulating balance; composed of the utricle and the saccule

senescence: postmaturational processes that lead to diminished homeostasis and increased vulnerability; used interchangeably with aging

senescent bone loss: slower loss phase that affects both men and women; associated with aging

senile plaque: accumulations of proteins surrounding deposits of β-amyloid protein

sensitization phase: initial phase of delayed hypersensitivity reaction; stimulated by entry of antigen via the skin and presentation of antigen by Langerhans cells, stimulating immune responses

sensitized: development of an immune response to an antigen by previous exposure

sensorineural hearing loss: permanent hearing loss, resulting from disease, trauma, or genetic inheritance of a defect in the cochlea nerve cells

sensory neurons: neurons that carry impulses from receptors to the distant targets of the brain and spinal cord; also known as afferent neurons

sepsis: a bacterial infection of the blood

septic shock: a condition of altered perfusion by shock as the result of overwhelming systemic infection, often with gram-negative bacteria (the endotoxin component) leading to inadequate perfusion of vital organs

septicemia: a problem of microorganisms gaining access to the blood and circulating throughout the body

seroconversion: development of antibodies to a particular antigen

serous exudate: a clear fluid that seeps out of the tissues

sex chromosome: known as X and Y; the genetic determinants of the sex of an individual

sex-linked: characteristics passed on by sex chromosomes; most often recessive traits; often linked to the X chromosome

shock: a state of inadequate blood flow to peripheral tissues

short tandem repeats (STR): unique lengths of DNA stretches in an individual

shunting: the movement of blood across the atria or ventricles of the heart

sickle cell anemia: single gene disorder resulting from a mutation of the sickle beta globin gene; characterized by sickled hemoglobin (HbS); autosomal recessive

sickle cell trait: heterozygous for a mutation of the sickle beta globin gene; carrier of the autosomal recessive trait

sidestream smoke: passive or secondhand smoke

signal transduction pathway: mechanism of cellular communication; initiated by binding of ligand to receptor and resulting in an action through subsequent communication events

signs: relating to disease, the observable or measurable expression of the altered health condition

single gene trait: characteristics passed on by the transmission of a single gene

sinoatrial (SA) node: the pacemaker of the heart, which generates a rhythmic impulse in the atria

soma: also known as a cell body; component of cell composed of cytoplasm and organelles responsible for specialized functions of the cell

somatic: relating to the soma, or body

somatic mutation: a mutation occurring in body cells, rather than gametes; not transmittable to subsequent generations

somatic mutation theory: stochastic theory of aging suggesting that the aging process is caused by impaired DNA repair, antioxidant defense, or errors in protein expression

somatic nervous system: voluntary nervous control in skeletal muscles

somatosensory modality: specific nature of the perception of various stimuli

Somogyi effect: the presence of rebound hyperglycemia as a reaction to insulin-induced hypoglycemia

spastic: increased muscle tone with exaggerated tendon reflexes

specificity theory: theory of pain suggesting that sensations of touch, warmth, cold, and pain involve specific receptors and pathways

spermatogonia: a primitive sperm cell

spinal muscular atrophy: condition that results from disuse because of impaired neural innervation to muscle tissue

sputum: expectorated material

squamocolumnar junction: area of the merger of squamous and columnar epithelium; also known as the transformation zone of the cervix

squamous epithelium: epithelium consisting of a single flattened layer of cells

stable cells: cells that stop regenerating when growth is complete but can resume regeneration if injured

staging: a process of classifying the extent or spread of the disease from the site of origin

stapes: one of three bones comprising the ossicle of the ear; also known as the stirrup

status asthmaticus: a state of bronchospasm that is not reversed by the patient's medications or other measures

steatorrhea: stool containing large amounts of fat; may be caused by absence of bile acids or gastrointestinal malabsorption

stem cells: highly undifferentiated units that have the potential to divide into daughter stem cells, which can then mature into more differentiated units with a specific function

stenosis: a problem in which narrowing of the valve occurs, making it unable to open adequately

stercobilin: bile pigment; provides the characteristic brown color of stool

stochastic theory: theory positing that aging is the result of cumulative cellular damage

storage fat: adipose that accumulates under the skin and around internal organs and is not required for physiologic functioning

strabismus: lack of coordination of extrinsic eye muscles; results in a condition known as "cross-eyed"

stress: the reactions of the body to forces of a deleterious nature that disturb homeostasis

stress incontinence: involuntary loss of urine via an exertional stimulus; may be associated with impaired sphincter control

stressor: any endogenous or exogenous force that causes stress

stroke: any clinical event, such as shock, cerebral hemorrhage, ischemia, or infarction, that leads to the impairment of cerebral circulation

stroke volume: the amount of blood pumped out of one ventricle of the heart in a single beat

stromal tissue: also called interstitial tissue; the connective tissue layer composed primarily of collagen, elastin, and glycoproteins

structure: the formation of the parts in the body; that is, how the body is put together

struvite: magnesium ammonium phosphate; common component of renal calculi

subacute: somewhere in duration and severity between acute and chronic

substantia gelatinosa: gray matter extending throughout the posterior horn of the spinal cord to the medulla oblongata

subthreshold: membrane potential less than that necessary for commitment to an action potential

sulci: fissures in the brain that provides anatomic divisions

superficial partial-thickness burns: formerly known as first-degree burns, these burns damage the epidermis

superinfection: when a new infection arises in addition to one that is already present

suppressor T lymphocytes: subset of T lymphocyte that inhibits humoral and cell-mediated responses

supraphysiologic: blood levels of substances much higher than would normally be expected

surfactant: a lipoprotein lubricant that coats the inner portion of the alveolus and promotes ease of expansion and repels fluid accumulation

sympathetic nervous system (SNS): component of the autonomic nervous system; also known as the thoracolumbar nervous system

symport: system of substances transported in the opposite direction

symptom: an indicator that is reported by an ill individual and is often considered a "subjective" manifestation

synapse: small gap or junction separating cells

syncope: loss of consciousness; fainting

syndactyly: fusion or incomplete separation of digit soft tissue

syndrome: a cluster of clinical manifestations and laboratory and other diagnostic tests that fit a recognizable, predictable pattern

syndrome of inappropriate antidiuretic hormone (SIADH): a condition of excessive production and release of ADH despite changes in serum osmolality and blood volume

synergistic: greater effect produced through two or more substances acting in concert than any one substance alone

syngeneic: graft from genetically identical individuals (e.g., monozygotic twins)

systemic: describes manifestations that present throughout the body and are not confined to a local area

systole: a heart contraction that forcefully moves blood out of the ventricles

systolic blood pressure: the amount of pressure exerted during contraction of the left ventricle and ejection of blood into the aorta

systolic failure: heart failure caused by a loss of contractile ability of the heart

T-cell receptor: receptor on T lymphocytes that bind to antigens, promoting a characteristically rapid immune response

T lymphocytes: type of white blood cell responsible for cell-mediated immunity; classified by function—helper, cytotoxic, and suppressor

telomerase: an enzyme that adds length to the telomere, the chromosomal "time clock"

teniae coli: longitudinal segments of smooth muscle in the large intestine; contractions produce haustra

teratocarcinomas: a combination of embryonic carcinomas and undifferentiated somatic (e.g., skin, muscle, bone, glands) tissues

teratogen: substances causing damage to a developing embryo or fetus

teratomas: benign tumors that arise from germ cells

tertiary prevention: rehabilitation of the patient after detection of disease

T_H: 1 class of CD4 helper T lymphocytes; activate macrophages, secrete chemokines and cytokines to attract macrophages; promote fusion of lysosomes with vesicles containing bacteria; and stimulate phagocytosis

T_H: 2 class of CD4 helper T lymphocytes; activate B cells to produce antibodies

thermal injury: damage caused by extremes of temperature

thermoreceptor: receptor that recognizes thermal sensation

thiazide diuretic: drug that increases urine output through prevention of NaCl reabsorption in the distal convoluted tubule

thoracolumbar nervous system: component of the autonomic nervous system; also known as the sympathetic nervous system

threshold potential: intracellular electrical potential stimulating an action potential

thrombocythemia: a condition of excess platelets in the blood

thrombocytopenia: abnormally low number of platelets

thromboembolus: a situation in which a thrombus breaks off within a vessel and travels to another location in the body; see also embolus

thrombosis: the formation of a blood clot

thrombus: a protective scab that is formed from dried exudate at the site of injury

thyrotoxic crisis: a sudden, severe worsening of hyperthyroidism that may result in death; also called a thyroid storm

thyrotoxicosis: the presence of excessive circulating thyroid hormone

tic: habitual repeated contraction of certain muscles

tidal volume (TV): the amount of air that is exhaled after passive inspiration; this is the volume of air going in and out of the lungs at rest; in adults, this volume is approximately 500 mL

tinnitus: ringing or whistling in the ears

tissue: groups of similar cell types that combine to form a specific function; the four major tissue types in the body include epithelium (skin), connective tissue (including blood, bone, and cartilage), muscle, and nerve

tonic: state of continuous muscle contraction

total lung capacity (TLC): the total amount of air in the lungs when they are maximally expanded; is the sum of the vital capacity and residual volume

toxigenicity: the ability of a pathogen to produce harmful toxins that increase host cell and tissue damage

trabecular network: the meshlike ocular structure responsible for the reabsorption of aqueous humor

transillumination: technique using a shining light to view accumulations of fluid

transcription: transfer of the genetic code from one type of ribonucleic acid to another; based on the nucleotide sequence of a complementary DNA template

transfer RNA (tRNA): involved in the production of proteins with specific amino acid arrangements through interaction with mRNA

transformation zone: area of the merger of squamous and columnar epithelium; also known as the squamocolumnar junction of the cervix

transient ischemic attack (TIA): a brief period of inadequate cerebral perfusion causing a sudden focal loss of neurologic function; full recovery of function usually occurs within 24 hours

translation: process involved in the production of protein from amino acids

translocation: exchange of a section of chromosome from one to another; often occurs during meiosis; able to be transferred to subsequent generations

transmembrane protein: protein extending through the plasma membrane, contacting both the intracellular and extracellular components

tremor: repetitive, often regular, oscillatory movements

trigone: triangular smooth area at the base of the bladder between the openings of the two ureters and the urethra; serves as a functional sphincter that prevents urine from moving in a retrograde manner back into the ureter from the bladder

trisomy: presence of three copies of a chromosome in place of the normal pair; the result of nondisjuncture

trophic: related to growth

tropism: a term used to describe the affinity of a primary tumor to a specific distant site

truncated: shortened

tuberculosis (TB): an infectious disease caused by an aerobic, rod-shaped bacterium (bacillus) called *Mycobacterium tuberculosis:*

tumor markers: substances that may be detected in cells or body fluids and can provide clues to the presence, extent, and treatment response of certain neoplasms

tumor suppressor genes: genes that prohibit overproliferation of cells and regulate apoptosis

turgor: fullness; evaluation made on skin to determine hydration status

two-point discrimination: discriminative pathway allowing the identification of an object based on touch or the location of skin touch in two different areas

tympanic membrane: located at the end of the ear canal opposite the external auditory meatus; structure marking the boundary of the middle ear; commonly known as the "ear drum"

tympanometry: measures the degree of movement of the tympanic membrane to identify middle ear fluid, perforation, or cerumen blockage of the ear canal

ulcer: circumscribed, open, craterlike lesion of the skin or mucous membranes

undernutrition: a lack of intake of nutrients most often related to inadequate calorie consumption, inadequate intake of essential vitamins and minerals, or problems with digestion, absorption, or distribution of nutrients in the body

universal precautions: a standard of health care that recognizes all blood and body fluid as potentially infected

unsaturated fatty acids: have one or more double bond and are not known to elevate blood cholesterol levels, are usually found in plant sources, and are often liquid at room temperature

urge incontinence: involuntary leakage of urine that is accompanied or immediately preceded by a strong urge to void; also known as overactive bladder

urgency: the need to urinate immediately

ureteroscopic stone removal: procedure used when calculi are located in the mid or distal portions of the ureters; calculi localization and removal is accomplished through a ureteroscope

urine: clear yellow fluid composed primarily of water, which contains a variety of water-soluble waste products

urine dipstick: tool used to perform biochemical analyses of urine

urine specific gravity: measurement of the concentration of particles in the urine, comparing the weight of urine to the weight of water

urticaria: sensation of itching

utricle: structural component of the semicircular canal

uveal-scleral outflow pathway: route of reabsorption of a small quantity of aqueous humor

vaccine: substance stimulating immunity through exposure to an antigen

Valsalva maneuvers: the generation of intra-abdominal pressure through inhalation, forcing the diaphragm and chest muscles against the glottis; provides stimulation of the vagus nerve

variable region: structure of antibody that allows binding to specific antigens

vascular response: the role of inflammation in increasing blood flow to the site of an injury

vasodilate: to widen the blood vessel, primarily at the capillary arteriole, allowing an increase in blood flow to the site

vector: a vehicle that harbors a pathogen and carries it to a host

venous stasis: stagnation of blood in the veins with reduced venous return

ventilation: the movement of air into and out of the trachea, bronchi, and lungs

ventilation–perfusion ratio: the relationship between inspired oxygen and the pulmonary circulation, which is responsible for transporting the oxygen to the heart to be pumped to the rest of the body; this is expressed as a ratio and is typically 0.8–0.9, where the rate of ventilation is usually slightly less than the rate of perfusion

ventral horns: anterior extensions of the spinal cord that contain efferent motor neurons

ventricles: four fluid-filled interconnecting cavities in the brain; site of cerebrospinal fluid storage and production

Virchow triad: three major factors are responsible for thrombus formation: vessel wall damage, excessive clotting, and alterations in blood flow, such as turbulence or sluggish blood movement

virions: particles released by cells infected by viruses, which can enter and infect other nearby cells

virulence: the potency of a pathogen indicated by the ratio of the number of cases of disease in a population compared with the number of people exposed to the microorganism

viruses: obligate intracellular parasites

viscosity: concentration or thickness

visual processing: coordination of visual images in the brain during the sequence of steps from visual receptor signaling to cognitive recognition

vital capacity (VC): the maximal amount of air that can be moved in and out of the lungs with forced inhalation and exhalation

vitamins: micronutrient organic substances that the body is unable to manufacture and therefore must consume; often classified according to solubility (fat or water soluble) or by metabolic function

volatile: tendency for a substance to vaporize; form of substance excreted by the lungs

Wallerian degeneration: degeneration of axons caused by crushing injury

wet (exudative) MD: macular degeneration characterized by the formation of new blood vessels under the retina and macula, known as choroidal neovascularization; macular damage caused by leakage of fluid and bleeding from new vessels, altering the shape of the macula and distorting central vision; also known as exudative macular degeneration

white matter: tissue of the central nervous system composed mainly of axons and dendrites

yeasts: unicellular forms of fungi that reproduce by budding

Index

Page numbers in italics denote figures; those followed by a *t* denote tables; those followed by a *b* denote boxes.

Osmotic pressure, 12, 192–193, 195
Osmotic swelling, 189
Ossicles, 263
Osteomas, 169
Osteopenia, 454, 460
Osteoporosis
  in aging, 458–462, *459*
    clinical manifestations, 459–460
    diagnosis of, 460–461
    pathophysiology, 458–459, 459t
    treatment, 461–462, 461t
  bone remodeling in, *460*
  menopausal in, 454
Otitis externa, 265
Otitis media, 265
  clinical manifestations of, 271, *272*
  defined, 271
  diagnostic criteria of, 271
  pathophysiology of, 271
  treatment of, 271
Otitis media with effusion (OME), 271, *272*
Otoacoustic emission (OAE), 267
Otosclerosis, 265
Ovarian cancer
  clinical manifestations of, 315
  diagnosis of, 315–316
  pathophysiology of, 314–315, *315*
  treatment of, 316
Ovary
  cross-section of, *306*
  function of, *306*
  polycystic disease of, *314*
Overactive bladder, 439
Overflow incontinence, 439
Overnutrition, 405t–406t, 406
Ovulation, 305
Ovulatory cycle, of endometrium, 307, *307*
Oxidative stress, 19
  cellular response to, *19*
Oxygen
  diffusion of, 331
  saturation of, 332
  transport of, 329, 331
Oxygen free radicals, 11
Oxygen saturation (SaO$_2$), 331
Oxyhemoglobin (HbO$_2$), 331
Oxytocin, 283t, 285, 304

P
P53 gene, 163
Pain, 254b, *255*, 434
  altered urinary function and, 427
  characterization of, 253
  classifications of, 256b
  control methods, 256b
  fibromyalgia. *See* Fibromyalgia
  management, 255
  theories
    gate control theory, 254
    neuromatrix theory, 254, 255
    pattern theory, 254
    specificity theory, 254
  treatment, 255, 256
Pallidotomy, 464
Pancreas
  endocrine, 471
  exocrine, 471
  islets of Langerhans, 471, *471*
Pancreatic amylase, 398t, 399
Pancreatic lipases, 398t, 402
Pandemic disease, defined, 5
Panhypopituitarism, 290
Pannus, 55, *55*
Pantothenic acid, 393t
Papanicolaou (Pap) smear, 28–29
Papilloma, 169
PAPP-A. *See* Pregnancy associated plasma
  protein-A (PAPP-A)
Paracentesis, 205, *206*
Paracrine pathway, 287, *287*
Paracrine signaling, 14
Paralytic ileus, 444
Paramyxovirus, 106t
Paraneoplastic syndromes, 167

Parasympathetic nervous system (PNS),
  229, *231*
Parathyroid hormone (PTH), 283t, 292t, 455
Paresthesia, 191, 225
Parietal cells, 397
Parkinson, James, Dr, 462
Parkinson disease (PD), 462–465
  brain changes in, 462, *462, 463*
  clinical manifestations, 462–464, *463*
  diagnosis, 464
  facial features of, 463, *464*
  treatment, 464–465
Partial pressure, during diffusion, 330–331
Passive diffusion, 399, *401*
Passive transport, 11–12
Pathogenesis, defined, 2
Pathogenic defense mechanisms, 101
Pathogenicity, 101
Pathogens, 101–108
  defined, 2
  factors affecting, 101
  types of, 101
Pathology, defined, 2
Pathophysiology
  applying, 4–5
  concept map, *4*
  conceptual approach in, 6
  defined, 2
  evidence-based practice, 5–6
Pattern theory, of pain, 254
PCI. *See* Percutaneous coronary intervention
  (PCI)
PCOS. *See* Polycystic ovary syndrome (PCOS)
PD. *See* Parkinson disease (PD)
Peak expiratory flow rate (PEFR), 349
Pedigrees, 140
PEEP. *See* Positive end-expiratory pressure
  (PEEP)
PEFR. *See* Peak expiratory flow rate (PEFR)
Pelvic inflammatory disease (PID), 312–313
  clinical manifestations of, *312*, 312–313
  diagnosis of, 313
  pathophysiology of, 312
  treatment of, 313
Pelvic muscles, 439
Penetrance, 132
Penicillin, allergies to, 77
Penicillin prophylaxis, 145
Penile erection, anatomic depiction of, *319*
Penis, 307, *308*
Pepsin, 397, 398t
Peptides, 217
Percutaneous coronary intervention (PCI), 380
Percutaneous nephrolithotomy, 439
Percutaneous transluminal coronary angioplasty
  (PTCA), 380
Perfluorochemical (PFC) liquids, 341
Perfusion, 47, 327
  alteration of, *367*, 367–372, 372t
    diagnosis of, 371, 372t
    excessive demands of, 370
    general manifestations of, 370–371
    treatment of, 371, 373t
  bowel, alteration in, 432–433
  defined, 359
  overview, 358
  with oxygenated blood, 359
  requirements for, 359
  urinary, alteration in, 425
  ventilation and, 455
Pericarditis, 92
Pericardium, 361
Perimenopause, 316
Peripheral nervous system, 227–233
  ANS, 227, 229, *230, 231*
  cranial nerves, 227, 228t
  injury to, 231, 232–233
  motor dysfunction, 233, 233b
  PNS, 229, *231*
  SNS, 227, 229, *230*
  spinal nerves, 227, 228t, *229*
Peripheral organs, of lymphatic system, 71
Peristalsis, 430, *431*
Peritoneal dialysis, 441–442
Peritonitis, *444*

Permanent cells, 45
Pernicious anemia, 58
Peroxisomes, 11
Petechiae, 371
Peyer's patches, 69t, 398
PFC. *See* Perfluorochemical (PFC) liquids
pH, 200
  buffer systems for, 201, 202
  renal regulation of, 202
Phagocytosis, 13, 36
Pharmacologic therapy, for hypertension,
  375, 376t
Phenotype, 131
Phenylalanine, 126t
Phenylketonuria (PKU), 130t, 403, *403*
Phlegm, 335
Phosphate, 191t, 422t, 455
  balance, altered, 190–191
Phospholipids, 10
Phosphorus, 395t, 406t
Photophobia, 121
Photoreceptors, 250t, 258, 259
Photosensitivity, 92
Physical injury, 18
Physiology, defined, 2
Pica, 409
PID. *See* Pelvic inflammatory disease (PID)
PIN. *See* Prostatic intraepithelial neoplasia
  (PIN)
Pinna, 262
Pinocytosis, 13
Pitting edema, 198, *200*
Pituitary gland, 282
PKD. *See* Polycystic kidney disease (PKD)
PKU. *See* Phenylketonuria (PKU)
Placenta, 93
Plaquenil, 93
Plasma
  buffer systems, 201
  inflammatory mediators in, 38–39, 38t
  membrane, 10, *10*
Platelet-activating factor, 38
Platelets, inflammatory mediators in, 38
Pleuritis, 92
Plexus, 227
Pneumocystis carinii, 340
Pneumocystis jiroveci, 86
Pneumonia
  clinical manifestations of, 341
  diagnosis of, 341
  pathophysiology of, 340–341
  treatment of, 342
Pneumothorax, 349
PNS. *See* Parasympathetic nervous system
  (PNS)
Poikilocytosis, 409
Polar head, 10
Polycystic kidney disease (PKD), 439–443,
  440–443
  categories of, 440
  diagnosis, 440–441
  pathophysiology, 440
  symptoms of, 440
  treatment of, 441–443
Polycystic ovary syndrome (PCOS), *313,*
  313–314, *314*
  clinical manifestations with, 314
  diagnosis of, 314
  pathophysiology of, 313
  treatment of, 314
Polydipsia, 473
Polygenic disorders, inheritance of, 135
Polygenic MHC molecule, 82
Polygenic traits, 131
Polymenorrhea, 316
Polymorphic MHC molecule, 82
Polymorphism, 131
Polymorphonuclear (PMN) leukocytes, 71
Polyneuropathy, 233
Polyphagia, 473
Polyuria, 294, 473
Pons, 220t
Portal circulation, 114, *114*
Portal hypertension, 204
Portal of entry, 110